The NeuroICU
BOARD REVIEW

NOTICE

Medicine is an ever-changing science. As new research and clinical experience broaden our knowledge, changes in treatment and drug therapy are required. The authors and the publisher of this work have checked with sources believed to be reliable in their efforts to provide information that is complete and generally in accord with the standard accepted at the time of publication. However, in view of the possibility of human error or changes in medical sciences, neither the editors nor the publisher nor any other party who has been involved in the preparation or publication of this work warrants that the information contained herein is in every respect accurate or complete, and they disclaim all responsibility for any errors or omissions or for the results obtained from use of the information contained in this work. Readers are encouraged to confirm the information contained herein with other sources. For example and in particular, readers are advised to check the product information sheet included in the package of each drug they plan to administer to be certain that the information contained in this work is accurate and that changes have not been made in the recommended dose or in the contraindications for administration. This recommendation is of particular importance in connection with new or infrequently used drugs.

The NeuroICU BOARD REVIEW

Editors

Saef Izzy, MD
Neurocritical Care Attending
Divisions of Stroke, Cerebrovascular, and Critical Care Neurology
Department of Neurology
Brigham and Women's Hospital
Research Associate, Massachusetts General Hospital
Instructor in Neurology, Harvard Medical School
Boston, Massachusetts

David P. Lerner, MD
Neurocritical Care Fellow
Departments of Neurology
Massachusetts General Hospital, Brigham and
Women's Hospital and Harvard Medical School
Boston, Massachusetts

Kiwon Lee, MD, FACP, FAHA, FCCM
Professor and Chief of Neurology
Director, Comprehensive Stroke Center
Director, Stroke and Critical Care Division
Director, Neuro Intensive Care Unit
Rutgers, The State University of New Jersey
Robert Wood Johnson Medical School
Robert Wood Johnson University Hospital
New Brunswick, New Jersey

New York   Chicago   San Francisco   Athens   London   Madrid   Mexico City
Milan   New Delhi   Singapore   Sydney   Toronto

The NeuroICU Board Review

3 4 5 6 7 8   QVS   24 23 22 21 20

ISBN 978-1-260-01100-5
MHID 1-260-01100-3

This book was set in Minion pro by Cenveo® Publisher Services.
The editors were Andrew Moyer and Regina Y. Brown.
The production supervisor was Catherine H. Saggese.
Production management was provided by Kritika Kaushik, Cenveo Publisher Services.

This book is printed on acid-free paper.

Contents

PART 4 SURGICAL CRITICAL CARE

Authors

Firas N. Abdulmajeed, MB, ChB
Clinical Fellow of Neurocritical Care
University of Virginia
University of Virginia Medical Center
Charlottesville, Virginia

Ahmad AbouLeila, MD
Clinical Fellow
Cleveland Clinic
Department of surgical critical care
Cleveland, Ohio

Max W. Adelman, MD
Internal Medicine Resident
Massachusetts General Hospital
Boston, Massachusetts

Avneep Aggarwal, MD
Department of General anesthesiology, Center for
    Critical Care
Cleveland Clinic
Cleveland, Ohio

Feras Akbik, MD, PhD
Neurology Resident
Massachusetts General Hospital
Brigham and Women's Hospital
Harvard Medical School
Boston, Massachusetts

Catherine S.W. Albin, MD
Neurology Resident
Department of Neurology
Massachusetts General Hospital
Brigham and Women's Hospital
Harvard Medical School
Boston, Massachusetts

Rami Algahtani, MD
Neurology Resident
Department of Neurology
George Washington University
Washington, DC

Fawaz Al-Mufti, MD
Assistant Professor of Neurology
Director of Interventional Neurology
    (Neuroendovascular Surgery)
Associate Director of Neurocritical Care
Rutgers University-Robert Wood Johnson University
    Hospital
New Brunswick, New Jersey

Anthony A. Amato, MD
Vice Chairman
Department of Neurology
Brigham and Women's Hospital
Boston, Massachusetts

Hassan Anbari, MD
Radiology Resident
Michigan State University College of Human Medicine,
    Southeast Michigan Campus
Providence-Providence Park Hospital
Southfield, Michigan

Yasir Azzawi, MD
Assistant Professor of Internal Medicine
Division of Gastroenterology
University of Massachusetts Medical School
Worcester, Massachusetts

Marc-Alain Babi, MD
Neurocritical Care Fellow
Division of Neuro-Critical Care, Department of
 Neurology
Duke University
Durham, North Carolina

Sanam Baghshomali, MD
Neurocritical Care Fellow
Department of Neurology
Hospital of University of Pennsylvania
Philadelphia, Pennsylvania

Oladi Bentho, MD
Departments of Anesthesia and Critical Care Medicine
Johns Hopkins University
Baltimore, Maryland

Matthew B. Bevers, MD, PhD
Neurocritical Care Attending
Department of Neurology
Divisions of Stroke, Cerebrovascular, and Critical Care
 Neurology
Brigham and Women's Hospital
Harvard Medical School
Boston, Massachusetts

Edward A. Bittner MD, PhD, MSEd, FCCM, FACE
*Program Director, Critical Care-Anesthesiology
 Fellowship*
Associate Director, Surgical Intensive Care Unit
Associate Professor of Anesthesia
Dept of Anesthesia, Critical Care and Pain Medicine
Massachusetts General Hospital
Harvard Medical School
Boston, Massachusetts

Somnath Bose, MD
Instructor of Anesthesiology
Department of Anesthesia Critical Care and Pain
 Medicine
Beth Israel Deaconess Medical Center
Boston, Massachusetts

Lawrence J. Brandt, MD, MACG, AGA-F, FASGE
Emeritus Chief
Division of Gastroenterology
Montefiore Medical Center/Albert Einstein College of
 Medicine
Bronx, New York

David Cachia, MD
Assistant Professor in Neuro-Oncology
Department of Neurosurgery
Medical University of South Carolina
Charleston, South Carolina

Xuemei Cai, MD
Neurocritical Care Attending
Department of Neurology
Tufts Medical Center
Boston, Massachusetts

Alyssa Y. Castillo, MD
Internal Medicine Resident
Massachusetts General Hospital
Boston, Massachusetts

Jan Claassen, MD, PhD, FNCS
Associate Professor of Neurology
*Head of Neurocritical Care and Medical Director of the
 Neurological Intensive Care Unit*
Department of Neurology
Columbia University College of Physicians and
 Surgeons
New York, New York

Caitlin Lee Cohen, MD
Internal Medicine Resident
Massachusetts General Hospital
Boston, Massachusetts

Neha S. Dangayach, MD
*Assistant Professor of Neurology, Neurosurgery, and
 Critical Care*
Icahn School of Medicine at Mount Sinai
Attending Physician, Neurocritical Care
Mount Sinai Hospital
New York, New York

Ali Daneshmand MD, MPH
Neurology Resident
Tufts Medical Center
Boston, Massachusetts

Mark Dannenbaum, MD
Assistant Professor of Neurosurgery
The Vivian L. Smith Department of Neurosurgery
The University of Texas Medical School at Houston
Houston, Texas

Abduljabbar Dheyab, MD
Second-Year Fellow
Pulmonary Critical Medicine
University of Massachusetts Medical School
Worcester, Massachusetts

Brian L. Edlow, MD
Neurocritical Care Staff,
Massachusetts General Hospital
Assistant Professor in Neurology
Harvard Medical School
Boston, MA

Christyn M. Edmundson, MD
Neuromuscular Fellow
Department of Neurology
Brigham and Women's Hospital
Massachusetts General Hospital
Boston, Massachusetts

Mohammad El-Ghanem, MD
Endovascular Neuroradiology Fellow
Department of Neurosurgery
Rutgers University School of Medicine
Newark, New Jersey

Steven K. Feske, MD
Associate Professor of Neurology
Harvard Medical School
Chief, Stroke Division
Brigham and Women's Hospital
Boston, MA

Laura A. Foster, MD
Neuromuscular Fellow
Department of Neurology
Brigham and Women's Hospital
Massachusetts General Hospital
Boston, Massachusetts

Rajan Gadhia, MD
Cerebrovascular Fellow
Department of Neurology
Massachusetts General Hospital, Brigham & Women's
  Hospital, Harvard Medical School
Boston, Massachusetts

James L. Gentry III, MD
Cardiovascular Fellow
Suzanne Tomsich Department of Cardiovascular
  Medicine
Heart and Vascular Institute, Cleveland Clinic
Cleveland, Ohio

Shivani Ghoshal, MD
Neurocritical Care Fellow
Department of Neurology
Columbia University Medical Center and Weill Cornell
  Medicine
New York, New York

David M. Greer, MD, MA, FNCS
Chair of the Department of Neurology
Boston Medical Center
Boston University School of Medicine
Boston, Massachusetts

Gaurav Gupta, MD
*Director, Cerebrovascular and Endovascular
  Neurosurgery*
Assistant Professor of Surgery
Rutgers University, Robert Wood Johnson Medical
  School
New Brunswick, New Jersey

Simon Hanft, MD
Director, Minimally Invasive Brain Tumor Surgery
Surgical Director, Pituitary Tumor Program
Assistant Professor, Neurosurgery
Rutgers Cancer Institute of New Jersey
Rutgers-Robert Wood Johnson Medical School
New Brunswick, New Jersey

Arnavaz Hajizadeh Barfejani, PharmD
Neurovascular Research Laboratory
Massachusetts General Hospital
Boston, Massachusetts

Mohammad I. Hirzallah, MD
Neurology Resident
Department of Neurology
University of Texas Health Science Center at Houston
Houston, Texas

Manhal Izzy, MD
Clinical Fellow
Division of Gastroenterology
Montefiore Medical Center/Albert Einstein College of
    Medicine
Bronx, New York

Saef Izzy, MD
Neurocritical Care Attending
Divisions of Stroke, Cerebrovascular, and Critical Care
    Neurology
Department of Neurology
Brigham and Women's Hospital
Research Associate, Massachusetts General Hospital
Instructor in Neurology, Harvard Medical School
Boston, Massachusetts

Christina Anne Jelly, MD, MS
Staff Anesthesiologist, Chief Resident
Department of Anesthesia, Critical Care and Pain
    Medicine
Massachusetts General Hospital
Boston, Massachusetts

Maurice Francis Joyce, MD.
Staff Anesthesiologist and Intensivist
LPG Anesthesia, Rhode Island Hospital, Warren Alpert
    Medical School of Brown University
Providence, Rhode Island

Stephen Katzen, MD
Neurosurgery Resident
Department of Neurosurgery
University of Texas Health Science Center at Houston
Houston, Texas

Barry Kelly, MD
Clinical Fellow
Department Critical Care Anesthesia
Beth Israel Deaconess Medical Center
Boston, Massachusetts

Erich L. Kiehl, MD
Cardiovascular Fellow
Suzanne Tomsich Department of Cardiovascular
    Medicine
Heart and Vascular Institute, Cleveland Clinic
Cleveland, Ohio

Menhel Kinno, MD, MPH
Advanced Cardiovascular Imaging Fellow
Bluhm Cardiovascular institute
Northwestern University - Feinberg School of Medicine
Chicago Illinois

Ryan S. Kitagawa, MD
Assistant Professor of Neurosurgery
Director of Neurotrauma
The Vivian L. Smith Department of Neurosurgery
University of Texas Health Science Center, University of
    Texas at Houston
Houston, Texas

Scott Kopec, MD
Associate Professor
Program Director of Pulmonary and Critical Care
    Medicine
University of Massachusetts Medical School
Worcester, Massachusetts

Jason Kovacevic, MD
Internal Medicine *Resident*
University of Massachusetts Medical School
Worcester, Massachusetts

Tobias B. Kulik, MD
Clinical Instructor
Fellow in Neurocritical Care
Washington University in St. Louis
St. Louis, Missouri

Monisha Kumar, MD
Assistant Professor
Department of Neurology, Neurosurgery and
    Anesthesiology, and Critical Care
Hospital of University of Pennsylvania
Philadelphia, Pennsylvania

Shouri Lahiri, MD
Neurocritical Care Attending
Departments of Neurology and Neurosurgery
Cedars-Sinai Medical Center
Los Angeles, California

Eugene C. Lai, MD, PhD
Department of Neurology
Houston Methodist
Houston, Texas

Andrew G. Lee, MD
Department of Ophthalmology
Houston Methodist
Houston, Texas

Kiwon Lee, MD, FACP, FAHA, FCCM
Professor and Chief of Neurology
Rutgers, The State University of New Jersey
Robert Wood Johnson Medical School
Department of Neurology
New Brunswick, New Jersey

Joshua Leibner, MD
Staff Neurologist
Martin Health Physicians Group
Stuart, Florida

Christopher Leon-Guerrero, MD
Assistant Professor in Neurology
Department of Neurology
Division of Stroke and Cerebrovascular Disease
George Washington University
Washington, DC

David P. Lerner, MD
Neurocritical Care Fellow
Departments of Neurology
Massachusetts General Hospital, Brigham and Women's Hospital and Harvard Medical School
Boston, Massachusetts

Andrew Martin, MD
Neurocritical Care Fellow
Department of Neurology
Columbia University Medical Center and Weill Cornell Medicine
New York, New York

Jose R. McFaline Figueroa, MD, PhD
Neurology Resident
Department of Neurology
Brigham and Women's Hospital
Massachusetts General Hospital
Harvard Medical School
Boston, Massachusetts

Kara R. Melmed, MD
Neurology Resident
Department of Neurology
Cedars-Sinai Medical Center
Los Angeles, California

Venu Menon, MD
Suzanne Tomsich Department of Cardiovascular Medicine
Heart and Vascular Institute, Cleveland Clinic
Director Cardiovascular Intensive Care Unit
Director of Cardiovascular Medicine
Fellowship, Professor of Medicine
Cleveland Clinic Lerner College of Medicine
Case Western Reserve University
Cleveland, Ohio

Ayman Mithqal, MD
Assistant Professor
Department of Radiology and Imaging
Division of Neuroradiology
University of Virginia
Charlottesville, Virginia

Barnett Nathan, MD
Professor of Neurology
Division of Neurocritical Care and Vascular Neurology
University of Virginia
Charlottesville, Virginia

Jamel Ortoleva, MD
Clinical Fellow
Surgical Critical Care
Beth Israel Deaconess Medical Center
Boston, Massachusetts

Mohamed Osman, MD
Neurocritical Care Fellow
Department of Neurosurgery
Zale Lipshy University Hospital, University of Texas Southwestern Medical Center
Dallas, Texas

Jay Patel, MD
Cardiovascular Medicine Fellow
Suzanne Tomsich Department of Cardiovascular Medicine
Heart and Vascular Institute, Cleveland Clinic
Cleveland, Ohio

Juan Perrone, MD
Clinical Fellow
Department of Anesthesia Critical Care and Pain Medicine
Massachusetts General Hospital
Harvard Medical School
Boston, Massachusetts

Swarna Rajagopalan, MD
Neurocritical Care Fellow
Department of Neurology
Hospital of University of Pennsylvania
Philadelphia, Pennsylvania

Kaitlin Reilly, MD
Neurocritical Care Fellow
Department of Neurology
Mount Sinai Hospital
New York, New York

Alexandra Reynolds, MD
Neurocritical Care Fellow
Department of Neurology
Columbia University Medical Center and Weill Cornell
    Medicine
New York, New York

Michael Reznik, MD
Neurocritical Care Fellow
Department of Neurology
Columbia University Medical Center and Weill Cornell
    Medicine
New York, New York

Lucia Rivera-Lara, MD
Neurocritical Care Attending
Department of Neurology
Johns Hopkins University
Baltimore, Maryland

Julia Ann Roberts, MD
Internal Medicine Resident
Massachusetts General Hospital
Boston, Massachusetts

Guy Rordorf, MD
Associate Professor of Neurology
Department of Neurology
Massachusetts General Hospital
Harvard Medical School
Boston, Massachusetts

Sudipta Roychowdhury, MD
Department of Surgery
Rutgers University, Robert Wood Johnson Medical
    School
New Brunswick, New Jersey

Daniel B. Rubin, MD, PhD
Neurology Resident
Brigham and Women's Hospital
Massachusetts General Hospital
Harvard Medical School
Boston, Massachusetts

Michael Rubin, MD, MA
Assistant Professor of Neurology and Neurotherapeutics
Neurological Surgery
University of Texas Southwestern Medical Center
Zale Lipschy University Hospital
Dallas, Texas

Nicole Ruopp, MD
Pulmonary Allergy, Sleep, and Critical Care Medicine
Boston Medical Center
Boston, Massachusetts

Jason L. Sanders, MD, PhD
Internal Medicine Resident
Massachusetts General Hospital
Boston, Massachusetts

Fernando Santos Pinheiro, MD
Fellow, Neuro-Oncology
Division of Medicine, Department of Neuro-Oncology
University of Texas MD Anderson Cancer Center
Houston, Texas

Vicki Sein, MD
Surgical Critical Care Fellow
Massachusetts General Hospital
Harvard Medical School
Boston, Massachusetts

Manan Shah, MD
Neurology Resident
Department of Neurology
University of Texas Health Science Center at Houston
Houston, Texas

Starane Anthony Shepherd, MD
Assistant Professor of Neurology
Section of Neurocritical Care
Department of Neurological Sciences
Rush University Medical Center
Chicago, Illinois

Faheem Sherriff, MD
Neurocritical Care Fellow
Department of Neurology
Massachusetts General Hospital
Brigham and Women's Hospital
Harvard Medical School
Boston, Massachusetts

Annesh B. Singhal, MD
Stroke Service, Cerebrovascular Attending
Department of Neurology
Massachusetts General Hospital and Harvard Medical
    School
Boston, Massachusetts

Stacy V. Smith, MD
Departments of Neurology and Ophthalmology
Houston Methodist
Houston, Texas

Abraham Sonny, MD
Anesthesiologist and Intensivist
Department of Anesthesia, Critical Care and Pain
    Medicine
Massachusetts General Hospital
Instructor in Anesthesia
Harvard Medical School
Boston, Massachusetts

Jamie Sparling, MD
Anesthesiology Resident
Massachusetts General Hospital
Harvard Medical School
Boston, Massachusetts

Matthew R. Summers, MD
Cardiovascular Medicine Fellow
Suzanne Tomsich Department of Cardiovascular
    Medicine
Heart and Vascular Institute, Cleveland Clinic
Cleveland, Ohio

Christa Swisher, MD
Assistant Professor of Neurology and Neurocritical Care
Assistant Medical Director
Inpatient Neuroscience Clinical Research Organization
Department of Neurology
Duke University
Durham, North Carolina

Zachary Threlkeld, MD
Neurocritical Care Fellow
Department of Neurology
Massachusetts General Hospital
Brigham and Women's Hospital
Harvard Medical School
Boston, Massachusetts

David W. Van Wyck, DO
Neurocritical Care Fellow
Division of Neuro-Critical Care, Department of
    Neurology
Duke University
Durham, North Carolina

Christopher Velez, MD
Gastroenterology Fellow
Division of Gastroenterology
Montefiore Medical Center/Albert Einstein College
    of Medicine
Bronx, New York

Sarah Wahlster, MD
Assistant Professor of Neurology
Division of Neurocritical Care, Department of
    Neurology
Harborview Medical Center
University of Washington
Seattle, Washington

Connie Wang
Anesthesiology Resident
Massachusetts General Hospital
Harvard Medical School
Boston, Massachusetts

Janice C. Wong, MD
Neuromuscular Fellow
Department of Neurology
Brigham and Women's Hospital
Massachusetts General Hospital
Boston, Massachusetts

Foreword

In the current era, it has become increasingly difficult to gauge the meaning of expertise in a clinical field. This is perhaps more true in the subspecialty of neurological intensive care than it is in other areas of neurology and neurosurgery. The intensivist is an activist, making decisions that integrate a tremendous amount of information and implementing solutions to a variety of problems that cross neurology, surgery, and general medicine. Therefore, this book project, which prepares readers for a number of certifications beyond neurological intensive care, is very welcome. By framing the learning experience through cases that are genuine or closely simulate real practice, the reader is brought along in a way that is meaningful and practical.

In keeping with the breadth of practice in this field, the material covered here is extraordinarily comprehensive but does not sacrifice depth. The knowledge base of each of the authors is on display and is clearly colored by true life experience in the ICU. Moreover, the answers to the questions posed for each case are logical and complete. When there is ambiguity, as there must be in critical care, this is acknowledged and the best course of action is outlined. I hope that readers, whether they are studying for the boards or trying to enhance their practice, will enjoy this book as much as I did.

Allan H. Ropper, MD
Executive Vice Chair,
Department of Neurology,
Brigham and Women's Hospital,
Boston, Massachusetts

Acknowledgments

We would like to make special recognition of the advisory panel that helped shape this work. Without their guidance, this board review book would not clearly, concisely and adequately cover all the topics of the neurocritical care, and other, board examinations.

To doctors: Christa Swisher (Duke University Medical Center), Dennis J. Beer (Newton Wellesley hospital), Fawaz Al-Mufti (Rutgers University, New Jersey Medical School), Galen V. Henderson (Brigham and Women's Hospital), Henrikas Vaitkevicius (Brigham and Women's Hospital), Lucia Rivera (Johns Hopkins University), Neha Dangayach (Mount Sinai Medical Center), Sahar Zafar (Massachusetts General Hospital), Steven K. Feske (Brigham and Women's Hospital), Santosh B. Murthy (Weill Cornell Medical Center), Sarah Wahlster (University of Washington), Shouri Lahiri (Cedars Sinai Medical Center), and Xuemei Cai (Tufts Medical Center).

We greatly appreciate your insightful feedback, recommendations, and commitment to developing a highly impactful reference.

Preface

Neurocritical care is a captivating, fast-growing subspecialty dedicated to the care and treatment of patients with the most severe nervous system diseases. Knowledge of neurology in conjunction with all critical care skills is needed to care for these patients. Because of the broad knowledge base required to practice neurocritical care, there is a lack of comprehensive and organized resources that describe the training curriculum or specific board preparation.

As we began to prepare for our own boards, we realized there was a large gap in the current materials available. We used the available educational resources at our Harvard Neurocritical Care Fellowship Program and invested the energy of nationwide fellows, residents, and junior faculty to generate a comprehensive question-and-answer book.

We have created this board review book to prepare you not only for the neurocritical care boards but also for the neurosurgery, emergency medicine, and surgical critical care boards! Readers will find that this book is not just about the brain, as it also covers the complexities of all organ failures and general critical care topics.

We designed this book to be a great resource and study guide to trainees rotating through neurocritical care units, including neurology and neurosurgery residents, as well as fellows from other subspecialties who are not familiar with core neurocritical care topics.

Given the lack of available curriculum, we created an advisory board composed of junior faculty from top facilities around the United States who have taken the board exam to review the questions and ensure that they mirror the board exam in quality, difficulty, and content. We have also gotten input from across the United States to ensure variance in different facility practices is addressed to not overwhelm your board preparation.

With over 700 questions and detailed answer explanation, all neurocritical care topics are covered. Although question-and-answer–based preparation works well for board review, we aspired for more. We hope that the 12 clinical cases at the end of the book can strengthen your understanding of critical care topics and prepare you further for practice in the neurologic intensive care unit.

"Wherever the art of medicine is loved, there is also a love of humanity." —Hippocrates

Saef Izzy, MD
David Lerner, MD
Kiwon Lee, MD

PART 1
Stroke and Neurocritical Care

1

Ischemic and Hemorrhagic Stroke

Rami Algahtani, MD and Christopher Leon-Guerrero, MD

Questions

1. A 72-year-old woman with a history of uncontrolled hypertension presents to the emergency department with a severe headache, blurry vision, and slurred speech. Initial blood pressure is 238/109 mm Hg. Emergent head computed tomography (CT) shows a cerebellar vermis hemorrhage measuring 4 cm with significant compression of the brainstem and encroachment of the fourth ventricle. Coagulopathy studies and platelets are normal. She is not taking any antithrombotic therapies. Shortly thereafter, she becomes obtunded and requires intubation. Which of the following treatments is most likely to improve outcome?

   A. Acute reduction in blood pressure
   B. Empiric platelet transfusion
   C. Emergent posterior decompressive craniotomy
   D. Hyperosmotic therapy
   E. Placement of an external ventricular drain (EVD)

2. A 59-year-old African American man with a history of hypertension presents to the emergency department with acute onset of headache, nausea, vomiting, right-sided weakness, and numbness. Initial blood pressure is 201/103 mm Hg. Initial Glasgow coma scale (GCS) score is 14. Emergent CT of the head shows a left thalamic intraparenchymal hemorrhage with intraventricular extension and no hydrocephalus. The calculated volume of the hematoma is 8 mL (based on the ABC/2 formula). Based on the data provided, what is this patient's intracerebral hemorrhage (ICH) score?

   A. 0
   B. 1
   C. 2
   D. 3
   E. 4

3. A 43-year-old man with a history of hypertension and atrial fibrillation was found in his apartment with left-sided weakness, rightward eye deviation, and severely slurred speech. He was last seen normal the day before while leaving work. Initial blood pressure is 167/93 mm Hg. A CT of the head shows hypoattenuation involving the entire right middle cerebral artery territory with associated cerebral edema, mass effect, and resultant 9-mm midline shift. Which of the following therapeutic interventions has been proven to improve functional outcomes and reduce mortality in the current acute settings?

   A. 3-Hydroxy-3-methylglutaryl-coenzyme-A (HMG-CoA) reductase inhibitors

   B. Hyperosmolar therapy

   C. Decompressive hemicraniectomy

   D. Systemic alteplase

   E. Intravenous heparin drip

4. A 62-year-old right-handed woman with a history of uncontrolled diabetes, hypertension, and hyperlipidemia is brought to the hospital with inability to speak, right-sided weakness, and leftward eye deviation. Her grandson recalls her being normal at dinner the night prior. Initial vitals are as follows: blood pressure 170/88 mm Hg, pulse rate 89, respiratory rate 18, and afebrile. CT of the head shows hypoattenuation involving the entire left middle cerebral artery distribution with associated cerebral edema and mass effect causing a 5-mm midline shift. She is admitted to the hospital. The next day, she becomes obtunded and requires intubation. Repeat exam is notable for new left-sided weakness. What is the most likely explanation for this finding?

   A. Charles Bonnet syndrome

   B. Kernohan notch phenomenon

   C. Foster-Kennedy syndrome

   D. Terson syndrome

   E. Anton syndrome

5. A 38-year-old man with a history of a cervical spine injury secondary to a car accident with resultant spastic quadriplegia and autonomic instability is admitted to the hospital with a severe headache. His systolic blood pressure fluctuates between 120 and 210 mm Hg as a result of the autonomic instability. On hospital day 2, he begins complaining of blurred vision and subsequently has a generalized tonic-clonic seizure. A magnetic resonance image (MRI) of the brain is obtained and demonstrates the following on the fluid-attenuated inversion recovery (FLAIR) sequence (see below). What is the most likely diagnosis?

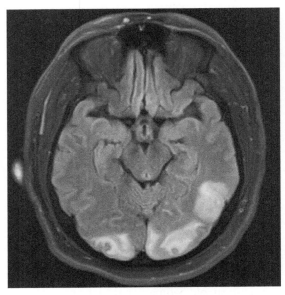

Axial view, T2-weighted, fluid-attenuated inversion recovery magnetic resonance image shows hyperintensity of the bilateral occipital lobes.

   A. Bilateral posterior cerebral artery strokes

   B. Basilar artery occlusion

   C. Posterior reversible encephalopathy syndrome

   D. Occipital subdural hematomas

   E. Thrombosis of the vein of Labbé

6. A 52-year-old woman with diabetes and hypertension (on lisinopril) presents to the emergency department with acute-onset right-sided weakness. CT of the head is negative for hemorrhage. She is treated with intravenous alteplase and admitted to the stroke unit. Fifteen minutes later, she is noted to have swelling around the right side of her lips and tongue. What is the most likely cause of the swelling?

   A. Perioral hemorrhage secondary to intravenous alteplase

   B. Angioedema

   C. Lemierre syndrome

   D. Dental abscess

   E. Anaphylaxis from a blood pressure medication

7. A 23-year-old African American man with sickle cell disease presents to the emergency department with acute-onset slurred speech and right-sided weakness concerning for a stroke. What is the most likely type of stroke in this case?

A. Ischemic stroke

B. Hemorrhagic stroke

C. Cerebral venous sinus thrombosis

D. Hypoperfusion-related stroke

E. Central nervous system vasculitis

8. A 32-year-old woman who is 2 weeks postpartum presents to the emergency department after a new-onset generalized tonic-clonic seizure. She is treated with intravenous lorazepam and intravenous fosphenytoin, resulting in cessation of her seizure. She becomes drowsy after the intravenous medications and is subsequently intubated for airway protection. An emergent head CT shows a longitudinal hyperdensity along the superior sagittal sinus with surrounding edema and small parenchymal hemorrhages. Her husband notes that she has been having headache, nausea, and blurry vision for the past 3 days. Her past medical history is significant for an unprovoked deep venous thrombosis. What is the next best step in management?

A. Lumbar puncture to measure opening pressure

B. Magnetic resonance venogram

C. Continuous electroencephalography (EEG)

D. Intravenous heparin infusion

E. Sending an antiphospholipid antibody panel

9. A 62-year-old man with a history of atrial fibrillation presents to the emergency department with acute-onset right-sided weakness and inability to speak. His symptoms started 45 minutes prior to arrival. Initial blood pressure is 172/82 mm Hg. Neurologic examination is notable for moderate expressive aphasia, right face and arm greater than leg weakness, right visual field deficit, and left gaze preference. Emergent head CT shows no evidence of bleeding. National Institutes of Health Stroke Scale (NIHSS) score is 8. He has no prior bleeding events. Which of the following is associated with improved functional outcomes?

A. Aspirin

B. CT angiogram

C. Intravenous alteplase

D. Intravenous heparin infusion

E. Warfarin

10. A 39-year-old woman with a history of systemic lupus erythematosus presented with new-onset psychosis. She was admitted to the medicine floor, and shortly thereafter, she was found to be minimally responsive and there is decreased movement on the left side than the right side of her body. She continues to worsen and requires intubation due to an inability to protect her airway. An emergent MRI of the brain shows multiple areas of subcortical ischemic stroke affecting bilateral hemisphere with more predominant right-sided involvement. She is noted to have nonblanching, deep bluish-red reticular skin lesions on the legs and body. Blood work showed erythrocyte sedimentation rate (ESR). ESR 93 mm/hr, C reactive protein (CRP) 189 mg/L, C3 and C4 <5 g/L, and antinuclear body (ANA) >1000 IU. Which of the following antibodies is most commonly associated with this condition?

A. Anti-ribonucleoprotein (RNP)

B. Anti-Ro and anti-La

C. Anti-Scl70

D. Antiphospholipid antibodies

E. Anti-gliadin

11. A 62-year-old man on dabigatran for stroke prevention in the setting of nonvalvular atrial fibrillation presents to the emergency department with a large putamen intraparenchymal hemorrhage. Which of the following is an effective reversal agent for dabigatran (direct thrombin inhibitor)?

A. Idarucizumab

B. Cryoprecipitate

C. Vitamin K

D. Andexanet alfa

E. Protamine sulfate

12. A 52-year-old patient with a history of recent dental surgery is brought to the emergency department by emergency medical services with acute-onset right-sided weakness and confusion. General examination is notable for a fever, a prominent cardiac murmur, and multiple linear hemorrhages underneath his nail beds. His NIHSS is 8 and his initial vitals are pertinent for tachycardia with heart rate of 112 beats/min and a blood pressure of 172/92 mmHg. Based on the most likely diagnosis, what is the most appropriate treatment?

A. Intravenous alteplase

B. Aspirin

C. Antibiotics

D. Levetiracetam

E. Intravenous Immunoglobulin therapy

13. An 85-year-old woman with progressive cognitive decline over the past few years presents with acute-onset left visual field deficit. Blood pressure on arrival is 125/72 mm Hg. A CT of the head is performed which demonstrates an intraparenchymal hemorrhage in the right occipital lobe. An MRI of the brain is obtained, and the susceptibility-weighted image (SWI) is shown below. What is the most likely cause of her intraparenchymal hemorrhage?

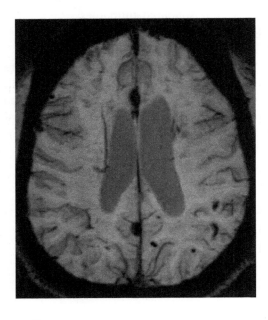

A. Cavernoma

B. Amyloid angiopathy

C. Metastatic lung cancer

D. Ruptured aneurysm

E. Moyamoya syndrome

14. A 62-year-old woman who was recently started on fluoxetine presents to the emergency department with acute-onset headache. A few minutes after arrival, she develops a tonic-clonic seizure. A CT of the head demonstrates isolated subarachnoid hemorrhage in the left intraparietal sulcus. CT angiography of the head is shown below. What is the most likely diagnosis?

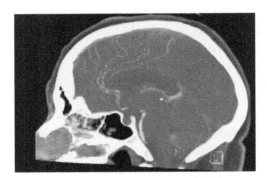

Reproduced with permission from Berkowitz AL. *Clinical Neurology and Neuroanatomy: A Localization-Based Approach.* New York, NY: McGraw-Hill, 2016.

A. Cerebral aneurysmal rupture

B. Reversible cerebral vasoconstriction syndrome

C. Meningoencephalitis

D. Moyamoya syndrome

E. Cavernoma with associated developmental venous anomaly

15. A 63-year-old woman with diabetes, hypertension, and smoking presents to the emergency department with right arm and leg weakness. Her symptoms started 2 days prior when she woke up. Her initial NIHSS score is 3. An MRI of the brain was obtained which shows a small infarct in the left corona radiata. She was started on aspirin therapy. A conventional cerebral angiogram was obtained and is shown below. Which treatment would be most appropriate for this patient?

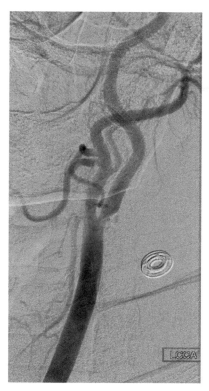

Digital subtraction angiogram with injection into the left common carotid artery.

A. Start clopidogrel in addition to aspirin therapy (dual antiplatelet therapy)

B. Start a heparin drip

C. Proceed with a carotid endarterectomy

D. Liberalize long-term blood pressure goals to >160/>100 mm Hg

E. Proceed with an extracranial-intracranial bypass surgery

16. Cerebral autosomal recessive arteriopathy with subcortical infarcts and leukoencephalopathy is caused by a mutation in which gene?

A. *NOTCH3*

B. *HTRA1*

C. *KRIT1*

D. *GLA*

E. *TREX1*

17. A 62-year-old man was brought to the emergency department via ambulance with speech difficulties and right-sided weakness. His last known normal was 2 hours prior to presentation. His NIHSS was 14 and notable for aphasia, left gaze deviation, and right hemiplegia. A CT of the head is negative for hemorrhage. Blood pressure is 162/84 mm Hg. He is not on any antithrombotics. Intravenous alteplase is administered. A CT angiogram of the head and neck is performed and is shown here. What is the next best step in management?

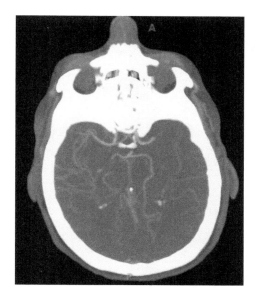

A. Heparin drip

B. Administration of intravenous tenecteplase

C. Consultation with neurosurgery for decompressive hemicraniectomy

D. Mechanical thrombectomy with stent retriever

E. Hyperosmotic therapy

18. A 49-year-old man with a history of hypertension presents with the "worst headache of his life." A CT of the head confirms subarachnoid hemorrhage. A CT angiogram reveals an 8-mm basilar artery aneurysm. He undergoes successful coiling of the artery. On postcoiling day 7, he is noted to be aphasic and unable to move his right arm. An emergent CT angiogram is obtained and is shown below. If the left middle cerebral artery was insonated by transcranial Doppler, what values would you expect to see?

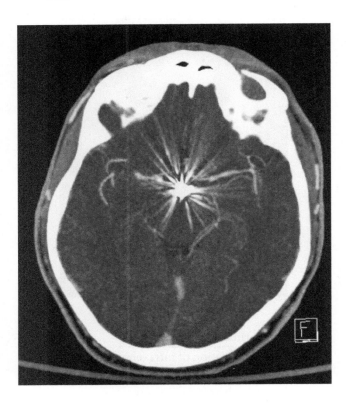

A. Elevated flow velocity and elevated Lindegaard ratio (middle cerebral artery velocity/internal carotid artery velocity)

B. Reduced flow velocity and elevated Lindegaard ratio

C. Elevated flow velocity and reduced Lindegaard ratio

D. Reduced flow velocity and reduced Lindegaard ratio

E. Normal flow velocity and normal Lindegaard ratio

19. A 54-year-old woman with no medical history presents to the emergency department with acute-onset right-sided weakness that started 1 hour prior to arrival. Initial vitals are as follows: temperature 39.2°C, blood pressure 172/98 mm Hg, heart rate 92, respiratory rate 12, and 100% oxygen saturations on room air. NIHSS is 6 for right-sided motor deficits. A CT of the head is negative for hemorrhage. Basic labs show a white blood cell of 12, hemoglobin of 7.2 g/dL, platelets of 11×10^3/microL, sodium of 140 mEq/L, potassium of 4.3 mEq/L, creatinine of 3.1 mg/dL, and glucose of 123 mg/dL. What is the most appropriate acute treatment?

A. Administer intravenous alteplase

B. Start intravenous fluids

C. Start plasma exchange transfusion

D. Give 2 units of platelets

E. Start a nicardipine drip

20. What is the most common segment involved in a spontaneous vertebral artery dissection?

A. Origin of the vertebral artery

B. V1 segment

C. V2 segment

D. Distal V3 segment

E. Junction of vertebral artery and basilar artery

Answers and Explanations

1. C. The 2015 American Heart Association Guildelines on management of intracerebral hemorrahge provide class 1 recommendation (level of evidence B) for management of cerebellar hemorrhage. In patients with clinical deterioration and evidence of brainstem compression due to a cerebellar hemorrhage, regardless of the largest diameter, decompressive surgery should be performed. The recommendations also advise against placement of an external ventricular drain prior to definitive surgical intervention (level III, class C).

Acute reduction in blood pressure has not been convincingly shown to improve outcomes. Specifically for this patient, neither the ATACH2 trial, as this is a posterior fossa hemorrhage, nor the INTERACT2 trial, as the patient requires emergent surgery, applies. Therapeutic hypothermia has not been proven to be effective in intraparenchymal hemorrhage. Platelet transfusion would not be indicated in someone with normal platelet levels, and even in patients on antiplatelet therapy, the evidence for empiric platelet transfusion is not supported. Hyperosmotic therapy may temporarily treat cerebral edema, but a more definitive intervention is needed.

2. B. The ICH score is a clinical grading scale and can be useful in estimating 30-day mortality. The scale ranges from 0 to 6, with 6 being associated with the highest mortality. One point is assigned for each of the following: age >80 years old, ICH volume >30 mL, associated intraventricular hemorrhage, and infratentorial location. One point is given for a Glasgow coma scale (GCS) of 5 to 12, and 2 points are given for a GCS of 3 to 4. The ICH score has been reevaluated, and the prognosis of ICH based on the initial study is substantially lower at moderate ICH scores (3-4), with a reduction of predicted mortality of 30% if there was limitation of do-not-resuscitate (DNR) orders.

The ICH Score

Component	Points	Total Points	30-Day Mortality (%)
Glasgow coma scale score			
3-4	2	5+	100
5-12	1		
13-15	0	4	97
ICH volume (mL)			
≥30	1	3	72
<30	0		
Intraventricular hemorrhage			
Yes	1	2	26
No	0	1	13
Age (years)			
≥80	1	0	0
<80	0		
Infratentorial origin			
Yes	1		
No	0		

(*Adapted from Hemphill JC 3rd, Bonovich DC, Besmertis L, Manley GT, Johnston SC. The ICH score: A Simple, reliable grading scole for intracerebral hemorrhage. Strake. 2001;32:891-897.*)

3. C. The patient has suffered a malignant right middle cerebral artery stroke with subsequent ischemic cerebral edema and mass effect, putting him in danger of transtentorial herniation and resultant death. Multiple randomized controlled trials (eg, DESTINY, HAMLET, DECIMAL) have shown up to a 50% reduction in mortality when decompressive hemicraniectomy is performed within the first 48 hours compared to maximum medical therapy.

The patient is beyond the 4.5-hour treatment window for intravenous alteplase. HMG-CoA reductase inhibitors are effective in secondary stroke prevention but have not been proven to reduce death or improve functional outcomes in the acute setting. Hyperosmolar therapy has not been proven to improve clinical outcomes.

4. **B.** The patient suffered a massive left middle cerebral artery stroke and is at risk of transtentorial herniation with the evolving cytotoxic edema. The typical clinical findings caused by transtentorial herniation include ipsilateral dilated pupil, contralateral hemiparesis (sometimes bilateral), and abnormal extensor posturing. In this case, the patient has developed ipsilateral (to the stroke) hemiparesis caused by the herniating uncus, resulting in compression of the contralateral cerebral peduncle against the tentorial edge. The ipsilateral weakness to the side of the stroke is a "false localizer" and is commonly referred to as the Kernohan notch phenomenon.

   Charles Bonnet syndrome, also known as visual release hallucination, can be seen in patients with partial or severe blindness and results in complex visual hallucinations. Foster-Kennedy syndrome is often caused by frontal lobe masses and results in ipsilateral optic atrophy and contralateral papilledema. Terson syndrome is intraocular hemorrhage associated with subarachnoid hemorrhage. It is thought to be caused by the sudden spike in intracranial pressure with aneurysmal rupture. Anton syndrome, or cortical blindness/visual agnosia, can occur with bilateral occipital damage. Patients are unaware of their visual deficit and confabulate visual scenes.

5. **C.** The clinical symptoms of headaches, blurred vision, and seizures in the setting of severe hypertension are common in posterior reversible encephalopathic syndrome (PRES) or reversible posterior leukoencephalopathy syndrome. Characteristic MRI findings consist of focal regions of confluent symmetric hemispheric vasogenic edema most commonly in the occipital and parietal lobes. The cause remains poorly understood. Failed autoregulation resulting in hyperperfusion and endothelial dysfunction/injury remains a popular theory. Other conditions commonly associated with PRES include eclampsia, renal failure, sepsis, autoimmune disorders, transplantation, and immunosuppressive therapies including cyclosporine and tacrolimus.

   Thrombosis of the vein of Labbé often results in temporal lobe hemorrhage or infarction and classically is associated headache and seizures. The fulminant, confluent, T2 hyperintense pattern on the brain MRI is inconsistent with an ischemic stroke. Subdural hematomas are extra-axial.

6. **B.** Angioedema reportedly occurs in 1.7% to 17% of patients treated with intravenous (IV) alteplase. Patients on angiotensin-converting enzyme inhibitors are at higher risk of developing angioedema after IV alteplase. The typical reaction is mild and transient. The hemi-swelling, contralateral to the ischemic hemisphere, is hypothesized to be due to loss of autonomic innervation on the hemiplegic/paretic side. Close monitoring of the patient's respiratory status and airway is essential. Patients who develop angioedema should be treated with histamine antagonists, such as ranitidine and diphenhydramine, along with corticosteroids.

   Lemierre syndrome is thrombophlebitis of the internal jugular vein and bacteremia often preceded by a recent oropharyngeal infection/abscess. The other choices are unlikely based on the history.

7. **B.** Roughly 11% of patients with sickle cell disease will have a stroke before the age of 20. Stroke subtype varies by age, with ischemia being the most common type in the first decade of life and after the age of 30. During the 20s, hemorrhage is more common than ischemia; in particular, subarachnoid hemorrhage related to a ruptured cerebral aneurysm is the most common subtype of hemorrhage.

   Management of acute stroke secondary to sickle cell disease can be challenging. Generally, thrombolytics and anticoagulation are avoided, yet may be considered on a case-by-case basis. Exchange transfusion is the best management to lower the percentage of sickle hemoglobin to ≤30% of total hemoglobin while maintaining the total hemoglobin level ≤10 g/dL.

8. **D.** Thrombosis of the dural sinus and/or cerebral veins is an uncommon form of stroke, representing 0.5% to 1% of all strokes. Multiple factors have been associated with cerebral venous thrombosis including hereditary or acquired thrombophilias, inflammatory conditions, transient conditions (eg, pregnancy and puerperium, dehydration, parameningeal infection), selected medications (eg, tamoxifen, steroids, intravenous immunoglobulin, oral contraceptives), and head trauma. Focal or generalized seizures occur in 40% of cases.

Anticoagulation is safe and effective in treating cerebral venous thrombosis, despite the presence of intracerebral hemorrhage, and should be started promptly whenever there is a high enough concern. A lumbar puncture would not be useful in this case, although opening pressure can be elevated in cerebral venous thrombosis. A hypercoagulable workup should be considered, including antiphospholipid antibodies; however, this would not be the most appropriate next step in management. A magnetic resonance venogram would be an appropriate test, but the patient already has evidence of cerebral venous sinus thrombosis and initiation of treatment should not be delayed. EEG and general anesthesia are appropriate in case of ongoing seizures, including subclinical seizures, but the seizure resolved after lorazepam and fosphenytoin.

9. **C.** This is a classic presentation of a stroke affecting the left middle cerebral artery (left middle cerebral artery syndrome). There is no evidence of hemorrhage on the head CT, and the NIHSS of 8 entails a moderate stroke burden. The patient is within the therapeutic window for systemic alteplase and should be treated with thrombolytics. This decision is supported by the NINDS trial, a randomized controlled trial comparing intravenous alteplase versus placebo. This trial showed that patients treated with intravenous alteplase within 3 hours of symptom onset were 30% more likely to achieve minor or no disability on disability scales at 90 days compared to placebo. In 2008, the ECASS trial, another large randomized controlled trial, demonstrated improved functional outcomes in patients treated with intravenous tissue plasminogen activator up to 4.5 hours after symptom onset with additional relative exclusion criteria of age >80 years old, presence of prior stroke and diabetes, and use of any anticoagulation.

The routine use of therapeutic anticoagulation is not recommended in acute strokes and should be reserved for select cases. Coumadin would be a reasonable antithrombotic for secondary stroke prevention in the setting of atrial fibrillation but not in the acute setting. Early administration of aspirin in ischemic stroke has been associated with reduction in recurrent stroke but is not associated with specifically improved functional outcomes. CT angiogram would be useful to screen for endovascular therapy cases, which could improve acute stroke patients' outcome in selected cases, but the CT angiogram alone does not improve functional outcomes.

10. **D.** This is a case of Sneddon syndrome, which is a rare noninflammatory thrombotic vasculopathy characterized by the combination of ischemic stroke with livedo reticularis, however as is the case with this patient livedo racemosa can also be present. Livedo racemosa is defined as a dusky erythematous to violaceous, large, irregular, mottling of the skin. Livedo racemosa may precede the onset of stroke by years and is located on limbs, trunk, buttocks, face, or the hands or feet. The cerebrovascular disease mostly occurs due to ischemia (transient ischemic attacks and cerebral infarct). The etiology is unknown, but it can be primary idiopathic or associated with a primary autoimmune disorder, including systemic lupus erythematosus and antiphospholipid antibodies. Up to 78% of patients with Sneddon syndrome test positive for antiphospholipid antibodies.

Anti-RNP antibodies are associated with mixed connective tissues disorders and systemic lupus erythematosus. Anti-Ro and anti-La antibodies are associated with various autoimmune conditions, in particular Sjögren disease and systemic lupus erythematosus. Anti-Scl70 antibodies are commonly associated with diffuse scleroderma. Anti-gliadin antibodies are associated with celiac disease.

11. **A.** Idarucizumab has been shown to be a fast and effective at reversing the anticoagulant effect of dabigatran (as assessed by percent reversal by measurement of dilute thrombin time or ecarin clotting time), based on the RE-VERSE AD study, in 88% to 98% of patients with elevated clotting times at baseline.

Cryoprecipitate is used for hemorrhagic conversion secondary to intravenous alteplase but would not work for a direct thrombin inhibitor. Vitamin K is given for warfarin-related hemorrhages; direct thrombin inhibitors are not vitamin K dependent. Andexanet alfa has been shown to be an effective reversal agent for factor Xa inhibitors such as rivaroxaban. Protamine sulfate is used for heparin reversal.

12. **C.** The patient in this vignette has infectious endocarditis. The majority of cases (80%) are caused by *Streptococci* and *Staphylococci*, and initiation of

antibiotics would be the most appropriate treatment. Common clinical findings including fever (80%), new murmur (48%), hematuria (25%), splenomegaly (11%), splinter hemorrhages (8%), Janeway lesions (5%), and Roth spots (5%). A randomized controlled trial studying aspirin 325 mg daily in patients with endocarditis showed no significant decrease in embolic events, and there was a trend toward increased rate of cerebral hemorrhage. Endocarditis can result in both hemorrhagic and ischemic strokes. In addition, the formation of mycotic aneurysms increases the risk for hemorrhage. Intravenous alteplase would not be appropriate in this setting. The patient has infective endocarditis, not nonbacterial/sterile/marantic endocarditis; thus, immunoglobulin therapy would not be appropriate therapy.

13. **B.** Cerebral amyloid angiopathy (CAA) is caused by β-amyloid deposits in the small arteries of the leptomeninges and cerebral cortex. It is the most common cause of lobar intraparenchymal hemorrhage in the elderly. Nearly 25% of patients with Alzheimer disease have advanced CAA, and less than half of patients with CAA meet criteria for Alzheimer disease. Despite the overlap, CAA remains a distinct clinical entity from Alzheimer disease. The image shown in the question depicts multiple cerebral microhemorrhages with a lobar pattern on a blood-sensitive sequence.

14. **B.** Reversible cerebral vasoconstriction syndrome (RCVS) classically presents with a severe "thunderclap" headache, with or without other acute neurologic symptoms, and diffuse segmental constriction of cerebral arteries. RCVS can be associated with both hemorrhagic and ischemic strokes. In particular, RCVS can be associated with convexity/sulcal subarachnoid hemorrhage, as in this case. Vascular imaging shows diffuse segmental constriction of cerebral arteries, which often normalizes within 3 months on repeat vascular imaging. Literature about the use of nimodipine, verapamil, and/or magnesium is controversial. Clinical and radiographic partial or complete recovery takes place within days to weeks after symptom onset.

15. **C.** The patient has symptomatic, severe, >70% proximal left internal carotid artery stenosis. She is an ideal candidate for carotid endarterectomy to prevent recurrent stroke based on the North American Symptomatic Carotid Endarterectomy Trial (NASCET) and the European Carotid Surgery Trial (ECST). Based on the NASCET results, the 2-year ipsilateral stroke risk for 70% to 99% symptomatic stenosis was 26% in the medical therapy alone group compared to 9% in the carotid endarterectomy and medical therapy group (P <.001) (absolute risk reduction, 17.0%; number needed to treat, 6). For 50% to 69% symptomatic stenosis, the 5-year rate of ipsilateral stroke was 22.2% in the medical therapy alone group compared to 15.7% in the carotid endarterectomy and medical therapy group (absolute risk reduction, 6.5%; number needed to treat, 15).

The rationale of liberalizing blood pressure to prevent hypoperfusion-related stroke in the setting of carotid disease has never been proven to be an effective long-term treatment to reduce the risk of recurrent stroke. One study has shown that tight blood pressure control (≤130/85 mm Hg) even in the setting of carotid occlusion was associated with a reduced risk of future stroke compared to patients with less well-controlled blood pressure (>130/85 mm Hg). Extracranial-intracranial bypass has never been proven to be effective in preventing future stroke in carotid disease even in the setting of complete carotid occlusion and confirmed hemodynamic cerebral ischemia identified by increased oxygen extraction fraction measured by positron emission tomography.

16. **B.** Cerebral autosomal recessive arteriopathy with subcortical infarcts and leukoencephalopathy (CARASIL) is characterized by cerebral small-vessel arteriopathy (nonhypertensive) with subcortical infarcts along with alopecia and spondylosis. Onset is usually in early adulthood. Mutations in the *HTRA1* gene are causative for this disease. Mutations in the *NOTCH3* gene are associated with cerebral autosomal dominant arteriopathy with subcortical infarcts and leukoencephalopathy (CADASIL). Patients with CADASIL often present with strokes in their 40s and 50s and have associated migraines. Mutations in *KRIT1* gene cause familial cerebral cavernous malformations. Mutations in the *GLA* gene cause Fabry disease; stroke can be the first presenting symptom of this disease. Mutations in *TREX1* cause retinal vasculopathy with cerebral leukodystrophy.

17. **D.** The patient has left middle cerebral artery syndrome with evidence of a left M1 division occlusion. Multiple randomized controlled trials support mechanical thrombectomy using mechanical stent retrievers in patients with a large-vessel occlusion. The American Heart Association currently recommends considering patients for intervention who can undergo recanalization within 6 hours from symptom onset. Recently announced DAWN trial showed that up to 24 hours after stroke onset, endovascular thrombectomy reduced poor outcome and disability in selected patients. Current trials are under way to determine if the time window for treatment can be expanded in selected cohort of acute stroke patients.

Heparin drip has never been proven as an effective treatment for acute large-vessel occlusions. Tenecteplase appears to be a promising treatment option for acute stroke based on a phase IIb trial. Multiple trials are currently under way to assess the efficacy of tenecteplase in acute ischemic stroke. Administration of tenecteplase after alteplase is not recommended. The patient may eventually need a hemicraniectomy and/or hyperosmotic therapy if the stroke continues to progress and result in significant cerebral edema; however, endovascular therapy should be considered first.

18. **A.** Transcranial Doppler can be used to screen and assess for cerebral vasospasm related to subarachnoid hemorrhage. The middle cerebral artery has been the most studied. In general, cerebral vasospasm result in an increase in flow velocities. Sensitivity and specificity vary depending on what thresholds are used. Mean flow velocities >120 cm/s are commonly considered abnormal. Mean flow velocities >200 cm/s often suggest severe vasospasm. In addition, the Lindegaard ratio (middle cerebral artery velocity/internal carotid artery velocity) can be used to assess for cerebral vasospasm. A Lindegaard ratio of <3 is usually considered normal. A Lindegaard ratio >6 can distinguish severe from moderate vasospasm.

19. **C.** The patient is presenting with thrombocytopenic thrombotic purpura (TTP). The classic pentad consists of thrombocytopenia, microangiopathic hemolytic anemia, neurologic symptoms, renal failure, and fever, but cases have been reported with isolated stroke as the presenting feature. *ADAMTS13* activity can be measured and is reduced in TTP. The treatment for TTP is plasma exchange transfusion.

Intravenous alteplase should not be administered because of the thrombocytopenia and high risk of bleeding. Platelet transfusion can potentially mediate pathologic thrombogenesis and should be avoided in most cases of TTP. Nicardipine and intravenous fluids are not immediately indicated in this case.

20. **D.** The most common site of injury is the distal V3 segment to the early portion of the V4 segment. This portion of the vertebral artery is relatively mobile and unfixed, making it susceptible to tearing by sudden motion and stretching. Arterial dissection is one of the most common identifiable causes of stroke in the young adult.

REFERENCES

Anderson CS, Heeley E, Hyang Y, et al. Rapid blood-pressure lowering in patients with acute intracerebral hemorrhage. *N Engl J Med.* 2013;368:2355-2365.
Back L, Nagaraja V, Kapur A, et al. Role of decompressive hemicraniectomy in extensive middle cerebral artery strokes: a meta-analysis of randomised trials. *Intern Med J.* 2015;45:711-717.
Baharoglu MI, Cordonnier C, Al-Shahi Salman R, et al. Platelet transfusion versus standard care after acute stroke due to spontaneous cerebral haemorrhage associated with antiplatelet therapy (PATCH): a randomised, open-label, phase 3 trial. *Lancet.* 2016;387:2605-2613.
Bardutzky J, Schwab S. Antiedema therapy in ischemic stroke. *Stroke.* 2007;38:3084-3094.
Bartynski WS. Posterior reversible encephalopathy syndrome, part 1: fundamental imaging and clinical features. *AJNR Am J Neuroradiol.* 2008;29:1036-1042.
Caplan CR. Dissections of brain-supplying arteries. *Nat Clin Pract Neurol.* 2008;4:34-42.
Chan KL, Dumesnil JG, Cujec B, et al. A randomized trial of aspirin on the risk of embolic events in patients with infective endocarditis. *J Am Coll Cardiol.* 2003;42:775-780.
Chaturvedi S, Bruno A, Feasby T, et al. Carotid endarterectomy—an evidence-based review. Report of the Therapeutics and Technology Assessment Subcommittee of the American Academy of Neurology. *Neurology.* 2005;65:794-801.
Chen JJ, Chang HF, Hsu YC, et al. Anton-Babinski syndrome in an old patient: a case report and literature review. *Psychogeriatrics.* 2015;15:58-61.
Ducros A. Reversible cerebral vasoconstriction syndrome. *Lancet Neurol.* 2012;11:906-917.
Egner, W. The use of laboratory tests in the diagnosis of SLE. *J Clin Pathol.* 2000;53:424-432.
Eilbert W, Singla N. Lemierre's syndrome. *Int J Emerg Med.* 2013;23:40.

Engelter ST, Fluri F, Buitrago-Tellez C, et al. Lift-threatening oroloingula angioedema during thrombolysis in acute ischemic stroke. *J Neurol.* 2005;252:1167-1170.

Hacke W, Kaste M, Bluhmki E, et al. Thrombolysis with alteplase 3 to 4.5 hours after acute ischemic stroke. *N Engl J Med.* 2008;359:1317-1329.

Hassan A, Lanzino G, Wijdicks EF, et al. Terson's syndrome. *Neurocrit Care.* 2011;15:554-558.

Hemphill JC 3rd, Bonovich DC, Besmertis L, et al. The ICH score: a simple, reliable grading scale for intracerebral hemorrhage. *Stroke.* 2001;32:891-897.

Hemphill JC 3rd, Greenberg SM, Anderson CS, et al. Guidelines for the Management of Spontaneous Intracerebral Hemorrhage: a guideline for healthcare professionals from the American Heart Association/American Stroke Association. *Stroke.* 2015;46:2032-2060.

Hoen B, Duval X. Infective endocarditis. *N Engl J Med.* 2013;368:1425-1433.

Kalashnikova LA, Nasonov EL, Stoyanovich LZ, et al. Sneddon's syndrome and the primary antiphospholipid syndrome. *Cerebrovasc Dis.* 1994;4:76-82.

Labauge P, Denier C, Bergametti F, et al. Genetics of cavernous angiomas. *Lancet Neurol.* 2007;6:237-244.

Lekoubou A, Phillippeau F, Derex L, et al. Audit report and systematic review of orolingual angioedema in post-acute stroke thrombolysis. *Neurol Res.* 2014;36:687-694.

Lerario A, Ciammola A, Poletti B, et al. Charles Bonnet syndrome: two case reports and review of the literature. *J Neurol.* 2013;260:1180-1186.

Logallo N, Kvistad CE, Thomassen L. Therapeutic potential of tenecteplase in the management of acute ischemic stroke. *CNS Drugs.* 2015;29:811-818.

Madden B, Chebl RB. Hemi-orolingual angioedema after tPA administration for acute ischemic stroke. *West J Emerg Med.* 2015;16:175-177.

Markus HS. Stroke genetics. *Hum Mol Genet.* 2011;20:R124-R131.

Massey EW, Schoenberg B. Foster Kennedy syndrome. *Arch Neurol.* 1984;41:658-659.

Morgenstern LB, Zahuranec DB, Sanchez BN, et al. Full medical support for intracerebral hemorrhage. *Neurology.* 2015;84:1739-1744.

National Institute of Neurological Disorders and Stroke rt-PA Stroke Study Group. Tissue plasminogen activator for acute ischemic stroke. *N Engl J Med.* 1995;333:1581-1588.

Parsons M, Spratt N, Bivard A, et al. A randomized trial of tenecteplase versus alteplase for acute ischemic stroke. *N Engl J Med.* 2012;366:1099-1107.

Pollack CV, Reilly PA, Eikelboom J, et al. Idarucizumab for dabigatran reversal. *N Engl J Med.* 2015;373:511-520.

Powers WJ, Clarke WR, Grubb RL Jr, et al. Extracranial-intracranial bypass surgery for stroke prevention in hemodynamic cerebral ischemia: the Carotid Occlusion Surgery Study randomized trial. *JAMA.* 2011;306:1983-1992.

Powers WJ, Clarke WR, Grubb RL Jr, et al. Lower stroke risk with lower blood pressure in hemodynamic cerebral ischemia. *Neurology.* 2014;82:1027-1032.

Powers WJ, Derdeyn CP, Biller J, et al. 2015 American Heart Association/American Stroke Association focused update of the 2013 guidelines for the early management of patients with acute ischemic stroke regarding endovascular treatment: a guideline for healthcare professionals from the American Heart Association/American Stroke Association. *Stroke.* 2015;46:3020-3035.

Qureshi AI, Plesch YY, Barsan WG, et al. Intensive blood-pressure lowering in patients with acute cerebral hemorrhage. *N Engl J Med.* 2016;375:1033-1045.

Rojas JC, Banerjee C, Siddiqui F, et al. Pearls & oysters: acute ischemic stroke caused by atypical thrombotic thrombocytopenic purpura. *Neurology.* 2013;80:e235-e238.

Rolfs A, Böttcher T, Zschiesche M, et al. Prevalence of Fabry disease in patients with cryptogenic stroke: a prospective study. *Lancet.* 2005;366:1794-1796.

Sandercock PA, Counsell C, Kane EJ. Anticoagulants for acute ischaemic stroke. *Cochrane Database Syst Rev.* 2015;3:CD000024.

Saposnik G, Barinagarrementeria F, Brown RD, et al. Diagnosis and management of cerebral venous thrombosis. *Stroke.* 2011;42:1158-1192.

Siegal DM, Curnutte JT, Connolly SJ, et al. Andexanet alfa for the reversal of factor Xa inhibitor activity. *N Engl J Med.* 2015;373:2413-2424.

Sloan MA. Detection of vasospasm following subarachnoid hemorrhage. In: Babikian VL, Wechsler LR, eds. *Transcranial Doppler Ultrasonography.* St. Louis, MO: Mosby-Year Book; 1993:105-127.

Verduzco LA, Nathan DG. Sickle cell disease and stroke. *Blood.* 2009;114:5117-5125.

Viswanathan A, Greenberg SM. Cerebral amyloid angiopathy in the elderly. *Ann Neurol.* 2011;70:871-880.

Wu S, Xu Z, Liang H. Sneddon's syndrome: a comprehensive review of the literature. *Orphanet J Rare Dis.* 2014;9:215.

Zhang CH, DeSouza RM, Kho JS, et al. Kernohan-Woltman notch phenomenon: a review article. *Br J Neurosurg.* 2016;26:1-8.

2
Subarachnoid Hemorrhage

Tobias B. Kulik, MD, Saef Izzy, MD, and David P. Lerner, MD

Questions

Questions 1-3

A 46-year-old African American woman with an extensive smoking history presents to the emergency department with the "worst headache" of her life that started abruptly 2 hours ago. Aside from a headache, she endorses mild nausea and "blurry vision." She denies a history of headache. Her blood pressure at the time of presentation is 220/110 mm Hg. On physical examination, a right third nerve palsy is found. An emergent head computed tomography (CT) is obtained and shown below.

1. Based on this description, what is the Hunt and Hess grade?

   A. 1
   B. 2
   C. 3
   D. 4
   E. 5

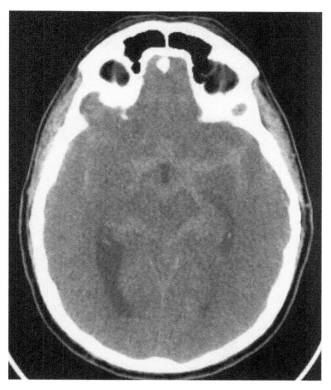

Head computed tomography: Axial noncontrast head CT at the level of the midbrain demonstrating diffuse subarachnoid hemorrhage left > right Sylvian fissure involvement. There are no areas of intraparenchymal or intraventricular hemorrhage.

2. You immediately consult the neurosurgical service. To deliver precise and objective information to your neurosurgical colleague, you determine the World Federation of Neurological Surgeons (WFNS) grade prior to initiating the call. Based on the earlier vignette, what is the patient's WFNS grade?

   A. 1
   B. 2
   C. 3
   D. 4
   E. 5

3. When talking to the consultant, you are asked about the patient's modified Fisher grade. The head CT is shown above. What is the patient's modified Fisher grade?

   A. 0
   B. 1
   C. 2
   D. 3
   E. 4

4. The American Heart Association recommends screening for unruptured intracranial aneurysms using noninvasive methods in whom?

   A. Two first-degree relatives with a known intracranial aneurysm
   B. One first-degree relative with a known intracranial aneurysm
   C. Patients with autosomal recessive polycystic kidney disease
   D. Patients below the age of 20 years

Questions 5-7

A 52-year-old Pacific Islander male presents to the emergency department at 11:00 P.M. with acute onset of the worst headache of his life, nausea, and vomiting. Symptoms started about 90 minutes ago during vigorous physical activity. He has been smoking about 1 pack per day for the last 30 years and has had a myocardial infarction. He does not take prescription medication, particularly no "blood thinners." On exam, the patient appears somnolent and has sluggish pupils bilaterally and a mild right hemiparesis. Lab work reveals mild leukocytosis, normal platelet count, and no coagulopathy. A head CT is obtained and shown below.

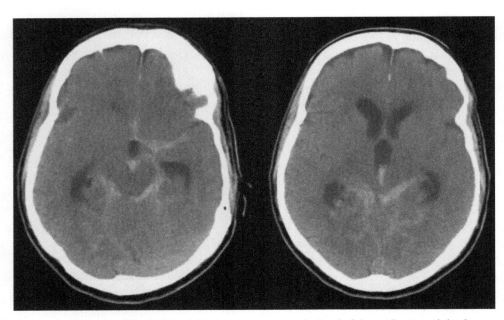

Head computed tomography (CT): Axial head CT with 2 consecutive cuts at the level of the midbrain and third ventricle shows diffuse subarachnoid hemorrhage (SAH) fissure with interventricular involvement.

5. What is the next best step in the management of this patient?

   A. Emergent placement of external ventricular drain (EVD)

   B. Obtain magnetic resonance angiogram (MRA) of the head

   C. Obtain digital subtraction angiogram

   D. Proceed to the operating room for open clipping of the aneurysm

   E. Transfuse platelets

6. Neurosurgery places an EVD for this patient, and a CT angiogram is performed demonstrating a left middle cerebral artery aneurysm. A digital subtraction angiogram is planned for the early morning to better characterize the aneurysm and for operative planning, and the patient is admitted to the neurointensive care unit. Management in the intensive care unit should include which of the following?

   A. Lowering the EVD to 0 mm H_2O and draining off cerebrospinal fluid

   B. Starting high dose intravenous dexamethasone

   C. Starting antihypertensives to maintain a mean arterial blood pressure <110 mm Hg

   D. Starting nimodipine 30 mg every 4 hours

   E. Starting an infusion of tranexamic acid (TXA)

7. Several hours later, a nurse informs you of deterioration in the patient's neurologic exam. You immediately assess the patient at the bedside and notice sonorous respirations and frank drainage of blood from the EVD. You are no longer able to wake the patient, and the blood pressure is now 220/140 mm Hg. What is the cause of the examination change?

   A. Severe vasospasm

   B. Hydrocephalus

   C. Aneurysmal rerupture

   D. Seizures

   E. EVD site–related bleeding

8. A patient with Hunt and Hess grade 2, modified Fisher grade 2 aneurysmal SAH is admitted to the intensive care unit overnight. The patient is started on the following medications: phenytoin, nimodipine, captopril, tranexamic acid infusion, and omeprazole. Which of the following statements is true regarding the medications?

   A. Phenytoin should be continued throughout the course of the vasospasm window.

   B. Nimodipine reduces the risk of vasospasm and delayed cerebral ischemia.

   C. Captopril is the blood pressure medication of choice for hypertension management.

   D. Short-term use of tranexamic acid may reduce early rebleeding rates and improve outcome.

   E. Proton pump inhibitors are more effective than H_2 blockers in reducing risk of gastrointestinal (GI) bleeding.

9. Which component of the classic triple-H therapy is considered the most effective therapy for a patient who has developed vasospasm?

   A. Hypertension

   B. Hypernatremia

   C. Hemodilution

   D. Hypervolemia

   E. Hypothermia

10. Which of the following raises concern for vasospasm following SAH?

    A. Apathy and abulia

    B. Electroencephalogram (EEG) with increase in the alpha-delta variability and left frontal lateralized periodic discharges at 0.5 Hz

    C. Elevation in mean velocities in all major cerebral vessels insonated on transcranial Doppler ultrasound and normal Lindegaard ratio

    D. Hypotension requiring vasopressors to maintain a mean arterial pressure of >65 mm Hg

11. Currently, consensus guidelines recommend the maintenance of euvolemia after aneurysmal SAH. Which of the following statements is true?

    A. Bedside assessment is the most sensitive assessment for volume status.

    B. Routine use of pulmonary artery catheters in hemodynamically stable patients is recommended.

    C. Fluid balance may not accurately reflect the intravascular volume.

    D. In a patient with sinus rhythm, stroke volume variability >5% predicts fluid responsiveness.

12. Which of the following statements about delayed cerebral ischemia (DCI) is true?

    A. Transcranial Doppler (TCD) ultrasound is the best test for diagnosing DCI.

    B. A normal digital subtraction angiogram excludes the diagnosis of DCI.

    C. Cerebral infarction occurs only in vascular territories affected by vasospasm.

    D. DCI is not completely understood but might be caused by microcirculatory dysfunction, cortical spreading depolarizations, and microthrombosis.

    E. Nimodipine has shown to reduce cerebral vasospasm and DCI.

13. A 70-year-old woman with hypertension is admitted to the intensive care unit from the emergency department for a Hunt and Hess grade 2, modified Fisher grade 2 SAH. She has an excruciating headache, which limits her ability to cooperate with examination and obtaining a history. As part of her admission evaluation, cardiac evaluation is completed. She is noted to have an elevation in troponin T of 1.17 ng/mL (normal <0.01 ng/mL). Electrocardiogram (ECG) is shown below, and a transthoracic echocardiogram is completed and demonstrates hypokinesis in the mid-inferolateral, anterolateral, and apical lateral segments. What is the cause of her cardiac abnormalities?

    A. Stunned cardiomyopathy

    B. Non–ST-segment elevation myocardial infarction (MI)

    C. ST-segment elevation MI

    D. Takotsubo cardiomyopathy

    E. Decompensated systolic heart failure

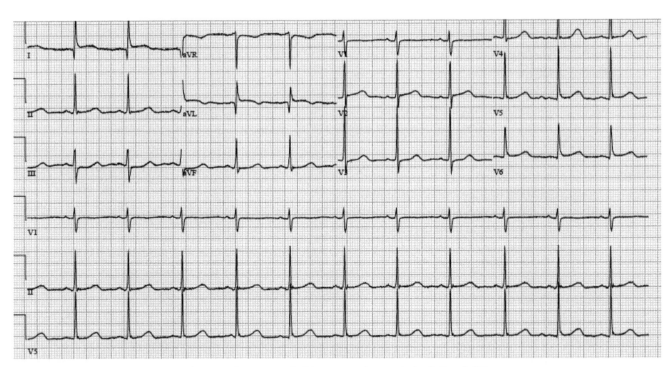

Electrocardiogram with ST-segment changes in leads I and aVL.

14. A 52-year-old African American woman presents to the emergency department with a severe headache that started abruptly 13 hours ago. Initially, she was reluctant to seek medical attention and hoping for the headache to resolve. However, after symptoms persisted throughout the night, her daughter insisted on her seeking medical attention. The patient denies any other neurologic symptoms. She denies a history of headaches and recreational drug use but has an extensive smoking history. A head CT scan is obtained immediately but fails to demonstrate any intracranial abnormality. What is the next best step in medical management?

A. Obtain brain magnetic resonance imaging (MRI)

B. Perform lumbar puncture

C. Admit for observation

D. Obtain digital subtraction angiography

E. Treat symptomatically and discharge from the emergency department

15. A 67-year-old white man is transferred to the neurointensive care unit from an outside hospital due to a concern for subarachnoid hemorrhage. He has acutely developed a severe headache but has no other neurologic deficits. He has smoked cigarettes in the past. His medical history is notable for hypertension. The physical exam is completely normal. You obtain a head CT, which is shown below. Which of the following statements is true?

A. Digital subtraction angiogram will likely show an aneurysm.

B. Patients will rarely have significant neurologic decompensation.

C. Hydrocephalus is a common complication.

D. This SAH pattern accounts for approximately 35% of all SAH.

E. Hypertension is one of the major risk factors for this SAH.

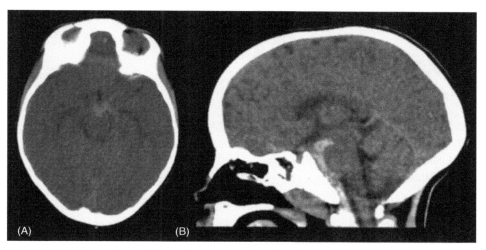

Noncontrast head CT (PMSAH) (A) axial view (B) sagital view. Reproduced with permission from Berkowitz AL. *Clinical Neurology and Neuroanatomy: A Localization-Based Approach.* New York, NY: McGraw-Hill, 2016.

16. A 65-year-old woman with hypertension and chronic obstructive pulmonary disease (COPD) presented to the emergency department; she was brought from her home by her husband because of a change in her mental status. In the emergency department, the patient had a reported tonic-clonic seizure that lasted for 2 minutes and stopped without medication. Her vitals just after the seizure were as follows: heart rate 96, blood pressure 196/82 mm Hg, and SpO_2 98% on room air. A head CT was obtained, which demonstrated a small amount of SAH on the cortical surface of the right posterior frontal lobe. A CT angiogram was completed and did not demonstrate any aneurysm. She was admitted, and an MRI of the brain was completed and is shown below (axial T2 fluid-attenuated inversion recovery sequence). What is the most likely cause of her cortical SAH?

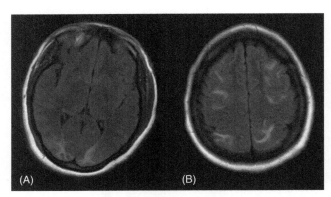

Reproduced with permission from Berkowitz AL. *Clinical Neurology and Neuroanatomy: A Localization-Based Approach.* New York, NY: McGraw-Hill, 2016.

A. Reversible vasoconstriction syndrome (RCVS)

B. Posterior reversible encephalopathy syndrome (PRES)

C. Cerebral venous thrombosis

D. Cerebral amyloid angiopathy

E. Occult trauma

17. A 55-year-old woman with lupus (on hydroxychloroquine) and hypertension presented to the emergency department via emergency medical services for loss of consciousness. She was intubated in the field and given agonal respirations. Workup in the emergency department revealed diffuse SAH, and an anterior communicating artery aneurysm was discovered on CT angiogram, which was later secured with endovascular coiling.

On hospital day 8, the patient had worsening of her examination with left face, arm, and leg weakness as well as mild dysarthria. Her transcranial Doppler (TCD) ultrasound results are listed below. Which of the following statements is true regarding the use of TCD ultrasound for cerebral artery vasospasm following aneurysmal SAH?

Blood Vessel	Transcranial Doppler Mean Velocity
R MCA	63
R ACA	–35
R PCA	45
R vertebral	36
L MCA	59
L ACA	–49
L PCA	50
L vertebral	39
Basilar	31

Transcranial Doppler ultrasound obtained via standard temporal and suboccipital approach. All values presented as velocity (cm/s).

Abbreviations: ACA, anterior cerebral artery; L, left; MCA, middle cerebral artery; PCA, posterior cerebral artery; R, right.

A. The anterior cerebral artery and vertebral artery are most reliable blood vessels for evaluating vasospasm via TCD.

B. TCD vasospasm (mean velocity >120 cm/s) typically correlates with clinical exam changes.

C. Lindegaard ratio can help evaluate the etiology of elevated mean velocities by comparing the middle cerebral artery and ipsilateral extracranial internal carotid artery velocities.

D. Following intra-arterial treatment with verapamil, TCD velocities will typically increase due to hyperemia.

18. A 57-year-old man with a Hunt and Hess grade 2, modified Fisher grade 3 aneurysmal SAH with a now-secured anterior communicating artery aneurysm is in the intensive care unit. On day 8, he is found to have a new hyponatremia on morning labs. While attempting to walk with physical therapy in the morning, he felt dizzy upon standing. His basic metabolic panel is remarkable for the following: sodium 131 mmol/L, potassium 3.2 mmol/L, and chloride 99 mmol/L. What is the next best step in management?

   A. Start fludrocortisone at 0.1 mg by mouth twice a day

   B. Start sodium chloride (NaCl) tablets 1 g by mouth 3 times a day

   C. Start fluid restriction of 1 L daily

   D. Give normal saline (0.9% NaCl) intravenous bolus

   E. Give desmopressin (DDAVP) 0.1 mg intravenous twice a day

19. A 61-year-old woman with a Hunt and Hess grade 3, modified Fisher grade 4 aneurysmal SAH who underwent successful coiling of a basilar artery aneurysm is currently in the intensive care unit. An external ventricular drain (EVD) is currently in place with normal intracranial pressure recordings and has remained open for drainage at a level of 5 cm above the tragus due to high cerebrospinal fluid (CSF) output and ongoing vasospasm. She is now day 11 post aneurysm rupture and has undergone intra-arterial therapy for symptomatic cerebral vasospasm on post-rupture days 6, 8, and 10 with improvement both angiographically and clinically. An angiogram completed prior to her most recent endovascular therapy is shown below. She again has worsening of her neurologic symptoms, and there is a discussion to start additional medical therapies. Which of the following statements is true?

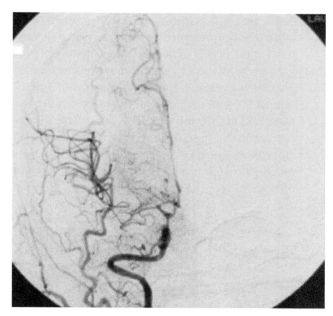

Digital subtraction angiogram: Anterior-posterior view of a right internal carotid artery injection. Severe proximal and distal vasospasm in the right middle cerebral and anterior cerebral artery. (Reproduced with permission from Lee K. *The NeuroICU Book.* New York, NY: McGraw-Hill; 2012.)

   A. Magnesium sulfate binds to voltage-dependent calcium channels, which in turn inhibits smooth muscle contraction and has failed to demonstrate vasospasm improvement.

   B. Milrinone is a phosphodiesterase III inhibitors with vasoconstricting and inotropic properties which associates with favorable outcome in SAH patients.

   C. Intraventricular instillation of nimodipine is superior to enteral nimodipine regarding outcome.

   D. Therapeutic hypothermia from 30°C to 32°C has been shown to increase cerebral blood flow.

   E. Raising the EVD to 15 can reverse delayed cerebral ischemia.

20. A 67-year-old African American woman with hypertension presented to the emergency department at the urging of her son for evaluation of progressive holocephalic, abrupt-onset headache with associated nausea and multiple episodes of emesis. A head CT was completed in the emergency department and is shown below. There was hemorrhage present in the suprasellar, prepontine cisterns and anterior craniocervical junction. Her exam was notable for stupor with inattention and limitation of upgaze. An EVD was placed with an elevated opening pressure and improvement in the patient's level of arousal. A diagnostic angiogram was completed the following day and is shown below. What is the most likely cause of the patient's SAH?

A. Right vertebral/anterior spinal artery aneurysm

B. Right vertebral artery dural fistula (dAVF)

C. Right vertebral artery arteriovenous malformation (AVM)

D. Cervical spinal cord cavernoma

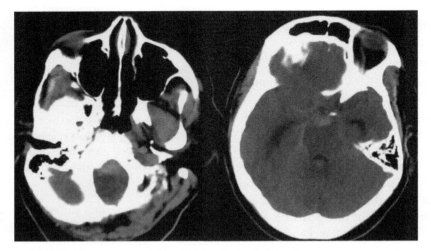

Head computed tomography (CT): Noncontrast axial head CT at the level of the foramen magnum and pons-midbrain junction.

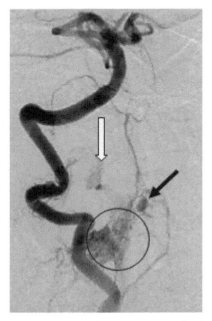

Digital subtraction angiogram: Selective injection of right vertebral artery.

21. A 58-year-old man was admitted to the intensive care unit following a Hunt and Hess grade 4, modified Fisher grade 4 aneurysmal SAH and underwent open clipping of a right middle cerebral artery aneurysm. He has remained in a minimally conscious state since admission with normal hemodynamics and minimal ventilator setting, but he is on continuous propofol infusion and has elevated intracranial pressures from a well-positioned EVD. Daily TCDs have been normal. He is also on continuous EEG monitoring, which has been reported as diffuse delta-theta slowing with a breech rhythm over the right hemisphere. He is now post-bleed day 10, and his quantitative EEG is shown below. What is the next best step in management?

A. Complete intravenous load of levetiracetam
B. Decrease rate of propofol infusion
C. Obtain "toxic-metabolic" workup with complete blood count, comprehensive metabolic panel, urinalysis, chest x-ray, blood cultures, ammonia, and thyroid-stimulating hormone
D. Raise the level of the EVD
E. Increase mean arterial pressure

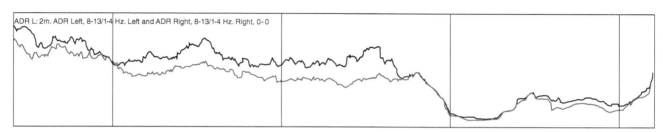

Quantitative electroencephalogram: Time lapse over the course of 4 hours. Black (*left*) and gray (*right*) with alpha-delta ratio over the course of time with sharp decrease in alpha delta ratio (ADR) in bilateral hemispheres.

Answers and Explanations

1. B. The Hunt and Hess scale is a widely used clinical grading system to predict prognosis and outcome in patients with SAH (Table 2-1). It is one of several available grading scales, is easy to use, but has been criticized for its interobserver variability. The scale ranges from 1 to 5. A lower score implies a better outcome and lower mortality.

2. A. The clinical grading system as proposed by the WFNS is easy to use, reliable, and depends less on subjective interpretation of clinical findings. It has been extensively validated. Grades range from 1 to 5 (Table 2-2) and are based on the Glasgow coma scale as well as the absence or presence of a motor deficit. The patient described in this question has a Glasgow coma scale score of 15, and therefore, the WFNS grade is 1.

3. D. The modified Fisher scale is a radiographic grading scale for subarachnoid hemorrhage (SAH) based on imaging findings on the initial head CT. It is derived from the original Fisher grading scale to account for the presence of thick cisternal blood and concomitant intraventricular hemorrhage. Grades range from 0 to 4, with a higher grade signifying a higher risk for the development of symptomatic vasospasm (Table 2-3). The figure for

Table 2-2. The World Federation of Neurological Surgeons (WFNS) Scale

Grade	Glasgow Coma Score	Motor Deficit
1	15	Absent
2	13-14	Absent
3	13-14	Present
4	7-12	Absent or present
5	3-6	Absent or present

Reproduced with permission from Drake CG, Hunt WE, Sano K, Kassell N, Teasdale G, Pertuiset B, et. al. Report of World Federation of Neurological Surgeons Committee on a Universal Subarachnoid Hemorrhage Grading Scale. J Neurosurg. 1988;68:985-86.

this case shows an axial, noncontrasted head CT with a focal, thick (>1 mm) SAH without an associated intraventricular component, and therefore, the patient's modified Fisher grade is 3.

4. A. In their 2015 guidelines, the American Heart Association recommends screening for unruptured intracranial aneurysms (IA) in the following situations:

- Families with 2 first-degree relatives with known IA
- Patients with a family history of IA

Table 2-1. Hunt and Hess Scale for Subarachnoid Hemorrhage

Hunt and Hess Grade	Description	Mortality (%)	Follow-Up Mortality (%)
1	Asymptomatic or minimal headache and slight nuchal rigidity	11	3
2	Moderate or severe headache, nuchal rigidity, no neurologic deficit other than cranial nerve palsy	26	3
3	Drowsiness, confusion, or mild focal deficit	37	9
4	Stupor, moderate to severe hemiparesis, possibly early decerebrate rigidity, and vegetative disturbance	71	24
5	Deep coma, decerebrate posturing, moribund appearance	100	71

Table 2-3. The Modified Fisher Scale

Grade	Criteria on Computed Tomography	Incidence of Symptomatic Vasospasm
0	No SAH; no IVH	0%
1	Focal or diffuse, thin SAH; no IVH	24%
2	Thin, focal or diffuse SAH; IVH	33%
3	Thick, focal or diffuse SAH; no IVH	33%
4	Thick, focal or diffuse SAH; IVH	40%

Abbreviations: IVH, intraventricular hemorrhage; SAH, subarachnoid hemorrhage.

Reproduced from Frontera JA, Claassen J, Schmidt JM et. al. *Prediction of symptomatic vasospasm after subarachnoid hemorrhage: the modified Fisher scale.* Neurosurgery 2006;59:21-27, with permission from Oxford University Press.

- Autosomal dominant polycystic kidney disease
- Type IV Ehlers-Danlos syndrome
- Microcephalic osteodysplastic primordial dwarfism

Screening can be considered in 1 first-degree relative and also in conditions associated with an increased occurrence of IA, such as coarctation of the aorta or bicuspid aortic valve.

5. **A.** Somnolence on exam is concerning for hydrocephalus. In this case, head imaging confirms mild ventriculomegaly, and therefore, an EVD should be placed immediately. Early hydrocephalus is seen in about 20% to 30% of patients with SAH and is frequently associated with a higher grade SAH and poor clinical condition. Delayed hydrocephalus, weeks to months after SAH, is much less frequently seen and associated with higher age, female gender, and intraventricular blood.

An MRA is not the diagnostic test of choice for SAH and would delay placement of an EVD. A digital subtraction angiogram will most likely be required during the patient's hospitalization but should not be the first imaging modality given its invasive nature. Prophylactic transfusion of platelets is not recommended per the Neurocritical Care Society's 2011 guidelines.

6. **C.** Until a causative aneurysm has been secured, either surgically or by using endovascular approaches, blood pressure control should be tight and aim at lowering the mean arterial blood pressure (MAP) to <110 mm Hg. Once the aneurysm is secured, the MAP goal can be relaxed. However, to maintain adequate cerebral perfusion, the blood pressure should not be lowered too aggressively.

Rebleeding in the first 24 to 72 hours is seen in 5% to 10% of patients and is one of the most feared

and potentially devastating conditions. Although guidelines cautiously recommend a short course of antifibrinolytics, such as transexamic acid, there are relative contraindications in patients including risk factors for thromboembolic events, particularly history of recent stroke, myocardial infarction, and venous thromboembolism.

It is common practice to start patients with SAH on levetiracetam even in the absence of overt seizure activity. Previously, phenytoin was commonly used, but data studying the effects of phenytoin on short-term functional and cognitive outcome demonstrated worse results in both of these domains. A short course (72 hours) of an anticonvulsant seems as effective as a longer course. Anticonvulsants should be continued outside the 3-day window with observed seizure activity or with evidence of electrographic seizures on electroencephalogram (EEG). Most advocate for keeping the EVD high or clamping it and only draining cerebrospinal fluid (CSF) when there is additional elevation in the intracranial pressure, because draining off large volumes of CSF may result in increased risk of aneurysmal rerupture. There is no role for steroids in the acute management of subarachnoid hemorrhage.

7. **C.** Aneurysmal rebleed is one of the most feared complications of SAH, associated with high morbidity and a mortality between 50% and 80%. The incidence is highest in the first 2 weeks postictus. However, patients are at maximal risk within the first 24 to 72 hours. The aim of all interventions and of the complex medical management is to prevent rebleeding. The only reliable way to reduce the risk of rebleeding is to repair a ruptured aneurysm as soon as possible. A recent study found the following independent predictors of aneurysmal rebleed:

- Known history of hypertension
- Diastolic blood pressure >90 mm Hg on admission
- Ictal loss of consciousness or seizures
- History of sentinel headaches
- Higher Fisher grade
- Presence of multiple aneurysms
- Irregular aneurysm surface

Seizures could explain a neurologic deterioration; however, they should not lead to drainage of frank blood from the EVD. A head CT should be obtained before starting a workup for nonconvulsive status epilepticus. EVD site–related bleeding should not cause that much frank blood to drain from the EVD. Sedating medications should be used sparingly as to not obscure neurologic assessment of the neurocritically ill patient. Worsening hydrocephalus could cause a change in mental status but should not cause frank blood to come out of the EVD, and lowering the EVD setting could help in such situations.

8. **E.** Although there is limited evidence for use of prophylactic antiepileptic medication in the setting of SAH and the AHA guidelines state that "administration of prophylactic anticonvulsants may be considered in the immediate post-hemorrhage period (Class IIB, Level of evidence B)," there are linkages between use of phenytoin and poor neurologic outcome. On further evaluation, longer periods of phenytoin prophylaxis use versus shorter periods (7 days vs 3 days) and are associated with no change in the rate of seizure and increased complications.

Nimodipine is a calcium channel blocker that has been approved by the US Food and Drug Administration (FDA) in 1989 for the reduction of neurologic symptoms associated with vasospasm and improvement of neurologic function after aneurysmal SAH, but it does not decrease the incidence of vasospasm. In the largest randomized controlled trial to date, patients on 60 mg every 4 hours (or 30 mg every 2 hours) nimodipine experienced a significantly lower risk of stroke and poor neurologic outcome.

Although blood pressure should be controlled prior to aneurysm obliteration, it is recommended to use a rapidly titratable agent (eg, nicardipine, labetalol, clevidipine). Although short-term treatment with tranexamic acid may reduce the early rebleeding rate, it has not demonstrated improvement in outcome.

A recent meta-analysis review demonstrated that proton pump inhibitors reduce the risk of clinically important GI bleeding and overt GI bleeding.

9. **A.** Originally, triple-H therapy was defined as hypertension, hypervolemia, and hemodilution; however, the current practice of triple-H therapy is highly variable. The overall goal of this approach is to improve cerebral hemodynamics. Several studies have shown an improved outcome for patients treated with hypertension, hemodilution, and hypervolemia. Recently, the practice of achieving prophylactic hypervolemia has fallen out of favor and been replaced by the maintenance of euvolemia. There is a general consensus that hypovolemia should be avoided. With triple-H therapy, the patient is at risk for cardiopulmonary failure, renal dysfunction, worsening of cerebral edema, and rupture of an unsecured aneurysm. Hypernatremia and hypothermia are not components of triple-H therapy.

Although there is not a general consensus on the components of tripe-H therapy, there are physiologic data that support euvolemic hypertension as the most likely component to increase cerebral blood flow after SAH.

10. **A.** Monitoring for vasospasm may take many modalities, including physical exam, transcranial Doppler ultrasound, EEG monitoring, and microdialysis/invasive monitoring. Of the examples in this question, the clinical exam changes of increased apathy and abulia are concerning for a potential anterior cerebral artery vasospasm. Although hypotension can worsen vasospasm, vasospasm does not result in hypotension. Transcranial Doppler ultrasound can assist with evaluation of potential vasospasm. Elevation in mean velocity can be consistent with vasospasm, but if there is global elevation and normal Lindegaard ratio, this is more likely due to cerebral hyperperfusion. EEG patterns that are related to vasospasm are decreased in the alpha-delta variability, although periodic discharges are associated with a worse overall outcome.

11. **C.** Understanding volume status is paramount to managing patients with SAH. Clinical evaluation of volume status is quite poor, and the assessment of hypovolemia has a sensitivity reported at 10%. Stroke volume variability as measured by arterial pressure–based cardiac monitoring has been useful in assessing volume status in SAH patients, but the stroke volume variability >9% is predictive of improvement with fluid challenge. Fluid balance management has been a strategy evaluated in the past. With the use of only fluid balance, as compared to blood volume measurements, there was an increased rate of severe hypovolemia. In patients who are hemodynamically stable, the use of a pulmonary artery catheter is not recommended.

12. **D.** Historically, delayed cerebral ischemia (DCI) was thought to be solely caused by large-vessel

vasospasm, resulting in a low-flow state downstream of the narrowed vessel, ultimately leading to ischemia and infarction. However, cerebral infarction sometimes occurs in the absence of demonstrable vasoconstriction or in territories remote from the affected vessel. While 70% of patients develop radiographically proven vasospasm, only 20% to 30% develop DCI.

A shift of interest has occurred in recent years. Aside from large-vessel narrowing, the research community now investigates microcirculatory dysfunction with loss of autoregulation, cortical spreading depolarization, and microthrombosis as elements of DCI. Although TCD is used commonly as a bedside test for evaluation of vasospasm there is substantial variability in the sensitivity, specificity, positive and negative predictive value depending on the vessel insonated.

Nimodipine does not significantly reverse angiographic vasospasm, but it has been shown to reduce risk of cerebral infarction and improves outcome after SAH.

13. C. Cardiac abnormalities are frequently seen after SAH and predominate in the early days after bleed. They are thought to reflect catecholamine-related myocardial injury.

Takotsubo cardiomyopathy, a condition characterized by apical ballooning on echocardiogram, is typically transient (Fig. 2-1). Stunned cardiomyopathy is similar to Takotsubo cardiomyopathy and thought to be due to catecholamine surge, but the echocardiogram can demonstrate atypical wall motion abnormalities. This patient's presentation is concerning for a primary cardiac event in addition to her SAH given that portions of the lateral wall are hypokinetic and there are ST-segment changes

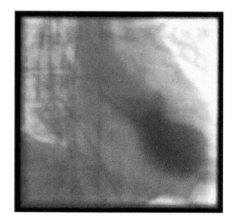

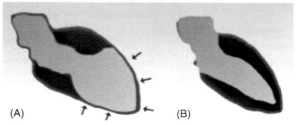

Figure 2-1 The upper image is a digital angiogram during left ventricular contraction. There is ballooning of the apex with stagnation of contrast while the base of the left ventricle contracts. (A) is a cartoon representation of the same apical ballooning phenomena, compared to (B) which is a normal presentation of ventricular contraction. Reproduced with permission from Lee K. *The NeuroICU Book.* McGraw-Hill, 2012.

in leads I and aVL, which are a single cardiac vascular territory. Troponin elevations are seen in up to 30% of patients. Although there are a number of ECG changes that can occur due to SAH, it is important to recall that patients can also have primary cardiac events. ECG changes described are ST elevations or depressions, T-wave inversions or peaked T waves, sinus tachycardia, and QT prolongation (Fig. 2-2).

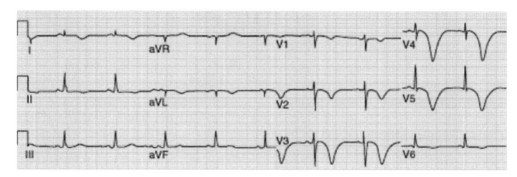

Figure 2-2 EKG shows T-wave inversions in V1-V6. Reproduced with permission from Lee K. *The NeuroICU Book.* McGraw-Hill, 2012.

14. **B.** A noncontrast head CT within 24 hours of symptom onset detects more than 95% of SAHs. If performed within 6 hours, the sensitivity and specificity to rule out aneurysmal SAH are 98.7% and 99.9%, respectively. If the initial head CT is normal and a strong suspicion for SAH remains, a lumbar puncture should be performed. The presence of xanthochromia in the cerebrospinal fluid, if assessed for spectrographically, is highly suggestive of SAH, whereas the absence practically rules out SAH during the first 2 weeks following symptom onset. MRI or digital subtraction angiography should not precede a lumbar puncture in the described case but may be warranted in a later stage depending on the clinical situation.

15. **B.** The noncontrast axial head CT shows the typical pattern for perimesencephalic subarachnoid hemorrhage (PMSAH). PMSAH commonly is a nonaneurysmal subset of SAH that occurs in approximately 10% of all patients with SAH. The radiographic pattern of PMSAH is relatively distinct, with hemorrhage located anterior to the midbrain or pons, with or without extension of blood around the brainstem, into the suprasellar cistern, or into the proximal Sylvian fissures. In PMSAH patients, digital subtraction angiogram will unlikely show an aneurysm, and patients rarely develop acute hydrocephalus in the first 1 to 2 days after bleed. In contrast to aneurysmal SAH, PMSAH patients have fewer in-hospital complications and have good outcome as well as normal life expectancy.

Smoking is a risk factor for perimesencephalic SAH. Compared with other types of SAH, patients with PMSAH are younger and less likely to be female or hypertensive. Alcohol consumption is not a recognized risk factor for PMSAH.

16. **B.** All of the conditions have been associated with cortical, or sulcal, SAH. In addition, antecedent trauma, PRES, septic emboli, septic aneurysms, Moyamoya disease, and coagulopathy can also cause a convexity pattern SAH. The patient's clinical history is most consistent with PRES given her confusion, seizure, and elevation in blood pressure.

17. **C.** Transcranial Doppler ultrasound (TCD) is a noninvasive, easily reproducible test that can be used to monitor for cerebral artery vasospasm following aneurysmal SAH and can be used for other disease evaluation, including emboli detection, brain death evaluation, and sickle cell disease evaluation. Although a good screening tool, TCD has limited sensitivity, specificity, and positive predictive value when compared to digital subtraction angiography (90%, 71%, and 57%, respectively). Early studies using TCD evaluated the diameter of blood vessels and the mean velocity, mean velocities >120 cm/s correlated with a decrease in blood vessel diameter by 50%. After intra-arterial treatment with verapamil, the blood vessel will be dilated and TCD velocities will detect lower mean velocities.

Our patient is an example that demonstrates that TCD can be normal despite the patient having angiographic and clinical vasospasm given the low specificity and positive predictive values of the testing. More importantly, there are limitations in the ability of TCD to detect vasospasm in major blood vessels other than the middle cerebral and basilar arteries. Although not present here, elevated velocities may not be a sign of vasospasm. At times, there can be hyperemia, resulting in increased velocities throughout. The advent of the Lindegaard ratio can be used to further evaluate elevation in velocities by comparing the mean velocity in the middle cerebral artery with that of the ipsilateral extracranial internal carotid artery.

Lindegaard ratio >3 and mean velocity >120 cm/s are correlated with clinical vasospasm (85%) and angiographic vasospasm (83.2%).

Mean Velocities (cm/s)	Lindegaard Ratio	Interpretation
<120	<3	Increased flow throughout the vascular system; "hyperemia"
>120	3-6	Mild-to-moderate vasospasm +/− hyperemia
>180	>6	Severe vasospasm

18. **D.** Hyponatremia is the most commonly encountered electrolyte abnormality in SAH, with a range of etiologies. The paramount clinical finding to assist with determining the etiology of hyponatremia is volume status. This patient has findings of orthostasis and likely hypovolemia. In cases of hypovolemic hyponatremia in SAH patients, cerebral salt wasting is the most likely etiology. Salt wasting

is due to abnormal release of natriuretic hormones resulting in excessive natriuresis. First-line therapy for treatment of cerebral salt wasting is to ensure and maintain euvolemia, so administration of a normal saline bolus is the most appropriate management step. Additional means of increasing sodium may be required including use of fludrocortisone and salt tablets, but these are not initial therapies. Fluid restriction is appropriate for the syndrome of inappropriate antidiuretic hormone secretion (SIADH), but this is not the likely cause of hyponatremia in this patient. The use of DDAVP is for management of hypernatremia, not hyponatremia, in the setting of diabetes insipidus.

19. **A.** Magnesium does bind to voltage-dependent calcium channels to inhibit smooth muscle contraction and may inhibit glutamate release (via a different mechanism). This has been studied in multiple trials for evaluation of improvement in outcome with SAH. The IMASH and MASH-2 trials failed to demonstrate improvement with magnesium sulfate infusion, and this has prompted a recommendation against use of magnesium sulfate in SAH.

   Milrinone is a phosphodiesterase III inhibitors which has vasodilating and inotropic properties. Few animal studies showed increased mean and peak blood flow velocity after milrinone. Limited human studies suggested the potential role of increased cardiac output in improving cerebral tissue perfusion independently of mean arterial pressure. Despite this effect, few underpowered studies showed angiographic improvement in vasospasm. At this point, limited data exist to support its use for the treatment of vasospasm.

   The use of intraventricular nimodipine has been used in the past and is now undergoing trials for evaluation of a sustained-release formulation. A randomized phase I/IIA study (NEWTON) demonstrated safety and tolerability of up to 800 mg of nimodipine instilled as a single dose and association with reduced delayed cerebral ischemia and rescue therapy. Further studies are needed to show superiority to enteral nimodipine.

   Limited data suggest that treating medical and radiographic refractory vasospasm as well as delayed cerebral ischemia with hypothermia, with targeted temperature of 32°C to 34°C, decreases cerebral blood flow and improves outcome in high-grade SAH. However, a large randomized trial, the Intraoperative Hypothermia for Aneurysm Surgery Trial, enrolled 1001 patients with "good-grade SAH" and showed no difference in neurologic outcome between hypothermic and normothermic groups 3 months after surgery.

   Limited case report–level data suggest that CSF diversion could decrease the risk of delayed cerebral ischemia after SAH. The authors postulated that using an aggressive lower EVD setting could improve cerebral perfusion and thus improve blood flow in microcirculation.

20. **A.** The etiology of the patient's SAH is from her cervical spine vascular lesion. The lesion that is easiest to identify is the prenidal aneurysm at the superior, medial aspect of the AVM (*black arrow* in figure). Perinidal aneurysms are associated with increased risk of bleeding associated with AVMs. Aneurysms associated with AVM are more prone to rupture due to higher flow, pressure, and shear stress. Although it can be difficult at times to ascertain the etiology of hemorrhage in the setting of complex vascular lesions, given there is only SAH that extends well outside of the region of the AVM (*circle*), the most likely cause of SAH is from the prenidal aneurysm. There is also a dAVF with supply from a radiculomeningeal branch from the right vertebral artery and the anterior spinal artery with venous drainage (draining vein depicted by *white arrow*) via the right paravertebral venous plexus. The complex tangle of vessels is the AVM, with supply from the right vertebral artery. Although AVMs can present with SAH, it is more common to present with concomitant intraparenchymal hemorrhage.

   Cavernomas typically present with seizure but can have intraparenchymal hemorrhage most commonly found in the supratentorial region, and they are typically solitary and would not present with diffuse SAH.

21. **E.** The patient presented with a high-grade SAH hemorrhage that places him at high risk for poor neurologic outcome (based on Hunt and Hess grade) and vasospasm (based on modified Fisher grade). Some centers advocate for use of continuous EEG for monitoring SAH patients. The quantitative EEG shown in the question demonstrates a decrease in the percent alpha variability, which has been associated with vasospasm and delayed

cerebral ischemia. There is a delay between EEG changes and clinical or radiographic changes in patients with decreased alpha variability. As a result, there is a potential window for medical optimization prior to surgical interventions, which would include a trial of increased mean arterial pressure. Although there is a risk of seizures given his SAH, the EEG does not demonstrate seizures or status epilepticus, and there is no role for levetiracetam. Although heavy sedation with propofol can result in burst suppression patterns, this is not what is demonstrated on the EEG and titration of propofol is not required if there are no other changes to the patient. An EEG can demonstrate findings consistent with metabolic encephalopathy (such as triphasic waves), but this is not demonstrated on quantitative EEG, and the loss of alpha variability is concerning for ischemia. Lowering the EVD could be a potential intervention for treatment of vasospasm and delayed cerebral ischemia.

REFERENCES

Alexandrov AV, ed. *Cerebrovascular Ultrasound in Stroke Prevention and Treatment.* New York, NY: Blackwell Publishing; 2008.

Alshamsi F, Belley-Cote E, Cook D, et al. Efficacy and safety of proton pump inhibitors for stress ulcer prophylaxis in crucially ill patients: a systematic review and meta-analysis of randomized trials. *Crit Care.* 2016;20:120.

Bergui M, Bradac GB. Uncommon symptomatic cerebral vascular malformations. *AJNR Am J Neuroradiol.* 1997;18:779-783.

Brown RD Jr, Weibers DO, Forbes GS. Unruptured intracranial aneurysms and arteriovenous malformations: frequency of intracranial hemorrhage and relationship of lesions. *J Neurosurg.* 1990;73:859-863.

Budohoski KP, Guilfoyle M, Helmy A, et al. The pathophysiology and treatment of delayed cerebral ischemia following subarachnoid hemorrhage. *J Neurol Neurosurg Psychiatry.* 2014;85:1343-1353.

Chumnanvej S, Dunn IF, Kim DH. Three-day phenytoin prophylaxis is adequate after subarachnoid hemorrhage. *Neurosurgery.* 2007;60:99-102.

Claassen J, Hirsch LJ, Kreiter KT, et al. Quantitative continuous EEG for detecting delayed cerebral ischemia in patients with poor-grade subarachnoid hemorrhage. *Clin Neurophysiol.* 2004;115:2699-2710.

Connolly ES Jr, Rabinstein AA, Charhaupoma R, et al. Guidelines for the management of aneurysmal subarachnoid hemorrhage. A guideline for healthcare professionals from the American Heart Association/American Stroke Association. *Stroke.* 2012;43:1711-1737.

D'Aliberti G, Talamonti G, Cenzato M, et al. Arterial and venous aneurysms associated with arteriovenous malformations. *World Neurosurg.* 2015;83:188-196.

Diringer MN. Management of aneurysmal subarachnoid hemorrhage. *Crit Care Med.* 2009;37:432-440.

Diringer MN, Bleck TP, Hemphill C, et al. Critical care management of patients following aneurysmal subarachnoid hemorrhage: recommendations from the Neurocritical Care Society's Multidisciplinary Consensus Conference. *Neurocrit Care.* 2011;15:211-240.

Drake CG, Hunt WE, Sano K, et al. Report of World Federation of Neurological Surgeons Committee on a Universal Subarachnoid Hemorrhage Grading Scale. *J Neurosurg.* 1988;68:985-986.

Dubosh NM, Bellolio MF, Rabinstein AA, et al. Sensitivity or early brain computed tomography to exclude aneurysmal subarachnoid hemorrhage: a systematic review and meta-analysis. *Stroke.* 2016;47:750-755.

Foreman B, Claassen J. Quantitative EEG for the detection of brain ischemia. *Crit Care.* 2012;16:2016.

Francoeur CL, Mayer SA. Management of delayed cerebral ischemia after subarachnoid hemorrhage. *Crit Care.* 2016; 20:277.

Fraticelli AT, Cholley BP, Losser MR, et al. Milrinone for the treatment of cerebral vasospasm after aneurysmal subarachnoid hemorrhage. *Stroke.* 2008;39:893-898.

Frontera JA, Claassen J, Schmidt JM, et al. Prediction of symptomatic vasospasm after subarachnoid hemorrhage: the modified Fisher scale. *Neurosurgery.* 2006;59:21-27.

Fugate JE, Rabinstein AA, Wijdicks EF, et al. Aggressive CSF diversion reverses delayed cerebral ischemia in aneurysmal subarachnoid hemorrhage: a case report. *Neurocrit Care.* 2012;17:112-116.

Fujii Y, Takeuchi S, Sasaki O, et al. Ultra-early rebleeding in spontaneous subarachnoid hemorrhage. *J Neurosurg.* 1996;84:35-42.

Germanwala AV, Huang J, Tamargo RJ. Hydrocephalus after subarachnoid hemorrhage. *Neurosurg Clin N Am.* 2010;21:263-270.

Gonzalez NR, Boscardin WJ, Glenn T, et al. Vasospasm probability index: a combination of transcranial Doppler velocities, cerebral blood flow and clinical risk factors to predict cerebral vasospasm after aneurysmal subarachnoid hemorrhage. *J Neurosurg.* 2007;107:1101-1112.

Greenberg M. *Handbook of Neurosurgery.* New York, NY: Thieme; 2006.

Gress DR, The Participants in the International Multi-Disciplinary Consensus Conference on the Critical Care Management of Subarachnoid Hemorrhage. Monitoring of volume status after subarachnoid hemorrhage. *Neurocrit Care.* 2011;15:270-274.

Hanggi D, Etminan N, Aldrich F, et al. Randomized, open-label, phase 1/2a study to determine the maximum tolerated dose of intraventricular sustained release nimodipine for subarachnoid hemorrhage. *Stroke.* 2017;48:145-151.

Hanggi D, The Participants in the International Multidisciplinary Consensus Conference on the Critical Care Management of Subarachnoid Hemorrhage. Monitoring and detection of vasospasm II: EEG and invasive monitoring. *Neurocrit Care.* 2011;15:318-323.

Hefzy HM, Bartynski WS, Boardman JF, et al. Hemorrhage in posterior reversible encephalopathy syndrome:

imaging and clinical features. *AJNR Am J Neuroradiol.* 2009;30:1371-1379.

Hoff RG, Rinkle GJ, Verweij BH, et al. Blood volume measurement after aneurismal subarachnoid hemorrhage. *Neurocrit Care.* 2008;8:391-397.

Hunt WE, Hess RM. Surgical risk as related to time of intervention in the repair of intracranial aneurysms. *J Neurosurg.* 1968;28(1):14-20.

Isotani E, Suzuki R, Tomita K, et al. Alterations in plasma concentrations of natriuretic peptides and antidiuretic hormone after subarachnoid hemorrhage. *Stroke.* 1994;25:2198-2203.

Kondziella D, Friberg CK, Wellwood I, et al. Continuous EEG monitoring in aneurysmal subarachnoid hemorrhage: a systematic review. *Neurocrit Care.* 2015;22:450-461.

Kumar G, Shahripour RB, Harrigan MR. Vasospasm on transcranial Doppler is predictive of delayed cerebral ischemia in aneurismal subarachnoid hemorrhage: a systematic review and meta-analysis. *J Neurosurg.* 2016;124:1257-1264.

Kurtz P, Helbok R, Ko SB, et al. Fluid responsiveness and brain tissue oxygenation augmentation after subarachnoid hemorrhage. *Neurocrit Care.* 2014;20:24-54.

Lindegaard KF, Nornes H, Bakke SJ, et al. Cerebral vasospasm diagnosis by means of angiography and blood velocity measurements. *Acta Neurochir (Wien).* 1989;100:12-24.

Marder CP, Narla V, Fink JR, et al. Subarachnoid hemorrhage: beyond aneurysms. *AJR Am J Roentgenol.* 2014;202:25-37.

Marupudi NI, Mittal S. Diagnosis and management of hyponatremia in patients with aneurysmal subarachnoid hemorrhage. *J Clin Med.* 2015;4:756-767.

Mees SMD, Algra A, Vandertop WP, et al. Magnesium for aneurysmal subarachnoid haemorrhage (MASH-2): a randomized placebo-controlled trial. *Lancet.* 2012;380:44-49.

Milikan CH. Cerebral vasospasm and ruptured intracranial aneurysm. *Arch Neurol.* 1975;32:433-439.

Murphy-Human T, Welch E, Zipfel G, et al. Comparison of short-duration levetiracetam with extended-course phenytoin for seizure prophylaxis after subarachnoid hemorrhage. *World Neurosurg.* 2011;75:269-274.

Naldech AM, Kreiter KT, Janjua N, et al. Phenytoin exposure is associated with functional and cognitive disability after subarachnoid hemorrhage. *Stroke.* 2005;36:583-587.

Nimodipine [package insert]. New Haven, CT: Bayer Pharmaceutical Corporation; 2005.

Pickard JD, Murray GD, Illingworth MD, et al. Effect of oral nimodipine on cerebral infarction and outcome after subarachnoid hemorrhage: British aneurysm nimodipine trial. *BMJ.* 1989;298:636-642.

Purykayastha S, Sorond F. Transcranial Doppler ultrasound: technique and application. *Semin Neurol.* 2012;32:411-420.

Rammos SK, Gardenghi B, Bortolotti C, et al. Aneurysms associated with brain arteriovenous malformations. *AJNR Am J Neuroradiol.* 2016;June 23. [Epub ahead of print]

Rots ML, van Putten MJ, Hoedemaekers CW, et al. Continuous EEG monitoring for early detection of delayed cerebral ischemia in subarachnoid hemorrhage: a pilot study. *Neurocrit Care.* 2016;24:207-216.

Seule M, Keller E. Hypothermia after aneurysmal subarachnoid hemorrhage. *Crit Care.* 2012;16(Suppl 2):A16.

Solanki C, Pandey P, Rao KV. Predictors of aneurysmal rebleed before definitive surgical or endovascular management. *Acta Neurochir (Wien).* 2016;158:1037-1044.

Starke RM, Connolly ES. Rebleeding after aneurysmal subarachnoid hemorrhage. *Neurocrit Care.* 2011;15:241-246.

Suarez J. Diagnosis and management of subarachnoid hemorrhage. *Continuum.* 2015;21:1263-1287.

Thompson BG, Brown RD, Amin-Hanjani S, et al. Guidelines for the management of patients with unruptured intracranial aneurysms. *Stroke.* 2015;46:268-400.

Treggiari MM, Deem S. Which H is the most important in triple-H therapy for cerebral vasospasm? *Curr Opin Crit Care.* 2009;15:83-86.

Van Gijn J, van Dongen KJ, Vermeulen M, et al. Perimesencephalic hemorrhage: a non-aneurysmal and benign form of subarachnoid hemorrhage. *Neurology.* 1985;35:493-497.

White H, Venkatesh B. Application of transcranial Doppler in the ICU: a review. *Intensive Care Med.* 2006;32:981-994.

Wong GKC, Chan MTV, Boet R, et al. Intravenous magnesium sulfate after aneurysmal subarachnoid hemorrhage: a prospective randomized piolet study. *J Neurosurg Anesth.* 2006;18:142-148.

3

Neurotrauma

Kaitlin Reilly, MD, Hassan Anbari, MD, and Neha S. Dangayach, MD

Questions

1. An 85-year-old woman with past medical history of hypertension and diabetes mellitus, not on insulin, suffered a witnessed fall. She tripped down a few stairs and struck her face against a concrete floor. She was brought in by her daughter who reported no loss of consciousness. The patient complained of some left hip pain on movement and had no other complaints. The emergency department (ED) attending physician would like to clear her spine clinically and is wondering if he should get a computed tomography (CT) of the cervical spine in this patient. Which of the following clinical characteristics should prompt cervical spine imaging for this patient?

   A. Age >65; dangerous mechanism or paresthesias in the extremities

   B. Age >65; dangerous mechanism or neck pain

   C. Age >80; dangerous mechanism or paresthesias in the extremities

   D. Regardless of age, dangerous mechanism or neck pain

2. A 45-year-old man was found unconscious by his neighbors at the bottom of a flight of stairs. When emergency medical technicians (EMTs) arrived at the scene, they found the patient covered in a pool of vomitus, mumbling incoherently and moving all his extremities spontaneously. He was placed in a C-collar and transported to the nearest level 1 trauma center. His head CT scan showed diffuse cortical subarachnoid hemorrhage (Fig. 3-1), and CT angiography (CTA) was negative for an underlying aneurysm. His cervical spine CT did not show any evidence of fractures or dislocation. His FAST scan was negative. His girlfriend reported alcohol abuse but no other past medical history or medications. The patient was admitted to the neuroscience intensive care unit neuroscience intensive care unit (NICU) for close monitoring. There is a discussion on rounds about use of nimodipine in subarachnoid hemorrhage. What is correct regarding this medication?

   A. Nimodipine is recommended for patients with aneurysmal subarachnoid hemorrhage but not traumatic subarachnoid hemorrhage.

   B. Nimodipine is recommended for patients with either aneurysmal or traumatic subarachnoid hemorrhage.

C. Prevention of vasospasm with nimodipine improves patient outcome in both aneurysmal and traumatic subarachnoid hemorrhage.

D. Nimodipine has been shown to worsen outcomes in patients with traumatic brain injury (TBI).

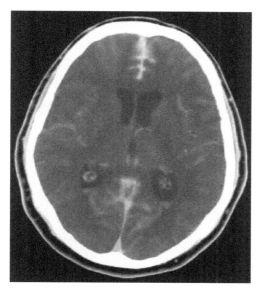

Figure 3-1 Axial view computed tomography of the head without contrast shows diffuse subarachnoid hemorrhage.

3. Which of the following statements is true about neuroprotective strategies in patients with moderate to severe TBI?

A. Early administration of steroids improves functional outcomes at 3 months.

B. Hypotension (systolic blood pressure [SBP] <85 mm Hg) is an independent predictor of poor outcomes.

C. The ProTECT III trial showed a benefit with progesterone over placebo.

D. Therapeutic temperature management at 32°C for 72 hours improves functional outcomes.

4. A 28-year-old man was admitted to your neurorehabilitation unit 8 weeks after a severe TBI. On exam, he demonstrates spontaneous eye opening but otherwise does not appear to react meaningfully to stimuli. His family asks if anything can be done to speed his recovery. Which of the following medications has been shown to improve recovery in TBI patients in a minimally conscious and persistently vegetative state?

A. Bromocriptine

B. Modafinil

C. Amantadine

D. Levodopa

5. A 22-year-old man is brought to the ED after a motorcycle crash. On exam, he was opening his eyes to painful stimuli and withdrawing all 4 extremities. Your medical student asks if it would be appropriate to give high-dose steroids to the patient. Which of the following is true about the CRASH trial?

A. Patients with severe TBI showed improved outcomes at 90 days after 48 hours of high-dose steroids on admission.

B. All-cause mortality at 2 weeks was higher in the group treated with steroids.

C. Six-month mortality was the same between the treatment and placebo groups.

D. Only severe TBI patients with a Glasgow coma scale (GCS) score <8 were included in the CRASH trial.

E. As a result of the trial, high-dose steroids are universally recommended for all patients with TBI.

6. A 19-year-old man is brought to the ED comatose after a high-speed motor vehicle accident. His head CT is shown in Figure 3-2. Which of the following interventions has been shown in a large randomized controlled trial to reduce intracranial pressure (ICP) and patients' ICU stay but worsen functional outcomes at 6 months?

   A. Hypothermia
   B. Bifrontal craniectomy
   C. Hypertonic saline
   D. ICP monitoring

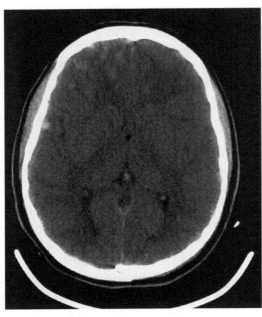

Figure 3-2 Axial view head computed tomography scan shows bifrontal contusions.

7. A 36-year-old woman who was involved in a high-speed motor vehicle crash had a depressed level of consciousness at the scene and was intubated. On arrival to the ED, she had a poor neurologic examination; the head CT is shown in Figure 3-3. An external ventricular drain (EVD) is placed. What is true about ICP monitoring?

   A. The use of an intraparenchymal monitor is preferred over an EVD in this patient's case.
   B. With normal ICP, there is no risk of herniation.

C. The use of intraventricular tissue plasminogen activator can clear the intraventricular hemorrhage more quickly than without use of a tissue plasminogen activator and will improve functional outcome.

D. No difference in mortality or unfavorable outcomes was seen between patients with ICP monitoring and patients followed only by neurologic exam and CT scans.

E. With her EVD, continuous drainage improves neurologic outcome.

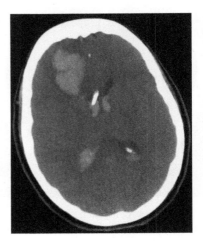

Figure 3-3 Axial view brain computed tomography without contrast demonstrates right frontal intraparenchymal hemorrhage with intraventricular extension and external ventricular drain in place.

8. A 44-year-old man is admitted to the surgical ICU after falling off a building. His GCS score is 4, and based on your assessment, invasive monitoring is indicated. Which method of invasive monitoring, when used to guide therapy in severe TBI patients, is more likely to result in a favorable patient outcome?

   A. ICP <20 mm Hg
   B. Brain tissue oxygenation (PbtO$_2$) with target >25 mm Hg
   C. Cerebral perfusion pressure (CPP) of 20 to 50 mm Hg
   D. Microdialysis monitoring with a goal lactate-to-pyruvate ratio (LPR) <25

9. An 18-year-old man presents to the ED 2 hours after a motor vehicle accident. His initial GCS score is 13; he appears drowsy and is having word-finding difficulties. His laboratory results, including platelet count, PT, and PTT, are within normal limits. His head CT is shown in Figure 3-4. Which of the following medications when given within 8 hours after a TBI with an intracranial hemorrhage demonstrated a tendency toward both decreased hematoma growth and decreased mortality?

A. Aminocaproic acid

B. Prothrombin complex concentrate (PCC)

C. Tranexamic acid

D. Activated factor VII

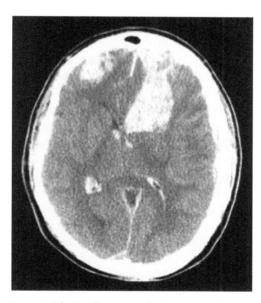

Figure 3-4   Axial view (brain window) computed tomography of the head without contrast demonstrates left more than right intraparenchymal hemorrhage with rightward midline shift and obliteration of anterior horn of the left lateral ventricle.

10. A 58-year-old man is admitted to the surgical ICU after falling down his basement stairs and striking his head on the concrete floor. The patient is opening his eyes to deep pain and extending in the right upper extremity. His initial CT (Fig. 3-5) shows a left temporal contusion and a small layering acute subdural hematoma, which remained stable on subsequent scans. Although there is no evidence that the patient has yet had a clinical seizure, given the location of his injury, there is significant concern for the development of seizures. To support this, a 2002 practice parameter from the American Academy of Neurology supported the use of which drug in acute severe TBI patients in order to prevent early posttraumatic seizures?

A. Phenobarbital

B. Phenytoin

C. Lacosamide

D. Levetiracetam

E. Valproic acid

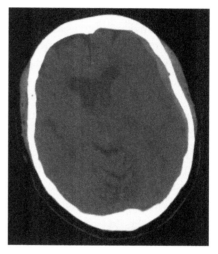

Figure 3-5   Computed tomography of the brain without contrast (subdural window) demonstrates a small acute left subdural hematoma with local mass effect and effacement of the sulci. There is minimal rightward midline shift.

11. Which of the following statements is true regarding the use of magnesium sulfate as a neuroprotective agent in patients with TBI?

A. Magnesium was shown to improve functional outcomes but not mortality in severe TBI.

B. Magnesium was shown to improve functional outcomes in low doses but worsen outcomes at high doses.

C. Magnesium was shown to worsen outcomes at low doses and increase mortality at high doses.

D. Magnesium was shown to increase mortality at both high and low doses.

12. The mother of an 18-year-old man with severe TBI asks what her son's chances are of having a meaningful recovery. You decide to use 1 of the 2 commonly used TBI prognosis calculators. Both the IMPACT (International Mission on Prognosis and Analysis of Clinical Trials) and CRASH (Corticoid Randomization after Significant Head Injury) models feature which 3 elements when determining prognosis after TBI?

    A. Age, GCS verbal score, CT classification

    B. Sex, GCS motor score, hemoglobin

    C. Age, GCS motor score, pupillary reactivity

    D. Age, GCS motor score, hemoglobin

13. A patient with a moderate TBI GCS (E2, M5, V3) develops fever on day 2 of ICU admission. Knowing that fever can cause secondary neurologic injury after a TBI, your resident asks if the patient should be cooled. Citing the most recent evidence, you make which of the following conclusions?

    A. The patient should be cooled within 48 hours of injury.

    B. The patient should be maintained at normothermia, but maintaining hypothermia may be harmful.

    C. The patient should be cooled to 32°C.

    D. The patient should be cooled within 2 hours after injury.

14. A 16-year-old boy is admitted to the surgical ICU at your local hospital after a motorcycle accident. His initial GCS score is 7. The pediatrician asks you for the most up-to-date guidelines regarding use of therapeutic hypothermia in pediatric TBI patients. Which of the following is correct?

    A. Therapeutic hypothermia to 32.5°C improved mortality in a randomized controlled trial of pediatric TBI patients.

    B. Therapeutic hypothermia to 32.5°C improves functional outcomes with no change in mortality in pediatric TBI patients.

    C. Therapeutic hypothermia was shown to be ineffective with a tendency toward higher mortality in pediatric TBI patients.

    D. Therapeutic hypothermia improves mortality in pediatric TBI but leaves survivors with worse functional outcomes.

15. An 18-year-old man with unknown history was evacuated from the scene of a motor vehicular accident. He was drowsy, appeared to be under the influence of alcohol, was not oriented to time, but was able to follow simple commands, and was moving all extremities spontaneously (GCS E3 M6 V5). EMTs placed him in a C-collar. On arrival to the ED, his initial SBP was in the 80s, and heart rate was 128 bpm with sinus tachycardia. Which resuscitation fluid should be used?

    A. Only hetastarch should be used for volume resuscitation in trauma patients

    B. Normal saline

    C. Albumin

    D. 3% sodium chloride

16. A 15-year-old boy is brought to the ED by emergency medical services after he is involved as a backseat, unrestrained passenger in a high-speed motor vehicle accident. On initial neurologic exam, his pupils are briskly reactive, and he opens his eyes to deep pain, withdraws with his left upper and lower extremities, and flexes with his right upper and lower extremities. A head CT reveals thin subarachnoid hemorrhage, global cerebral edema, and hypodensities consistent with a contusion in the bilateral inferior frontal lobes, more prominent on the left. He is intubated and admitted to the pediatric ICU where an ICP monitor is inserted, revealing an ICP sustained above 30 mm Hg. He is treated with sedation and given a bolus of mannitol without significant improvement in his ICP. Which of the following interventions has been shown in a prospective study to reduce ICP and improve CPP in this scenario?

    A. Increase sedation

    B. Therapeutic hypothermia

    C. Continuous infusion of 3% hypertonic saline

    D. Continuous magnesium infusion

17. An 85-year-old woman on aspirin for coronary artery disease is brought to the ED with a 3-month history of progressive confusion. A head CT is obtained, which shows a 2.5-cm-thick right frontoparietal chronic subdural hematoma (Fig. 3-6). She is seen by neurosurgery and recommended for evacuation of the hematoma via a burr hole. Which single intervention was shown in a randomized controlled trial to reduce recurrence of a subdural hematoma after burr hole drainage?

    A. Seizure prophylaxis with phenytoin

    B. Administration of tranexamic acid

    C. Placement of a surgical drain

    D. Platelet transfusion to reverse antiplatelet effect of aspirin

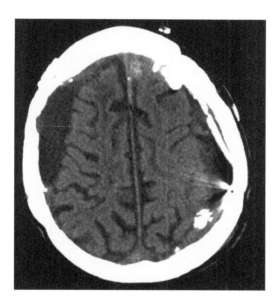

Figure 3-6 Axial computed tomography of the brain without contrast demonstrates hypodense right extra-axial fluid collection with 2.2-cm thickness in the right frontoparietal region with local mass effect related to chronic subdural hematoma. Note linear calcifications along the inner table of the left frontoparietal bone related to resolved old subdural hemorrhage.

18. A 24-year-old man is brought to the ED after sustaining multiple gunshot wounds. After initial resuscitation, he is found to have flaccid paraplegia with preserved sensation. A CT image shows a bullet lodged in T4 vertebral body, causing fracture and anterior compression of the spinal cord. After decompression surgery, which single feature, either of the history or exam, would suggest the best prognosis for recovery of motor function after presenting with a complete motor injury?

    A. Violent mechanism of injury

    B. Sacral sparing

    C. Sensory perseveration

    D. Young age

19. A 25-year-old man is admitted to the surgical ICU after being struck in the head with a baseball bat. His initial head CT shows an atlanto-occipital dissociation and a hairline fracture through the occipital bone. What vascular complication is he at risk for acutely?

    A. Vertebral dissection

    B. Venous sinus thrombosis

    C. Dural arteriovenous fistula

    D. Epidural hematoma formation

    E. Carotid-cavernous fistula

20. A 65-year-old man is found at the base of stairwell. He is brought to the ED with flaccid quadriplegia in a C-collar and sensory involvement to the C6 dermatome. While in the ED, he develops lethargy, skew deviation, and left facial numbness, dysarthria, and difficulty managing his secretions. What is the next step in management?

    A. Administer high-dose methylprednisolone stat

    B. Obtain CT scan of the entire spine

    C. Endotracheal intubation and stat CT of the cervical spine, CT of the brain, and CTA of the head and neck

    D. Talk to family about code status, and institute comfort measures

    E. Treat the patient with intravenous tissue plasminogen activator

21. An approximately 50-year-old unidentified man was found in a park by bystanders after they heard a single gunshot. He was found alone with agonal respirations and a firearm near him. EMS was called, and they noted active bleeding from his right parietal region of his head, GCS score of 3, and no other trauma. He was intubated in the field and brought to the ED for further evaluation. A head CT was completed and is shown in Figure 3-7. Which of the following statements is most correct about penetrating head trauma?

A. Prognosis is better for penetrating head trauma than blunt head trauma.

B. Extensive debridement of the scalp and bony wound should be undertaken, and accessible intraparenchymal bone and bullet fragments should be removed.

C. Antibiotic prophylaxis with vancomycin should be started.

D. Retained fragments in eloquent cortex increase the risk of epilepsy following penetrating head trauma.

E. The subarachnoid hemorrhage demonstrated on the CT commonly leads to vasospasm and worse outcome.

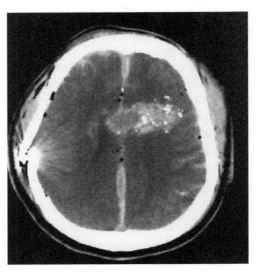

Figure 3-7 Axial view computed tomography scan of the head without contrast shows diffuse cortical subarachnoid, parafalcine, and left frontal lobe hemorrhage. Note the bullet entry injury in the right parietal bone with minimal displacement and multiple bone and bullet fragments in left more than right frontal lobes.

Answers and Explanations

1. **A.** The question of cervical spine imaging versus clinical clearance needs to be answered early in triaging trauma patients. Patients with a depressed level of consciousness or an unclear mechanism of injury should be maintained in a hard cervical collar until formal imaging can be obtained. However, many low-risk patients can be cleared clinically without the need for cervical imaging.

    The Canadian Cervical Spine Rules are extremely sensitive (correctly identifying cervical spine injury in 161 of 162 cases with 99% sensitivity) for identifying low-risk cases in awake patients with a normal mental status who do not require radiography (Table 3-1). In addition to the above criteria, patients must also have a low-risk factor, including a low-risk rear-end car accident, being comfortably seated in the ED, absence of midline cervical spine tenderness, or delayed onset of neck pain. The patient must then have a range of motion of 45° horizontally in both directions. If a high-risk factor is present, a low-risk factor is absent, or there is limited range of motion, an x-ray of the cervical spine is indicated.

Table 3-1. NEXUS Criteria and the Canadian Cervical Spine (C-Spine) Rules

NEXUS Criteria	Canadian C-Spine Rules
No posterior midline C-spine tenderness	*Step 1*
	Any high-risk factor that mandates radiography?
No evidence of intoxication	
Normal level of alertness	• Age ≥65
No focal neurologic deficit	• Dangerous mechanism
	• Paresthesias in extremities
No painful distracting injuries	*Step 2*
	Any low-risk factor that allows safe assessment of range of motion?
No evidence of intoxication	
Normal level of alertness	• Simple rear-end motor vehicle collision
No focal neurologic deficit	• Being comfortably seated in the emergency department
No painful distracting injury	• Ambulatory at any time
	• Absence of midline C-spine tenderness or delayed-onset neck pain
	Step 3
	Able to rotate neck actively?
	• 45° to left and right
Interpretation	*Interpretation*
Only if all criteria are present, C-spine radiography is NOT indicated	If answer to step 1 is yes, then radiography is needed. If answers to steps 2 and 3 are yes, then no radiography is needed.
Sensitivity: 90.7%	Sensitivity: 99%

2. **A.** The use of nimodipine in traumatic brain injury (TBI) was first studied in the early 1990s in the HIT 1 and HIT 2 trials, which demonstrated no improvement in patients treated with nimodipine. However, a subgroup analysis of patients with traumatic subarachnoid hemorrhage (SAH) demonstrated a trend toward improvement. This was further studied in the HIT 3 trial, which showed improvement in a small group of patients. The follow-up HIT 4 trial intended to confirm these findings, but instead showed an increase in poor outcomes in patients treated with nimodipine. A meta-analysis of traumatic SAH patients (with pooled data from the HIT 1, 2, and 4 studies) included 1074 patients. Poor outcome was similar in patients treated with nimodipine (39%) and those treated with placebo (40%); odds ratio was 0.88 (95% confidence interval [CI], 0.51-1.54), and there was no difference in mortality between the 2 groups. Thus, it is no longer recommended that patients with traumatic SAH receive nimodipine. Nimodipine, however, does improve functional outcomes at 3 months in patients with aneurysmal SAH and has been the standard of care since the 1980s.

3. **B.** Hypotension during the first 24 hours of TBI is an independent predictor of poor outcomes and should be avoided. As early as 1989, Klauber and colleagues reported a mortality of 35% in patients

admitted with an SBP <85 mm Hg, compared with only 6% in patients with a higher SBP. Additionally, hypotension has been shown to correlate with diffuse brain swelling. Maintaining normotension helps preserve cerebral perfusion pressure and cerebral blood flow. The Brain Trauma Foundation guidelines do not recommend administration of steroids. Although experimental models had demonstrated a potential neuroprotective effect of progesterone in TBI, in a large randomized controlled trial, ProTECT III, there was no reported difference in the primary outcome of neurologic improvement as measured by the extended Glasgow coma scale at 6 months.

4. **C.** To date, amantadine is the only medication that has shown recovery benefit in TBI patients with disorders of consciousness. In a multicenter, placebo-controlled trial, amantadine was administered 4 to 16 weeks after a severe TBI in patients with minimally conscious and persistently vegetative state over a period of 4 weeks and demonstrated improvement in the 6 cognitive domains assessed by the Disability Rating Scale. The mechanism of action of amantadine is unclear. It is thought to act as central neurostimulant through its work as an *N*-methyl-D-aspartate (NMDA) receptor agonist.

    Modafinil was studied in 2 randomized clinical trials that evaluated fatigue and daytime sleepiness: one study with a cohort of 20 patients showed benefit in alleviating excessive daytime sleepiness, and the other study of 53 TBI patients did not show a difference in outcomes.

5. **B.** The CRASH trial studied 10,008 TBI patients with within 8 hours of injury and with a GCS <14. The study compared high-dose methylprednisolone administered over a 48-hour period with placebo. Primary outcomes were death within 2 weeks of injury and death or disability at 6 months. The results showed that patients treated with steroids had overall higher mortality at 2 weeks compared to those treated with placebo (1052 [21.1%] vs 893 [17.9%] deaths; relative risk, 1.18 [95% CI, 1.09-1.27]; $P = .0001$), even when adjusting for severity of initial injury. The follow-up measure of 6-month mortality was also higher in the steroid-treated patients (21.1% vs 17.9%, $P = .0001$). As a result, empiric treatment with steroids is no longer recommended.

6. **B.** The DECRA (Decompressive Craniectomy in Diffuse Traumatic Brain Injury) trial randomized patients with diffuse TBI and refractory intracranial hypertension to values >20 mm Hg for more than 15 minutes within a 1-hour period who were refractory to first-tier therapies to receive either bifrontal craniectomy or medical therapy. The study demonstrated that although ICP was better controlled and patients had fewer ICU days in the bifrontal craniectomy group, the overall functional outcomes were worse. These results were similar to the more recent RESCUEicp trial, which combined the use of hemicraniectomy or bifrontal craniectomy as a last-tier attempt to control refractory ICP in patients with diffuse TBI and found lower mortality with worse functional outcomes among survivors.

7. **D.** In December 2012, the Global Neurotrauma Research Group published a multicenter, controlled trial conducted in Bolivia and Ecuador of ICP monitoring in severe TBI patients that showed there was no improvement in outcome with ICP monitoring and ICP-guided management when compared to medical management based on CT scans and changes in neurologic exam. This trial randomized 324 patients to either ICP-guided therapy (n = 157) or imaging/clinical examination–guided therapy (n = 167) and found similar rates of death (39% vs 44%) and unfavorable outcomes (17% vs 17%) in both groups. As a result of this study, the current 2016 Brain Trauma Foundation guidelines no longer recommend routine ICP monitoring in all salvageable patients with severe TBI and an abnormal CT scan; rather, they include a Level IIB recommendation to manage severe TBI patients using information from ICP monitoring to reduce in-hospital and 2-week mortality, which is based on results of a meta-analysis. ICP monitoring can be completed with a number of devices, and in this patient's case, the use of an EVD is favored over a intraparenchymal monitor given there is moderate intraventricular hemorrhage and an EVD will allow for clearance of the blood product. Although intraventricular tissue plasminogen activator is safe to administer, the most recent data from the CLEAR III study have not demonstrated clinical benefit. With EVDs, there is still ongoing discussions on what is the most appropriate means of cerebrospinal fluid (CSF) diversion—intermittent or continuous. In those with severe TBI, an overall lower ICP and

less time above 20 mm Hg occur when there is continuous drainage of CSF, but this has yet to yield findings of clinical benefit.

8. **B.** Although randomized controlled trial data are not available, a systematic review combining 4 studies dated from 2003 to 2010 analyzing 491 patients found that 61% of patients who received $PbtO_2$-based therapy had a favorable outcome compared to just 42% of patients receiving ICP/CPP-based therapy. The 2016 Brain Trauma Foundation guidelines further support targeting a $PbtO_2$ >25 mm Hg as well as an ICP <22 mm Hg and a CPP of 60 to 70 mm Hg.

9. **C.** The CRASH-2 intracranial bleeding study examined 270 trauma patients with significant extracranial bleeding and TBI. Half received tranexamic acid within 8 hours, and half received placebo. Hematoma growth averaged 6 mL in the treated group and 8 mL in the placebo group, whereas there were 14 deaths in the treated group and 24 in the placebo group. Neither of these end points met statistical significance and will be studied further in the CRASH-3 trial. Neither PCC nor activated factor VII is indicated because the patient is not in a coagulopathic state. The guidelines for management of severe traumatic head injury do not give recommendations on treatment with tranexamic acid, as more data is needed.

10. **B.** Acute symptomatic seizures may occur as a result of severe TBI. These posttraumatic seizures (PTS) are classified as *early* when they occur within 7 days of injury or *late* when they occur 7 or more days after injury. Posttraumatic epilepsy (PTE) is defined as recurrent seizures more than 7 days following injury. The risk factors for early PTS include GCS score of ≤10; immediate seizures; posttraumatic amnesia lasting longer than 30 minutes; linear or depressed skull fracture; penetrating head injury; subdural, epidural, or intracerebral hematoma; cortical contusion; age ≤65 years; and chronic alcoholism.

The 2002 practice parameter from the American Academy of Neurology, produced by pooling available class I studies, supported a significantly lower rate of PTS within 7 days of injury in severe TBI patients treated with phenytoin. Small prospective trials conducted later suggest levetiracetam may be equivalent.

11. **C.** In a randomized controlled trial of magnesium sulfate, 499 patients with moderate to severe TBI were randomized into 1 of 2 doses of magnesium or placebo within 8 hours of injury and continued on treatment for 5 days. Although animal data suggested it would have neuroprotective effects, the study demonstrated poor outcomes (a composite of mortality, seizures, functional measures, and neuropsychological tests 6 months after injury) with magnesium compared to placebo at a low dose and high mortality rate compared to placebo at a higher dose in an intent-to-treat analysis.

12. **C.** Both the IMPACT and CRASH prognostic models have been validated in large datasets for determination of prognosis after TBI. Both use a combination of age, GCS motor score, pupillary reactivity, CT classification, and presence or absence of traumatic subarachnoid hemorrhage as a core part of the model (Table 3-2). The IMPACT model also uses laboratory data, such as blood glucose and hemoglobin, as part of its model.

Table 3-2. The IMPACT and CRASH Head Injury Prognostic Models

IMPACT	CRASH
Core	Country
Age (14-99 years)	Age (<40-99 years)
GCS motor score (1-6)	GCS total score (3-15)
Pupils (bilateral, unilateral, unreactive)	Pupils (bilateral, unilateral, unreactive)
	Major extracranial injury?
Core + CT	**CT Scan**
Hypoxia (yes/no)	Presence of petechial hemorrhage (yes/no)
Hypotension (yes/no)	Obliteration of third ventricle/basal cistern (yes/no)
CT classification (diffuse injury I-IV, unevacuated or evacuated mass lesion)	Subarachnoid hemorrhage (SAH; yes/no)
Traumatic SAH (yes/no)	Midline shift (yes/no)
Epidural mass on CT (yes/no)	Nonevacuated hematoma (yes/no)
Core + CT + Labs	
Glucose (3-20 mmol/L)	
Hemoglobin (6-17 g/dL)	

Abbreviations: CT, computed tomography; GCS, Glasgow coma scale.

13. **B.** The Eurotherm trial is a large, multicenter, randomized controlled trial that compared the use of therapeutic hypothermia with a target temperature between 32°C and 35°C in addition to standard medical therapy versus medical therapy alone. The study enrolled TBI patients with at least elevation in ICP of >20 mm Hg for at least 5 minutes, and found no benefit to standard ICP management interventions. In fact, outcomes as measured by the Extended Glasgow Outcome Scale (GOSE) at 6 months found worse outcomes for patients in the hypothermia group compared with standard management. Based on the 2016 TBI guidelines, early (within 2.5 hours) or short-term (48 hours after injury) prophylactic hypothermia is not recommended to improve outcomes in patients with diffuse injury (Level IIB) brain trauma. The exact duration for which normothermia should be maintained after moderate to severe TBI is still unclear and will require further studies.

14. **C.** Although animal models of TBI had suggested a neuroprotective effective of moderate hypothermia. The Hypothermia Pediatric Head Injury Trial showed no functional improvement in pediatric TBI patients and, in fact, showed trend toward higher mortality in the hypothermia group (21% vs 12%, $P = .06$).

15. **B.** Post hoc analysis of the SAFE trial (Saline versus Albumin Fluid Evaluation) compared saline with albumin as a resuscitation fluid in ICU patients showed higher mortality among TBI patients who received albumin by a statistically significant margin (42% vs 22%). Isotonic fluids should be used in hypotensive patients. Hetastarch has been shown to be associated with worse renal function and mortality, and it should be avoided in the resuscitation of trauma patients.

16. **C.** A small prospective trial studying 10 pediatric patients with severe TBI and refractory intracranial hypertension treated for prolonged periods (average of 7 days) with continuous 3% hypertonic saline infusion demonstrated sustained efficacy in lowering ICP and medical tolerability, despite serum sodium that rose to as high at 170 mEq. There is no literature to support the superiority of mannitol over 3% hypertonic saline in severe pediatric TBI. Hypothermia and magnesium have not been shown to improve outcomes after TBI. Although hypothermia and increase sedation can decrease the ICP, it also will lower the mean arterial pressure, which may require use of vasoactive medications.

17. **C.** A single-center, randomized controlled trial of chronic subdural hematoma patients referred for burr hole drainage demonstrated decreased risk of recurrence with placement of a surgical drain (9% recurrence rate in drain arm vs 24% recurrence rate in standard arm). There was also a statistically significant difference in 6-month mortality (8% vs 18%) in patients for whom a drain was placed after evacuation.

18. **B.** Analysis of a large registry of spinal cord injury patients from the 1990s found that patients with complete motor injury and sensory perseveration were more likely to make a motor recovery if sacral sparing was present on initial exam (53% vs 13% in those without sacral sparing; $P < .001$). Violent mechanism of injury was associated with a poorer chance of recovery.

19. **B.** Through a combination of endothelial injury and static flow due to compression of the sinus, skull base fractures such as occurred in this patient increase the risk of venous sinus thrombosis, a potentially devastating complication. In a prospective cohort study including 541 patients with skull base fractures; 113 patients (21%) underwent venous imaging, of whom 38 patients (34%) exhibited cerebral venous sinus thrombosis; and 19 patients (17%) had external compression of the sinus. The use of CT venogram has been evaluated, and skull fractures that extended into the transverse, sigmoid, or jugular bulb petrous temporal bone had a higher risk of sinus thrombosis than skull fractures extending into the superior sagittal sinus. This finding supports the consideration of venous imaging in all patients with skull base fractures.

20. **C.** When evaluating a patient with suspected cervical spine injury, it is important to recognize concomitant vessel injury. Although the worsening of the patient's symptoms is likely due to a new ischemic stroke, the primary evaluation in a patient is stability of ABCs (airways, breathing,

and circulation). In this case, the patient has sustained an anterior subluxation of C5/6, which put him at risk for vertebral artery dissection. The presenting symptom of flaccid quadriplegia is due to acute spinal cord compression. The symptoms he developed while waiting in the ED are due to extension of vertebral artery dissection and impending basilar thrombosis, which is now his most life-threatening condition. Although treatment of ischemic stroke due to cervical artery dissection is safe, permitted the dissection does not involve the aorta or the intracranial portions of the vessels, the patient may not be a candidate for tissue plasminogen activator administration given his trauma burden.

In the setting of trauma, administration of high-dose steroids was studied in the NASCIS studies (National Acute Spinal Cord Injury Studies I-III). Based on the results of NASCIS I and II, high-dose steroids were recommended by the American Association of Neurological Surgeons (AANS) for acute spinal cord injury and were the standard of care for much of the 1990s. However, the larger NASCIS III trial, along with reanalysis of the NASCIS II trial accounting for functional neurologic outcomes, argued the intervention was not effective and potentially increased mortality. Thus, it is no longer the recommendation of the AANS.

21. D. Penetrating head trauma has limited data compared with nonpenetrating head trauma, and most of the literature and treatment paradigms are coming from military interventions. The prognosis for penetrating head trauma is worse than for nonpenetrating head trauma. A common finding on imaging is the presence of blood product including within the subarachnoid space. This type of hemorrhage is due to vascular injury, and although there is risk of cerebral vasospasm as with typical aneurysmal subarachnoid hemorrhage, there is no difference in outcomes in patients with vasospasm. In this case, there are retained fragments, and this places the patient at higher risk for intracranial infection, which should be treated with prophylactic antibiotics. The common infections are skin flora including *Staphylococcus aureus*, but gram-negative organisms can also cause infection. Therefore, broad-spectrum antibiotic therapy with a cephalosporin, vancomycin, and aerobic coverage

(e.g. metronidazole) is considered mainstay therapy. Removal of fragments typically results in worse functional outcomes, and their removal requires careful surgical decisions. Finally, retained fragments in eloquent cortex increases the risk of epilepsy following penetrating head trauma. Studies showed that approximately 50% of TBI patients, who have suffered injury for more than 15 years will have epilepsy.

REFERENCES

Allen GS, Ahn HS, Preziosi TJ, et al. Cerebral arterial spasm: a controlled trial of nimodipine in patients with subarachnoid hemorrhage. *N Engl J Med.* 1983;308:619-624.

Andrews PJ, Sinclair HL, Rodriguez A, et al. Hypothermia for intracranial hypertension after traumatic brain injury. *N Engl J Med.* 2015;373:2403-2412.

Bastion R, de Louvois J, Brown EM, et al. Use of antibiotics in penetrating craniocerebral injuries. Infection in Neurosurgery Working Party of British Society for Antimicrobial Chemotherapy. *Lancet.* 2000;355:1813-1817.

Bowers CA, Kundu B, Hawryluk GWJ. Methylprednisolone for acute spinal cord injury: an increasingly philosophical debate. *Neural Regen Res.* 2016;11:882-885.

Carney N, Totten AM, O'Reilly C, et al. Guidelines for the Management of Severe Traumatic Brain Injury, Fourth Edition. *Neurosurgery.* 2016;10:1-10.

Chang BS, Lowenstein DH. Practice parameter: antiepileptic drug prophylaxis in severe traumatic brain injury Report of the Quality Standards Subcommittee of the American Academy of Neurology. *Neurology.* 2003;60:10-16.

Chesnut RM, Temkin N, Carney N, et al. A trial of intracranial-pressure monitoring in traumatic brain injury. *N Engl J Med.* 2012;367:2471-2481.

Cooper DJ, Rosenfeld JV, Murray L, et al. Decompressive craniectomy in diffuse traumatic brain injury. *N Engl J Med.* 2011;364:1493-1502.

CRASH-2 Collaborators (Intracranial Bleeding Study). Effect of tranexamic acid in traumatic brain injury: a nested randomised, placebo controlled trial (CRASH-2 Intracranial Bleeding Study). *BMJ.* 2011;343:d3795.

CRASH Trial Collaborators. Predicting outcome after traumatic brain injury: practical prognostic models based on large cohort of international patients. *BMJ.* 2008;336:425.

Delgado Almandoz JE, Kelly HR, Schaefer PW, et al. Prevalence of traumatic dural venous sinus thrombosis in high-risk acute blunt head trauma patients evaluated with multidetector CT venography. *Radiology.* 2010;255:570-577.

Giacino JT, Whyte J, Bagiella E, et al. Placebo-controlled trial of amantadine for severe traumatic brain injury. *N Engl J Med.* 2012;366:819-826.

Guidelines for the management of penetrating brain injury. *J Trauma.* 2001;51(2 Suppl):S3-S6.

Hanley DF, Lane K, McBee N, et al. Thrombolytic removal of intraventricular haemorrhage in treatment of severe stroke:

results of the randomized, multicenter, multiregional, placebo-controlled CLEAR III trial. *Lancet.* 2017;389: 603-611.

Hoffman JR, Wolfson AB, Todd K, et al. Validity of a set of clinical criteria to rule out injury to the cervical spine in patients with blunt trauma. National Emergency X-Radiography Utilization Study Group. *N Engl J Med.* 2000;343:94-99.

Hutchinson PJ, Kolias AG, Timofeev IS, et al. Trial of decompressive craniectomy for traumatic intracranial hypertension. *N Engl J Med.* 2016;375:1119-1130.

Hutchison JS, Ward RE, Lacroix J, et al. Hypothermia therapy after traumatic brain injury in children. *N Engl J Med.* 2008;358:2447-2456.

Jha A, Weintraub A, Allshouse A, et al. A randomized trial of modafinil for the treatment of fatigue and excessive daytime sleepiness in individuals with chronic traumatic brain injury. *J Head Trauma Rehab.* 2008;23:52-63.

Kaiser PR, Valko P, Werth E, et al. Modafinil ameliorates excessive daytime sleepiness after traumatic brain injury. *Neurology.* 2010;75:1780-1785.

Kazim SF, Shamim MS, Tahir MZ, et al. Management of penetrating brain injury. *J Emerg Trauma Shock.* 2011;4:395-402.

Kordestani RK, Counelis GJ, McBride DQ, et al. Cerebral arterial spasm after penetrating craniocerebral gunshot wounds: transcranial Doppler and cerebral blood flow findings. *Neurosurgery.* 1997;41:351-359.

Khanna S, Davis D, Peterson B, et al. Use of hypertonic saline in the treatment of severe refractory posttraumatic intracranial hypertension in pediatric traumatic brain injury. *Crit Care Med.* 2000;28:1144-1151.

Lissauer ME, Chi A, Kramer ME, et al. Association of 6% hetastarch resuscitation with adverse outcomes in critically ill trauma patients. *Am J Surg.* 2011;202:53-58.

Marino RJ, Ditunno JF, Donovan WH, et al. Neurologic recovery after traumatic spinal cord injury: data from the Model Spinal Cord Injury Systems. *Arch Phys Med Rehabil.* 1999;80:1391-1396.

Myburgh J, Cooper DJ, Finfer S, et al. Saline or albumin for fluid resuscitation in patients with traumatic brain injury. *N Engl J Med.* 2007;357:874-884.

Nangunoori R, Maloney-Wilensky E, Stiefel M, et al. Brain tissue oxygen-based therapy and outcome after severe traumatic brain injury: a systematic literature review. *Neurocrit Care.* 2012;17:131-138.

Nwachuka EL, Ouccio AM, Fetzick A, et al. Intermittent versus continuous cerebrospinal fluid drainage management in adult severe traumatic brain injury. *Neurocrit Care.* 2014;20:49-53.

Roberts I, Yates D, Sandercock P, et al. Effect of intravenous corticosteroids on death within 14 days in 10008 adults with clinically significant head injury (MRC CRASH trial): randomised placebo-controlled trial. *Lancet.* 2004; 364:1321-1328.

Roozenbeek B, Lingsma HF, Lecky FE, et al. Prediction of outcome after moderate and severe traumatic brain injury: external validation of the IMPACT and CRASH prognostic models. *Crit Care Med.* 2012;40:1609.

SAFE Study Investigators. A comparison of albumin and saline for fluid resuscitation in the intensive care unit. *N Engl J Med.* 2004;350:2247-2256.

Santarius T, Kirkpatrick PJ, Ganesan D, et al. Use of drains versus no drains after burr-hole evacuation of chronic subdural haematoma: a randomised controlled trial. *Lancet.* 2009;374:1067-1073.

Shen L, Wang Z, Su Z, et al. Effects of intracranial pressure monitoring on mortality in patients with severe traumatic brain injury: a meta-analysis. *PLoS One.* 2016;11:e0168901.

Steyerberg EW, Mushkudiani N, Perel P, et al. Predicting outcome after traumatic brain injury: development and international validation of prognostic scores based on admission characteristics. *PLoS Med.* 2008;5:e165.

Stiell IG, Clement CM, McKnight RD, et al. The Canadian C-spine rule versus the NEXUS low-risk criteria in patients with trauma. *N Engl J Med.* 2003;349:2510-2518.

Szaflarski JP, Sangha KS, Lindsell CJ, et al. Prospective, randomized, single-blinded comparative trial of intravenous levetiracetam versus phenytoin for seizure prophylaxis. *Neurocrit Care.* 2010;12:165-172.

Temkin NR, Anderson GD, Winn HR, et al. Magnesium sulfate for neuroprotection after traumatic brain injury: a randomised controlled trial. *Lancet Neurol.* 2007;6:29-38.

Temken NR, Dikmen SS, Winn HR. Post-traumatic seizures. In: Eisenberg HM, Aldrich EF, eds. *Management of Head Injury.* Philadelphia, PA: W.B. Saunders; 1991:425-435.

Vergouwen MD, Vermeulen M, Roos YB. Effect of nimodipine on outcome in patients with traumatic subarachnoid haemorrhage: a systematic review. *Lancet Neurol.* 2006;5: 1029-1032.

Wright DW, Yeatts SD, Silbergleit R, et al. Very early administration of progesterone for acute traumatic brain injury. *N Engl J Med.* 2014;371:2457-2466.

Zinkstok SM, Vergouwen MDI, Engelter ST, et al. Safety and functional outcome of thrombolysis in dissection-related ischemic stroke: a meta-analysis of individual patient data. *Stroke.* 2011;42:2515-2520.

4

Epilepsy

Joshua Leibner, MD and Christa Swisher, MD

Questions

1. A 48-year-old man with little known past medical history presents to the emergency department (ED) in status epilepticus with an ongoing generalized tonic-clonic seizure that started 14 minutes ago. With emergency medical services (EMS), he received 4 mg of intravenous (IV) lorazepam. He arrives in the ED, and you plan to repeat a second dose of lorazepam. Following the second lorazepam dose, there is still ongoing rhythmic movements of the right arm and leg. The patient is stuporous with sonorous respirations; he keeps his eyes closed to noxious stimulation, makes incomprehensible sounds, and withdraws to noxious stimulation with the left arm and leg; however, there is no response to noxious stimulation in the right hemibody. Vitals include a heart rate of 102 bpm, blood pressure of 98/68 mm Hg, and oxygen saturation of 82% on 6 L nasal cannula. What is the next best step in management of the patient?

   A. Intubate the patient
   B. Obtain telemetry/electrocardiogram (ECG) monitoring
   C. Obtain finger stick glucose
   D. Prolonged electroencephalography (EEG) monitoring
   E. Give 1 liter normal saline bolus

2. A 72-year-old woman is 4 days status post left temporal glioblastoma multiforme resection. Since the operation, she has been encephalopathic. On examination, her vital signs are stable. She is alert and oriented to person and talking about her deceased husband. Since surgery, she has had right superior quadrantanopsia and right arm weakness, but her change in mental status has been fluctuating. What would be the appropriate action to take?

   A. Administer 2 mg of IV lorazepam
   B. EEG monitoring
   C. Attribute symptoms to postoperative delirium and continue to clinically monitor
   D. Magnetic resonance imaging (MRI) of the brain
   E. Treat for a urinary tract infection (UTI)

3. A 51-year-old woman with a history of epilepsy is post-op day 2 of an anterior cervical discectomy and fusion. She complains of intense pain radiating around her abdomen that started the day after surgery. You obtain basic labs, and her amylase and lipase are 423 Units/L and 789 Units/L, respectively. Which antiepileptic medication is most likely to cause this problem?

   A. Valproic acid
   B. Phenytoin
   C. Topiramate
   D. Carbamazepine
   E. Lamotrigine

4. A 63-year-old man with a right parietal intracranial hemorrhage (measuring approximately 35 mL) is experiencing a decline in status. His Glasgow coma scale (GCS) score on presentation was 8; however, on day 2 of admission, his GCS declines to 5. A stat head computed tomography (CT) scan is performed without a change in the size of the bleed. What would be the next recommended course of action?

   A. Routine EEG
   B. Administer 2 mg of IV lorazepam
   C. Prolonged EEG monitoring
   D. Load 20 mg/kg of phenytoin
   E. Clinically monitor symptoms

5. A 63-year-old man with known focal epilepsy as a result of a prior right middle cerebral artery (MCA) stroke is admitted for focal status epilepticus. He was taking levetiracetam 1500 mg twice a day at home. He has been treated with 2 doses of 4 mg of IV lorazepam and a phenytoin load of 20 mg/kg IV, and he is now intubated. His vital signs are stable, and he has a GCS score of 7. Examination is notable for a left gaze deviation and rhythmic left arm and leg jerking. What would be the next course of action?

   A. Administer another 4 mg of IV lorazepam
   B. Load 20 mg/kg of levetiracetam
   C. Prolonged EEG
   D. Initiate a midazolam infusion with a loading dose
   E. MRI of the brain

6. A 39-year-old man is admitted to the medical intensive care unit (ICU) with ascending cholangitis. He remains persistently altered and is unable to say where he is or what his name is. He talks incoherently, making frequent paraphasic errors. His neurologic examination other than his mental status is otherwise unremarkable. CT of the head is performed, which shows no acute intracranial structural abnormalities. A routine EEG is performed and is shown below. Which of the following should be done based on the EEG finding?

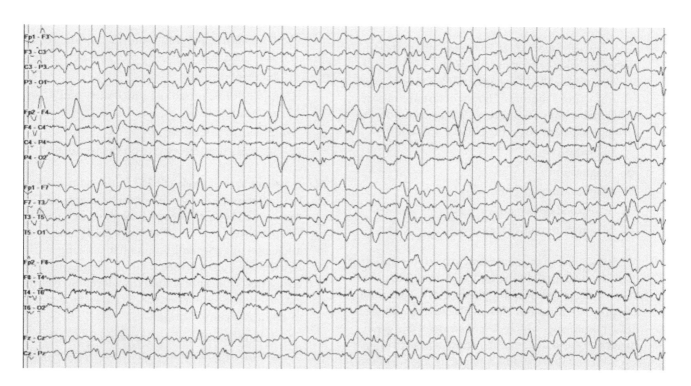

A. Load phenytoin 20 mg/kg IV

B. Administer lorazepam 2 mg IV

C. Obtain ammonia and liver function tests

D. Order MRI of the brain

E. Intubate and start a midazolam infusion

7. A 63-year-old man presents with 3 generalized tonic-clonic seizures over 20 minutes. He has a known history of alcohol abuse, and your suspicion is high that he is in alcohol withdrawal. An ED physician tells you his last drink was 7 hours ago, so these cannot be alcohol withdrawal seizures. How long after the last drink are alcohol withdrawal seizures usually seen?

    A. 2 to 10 hours

    B. 6 to 48 hours

    C. 24 to 72 hours

    D. 3 to 5 days

8. A 25-year-old woman is 33 weeks pregnant and diagnosed with eclampsia. An urgent ICU neurology consult is called for a generalized tonic-clonic seizure lasting 3 minutes. Her mental status returns to normal within 10 minutes. What would be the correct treatment given the clinical scenario?

    A. Phenytoin

    B. Magnesium

    C. Magnesium plus phenytoin

    D. Scheduled diazepam

    E. Magnesium plus diazepam

9. A 53-year-old man is in refractory status epilepticus. He was initially treated with multiple doses of lorazepam followed by phenytoin, lacosamide, and propofol infusion. He was placed on prolonged EEG monitoring, which demonstrates 4-Hz generalized spike and wave activity consistent with ongoing nonconvulsive status epilepticus. He was then started on midazolam infusion; however, the EEG has remained unchanged. Which of the following is the next most appropriate treatment for refractory status epilepticus, and what changes would you like to see on the EEG?

    A. Levetiracetam 20 mg/kg causing cessation of seizure activity on EEG

    B. Electroconvulsive therapy (ECT) causing a break in seizure activity on EEG

    C. Pentobarbital infusion titrated until discharges are less than 3 Hz

    D. Pentobarbital infusion titrated until burst suppression

    E. IV solumedrol causing seizure cessation on EEG

10. A 58-year-old man is currently in the ICU for status epilepticus. He was started on propofol 5 days ago with increasing doses required to maintain seizure cessation. He has been seizure free for the last 12 hours on prolonged EEG monitoring. Propofol is currently infusing at 90 µg/kg/min. You are called to the bedside for a drop in heart rate to 33 bpm and desaturations. An arterial blood gas (ABG) demonstrates a severe metabolic acidosis. A third vasopressor has to subsequently be added for resistant hypotension. The patient's heart rate is persistently in the 30s. What would be the next best course of action?

    A. Discontinue propofol immediately and switch to midazolam

    B. Increase propofol

    C. Discontinue propofol immediately and monitor EEG

    D. Obtain CT of the head

    E. Increase respiratory rate on the ventilator

11. A patient arrives from the ED to the neuroscience ICU after presenting with status epilepticus. He was treated with IV benzodiazepines followed by IV phenytoin into a left antecubital IV. He is no longer seizing. Several hours after arriving in the ICU, he develops a severe, painful, edematous, blistering rash with a purple/red discoloration over the entire left hand into the wrist. What is the best way to avoid this complication?

    A. Administration of the medication via a central venous line

    B. Slower infusion

    C. Administration of fosphenytoin rather than phenytoin

    D. Concomitant administration with aspirin

    E. Flushing the IV tubing to ensure the IV was in the vein

12. An 83-year-old man with mild Alzheimer dementia is admitted to the internal medicine service for a UTI requiring IV antibiotics. Overnight, a rapid response is called due to a generalized tonic-clonic seizure. He has no history of seizures. He is subsequently transferred to the neuroscience ICU for closer monitoring. A stat CT of the head is obtained, which shows no acute intracranial process. He is given 1500 mg of levetiracetam. Twelve hours later, the patient remains encephalopathic. He is oriented to person only, difficult to arouse, and frequently staring to his right. He is unable to name objects, and his wife reports that this is well below his baseline mental status prior to the seizure. What would you do next?

  A. Obtain MRI of the brain

  B. Administer lorazepam 2 mg

  C. Administer haloperidol for agitation

  D. EEG monitoring

  E. Give another loading dose of levetiracetam

13. A 19-year-old woman with a history of bipolar disorder is admitted to the neuro-ICU after developing seizures and worsening hallucinations. Three days after admission, she develops dyskinesias. An EEG is obtained and is shown below. What is the most likely diagnosis?

  A. Bipolar disorder with psychosis

  B. Creutzfeldt-Jakob disease

  C. Anti-NMDA (*N*-methyl-D-aspartate) receptor encephalitis

  D. Nonconvulsive status epilepticus

  E. Wilson disease

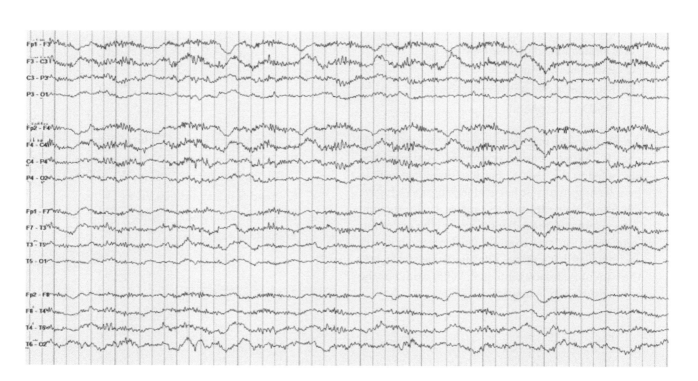

14. A previously healthy 41-year-old man is admitted to the neuro-ICU after presenting with 2 days of confusion, agitation, and a tonic-clonic seizure. An EEG is obtained, which is shown below. What is the most likely diagnosis?

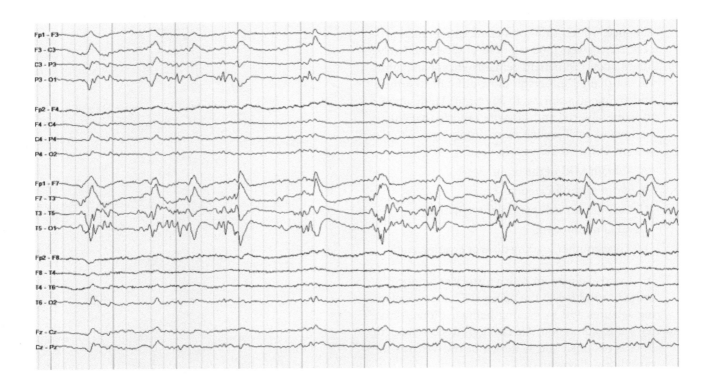

    A. Herpes simplex virus (HSV) encephalitis
    B. Creutzfeldt-Jakob disease
    C. Bacterial meningitis
    D. Nonconvulsive status epilepticus
    E. NMDA encephalitis

15. An 86-year-old man is admitted to the neuroscience ICU after a complete right MCA stroke. You are called to the bedside because the nurse notices he is having rhythmic left arm jerking and left gaze deviation. You administer 2 mg of IV lorazepam. After 5 minutes, the patient is still having forced left gaze deviation and continuous rhythmic left arm and now left leg jerking. Vital signs are stable, and the patient is already intubated. What would be the next best step in management?

    A. Administer 4 mg of IV lorazepam
    B. Administer 4 mg of IV lorazepam followed by fosphenytoin 20 PE/kg IV
    C. Load fosphenytoin 20 PE/kg IV
    D. Obtain stat head CT scan
    E. Obtain a stat EEG

Answers and Explanations

1. **A.** The patient presents in status epilepticus. First-line management was completed by EMS with an appropriate dose of the benzodiazepine (eg., lorazepam). The initial and second dose of lorazepam have not stopped the clinical seizure activity. The patient's current mental status is likely due to ongoing seizure and sedation following benzodiazepine administration. Reevaluation of the patient's airway, breathing, and circulation should be done at the time of presentation. In this patient's case, he is not protecting his airway and requires intubation. Although the patient will need telemetry monitoring, glucose check, and treatment if hypoglycemic or hyperglycemic, the need to secure a stable airway is paramount. Not included as an option is use of a second antiepileptic agent, which will also need to be completed.

Initial Common Steps in the Management of Status Epilepticus Immediate Treatment

Preserve airway and oxygenation
Secure IV access with preferably two peripheral lines
Check vitals including oxygen saturation—treat hypotension with fluid and vasopressors if necessary (central line)
Measure fingerstick blood glucose. If <60 mg/dL, administer 1 amp $D_{50}W$
$D_{50}W$ 50 mL IV and thiamine 100 mg IV unless adequate glucose known

Reproduced with permission from Lee K. *The NeuroICU Book*. New York, NY: McGraw-Hill; 2012.

2. **B.** This patient has signs of encephalopathy with a high risk for postoperative seizures, so an EEG should be performed. It would be incorrect to assume the patient is seizing and treat the patient without any evidence for seizures. While this may be postoperative delirium, further workup of the patient's persistent symptoms is warranted given she is 4 days post-op with persistent symptoms. Although a computed tomography (CT) of the head would be warranted to examine the operative cavity for bleeding, it would be unnecessary to get an MRI of the brain immediately. Investigation for toxic and metabolic causes of delirium would be warranted, but treating for UTI without evidence of it would be incorrect.

3. **A.** Valproic acid can, in rare cases, cause a life-threatening pancreatitis. Valproic acid–induced pancreatitis is a US Food and Drug Administration (FDA) boxed warning. This can occur at the start of therapy or following years of use. It has been reported in both children and adults. Symptoms suggestive of pancreatitis include abdominal pain, nausea, vomiting, and/or anorexia. Treatment is supportive, and valproic acid should be discontinued if pancreatitis is diagnosed.

4. **C.** Subclinical nonconvulsive seizures are frequently seen in the neurologic intensive care unit (ICU) setting. Approximately 20% of critically ill patients undergoing EEG monitoring will have nonconvulsive seizures or nonconvulsive status epilepticus. Up to 92% of seizures in patients with acute brain injury are nonconvulsive, necessitating the need for EEG monitoring to establish the diagnosis. Routine EEGs (recording under 1 hour) detect less than 50% of seizures that will eventually be detected in critically ill patients. Therefore, prolonged EEG monitoring would be warranted in this scenario. Although a benzodiazepine trial can be considered, a better diagnostic decision would be to obtain EEG monitoring. Monitoring after a decline in examination or treating with an antiepileptic drug (AED) would not be correct in this case.

5. **D.** This patient is in refractory status epilepticus (RSE), defined by the Neurocritical Care Society as "SE [status epilepticus] that does not respond to the standard treatment regimen, such as an

initial benzodiazepine followed by another AED." The next course of action after multiple doses of a benzodiazepine and a loading dose of an AED would be to start an infusion of either midazolam or propofol. A loading dose of a second AED, such as valproic acid or phenobarbital, can be considered prior to infusion; however, this patient is already on a high dose of levetiracetam at home, and little benefit would be achieved with reloading this medication. Prolonged EEG monitoring is recommended; however, it is clear that the patient remains in convulsive status epilepticus and therefore should continue to be treated with AEDs. It is of upmost importance to stop the patient's seizures. EEG monitoring should commence as soon as possible to evaluate for the presence of nonconvulsive seizures. Treating with another dose of a benzodiazepine is unlikely to help after the patient has already received 8 mg. CT of the head would be important to obtain early in the presentation; however, MRI of the brain is unnecessary at this time in someone with a known history of epilepsy.

6. **C.** The EEG demonstrated generalized periodic discharges (GPDs) with a triphasic morphology, which in the right clinical setting could be consistent with a toxic metabolic dysfunction. Given that the patient has ascending cholangitis, he is at high risk for liver failure and hyperammonemia. GPDs with triphasic morphology are high-amplitude generalized discharges that are often frontally predominant. Morphology consists of a low-amplitude negative phase followed by a large positive phase followed by a final negative phase that typically has the longest duration compared to the others. An anterior-posterior "time lag" can often be seen. These are typically seen with toxic or metabolic encephalopathies (such as hepatic or uremic)

but may be seen with other etiologies. Previously thought to be benign, it is now know that GPDs with triphasic morphology have been associated with nonconvulsive seizures and nonconvulsive status epilepticus in some cases.

7. **B.** Alcohol withdrawal seizures can take place early in the course. A single seizure or flurry of generalized tonic-clonic seizures can be seen in the first 6 to 48 hours after the patient's last drink. Hallucinations commonly occur around this time as well. Delirium tremens symptoms including delirium, agitation, tachycardia, hypertension, and fever typically do not occur until 2 to 4 days after the last drink.

8. **B.** The Eclampsia Trial Collaborative Group conducted a seminal trial of magnesium sulfate versus diazepam or phenytoin in eclampsia. Magnesium sulfate was significantly more effective than diazepam or phenytoin. There would not be any indication to add an AED or benzodiazepine after one eclamptic seizure. Recurrent eclamptic seizures will often require the addition of a benzodiazepine.

9. **D.** The patient has refractory status epilepticus, which can complicate up to 20% of all patients with status epilepticus. High-dose barbiturates are used because they appear to offer greater effectiveness in seizure control. Pentobarbital would be the best next treatment and should be titrated up until burst suppression in refractory status epilepticus. Pentobarbital is usually started with a bolus followed by a continuous infusion. The other choices would not be the next best treatment in refractory status epilepticus, although ECT and steroids can be used in some cases of super-refractory status epilepticus.

Continuous IV Infusion Therapies Used in RSE Medications

1. Continuous IV midazolam infusion
- Loading Dose: 0.2 mg/kg. Repeat 0.2-0.4 mg/kg boluses every 5 min until seizure stops, up to a maximum total loading dose of 2 mg/kg
- Continuous IV: Initial infusion rate 0.1 mg/kg. Usual maintenance rate 0.05 mg/kg.
- Dose Range: 0.05-2.9 mg/kg/h. For breakthrough seizures, an additional bolus can be given and the continuous IV rate should be increased by approximately 20%.
- Time to Stop Status Epilepticus: Minutes, usually less than 1 h.
- Duration of Antiepileptic Effect: Minutes to hours.
- Elimination Half-Life: 1.5-3.5 h initially. With prolonged use, tolerance, tachphylaxis, and significant prolongation of half-life can occur.
- Main side Effect: Sedation of minutes to several hours and a possible day if prolonged use, respiratory depression, hypotension.

2. Continuous IV Propofol Infusion
- Loading Dose: 1 mg/kg. Repeat 1-2 mg/kg boluses every 5 min until seizure stops, up to a maximum loading dose of 10 mg/kg. Initial continuous IV rate: 2 mg/kg/h.
- Continuous IV Dose Range: 1-15 mg/kg/h. Do not exceed 5 mg/kg/h for >48 h due to risk of propofol infusion syndrome.
- Time to Stop Status Epilepticus: Usually <10 min.
- Contraindications: Allergy to soybean oil, egg lecithin, or glycerol. Use with caution in combination with carbonic anhydrase inhibitors, including zonisamide and topiramate, because of the risk of refractory acidosis.
- Main Side Effects: Sedation, large lipid load requiring adjustment of caloric intake, occasional pancreatitis, dose-dependant hypotension, potential fatal multiorgan failure and "propofol infusion syndrome" (metabolic acidosis, rhabdomyolysis, and circulatory colapse) with high dose or prolonged use.
- Monitor: CPK, triglycerides, amylase/lipase, blood gases, and lactic acid. Consider cardiovascular monitoring.

3. Continuous IV Pentobarbital Infusion
- Loading Dose: 5 mg/kg. Repeat 5 mg/kg boluses until seizure stops.
- Maximum Bolus Rate: 25-50 mg/min.
- Continuous IV Dose Range: Initial infusion rate 1 mg/kg/h. Usual maintenance range 0.5-10.0 mg/kg/h, traditionally titrated to suppression burst on EEG.
- Elimination Half-Life: 15-60 h.
- Main Side Effect: Prolonged coma (usually days after infusion stopped), hypotension (usually requires vasopressors), myocardial depression, immune suppression, ileus, allergy including Stevens-Johnson syndrome.
- Target Serum Levels: See phenytoin. Serum phenytoin levels should be measured >2 h after IV or >4 h after IM infusion to allow complete conversion to phenytoin.

Abbreviations: CPK, creatine phosphokinase; EEG, electroencephalogram; RSE, refractory status epilepticus.

Reproduced with permission from Lee K. *The NeuroICU Book.* New York, NY: McGraw-Hill; 2012.

10. A. The patient likely has propofol infusion syndrome (PIS). This syndrome typically occurs with higher doses of propofol (>60-70 µg/kg/min) used for longer periods of time (>48 hours). Symptoms of PIS include:

- Cardiac: tachycardia, bradycardia, heart failure, and cardiovascular collapse
- Electrolytes changes: hyperkalemia, severe metabolic acidosis, and hyperlipidemia
- Rhabdomyolysis and renal failure

Mortality can be very high (up to 33%). Onset of symptoms typically occurs within 4 days of initiation. The mechanism is unknown. Given the high doses of propofol needed to control the patient's seizures, it would be difficult to withdraw propofol completely without adding a different medication such as midazolam.

11. A. The description of a distal, swollen, painful rash with purple discoloration depicts purple glove syndrome due to the IV administration of phenytoin. This is an uncommon reaction to IV infusion of phenytoin that usually develops within the first 24 hours of infusion. It presents with peripheral edema, blistering, pain, and discoloration of the extremity that received IV phenytoin. Treatment may require surgical intervention. Extravasation is not always present, and extravasation of phenytoin does not necessarily result in purple glove syndrome. Use of a large-bore cannula or central line for phenytoin administration can decrease the incidence of purple glove syndrome. Although slower administration rates may reduce the risk of purple glove syndrome, the best method of avoidance is to administer phenytoin via a central line. Although the risk of purple glove syndrome is less with fosphenytoin, cases of purple glove syndrome have been reported with fosphenytoin.

12. **D.** The patient has a risk of seizures from his dementia. He had a single generalized seizure and has not returned back to his baseline functioning after 14 hours. There may be other confounding factors to his mental status such as his UTI; however, EEG monitoring would be warranted to rule out subclinical seizures given the persistent change in mental status 14 hours after the seizure.

13. **C.** The EEG demonstrates extreme delta brush as evidenced by background delta slowing with overriding fast beta activity. This can be a unique EEG pattern in adults with NMDA encephalitis. Although not always present in patients with anti-NMDA receptor encephalitis, the presence of extreme delta brush is associated with a more prolonged illness. The patient's symptoms of seizures, hallucinations, and dyskinesias can all be seen with NMDA encephalitis. Her past history of bipolar disorder may be a misdiagnosis, as NMDA encephalitis can sometimes initially be mistaken for psychiatric disease.

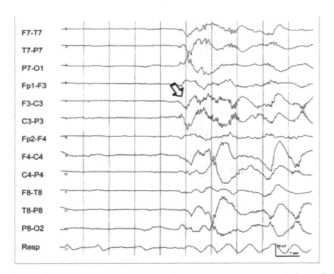

Reproduced with permission from Laoprasert P., *Atlas of Pediatric EEG*, New York, NY: McGraw-Hill, 2011.

14. **A.** The EEG demonstrates left temporal lateralized periodic discharges, which is the most likely finding in HSV encephalitis. Generalized periodic discharges can sometimes be seen with Creutzfeldt-Jakob disease. Although lateralized periodic discharges can be seen with NMDA encephalitis, this patient was previously healthy, and the clinical scenario is more indicative of HSV encephalitis. The EEG does not demonstrate status epilepticus.

15. **B.** The clinical scenario is consistent with an ongoing seizure that is now status epilepticus. The seizure did not abort with 2 mg of an IV benzodiazepine; however, another dose of a benzodiazepine should be given.

Per the Neurocritical Care Society guidelines on status epilepticus, all patients should receive emergent initial therapy (lorazepam chosen in this case) and urgent control therapy (fosphenytoin chosen in this case). The recommended initial dosing of lorazepam is 0.1 mg/kg IV up to 4 mg per dose. This may be repeated in 5 to 10 minutes. Per these guideline, emergent initial therapy is always followed by urgent control therapy. For patients who respond to emergent initial therapy, urgent control therapy is needed to maintain seizure control. For patients who do not respond to emergent initial therapy, urgent control therapy is needed to attain seizure cessation. EEG and head CT may eventually be needed, but aborting status epilepticus is the priority. The patient must be clinically stable before being transported to CT. Prolonged EEG monitoring is necessary for the management of status epilepticus to rule out nonconvulsive status epilepticus after convulsive status epilepticus is stopped.

REFERENCES

Brigo F, Storti M. Triphasic waves. *Am J Electroneurodiagnostic Technol.* 2011;51:16-25.

Brophy GM, Bell R, Claassen J, et al. Guidelines for the evaluation and management of status epilepticus. *Neurocrit Care.* 2012;17:3-23.

Chapman SA, Wacksman GP, Patterson BD. Pancreatitis associated with valproic acid: a review of the literature. *Pharmacotherapy.* 2001;21:1549-1560.

Claassen J, Hirsch LJ, Emerson RG, et al. Treatment of refractory status epilepticus with pentobarbital, propofol, or midazolam: a systematic review. *Epilepsia.* 2002;43:146-153.

Claassen J, Riviello JJ Jr, Silbergleit R. Emergency neurological live support: status epilepticus. *Neurocrit Care.* 2015;23(Suppl 2):S136-S142.

Earnest MP, Marx JA, Drury LR. Complications of intravenous phenytoin for acute treatment of seizures. Recommendations for usage. *JAMA.* 1983;249:762-765.

Eclampsia Trial Collaborative Group. Which anticonvulsant for women with eclampsia? Evidence from the Collaborative Eclampsia Trial. *Lancet.* 1995;345:1455-1463.

Food and Drug Administration. Depakene (valproic acid) capsules and oral solution. Food and Drug Administration Approved Labeling. Maryland. 2011. https://www.accessdata.fda.gov/drugsatfda_docs/label/2011/018081s046_18082s031lbl.pdf. Accessed June 5, 2017.

Fountain NB, Waldman WA. Effects of benzodiazepines on triphasic waves: implications for non-convulsive status epileptics. *J Clin Neurophysiol.* 2001;18:345-352.

Fudickar A, Bein B. Propofol infusion syndrome: update of clinical manifestation and pathophysiology. *Minerva Anesthesiol.* 2009;75:339-344.

Kim YS, Jung HS, Lee ST, et al. Prognostic value of initial standard EEG and MRI in patients with herpes simplex encephalitis. *J Clin Neurol.* 2016;12:224-229.

Martins WA, Palmini A. Periodic lateralized epileptiform discharges (PLEDs) in herpetic encephalitis. *Arq Neuropsiquiatr.* 2015;73:1046.

Ney JP, van der Goes DN, Nuwer MR, et al. Continuous and routine EEG in the intensive care: Utilization and outcomes, United States 2005-2009. *Neurology.* 2013;81:2002-2008.

Nuwer MR. Electroencephalograms and evoked potentials. Monitoring cerebral function in the neurosurgical intensive care unit. *Neurosurg Clin N Am.* 2994;5:647-659.

O'Brien TJ, Cascino GD, So EL, et al. Incidence and clinical consequence of the purple glove syndrome in patients receiving intravenous phenytoin. *Neurology.* 1998;51:1034-1039.

Rossetti AO, Milligan TA, Vulliemoz S, et al. A randomized trial for the treatment of refractory status epilepticus. *Neurocrit Care.* 2011;14:4-10.

Schmitt SE, Pargeon K, Frechette ES, et al. Extreme delta brush: a unique EEG pattern in adults with anti-NMDA receptor encephalitis. *Neurology.* 2012;79:1094-1100.

Sibai BM. Magnesium sulfate prophylaxis in preeclampsia: lessons learned from recent trials. *Am J Obstet Gynecol.* 2004;190:1520-1526.

Vespa PM, Nenov V, Nuwer MR. Continuous EEG monitoring in the intensive care unit: early findings and clinical efficacy. *J Clin Neurophysiol.* 1999;16:1-13.

Victor M, Brausch C. The role of abstinence in the genesis of alcohol epilepsy. *Epilepsia.* 1967;8:1-20.

5

Neuromuscular Diseases

Christyn M. Edmundson, MD, Laura A. Foster, MD, Janice C. Wong, MD, and Anthony A. Amato, MD

Questions

1. A 38-year-old woman with generalized myasthenia gravis who has been well controlled on low-dose prednisone presents to the emergency department with symptoms of abdominal pain, fever, and dysuria. Over the next 12 hours, she develops dyspnea and is admitted to the intensive care unit (ICU) for further monitoring. On arrival to the ICU, the patient's speech is hypophonic and staccato, and she has marked weakness of neck flexion. Negative inspiratory force (NIF; also known as maximal inspiratory pressure [MIP]) is 15 cm H_2O, and vital capacity (VC) is 10 mL/kg. Arterial partial pressure of carbon dioxide (PcO_2) is 38 mm Hg and arterial partial pressure of oxygen (PO_2) is 92 mm Hg. What is the most appropriate next step in management of this patient?

   A. Urgently administer 2 mg of intravenous (IV) pyridostigmine

   B. Urgently administer 1000 mg of IV methylprednisolone

   C. Urgently administer 0.4 mg/kg of IV immunoglobulin (IVIG)

   D. Proceed with endotracheal intubation

   E. Continue to observe the patient, monitoring NIF and VC every 2 to 4 hours

2. A 62-year-old man with diabetes, end-stage renal disease on hemodialysis, and recently diagnosed generalized myasthenia gravis is directly admitted to the hospital for progressively worsening diplopia, difficulty climbing stairs, frequent choking while eating or drinking, and dyspnea. Home medications include pyridostigmine 60 mg 3 times a day (TID). He was previously prescribed prednisone 10 mg daily but has not started taking this medication. On examination, he has right greater than left ptosis and proximal arm and leg weakness. NIF (also known as MIP) is –35 cm H_2O, and VC is 25 mL/kg. What is the most appropriate treatment for this patient?

   A. Start prednisone 80 mg orally (PO) daily

   B. Start methylprednisolone 1000 mg IV daily for 3 days

   C. Increase pyridostigmine to 120 mg TID

   D. Initiate a course of IVIG

   E. Initiate a course of plasmapheresis

3. A 31-year-old woman with a history of Graves disease and recently diagnosed ocular predominant myasthenia gravis presents to the emergency department with diarrhea and weakness. Examination is notable for generalized weakness, diffuse fasciculations, and bradycardia. Ptosis is absent, and extraocular movements are intact, but her pupils are small and sluggishly reactive. What is the most likely cause of the patient's symptoms?

   A. Thyrotoxicosis

   B. Myasthenic crisis

   C. Cholinergic crisis

   D. Miller Fisher variant of Guillain-Barré syndrome

   E. Electrolyte abnormality due to diarrhea

4. A 61-year-old man with a 40-pack-year smoking history has experienced several months of weight loss and hemoptysis. He subsequently develops arm and leg weakness, difficulty initiating rapid movements, and progressive dyspnea. He is admitted to the ICU for respiratory decline. On examination, he has weakness of shoulder abduction, hip flexion, and neck flexion and extension. Reflexes are reduced. Muscle strength and reflexes improve markedly with repeated testing. Which serologic test is most likely to provide a diagnosis for this patient?

   A. Anti–voltage-gated potassium channel antibodies

   B. Anti–voltage-gated calcium channel antibodies

   C. Anti-Hu antibodies

   D. Anti–acetylcholine receptor antibodies

   E. Anti–muscle specific kinase antibodies

5. A 30-year-old woman presents with severe shortness of breath. The previous evening, she sampled homemade sausage at a friend's dinner party. Several hours later, she developed progressively worsening blurred vision, dry mouth, and hoarseness. Examination reveals bilateral ptosis, dilated pupils, facial weakness, and diminished deep tendon reflexes. She is admitted to the ICU for further monitoring and treatment. Which pattern of abnormalities is most likely on electromyography (EMG)/nerve conduction studies (NCS)?

   A. Normal sensory nerve conduction studies, low compound motor action potential (CMAP) amplitudes, decremental CMAP response to slow repetitive stimulation, incremental CMAP response to fast repetitive stimulation

   B. Normal sensory conduction studies, low CMAP amplitudes, incremental CMAP response to slow repetitive stimulation, incremental CMAP response to fast repetitive stimulation

   C. Absent sensory responses, normal CMAP amplitudes, decremental CMAP response to slow repetitive stimulation, incremental CMAP response to fast repetitive stimulation

   D. Absent sensory responses, low CMAP amplitudes, no change in CMAP amplitude with fast or slow repetitive stimulation

6. A 76-year-old man with a history of hypertension presented to the hospital with confusion, fevers, headache, and nuchal rigidity. During admission, he developed flaccid paralysis and hypoxemia requiring intubation. Cerebrospinal fluid (CSF) testing revealed lymphocytic pleocytosis and elevated protein; bacterial culture was negative. With supportive care and appropriate disease-specific treatment, the patient's systemic symptoms gradually improved, but he could not be weaned from the ventilator. Electrodiagnostic studies were performed approximately 3 weeks after intubation. NCS showed motor responses with severely reduced amplitudes but normal conduction velocities and normal sensory responses. Needle EMG showed abundant spontaneous activity and reduced motor unit recruitment but no myopathic-appearing motor units. What is the most likely diagnosis?

   A. Critical illness myopathy

   B. West Nile virus–induced poliomyelitis

   C. Adult-onset Pompe disease

   D. Critical illness polyneuropathy

   E. Acute inflammatory demyelinating polyneuropathy

7. How would a patient with myasthenia gravis be expected to respond to neuromuscular blocking agents?

   A. The patient would display increased sensitivity to both depolarizing and nondepolarizing neuromuscular blocking agents.

   B. The patient would display decreased sensitivity to both depolarizing and nondepolarizing neuromuscular blocking agents.

   C. The patient would display increased sensitivity to depolarizing neuromuscular blocking agents and decreased sensitivity to nondepolarizing neuromuscular blocking agents.

   D. The patient would display variable sensitivity to depolarizing neuromuscular blocking agents and increased sensitivity to nondepolarizing neuromuscular blocking agents.

8. A 45-year-old man (weighing 100 kg) presents to the emergency department complaining of numbness and tingling in his feet that has been spreading to his legs and arms over the past 2 days and inability to walk. On exam, he cannot whistle and has marked weakness in his arms and legs (elbow flexion and knee extension are less than antigravity). Reflexes are absent. Vibration and proprioception are severely reduced in the toes and ankles. He is admitted to the ICU, and his respiratory parameters are monitored every 4 hours. Which of the following would be the *first* indication for prompt intubation and mechanical ventilation?

   A. NIF of –80 cm H_2O
   B. Mean expiratory pressure (MEP) of 100 cm H_2O
   C. VC of 900 mL
   D. Oxygen saturation of 88% on room air
   E. P_{CO_2} of 55 mm Hg on arterial blood gas

9. A 42-year-old man developed double vision and ptosis a few days ago. He decided to come to the emergency department after spilling his coffee, cutting himself while shaving, and tripping on the stairs. He continues to feel unsteady while walking. On examination, he has limited adduction of both eyes and limited abduction of the left eye. He has facial weakness, mild weakness of hip flexion, absent reflexes, limb dysmetria, and an ataxic gait. Which of the following serum antibodies are most likely to be present?

A. Acetylcholine receptor
B. GAD
C. GD1a
D. GM1
E. GQ1b

10. In patients with Guillain-Barré syndrome, which of the following have been shown to be predictors of the development of respiratory insufficiency requiring mechanical ventilation?

   A. Days between onset of weakness and admission and presence of facial, bulbar, neck, and/or shoulder girdle weakness.

   B. Antecedent upper respiratory tract infection and presence of leg weakness

   C. Antecedent upper respiratory tract infection and presence of facial and/or bulbar weakness

   D. Chronic pulmonary disease and presence of facial and/or bulbar weakness

   E. Days between onset of weakness and admission and antecedent upper respiratory tract infection

11. A 35-year-old man recovered from a flu and then developed a prickly sensation throughout his arms and legs. A couple of days later, he was unable to climb stairs. On exam, in addition to symmetric distal weakness and sensory deficits, he has tachycardia and absent reflexes. Which of the following additional symptoms is most consistent with a diagnosis of Guillain-Barré syndrome?

   A. Urinary incontinence
   B. Lightheadedness upon standing
   C. Weakness on the right much more than left
   D. Muscle twitching
   E. Tea-colored urine

12. A 65-year-old man who was diagnosed with amyotrophic lateral sclerosis (ALS) 3 years ago presented to the emergency department for dyspnea. While in the emergency department, he wrote on a white board, "not ready to die." He was promptly sedated, intubated, and mechanically ventilated. He was admitted to the ICU, and workup has revealed his respiratory failure is due to his ALS and he will not wean from the ventilator. During brief sedation breaks for neurochecks, he follows commands, and other features of the neurologic examination are

comparable to clinic examination 3 months ago. At his last clinic visit 3 months ago, his cognition was intact, and he had significant bulbar weakness (dysarthria and dysphagia) and a decline in his pulmonary function tests to a forced vital capacity (FVC) of 30%. After discussion with his primary neurologist and his wife (who is his medical power of attorney/healthcare proxy), he decided against tracheostomy and mechanical ventilation and signed a do not resuscitate and/or intubate (DNR/DNI) order. Tracheostomy is indicated for definitive management of respiratory failure. What is the most appropriate next course of action?

- A. Ask the patient's wife to consent for a tracheostomy
- B. Wean sedation, explain the pros and cons of tracheostomy, and ask the patient whether he would like a tracheostomy
- C. Because of his previous DNR/DNI order, initiate palliative sedation protocol and extubate
- D. Because his ventilatory function could improve in the short-term, perform ventilatory weaning trials according to ICU protocol
- E. Request an ethics consultation

13. A 37-year-old man was admitted for status asthmaticus for which he required intubation with use of neuromuscular blocking agents due to dyssynchrony with the ventilator and treatment with high-dose intravenous corticosteroids. After 10 days, despite evidence of intact mental status (eg, opening eyes to command), he continued to fail extubation and was unable to move his extremities on command. Creatine kinase (CK) level was moderately elevated. What are the most likely NCS findings?

- A. Normal CMAP amplitude, normal sensory nerve action potential (SNAP), decrement on repetitive nerve stimulation
- B. Mildly (>80% of normal) reduced CMAP amplitude, prolonged SNAP peak latency, and decreased SNAP amplitude, no decrement on repetitive nerve stimulation
- C. Mildly (>80% of normal) reduced CMAP amplitude, normal SNAP, decrement on repetitive nerve stimulation

- D. Markedly (<80% of normal) reduced CMAP amplitude, normal SNAP, no decrement on repetitive nerve stimulation
- E. Markedly (<80% of normal) reduced CMAP amplitude, absent SNAP, decrement on repetitive nerve stimulation

14. A 65-year-old man underwent a prolonged open-heart surgery involving median sternotomy. Preoperatively, he did not have any sensory deficits or focal weakness. Immediately postoperatively, he noted numbness in the left medial hand and forearm and severe weakness in his left hand. NCS performed 3 weeks later showed moderately reduced ulnar digital SNAP, but normal median digital SNAP. Both ulnar abductor digiti minimi (ADM) and median abductor pollicis brevis (APB) CMAP amplitudes were reduced. Concentric needle EMG showed abnormal spontaneous activity in the form of positive sharp waves and fibrillation potentials and reduced motor unit recruitment in the ADM, APB, and extensor indicis proprius (EIP) muscles. What is the most likely diagnosis?

- A. Ulnar neuropathy and carpal tunnel syndrome
- B. Lower trunk injury
- C. C8 nerve root injury
- D. Motor neuron disease
- E. Middle trunk injury

15. A 36-year-old woman presented to the emergency department with shortness of breath and required intubation for respiratory acidosis. Her family members noted that she has been experiencing dyspnea, difficulty with climbing stairs, and some muscle pain in the past few years. CK level was within normal limits. NCS were normal. On EMG, there were myotonic discharges in paraspinal muscles, and motor unit potentials appeared myopathic with small-amplitude and short-duration morphology and early recruitment. What additional targeted test may be helpful in the diagnosis?

- A. *C9orf72* gene mutation
- B. Antinuclear antibody
- C. Dried blood spot to assess for α-glucosidase activity
- D. Dystrophin analysis for Becker muscular dystrophy
- E. Limb girdle muscular dystrophy 1 genetic panel

16. A 78-year-old woman was found on the ground and pulseless and was resuscitated with return of circulation. The patient did not undergo cooling following cardiac arrest given profound hemodynamic instability requiring multiple pressors to maintain adequate perfusion. Neurology is consulted to assist with prognostication. A median nerve somatosensory evoked potential (SSEP) study is ordered to help with prognostication. N20 (cortical) responses were bilaterally absent. In this patient, what is the earliest time in which this SSEP response can help predict poor prognosis after anoxic brain injury?

    A. 12 hours

    B. 24 hours

    C. 48 hours

    D. 72 hours

    E. Undetermined

17. A 55-year-old man underwent abdominal surgery with general anesthesia. During this surgery, he developed muscle rigidity, myoglobinuria, and abnormal vital signs including temperature of 102°C, oxygen saturation of 80%, and heart rate of 130 bpm with an irregular rhythm. Which of the following statements about his diagnosis is true?

    A. Muscle biopsies often reveal rimmed vacuoles in muscle fibers.

    B. Serum CK is normal during these episodes.

    C. Hypokalemia usually is found during these episodes.

    D. Only 1 gene has been found to be associated with this condition.

    E. Individuals with central core myopathy are at higher risk for this condition.

18. A 70-year-old woman presented with status epilepticus secondary to a traumatic subdural hematoma, requiring intubation and sedation with propofol. Several days after admission, she was found to have darkened urine. Further workup included CK levels of 5500 Unit/L, metabolic acidosis, hyperkalemia, and acute renal failure. What medication was most likely responsible for this presentation?

    A. Phenytoin

    B. Levetiracetam

    C. Propofol

    D. Midazolam

    E. None of the above

19. A 44-year-old man with a history of depression was found lying on the ground next to an emptied bottle of insecticide. He was unresponsive and required intubation. On admission, exam included bradycardia, increased respiratory secretions, diaphoresis, small reactive pupils, and weak limbs. Which of the following is an electrodiagnostic test finding that is often found in this condition?

    A. Reduced CMAP amplitude

    B. Slow CMAP conduction velocity

    C. Prolonged sensory nerve action potential (SNAP) peak latency

    D. Rapid repetitive stimulation with incremental response

    E. Slow repetitive stimulation with decremental response

Answers and Explanations

1. **D.** This patient is presenting with manifest myasthenic crisis, defined as worsening of myasthenic weakness requiring intubation or noninvasive ventilation to avoid intubation. Her abrupt symptomatic deterioration and respiratory parameters warrant intubation. In patients with markers of respiratory compromise, elective intubation is preferred over emergent intubation in response to abrupt respiratory collapse. Clinical features of impending respiratory failure in myasthenia gravis include shortness of breath, tachypnea, paradoxical breathing or use of accessory muscles, marked neck flexion weakness, and staccato speech or speaking in shortened sentences.

   In neuromuscular disorders, the "20/30/40" formula suggests mechanical ventilation should be considered in patients with the following respiratory parameters:

   - VC <20 mL/kg
   - NIF (also called MIP) < –30 cm H_2O
   - Maximal expiratory pressure <40 cm H_2O or >30% or more decline in these measurements on serial testing
   - Some experts use a more stringent cutoff of VC <15 mL/kg and NIF (or MIP) < –20 cm H_2O when considering elective intubation.

   Note that patients with weak bulbar muscles may be unable to form an adequate seal around the spirometer, making accurate measurements difficult. Positive-pressure ventilation may be considered in some myasthenic patients to avoid intubation during treatment of a myasthenic crisis.

   Hypercapnia and hypoxemia are relatively late findings in the course of neuromuscular respiratory failure, and this patient's normal arterial Po_2 and Pco_2 should not delay intervention.

   Pyridostigmine is typically discontinued during a myasthenic crisis, as it may worsen respiratory secretions. IV pyridostigmine is primarily used in stable myasthenic patients undergoing elective surgery.

   IVIG and plasmapheresis (PLEX) are rapid therapies for the treatment of myasthenic crisis, but treatment with these therapies should be initiated after the patient's respiratory compromise has been addressed. High-dose corticosteroids (prednisone 60-80 mg/d) are frequently initiated during a myasthenic crisis to ensure a sustained clinical response. However, because corticosteroids may cause transient worsening of myasthenic weakness, it may be appropriate to wait several days after starting IVIG or PLEX to initiate high-dose corticosteroid therapy.

2. **E.** This patient is presenting with impending myasthenic crisis. Impending myasthenic crisis is defined as rapid clinical worsening of myasthenia gravis that could lead to manifest crisis in days to weeks. Manifest myasthenic crisis is defined as worsening of myasthenic weakness requiring intubation or noninvasive ventilation to avoid intubation. Impending and manifest myasthenic crisis with respiratory or bulbar symptoms are emergent situations, and both require urgent management. In addition to admission to an intensive care or step-down unit for respiratory monitoring and/or support, patients should be treated urgently with IVIG or PLEX. The choice between these therapies is determined by availability and patient comorbidities. Contraindications for IVIG include renal failure (as in this patient's case) and hypercoagulable states. Contraindications to PLEX include sepsis due to hemodynamic issues and bacterial colonization of plasmapheresis catheters. Clinical trials suggest that IVIG and PLEX are both effective in the treatment of myasthenic crisis.

3. **C.** Although rare, deterioration in myasthenia gravis can be caused by cholinergic crisis. This is most often seen in patients with worsening myasthenic symptoms for whom the dose of pyridostigmine is gradually escalated to the point of

overdose, contributing to generalized weakness. Characteristic signs and symptoms of cholinergic crisis include miosis, excess pulmonary secretions, muscle fasciculations, abdominal cramping and diarrhea, diaphoresis, and bradycardia. Treatment of cholinergic crisis consists of respiratory support with discontinuation of pyridostigmine, in addition to treatment of possible concomitant myasthenic exacerbation.

In the patient described in this question, bradycardia, fasciculations, and miosis, as well as the symptom of diarrhea, support a diagnosis of cholinergic crisis. Thyrotoxicosis is likely associated with tachycardia rather than bradycardia. Miller Fisher variant of Guillain-Barré syndrome is marked by the triad of ataxia, areflexia, and oculomotor weakness, which is not seen in this patient.

4. **B.** This patient likely has Lambert-Eaton myasthenic syndrome (LEMS). In older adults, LEMS is frequently a paraneoplastic disorder associated with small-cell lung cancer. In younger adults or children, LEMS is more often a primary autoimmune disorder without a detectable underlying malignancy. Antibodies directed against presynaptic voltage-gated calcium channels (VGCC) are detected in the majority of LEMS patients.

Transient improvement in strength and reflexes with exercise is a characteristic of presynaptic disorders of neuromuscular transmission, such as LEMS. This is the clinical correlate of the incremental response seen with rapid repetitive stimulation on electrodiagnostic testing (increased amplitude of motor responses with rapid repetitive nerve stimulation). Repeated firing of the motor nerve results in an accumulation of calcium in the presynaptic nerve terminal that is sufficient to overcome the decreased density of presynaptic VGCCs.

Treatment of LEMS may include the identification and treatment of an underlying neoplasm, pharmacologic treatment with pyridostigmine or 3,4-diaminopyridine (3,4-DAP), or sometimes immunotherapy (eg, corticosteroids, IVIG, PLEX).

Anti–voltage-gated potassium channel antibodies are typically associated with Isaacs syndrome (nerve hyperexcitability causing cramps, fasciculations, and stiffness) and Morvan syndrome (Isaacs syndrome plus encephalitis). Anti-Hu antibodies and ANNA-1 (antineuronal nuclear antibody type 1) cause a variety of paraneoplastic syndromes, including sensory neuronopathy, cerebellar degeneration, and limbic encephalitis. Anti-Hu antibodies and their associated syndromes frequently coexist with LEMS and VGCC antibodies. Anti–acetylcholine receptor antibodies and anti–muscle specific kinase (MuSK) antibodies are associated with myasthenia gravis.

5. **A.** This patient's clinical presentation is most consistent with foodborne botulism acquired from improper preparation of cured meat. Botulism can also be acquired from improperly canned foods or through wounds in adults. Infantile botulism is caused by bacterial colonization of the gastrointestinal tract after exposure to clostridial spores via honey ingestion or environmental exposure.

Botulism toxin causes presynaptic dysfunction at the neuromuscular junction by interfering with acetylcholine release. Sensory nerves are not affected. On electrodiagnostic testing, CMAPs are reduced at baseline. Decrement in CMAP amplitude is seen with slow repetitive stimulation (2-5 Hz), and the classic increment in CMAP amplitude is seen with fast repetitive stimulation (>20 Hz). Thus, electrodiagnostic studies can provide diagnostic support for botulism and classically demonstrate normal sensory studies, low CMAP amplitudes, decremental CMAP response with slow repetitive stimulation, and incremental CMAP response with high-frequency repetitive stimulation. A similar pattern is seen in other presynaptic disorders, such as LEMS. Gold standard for diagnosis of botulism is a mouse bioassay, although the sensitivity of this test is approximately 45%.

6. **B.** This patient likely suffered from a polio-like illness caused by West Nile virus. Meningoencephalitis and acute flaccid paralysis caused by West Nile virus may present simultaneously, as in this patient.

This patient's electrodiagnostic studies are consistent with a subacute motor neuronopathy, as may be seen in West Nile virus infection. Low-amplitude motor responses with preserved sensory responses on electrodiagnostic studies suggest either a disorder of motor neurons or a process affecting the nerves proximal to the dorsal root ganglion (such as a polyradiculopathy, which is not an answer choice). Reduced motor unit recruitment and the absence of small, myopathic-appearing motor units suggest a neurogenic rather than myopathic process. Notably, large-amplitude, long-duration ("neurogenic-appearing") motor units resulting from denervation followed by reinnervation do not appear until several months after injury.

In critical illness polyneuropathy, sensory studies would be abnormal. In critical illness myopathy, myopathic motor units would be expected. In acute inflammatory demyelinating polyneuropathy (AIDP; or Guillain-Barré syndrome), absent sensory responses and slowed motor conduction velocities would be expected. Although there is an isolated axonal and motor form of Guillain-Barré syndrome (acute motor axonal neuropathy), it is less likely than West Nile–induced flaccid paralysis in this patient given his concomitant encephalopathy. In adult-onset Pompe disease, spontaneous activity, classically including myotonic discharges, may be present, but myopathic motor units would also be expected.

7. **D.** Depolarizing and nondepolarizing neuromuscular blocking agents (NMBAs) have different mechanisms of action. Depolarizing NMBAs, such as succinylcholine, are postsynaptic acetylcholine (ACh) receptor *agonists*. These agents induce continuous end plate depolarization, resulting in an initial muscle contraction, followed by muscle relaxation as the end plate cannot repolarize. Nondepolarizing NMBAs, such as cisatracurium and vecuronium, are *competitive antagonists* of postsynaptic ACh receptors. These agents bind to ACh receptors but do not induce the channel opening required for end plate depolarization. Rather, they prevent ACh from binding at the same receptor site.

In myasthenia gravis, the density of ACh receptors is decreased. Myasthenic patients are exquisitely sensitive to nondepolarizing agents (competitive antagonists) because a lower concentration of drug is required to occupy a critical proportion of receptor sites. In contrast, myasthenic patients typically demonstrate resistance to depolarizing agents (agonists) because the decrease in ACh receptors reduces the drug's ability to effectively cause end plate depolarization. However, cholinesterase inhibitors, such as pyridostigmine, can slow the metabolism of depolarizing agents (succinylcholine), prolonging and enhancing their effect. Thus, in practice, myasthenic patients may display increased or decreased sensitivity to depolarizing NMBAs.

ACh receptors are upregulated in several circumstances, such as muscle denervation, disuse atrophy, or prolonged use of NMBAs. These patients display decreased sensitivity to nondepolarizing NMBAs (a greater amount of drug is needed to occupy the same proportion of receptor sites) and increased sensitivity to depolarizing NMBAs (more receptors are available to participate in end plate depolarization).

8. **C.** VC less than 2000 mL in a patient with acute inflammatory demyelinating neuropathy weighing 100 kg is an indication for mechanical ventilation. Hypoxemia and hypercarbia are later findings. Therefore, spirometry should be monitored at frequent intervals to assess for respiratory failure and need for intubation. In neuromuscular disorders, the 20/30/40 formula suggests mechanical ventilation should be considered in patients with the following respiratory parameters:

- VC <20 mL/kg
- NIF (also called MIP) < –30 cm H_2O
- MEP <40 cm H_2O or >30% or more decline in these measurements on serial testing

Some experts use a more stringent cutoff of VC <15 mL/kg and NIF (or MIP) < –20 cm H_2O when considering elective intubation.

Note that patients with weak bulbar muscles may be unable to form an adequate seal around the spirometer, making assessment technically difficult. Elective intubation should also be considered in patients with bulbar dysfunction and aspiration. Positive-pressure ventilation should not be applied to patients with Guillain-Barré syndrome, as they are likely to decline further and require intubation.

9. **E.** Miller Fisher syndrome is a variant of Guillain-Barré syndrome characterized by ataxia, areflexia, and ophthalmoplegia. Approximately 85% of patients have serum GQ1b IgG antibodies. Acetylcholine receptor antibodies are associated with myasthenia gravis, GAD antibodies with stiff person syndrome, and both GD1a and GM1 antibodies with acute motor axonal neuropathy.

10. **A.** In patients with Guillain-Barré syndrome, days between onset of weakness and admission and presence of facial, bulbar, neck, and/or shoulder girdle weakness are associated with need for

mechanical ventilation. Patients with a faster decline are more likely to require mechanical ventilation, and those with weakness in the facial/bulbar region and/ or muscles that are innervated by the same cervical roots as the diaphragm (neck flexion/extension and shoulder girdle) are more likely to require mechanical ventilation. Antecedent respiratory/pulmonary disease (either chronic or acute) has not been shown to increase likelihood of respiratory failure.

Predictors of poorer prognosis (including inability to walk) at 6 months are as follows:

- Age
- Preceding diarrhea
- Severe extremity weakness at hospital admission and at 1 week

11. **B.** Autonomic instability is common in acute inflammatory demyelinating polyneuropathy (AIDP), the most common variant of Guillain-Barré syndrome, manifesting as hypotension/hypertension, bradycardia/tachycardia, arrhythmias, ileus, and anhidrosis. Urinary retention may also be a symptom of autonomic instability, but urinary incontinence is less common and should prompt consideration of alternative diagnosis and perhaps workup of cauda equina syndrome. As an aside, autonomic instability and respiratory dysfunction are more common in AIDP than chronic inflammatory demyelinating polyneuropathy (CIDP) and may be useful distinguishing features if clinical progression is ambiguous. Although tachycardia and hypotension could be symptoms of a coexisting infection in patients with AIDP, these signs may ultimately be attributed to AIDP itself.

About 50% of patients with AIDP develop facial weakness. Fasciculations, sometimes described by patients as muscle twitching, are a sign of denervation, which is indicative of a more chronic, axonal process than the acute demyelination of AIDP. Hemiparesis is more likely to be a central process, such as myelopathy or stroke. Myoglobin is released from damaged muscle, along with creatine kinase, and results in very dark-colored urine (tea- or Coca Cola–colored urine). Myoglobinuria is associated with disorders of lipid and glycogen metabolism such as carnitine palmitoyltransferase deficiency and McArdle disease.

12. **B.** In general, competent patients are allowed to change their preferences regarding life-sustaining therapy at any time. A competent patient's explicit informed request for mechanical ventilation should be honored, regardless of prior orders or documentation. Note that writing "not ready to die" is not equivalent to requesting mechanical ventilation and, ideally, should have been clarified further prior to intubation.

Respiratory failure is a known complication of ALS and is a common cause of death. Dyspnea can be treated pharmacologically in patients with ALS, relieving distress. A benefit of hospice is that providers who know the patient's end of life preferences visit the home or care facility to intervene when patients become uncomfortable, avoiding the commotion and invasive interventions of the emergency department.

Healthcare providers should seek the input of a patient's healthcare proxy only if the patient is unable to speak for himself or herself. Because of the ambiguity regarding whether the patient changed his end-of-life preferences before intubation, palliative extubation is premature. A patient with a significantly reduced FVC cannot be expected to wean from mechanical ventilation. Although an ethics consultation could be helpful, getting the patient's direct input is the best next step.

13. **D.** This patient has critical illness myopathy (CIM), or acute quadriplegic myopathy (AQM). Patients in the ICU may develop CIM, critical illness polyneuropathy (CIP), or both. Risk factors for CIM include:

- High-dose corticosteroids
- Nondepolarizing NMBAs
- Sepsis and multiorgan failure

In both CIM and CIP, patients have weakness in extremities, trunk, and respiratory muscles. In both, there are reduced or absent muscle reflexes. It is difficult to distinguish between CIM and CIP clinically, but CK level and NCS/EMG findings can help. With an elevated CK level, the diagnosis is more likely CIM.

The typical NCS findings in CIM are markedly (<80% of normal) reduced CMAP amplitude with normal distal latency and conduction velocity. SNAPs are typically normal or mildly reduced, although it is possible that SNAPs are more reduced in the setting of coexistent neuropathy or may be difficult to obtain with extremity edema.

There should not be decrement on repetitive nerve stimulation for CIM as this is not a neuromuscular junction disorder. Thus, markedly reduced CMAP amplitude, preserved SNAPs, and no decrement on repetitive nerve stimulation are most consistent with the clinical picture of CIM. EMG in CIM can show abnormal spontaneous activity (ie, fibrillation potentials and positive sharp waves), but these can also be seen in CIP; usually, patients are not able to generate motor units, but if motor unit potentials are generated, they are typically myopathic (ie, early recruitment of small-amplitude, short-duration, polyphasic motor unit potentials), which can help differentiate from CIP.

Electrodiagnostic Findings in CIP	Electrodiagnostic Findings in CIM
Axonal sensorimotor neuropathy	1. Reserved sensory response 2. Reduced motor response (CMAP <80%) 3. Normal repetitive nerve stimulation 4. EMG with short-duration, low-amplitude motor unit potential with early or normal recruitment of motor unit action potential

14. **B.** Patients undergoing median sternotomies can develop injuries of the brachial plexus, which can be at risk for stretching during these procedures. The clinical and EMG/NCS findings are consistent with a lower trunk lesion. In a lower trunk lesion, there is weakness of hand and wrist muscles in the C8 and T1 myotomes, such as the ADM, APB, and EIP. ADM is ulnar innervated, APB is median innervated, and EIP is radial innervated. It is important to note the involvement of the EIP to differentiate a lower trunk lesion from a medial cord lesion in which there is sparing of radial-innervated muscles. In a lower trunk lesion, sensory loss is expected in the C8 and T1 dermatomes (medial hand and forearm). The ulnar SNAP is abnormal, as the ulnar sensory nerve to the fifth digit is derived from the C8 root and lower trunk. The median SNAP is not affected, as the median sensory nerve to the second and third digits is derived from C6 and C7 roots and upper and middle trunks.

This is not a combined ulnar and median neuropathy; if reduced median APB CMAP is due to carpal tunnel syndrome, the median SNAP is also expected to be abnormal. Combined ulnar and median neuropathy also does not explain involvement of the EIP muscle. This is not a nerve root injury given the abnormal SNAPs. In nerve root injuries, the lesion is proximal to the dorsal root ganglia, so SNAPs are expected to be preserved. The clinical presentation of acute-onset focal weakness and numbness after surgery is not typical of motor neuron disease. This is not a middle trunk injury, in which there is involvement of C7-innervated muscles (such as triceps and wrist extensors) with preservation of C8- or T1-innervated muscles (such as APB and ADM). In a middle trunk lesion, reduced amplitude of the median to third digit SNAP may be seen. Furthermore, middle trunk injuries are unlikely to occur in isolation.

15. **C.** The presentation is most consistent with adult-onset Pompe disease (also called acid maltase deficiency, glycogenosis type II, or α-glucosidase deficiency). Pompe disease is an autosomal recessive disorder in which there is decreased activity of lysosomal α-glucosidase. Adult-onset Pompe disease typically presents in the second to sixth decades with gradually progressive proximal weakness, and ventilatory muscles are often affected. Adult-onset Pompe disease can present with respiratory failure requiring noninvasive positive-pressure ventilation or intubation and/or difficulty to wean from ventilation. CK levels can be elevated or normal in adult-onset Pompe disease. EMG may reveal myotonic discharges, especially in paraspinal muscles. Diagnostic testing includes dried spot test for α-glucosidase activity, confirmatory testing with α-glucosidase activity in fibroblasts or muscle tissue, and genetic testing. Muscle biopsy can reveal vacuoles with glycogen in muscle fibers, although it may be nonspecific in adult-onset cases.

Other tests help confirm diagnoses of disorders that can be associated with weakness and respiratory difficulty, but are not consistent with the case. ALS is a neurodegenerative disease with involvement of anterior horn cells and the corticospinal tract, which may have bulbar or limb onset and upper and/or lower motor neuron signs. *C9orf72* mutation is present in some cases of familial ALS and/or frontotemporal dementia, but this case is not consistent with ALS given the myopathic EMG changes. Rather, motor unit potentials in ALS often show evidence of chronic denervation/reinnervation changes (ie, large-amplitude, long-duration, and/or polyphasic motor unit potentials) secondary to lower motor neuron degeneration. Antinuclear antibody may be elevated for some of the idiopathic inflammatory myopathies, such as polymyositis, but CK should be elevated in polymyositis. Dystrophin analysis is helpful for diagnosis of Becker muscular dystrophy, but CK should be elevated in Becker muscular dystrophy. It would also be rare for a woman to have clinical manifestations of Becker muscular dystrophy; Becker muscular dystrophy is an X-linked recessive disorder in inheritance, so women may be carriers of the dystrophin mutation, of which a minority manifest clinical symptoms. Limb girdle muscular dystrophy 1 (LGMD1, autosomal dominant) is unlikely to present with severe respiratory failure, although some types of LGMD2 can have respiratory difficulty such as LGMD2A and LGMD2Q.

16. **B.** Typically, SSEP studies involve stimulation at the median nerve and measurement of various potentials, including those over the brachial plexus (Erb's point, which is the reference point), cervical region (N13), and cortical region (N20). After anoxic injury, absence of N20 (cortical) responses on SSEP study can predict poor outcome at 24 hours or more after cardiopulmonary resuscitation. For absence of N20 responses to be a reliable finding, brachial plexus and cervical potentials must be present.

17. **E.** This patient developed malignant hyperthermia (MH), which can be triggered by exposure to some types of general anesthesia, including inhalational anesthetics and succinylcholine. Some patients with MH have mutations in the ryanodine receptor gene, which also cause central core myopathy, but there are other genes that are associated with increased MH risk. Lab abnormalities during MH episodes include highly elevated CK (can have associated renal failure from myoglobinuria), respiratory and metabolic (lactic) acidosis, and hyperkalemia. Muscle biopsies reveal central cores on NADH stain. Muscle fiber rimmed vacuoles are not typical of MH, but rather of inclusion body myositis.

18. **C.** This patient developed propofol-induced rhabdomyolysis, in which there is underlying necrotizing myopathy of skeletal muscle, often including cardiac muscle. Clinical findings include myoglobinuria (which, in turn, causes renal failure), highly elevated CK, myocardial injury with increased troponin levels, metabolic acidosis, and hyperkalemia. It would be rare for phenytoin, levetiracetam, or midazolam to be associated with rhabdomyolysis, although there have been isolated case reports. Phenytoin can be associated with a hypersensitivity reaction in which there is elevated CK, myalgia, and proximal weakness.

19. **E.** The clinical scenario (likely a suicide attempt with ingestion of insecticide) and clinical syndrome (cholinergic toxidrome) are most suggestive of acute organophosphate toxicity, in which there is inactivation of acetylcholinesterase at synapses in the peripheral and central nervous systems. In acute organophosphate toxicity, CMAPs usually are normal at rest and show decremental response with both slow and rapid repetitive nerve stimulation. SNAPs should not be affected by acute organophosphate toxicity. However, some patients may develop a sensorimotor axonal polyneuropathy several weeks after organophosphate toxicity, in which case CMAP and SNAP amplitudes would be reduced.

REFERENCES

Amato AA, Russell JA, eds. *Neuromuscular Disorders* (2nd ed). New York, NY: McGraw-Hill Education; 2016.

Butterworth JF, Mackey DC, Wasnick JD, eds. *Morgan & Mikhail's Clinical Anesthesiology* (5th ed.). New York, NY: The McGraw-Hill Companies; 2013.

Chaudhuri A, Behan PO. Myasthenic crisis. *QJM.* 2009;102(2): 97-107.

Daroff RB, Jankovic J, Mazziotta JC, Pomeroy SL, eds. *Bradley's Neurology in Clinical Practice* (7th ed.). New York, NY: Elsevier; 2016.

DeJesus-Hernandez M, Mackenzie IR, Boeve BF, et al. Expanded GGGGCC hexanucleotide repeat in noncoding region of C9ORF72 causes chromosome 9p-linked FTD and ALS. *Neuron.* 2011;72(2):245-256.

Graham JG, Pye IF, McQueen IN. Brachial plexus injury after median sternotomy. *J Neurol Neurosurg Psychiatry.* 1981;44(7):621-625.

Harney J, Glasberg MR. Myopathy and hypersensitivity to phenytoin. *Neurology.* 1983;33(6):790-791.

Hers HG. Alpha-glucosidase deficiency in generalized glycogen storage disease (Pompe's disease). *Biochem J.* 1963;86: 11-16.

Hobson-Webb LD, Dearmey S, Kishnani PS. The clinical and electrodiagnostic characteristics of Pompe disease with post-enzyme replacement therapy findings. *Clin Neurophysiol.* 2011;122(11):2312-2317.

Kishnani PS, Steiner RD, Bali D, et al. Pompe disease diagnosis and management guideline. *Genet Med.* 2006;8(5):267-288.

Lacomis D. Myasthenic crisis. *Neurocrit Care.* 2005;3(3): 189-194.

Lancaster E. Paraneoplastic disorders. *Continuum (Minneap Minn).* 2015;21(2 Neuro-oncology):452-475.

Latronico N, Bolton CF. Critical illness polyneuropathy and myopathy: a major cause of muscle weakness and paralysis. *Lancet Neurol.* 2011;10(10):931-941.

Leis AA, Stokic DS, Webb RM, Slavinski SA, Fratkin J. Clinical spectrum of muscle weakness in human West Nile virus infection. *Muscle Nerve.* 2003;28(3):302-308.

Martyn JA, White DA, Gronert GA, Jaffe RS, Ward JM. Up-and-down regulation of skeletal muscle acetylcholine receptors. Effects on neuromuscular blockers. *Anesthesiology.* 1992;76(5):822-843.

McCarthy TV, Quane KA, Lynch PJ. Ryanodine receptor mutations in malignant hyperthermia and central core disease. *Hum Mutat.* 2000;15(5):410-417.

Preston DC, Shapiro BE, eds. *Electromyography and Neuromuscular Disorders: Clinical-Electrophysiologic Correlations* (3rd ed). New York, NY: Elsevier; 2013.

Rabinstein AA. Acute neuromuscular respiratory failure. *Continuum (Minneap Minn).* 2015;21(5 Neurocritical Care):1324-1345.

Ropper AH, Samuels MA, Klein JP, eds. *Adams and Victor's Principles of Neurology* (10th ed.). New York, NY: McGraw-Hill Education; 2014.

Sakakibara R, Uchiyama T, Kuwabara S, et al. Prevalence and mechanism of bladder dysfunction in Guillain-Barre syndrome. *Neurourol Urodyn.* 2009;28(5):432-437.

Sanders DB, Wolfe GI, Benatar M, et al. International consensus guidance for management of myasthenia gravis: executive summary. *Neurology.* 2016;87(4):419-425.

Shepherd S, Batra A, Lerner DP. Review of critical illness myopathy and neuropathy. *Neurohospitalist.* 2017;7(1):41-48.

Stelow EB, Johari VP, Smith SA, Crosson JT, Apple FS. Propofol-associated rhabdomyolysis with cardiac involvement in adults: chemical and anatomic findings. *Clin Chem.* 2000;46(4):577-581.

Strazis KP, Fox AW. Malignant hyperthermia: a review of published cases. *Anesth Analg.* 1993;77(2):297-304.

Tecellioglu M, Kamisli O. Familial Pompe disease. *Med Arch.* 2015;69(5):342-344.

Unlu Y, Velioglu Y, Kocak H, Becit N, Ceviz M. Brachial plexus injury following median sternotomy. *Interact Cardiovasc Thorac Surg.* 2007;6(2):235-237.

van Koningsveld R, Steyerberg EW, Hughes RA, et al. A clinical prognostic scoring system for Guillain-Barre syndrome. *Lancet Neurol.* 2007;6(7):589-594.

Veatch RM, ed. *Medical Ethics* (2nd ed.). Sudbury, MA: Jones and Bartlett Publishers; 1997.

Wadia RS, Chitra S, Amin RB, Kiwalkar RS, Sardesai HV. Electrophysiological studies in acute organophosphate poisoning. *J Neurol Neurosurg Psychiatry.* 1987;50(11): 1442-1448.

Walgaard C, Lingsma HF, Ruts L, et al. Prediction of respiratory insufficiency in Guillain-Barre syndrome. *Ann Neurol.* 2010;67(6):781-787.

Wijdicks EFM, ed. *The Practice of Emergency and Critical Care Neurology.* Oxford, United Kingdom: Oxford University Press; 2010.

Zandbergen EG, Hijdra A, Koelman JH, et al. Prediction of poor outcome within the first 3 days of postanoxic coma. *Neurology.* 2006;66(1):62-68.

6

Neurologic Infectious Diseases

Firas N. Abdulmajeed, MB, ChB, Ayman Mithqal, MD, and Barnett Nathan, MD

Questions

Questions 1 and 2

A 42-year-old woman was transferred to the intensive care unit (ICU) from the psychiatry ward for fevers, fluctuation of blood pressure, tachycardia, and a seizure. There was a concern for her ability to protect her airway, and she was intubated. Her admission note states that she was admitted due to hallucinations, disorganized thinking, catatonic features, and echolalia.

1. What is the likely cause of her initial presentation?
   A. Zika virus
   B. West Nile encephalitis
   C. Anti-NMDA (*N*-methyl-D-aspartate) encephalitis
   D. Serotonin syndrome
   E. Malignant hyperthermia

2. What is your next step in the workup of the proposed diagnosis?
   A. Serum collection for viral testing
   B. Lumbar puncture for viral testing
   C. Transvaginal ultrasound

D. Abdominal computed tomography (CT) scan
E. Transesophageal echocardiography

3. A 43-year-old woman presented to the emergency department (ED) with 12 hours of headache, neck stiffness, and fevers, and 1 minute of generalized rhythmic body shaking with loss of consciousness on the way to the ED. She returned to normal baseline but continues to have a headache and fever. You attend to her bedside and find that the ED intern is scrubbing in to perform a lumbar puncture (LP) after starting her on the appropriate antibiotics. His senior resident who is standing there asks you if it is okay to perform the LP. How should you reply?
   A. Defer lumbar puncture until a brain magnetic resonance imaging (MRI) with contrast is completed.
   B. Defer lumbar puncture as there is no need, given the diagnosis of meningitis is already made.
   C. Defer lumbar puncture until after a non-contrast head CT is completed, and continue antibiotics in the interval.

D. Proceed with the lumbar puncture at this time.

E. Defer lumbar puncture until after a noncontrast head CT in obtained, and discontinue the antibiotics until after the procedure.

4. An 18-year-old woman who works in a book store in her home town of Atlanta, Georgia, presents to the ED. She exercises regularly and hikes with friends on occasion. She presented to an urgent care center last week with a 3-day history of headache, fever, and maculopapular rash that covered part of her trunk initially, and it was thought to be cellulitis. She was started on a 3-day course of an antibiotic but cannot remember its name, and she was sent home. The rash progressed to involve her whole trunk, palms, and soles; then 2 days later, she presented to the ED with a tonic-clonic seizure. She is obtunded, with a temperature of 102°F, respiratory rate of 26, heart rate of 110 bpm, oxygen saturation of 95% on 2-L nasal cannula. She localizes in all 4 extremities. Noncontrast CT was performed, and it was followed by an LP. Cerebrospinal fluid (CSF) showed the following: white blood cells (WBC) of 82 cells/high-power field with lymphocytic predominance, protein 135 mg/dL (normal <50 mg/dL), and glucose normal. Complete blood count showed WBC of 11.2×10^9 cells/L and platelet count of 98×10^3 cells/μL. Basic metabolic panel was significant for Na of 129 mEq/L. What is the most appropriate next step in the management of this patient?

A. Acyclovir 10 mg/kg intravenous every 8 hours

B. Doxycycline 100 mg oral every 12 hours

C. Penicillin G benzathine 2.4 million units intramuscular once

D. Metronidazole 500 mg oral every 8 hours

E. No antimicrobial is effective against the organism causing this disease

5. A 42-year-old man from Palm Beach, Florida, presented to the hospital with weakness that started in his legs one day prior to presentation. He had absent patellar reflexes. His weakness worsened acutely, and pulmonary mechanics were ordered.

His negative inspiratory force (NIF) was –15 cm H_2O, and vital capacity was 10 mL/kg. Because of his pulmonary mechanics and concern for impending respiratory failure, he was intubated in the ED. When interviewing his fiancé, she mentioned that he had a low-grade fever, some maculopapular pruritic rash, joint pain in his hands and feet, and conjunctivitis a few days ago. What do you suspect is the diagnosis?

A. West Nile meningitis

B. Myasthenia gravis

C. Guillain-Barré syndrome precipitated by Zika virus

D. Guillain-Barré syndrome precipitated by *Campylobacter jejuni*

E. NMDA encephalitis

6. What are the dose and duration of intravenous (IV) dexamethasone when initiating treatment for bacterial meningitis in developed countries?

A. 0.15 mg/kg IV every 6 hours for 4 days

B. 0.4 mg/kg IV every 12 hours for 4 days

C. 1 mg/kg IV every 6 hours for 2 to 4 days

D. 1 mg/kg IV every 8 hours for 7 days

E. 2 mg/kg IV every 6 hours for 7 days

7. A 34-year-old man presented to the ICU unresponsive and intubated after he was assaulted with a baseball bat in a bar fight. His noncontrast head CT showed a skull base fracture. What common pathogens is he prone to as a result of his trauma?

A. *Staphylococcus aureus*, coagulase-negative *Staphylococcus*, aerobic gram-negative bacilli (including *Pseudomonas aeruginosa* and *Acinetobacter baumannii*)

B. *Streptococcus pneumoniae, Haemophilus influenzae,* β-hemolytic streptococci

C. *Streptococcus agalactiae, Escherichia coli, Listeria monocytogenes, Klebsiella* species

D. Coagulase-negative *Staphylococcus, S aureus, Propionibacterium acnes*

E. *Neisseria meningitidis, S pneumoniae*

Questions 8 and 9

A 57-year-old woman with a history of poorly controlled hypertension and tobacco abuse presented 2 weeks ago with a Hunt and Hess grade 4, Fisher grade 4 subarachnoid hemorrhage due to a large left anterior communicating artery aneurysm rupture. The aneurysm was secured following endovascular coiling on the day of admission. An external ventricular drain (EVD) was placed at the time of admission given findings of hydrocephalus on head CT. On day 14 of hospitalization, the patient became more obtunded and had a fever of 38.9°C. Her WBC on labs changed from 7.5 to 14.6×10^9 cells/L with neutrophilic predominance. CSF that was sent from the EVD showed WBC count of 13,000 cells/μL, red blood cell (RBC) count of 21,000 cells/μL, glucose of 30 mg/dL, and protein of 190 mg/dL. MRI with diffusion-weighted imaging (DWI) and corresponding apparent diffusion coefficient (ADC) are shown in Figure 6-1.

8. What is the treatment of choice?
   A. Start ceftriaxone, metronidazole, and vancomycin pending the culture results.
   B. Start ceftriaxone and vancomycin pending the culture results.
   C. Start meropenem or cefepime and vancomycin pending the culture results.
   D. Start metronidazole, doxycycline, and Zosyn (piperacillin and tazobactam).
   E. Remove the EVD; no antibiotics are needed.

9. When should the CSF be rechecked for response, and what is the duration of antibiotic therapy?
   A. Check CSF daily until there is a decreasing WBC count and treat for 14 days
   B. Check CSF on day 5 and treat for 14 days
   C. Check CSF on day 5 and treat for 21 days
   D. Check CSF on day 14 and treat for 28 days
   E. None of the above

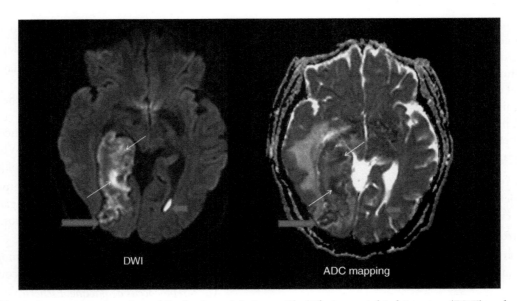

Figure 6-1   Magnetic resonance imaging of the brain, axial view, with diffusion-weighted imaging (DWI) and corresponding apparent diffusion coefficient (ADC) mapping, shows diffuse right lateral ventricle ependymal diffusion restriction (*thin arrows*). There is also a focus of diffusion restriction seen in the dependent portion of the left lateral trigon (short *thick arrow*), and extraventricular extension is again seen (*long thick arrow*).

10. When would it be appropriate to use intrathecal gentamycin/tobramycin or amikacin to treat gram-negative bacterial ventriculitis?

   A. When CSF is not sterile by day 5 to 7

   B. When CSF is not sterile by day 3

   C. When CSF is sterile by day 5

   D. All the time

   E. There is no utility of using this therapy

Questions 11 and 12

A 35-year-old man served in the US Army in Iraq a few years ago, and as part of his campaign, he was in contact with stray dogs. He was admitted to the ICU following a reported generalized tonic-clonic seizure and intubation for airway protection. His head CT showed a cyst with daughter cysts in solid matrix.

11. What is the causative organism?

   A. *Echinococcus granulosus*

   B. Cysticercosis

   C. *Trichinella spiralis*

   D. CNS lymphoma

   E. None of the above

12. What is the ultimate treatment for this brain lesion?

   A. Albendazole alone without surgical intervention

   B. Albendazole plus puncture, aspiration, injection, and reaspiration

   C. Albendazole plus either modified catheterization or surgery

   D. Metronidazole plus modified catheterization or surgery

   E. Observation

Questions 13 and 14

You were called by the intern on service for your neuro-ICU with a new admission. She told you about a 22-year-old vegetarian woman who presented to the ED with new-onset seizures. The woman was treated with IV lorazepam and was intubated for airway protection. She has no past medical or surgical history. The patient is not a smoker and drinks alcohol occasionally. She just moved from Mexico 9 months ago and has never had a seizure in the past. CT of the head is done and is shown in Figure 6-2.

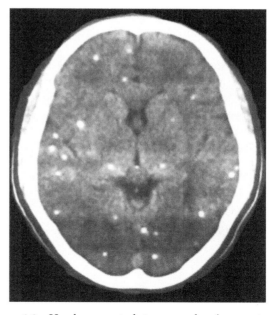

Figure 6-2 Head computed tomography (noncontrasted axial): multiple, bilateral, calcified lesions are seen through hemispheres. Reproduced with permission from Ropper AH, Samuels MA, Klein JP. *Adams and Victor's Principles of Neurology*, 10th edition. New York, NY: McGraw-Hill, 2014.

13. What is the most likely diagnosis?

   A. Toxoplasmosis

   B. Lymphoma

   C. Cysticercosis

   D. Glioblastoma

   E. Meningioma

14. What step can be taken to minimize the major side effect of the medical treatment for this patient?

   A. Use corticosteroids

   B. Cut the dose of antiparasitic therapy to half

   C. Stop the antiparasitic treatment permanently

   D. Plan a biopsy to confirm the diagnosis

   E. Use scheduled mannitol during induction therapy

15. A 65-year-old woman is admitted to the neuro-ICU with fluctuating mental status over the past 2 weeks. She presented to the ED with fever and stiff neck. The exam demonstrated bilateral facial nerve palsy. As you are reading through her outpatient chart, you notice that the electrocardiogram (ECG) shown in Figure 6-3 was done 4 months ago. What is your likely diagnosis?

    A. West Nile meningitis
    B. Rocky Mountain spotted fever
    C. Lyme disease
    D. Malaria
    E. Tuberculosis

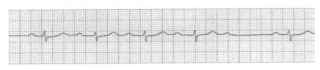

Figure 6-3 Electrocardiogram showing prolongation of PR interval and single nonconducted P wave.

16. A 27-year-old man with human immunodeficiency virus (HIV) diagnosed 3 years ago, who is intermittently taking highly active antiretroviral therapy (HAART) due to noncompliance, was found down on the ground by his neighbor, who did not know how long he had been like that. En route to the hospital, emergency medical services intubated the patient. CT of the head was negative for space-occupying lesion, and LP performed in the ED showed opening pressure of 52 mL, WBC of 42 predominantly mononuclear cells, protein of 70 mg/dL, and glucose of 35 mg/dL. You suspect cryptococcal meningitis. Which of the following stains may be most useful in diagnosis?

    A. Congo red
    B. Giemsa stain
    C. Wrights and Field stain
    D. India ink
    E. None of the above

17. In cryptococcal meningitis, what is a predictor of death in the initial few weeks of treatment?

    A. CSF antigen titer >1:256
    B. CSF WBC count <20 cells/μL
    C. Blood glucose of 200 mg/dL and above
    D. WBC within normal range
    E. Thrombocytopenia

18. A 54-year-old man who has history of intravenous drug abuse is admitted to the medical ICU for septic shock. His initial blood cultures are growing *Staphylococcus aureus*. The patient is intubated, mechanically ventilated, on norepinephrine, and being treated with vancomycin and piperacillin/ tazobactam. He has a transthoracic echocardiography (TTE) that is scheduled for today. On waking the patient for an examination, the nurse noticed right arm and leg weakness, which is new, compared to his last examination 2 hours prior. His coagulation laboratory tests are normal, platelets are normal, and a bedside blood glucose check is 129 mg/dL. CT was unremarkable. MRI of the brain was done and is shown in Figure 6-4. National Institutes of Health Stroke Scale (NIHSS) examination results are listed below. What is the next best step in management for the patient?

NIHSS Examination

Level of consciousness – 1
Answering questions – 1 (due to intubation)
Right arm weakness – 1
Right leg weakness – 1
Dysarthria – Untestable
TOTAL SCORE: 4

A. Give tissue plasminogen activator (tPA)

B. Give tPA and consult neurointervention for mechanical thrombectomy

C. Consult neurointerventional for mechanical thrombectomy

D. Continue antibiotic coverage, obtain a stat transesophageal echocardiography, and obtain thoracic surgery consult if positive for valve vegetation

E. Continue antibiotic coverage pending scheduled TTE

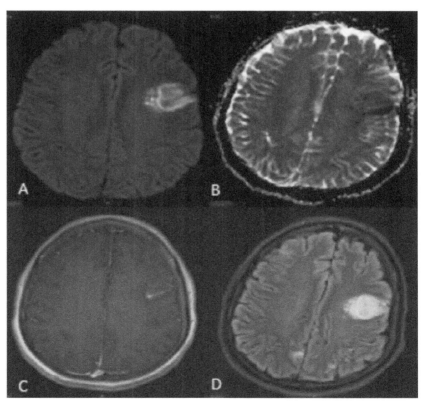

Figure 6-4 Magnetic resonance imaging of the brain, axial view. **A.** Diffusion-weighted imaging sequence shows left frontal hyperintensity, which correlated with apparent diffusion coefficient hypodensity shown in **B.** Panel **C** shows postcontrast mild enhancement in the left frontal region and increased fluid-attenuated inversion recovery hyperintensity signals in the same region shown in **D.**

19. A 63-year-old man underwent a transsphenoidal hypophysectomy that was complicated by uncontrolled blood glucose, which required an insulin drip and monitoring in the neuro-ICU. He was sent to a step-down unit on postoperative day 3 and was doing well until postoperative day 6, when he started complaining of severe facial pain associated with some intermittent epistaxis. This morning, he was brought to the neuro-ICU after the rapid response team evaluated him on the floor for fever, tachycardia, elevated WBC, and altered mental status. You intubate him for airway protection and obtain a broad infectious workup including a CT of the head and sinuses, which is shown in Figure 6-5. What is the next step in evaluation?

A. Order MRI

B. Consult ENT (ear, nose, and throat) for early nasal endoscopy with biopsies of affected tissues

C. No need for further diagnostic studies; start empiric vancomycin, cefepime, and amphotericin B

D. Repeat CT in 1 to 2 days

E. None of the above

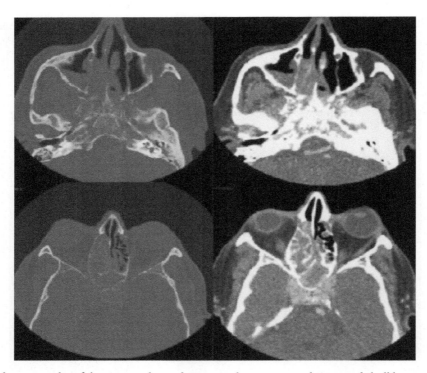

Figure 6-5   Computed tomography of the sinuses shows destructive bony paranasal sinus and skull base erosive process with soft tissue thickening.

20. A 71-year-old man with history of diabetes mellitus, end-stage renal disease treated with hemodialysis 3 times a week, hypertension, and myelodysplasia presented to the ED for the third time this month with a chief complaint of back pain. The ED calls you this time because his temperature is 38.6°C, WBC is within normal limits, erythrocyte sedimentation rate is 62 mm/hr, and C-reactive protein is 116 mg/L, and he is expressing some right lower extremity weakness. While you are examining his back, he expresses severe tenderness at the L3-4 area. MRI was done and is shown in Figure 6-6. Which of the following is the next step of management?

A. Start antibiotics immediately, and cover with vancomycin and cefepime

B. Obtain 2 sets of blood cultures and start IV vancomycin and IV metronidazole

C. Obtain 2 sets of blood cultures and start IV vancomycin and IV ceftriaxone

D. Obtain fine-needle aspiration (FNA) of the abscess before starting antibiotic coverage; start IV vancomycin and IV ceftriaxone

E. Obtain FNA of the abscess before starting antibiotic coverage; start IV vancomycin, OV ceftriaxone, and IV metronidazole

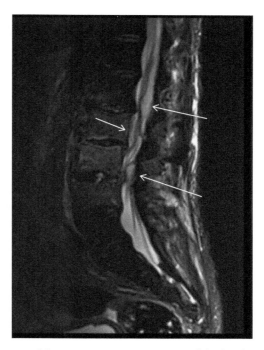

Figure 6-6 Magnetic resonance imaging of the lumbar spine (sagittal lumbosacral short tau inversion recovery T1 before and after gadolinium): Arrows demonstrate areas of concern with extradural lesions.

Answers and Explanations

1. **C.** Anti-NMDA encephalitis patients may present with prodromal headache, fever, or a viral-like process, followed in a few days by a multistage progression of symptoms that include prominent psychiatric manifestations (anxiety, agitation, bizarre behavior, hallucinations, delusions, disorganized thinking); isolated psychiatric episodes may rarely occur at initial onset or at relapse. Other symptoms may also include insomnia, memory deficits, seizures, decreased level of consciousness, stupor with catatonic features, frequent dyskinesias (orofacial, choreoathetoid movements, dystonia, rigidity, opisthotonic postures), autonomic instability (hyperthermia, fluctuations of blood pressure, tachycardia, bradycardia, cardiac pauses, and sometimes hypoventilation requiring mechanical ventilation), and language dysfunction (diminished language output, mutism). Echolalia is often noted in the early stages or in the recovery phase of the disorder.

2. **C.** Anti-NMDA encephalitis should be suspected with this clinical presentation. Transvaginal ultrasound should be done next to exclude ovarian malignancy because there is a high association between NMDA encephalitis and ovarian teratoma, but this is not necessarily present. Although the diagnosis is confirmed with detection of immunoglobulin (Ig) G antibodies to the GluN1 (also known as the NR1) subunit of the NMDA receptor in the serum or cerebrospinal fluid (CSF), there are additional common findings:

   - CSF lymphocytic pleocytosis with or without oligoclonal bands
   - Electroencephalography (EEG) with infrequent epileptic discharges, but frequent slow, disorganized activity that does not correlate with most abnormal movements (delta brush)
   - Brain magnetic resonance imaging (MRI) that is often normal or shows transient fluid-attenuated inversion recovery (FLAIR) or contrast-enhancing abnormalities in cortical (brain, cerebellum) or subcortical regions (hippocampus, basal ganglia, white matter)

3. **C.** Based on observations and in agreement with the 2004 Infectious Diseases Society of America (IDSA) guidelines for the management of bacterial meningitis, a CT scan of the head prior to obtaining LP should be performed in adult patients with suspected bacterial meningitis who have 1 or more of the following risk factors:

   - Immunocompromised state (eg, human immunodeficiency virus [HIV] infection, immunosuppressive therapy, solid organ or hematopoietic stem cell transplantation)
   - History of central nervous system (CNS) disease (mass lesion, stroke, or focal infection)
   - New-onset seizure (within 1 week of presentation)
   - Papilledema
   - Abnormal level of consciousness
   - Focal neurologic deficit

   However, it has been suggested that a normal CT scan does not always mean that performance of an LP is safe and that certain clinical signs of impending herniation (eg, deteriorating level of consciousness, particularly a Glasgow coma scale score <11; brainstem signs including pupillary changes, posturing, or irregular respirations; or a very recent seizure) may be predictive of patients in whom an LP should be delayed.

   Timing of starting antibiotics has been correlated with outcome in meningitis patients; early initation results in improved outcome. Antibiotics should not be delayed until a CT scan of the head and LP are performed, which might take some time.

4. **B.** This patient has the classic presentation of Rocky Mountain spotted fever (RMSF), which is

transmitted via *Dermacentor andersoni* tick in the United States and is caused by *Rickettsia rickettsii*. RMSF presents with early gradual or abrupt symptoms, which include fever, headache, and rash, in a person with a history of a tick bite, and malaise, myalgias, and arthralgias. However, all of these diagnostic clues are rarely identified on the initial patient encounter, leading to delays in appropriate therapy. In fulminant cases of RMSF, death may occur as early as 5 days. Poor outcomes have been associated with delay of appropriate antibiotics. Some patients, especially children, may also have prominent abdominal pain that may be severe.

If an LP is performed in a patient with RMSF, CSF analysis usually shows a WBC count of <100 cells/μL with either a polymorphonuclear or lymphocytic predominance. Moderately elevated protein (100-200 mg/dL) and a normal glucose level are common. These findings may not help distinguish RMSF from meningococcal disease. Doxycycline 200 mg/d divided in 2 doses is the treatment of choice in nonpregnant women. Treatment should continue for 3 days after the patient's fever subsides. Chloramphenicol is an alternative antibiotic; however, doxycycline is still superior due to the difficulty of obtaining chloramphenicol, which could cause gray baby syndrome if given in the third trimester.

5. **C.** Two studies have shown the connection between Zika virus and Guillain-Barré syndrome (GBS). A retrospective study in Colombia evaluated 68 patients with GBS between Fall 2015 and Spring 2016, and a case-control study in French Polynesia evaluated the association between GBS and Zika virus infection during the 2013 to 2014 outbreak. The management plan for this patient should include considering starting intravenous immunoglobulin (IVIG) or plasmapheresis and advising against unprotected sexual relations.

6. **A.** Steroids can reduce the inflammation caused by infection. Research on the use of corticosteroids in addition to antibiotics has had conflicting results. Some studies have shown that they reduce risk of hearing loss and neurologic complications, and other studies have shown reduction in mortality rates. The current recommendation is to start steroids just before or in conjunction with antibiotic therapy in selected meningitis patients, including

children >6 weeks old with *Haemophilus influenzae* and *Streptococcus pneumoniae* and adults with positive CSF Gram stain.

When indicated, dexamethasone is given 15 to 20 minutes before or at the time of antibiotic administration. Two-dose regimens are recommended: 0.15 mg/kg every 6 hours for 4 days in the developed world, based on the IDSA guidelines, and 0.4 mg/kg every 12 hours for 4 days in the developing world, based on the Vietnamese trial. Adjunctive dexamethasone should *not* be given to adults who have already received antimicrobial therapy because it is unlikely to improve patient outcomes. The other doses were not agreed on and/or tested.

7. **B.** Fractures of the base of the skull make patients prone to developing infections with *Streptococcus pneumoniae*, *Haemopholius influenzae*, and β-hemolytic streptococci. The common organisms related to penetrating head trauma and shunt related infections are: *Staphylococcus aureus*, *Pseudomonas* coagulase-negative *Staphylococcus*, and aerobic gram-negative bacilli (including *P aeruginosa* and *Actinomyces baumannii*). *Staphylococcus agalactiae*, *Escheria coli*, *Listeria monocytogenes*, and *Klebsiella* species are common pathogens associated with infants less than 1 month of age. Although *Neiseria meningitidis* and *S pneumoniae* are the most common causes of meningitis in adults, they are not associated with skull base fractures.

8. **C.** The patient has ventriculitis. There are many causes of ventriculitis, including trauma (complicating CSF leak), following placement of ventricular drains or shunt, ruptured abscess, or immunocompromised host. Ventriculitis can be a complication of intraventricular surgery, intrathecal chemotherapy, or meningitis. Ventricular catheter-related ventriculitis ranges from 0% to 22%. Gram-negative meningitis followed by *Staphylococcus* infections are the most frequent types of infection associated with pyogenic ventriculitis. Gram-positive cocci consistent with skin flora are the most commonly isolated organisms associated with ventricular catheter-related ventriculitis.

Decisions on the choice of a specific antimicrobial agent are based on knowledge of relative penetration into CSF in the presence of meningeal inflammation.

In this patient, we should consider an antibiotic to cover gram-positive cocci including methicillin-resistant *Staphylcoccus aureus* (MRSA) and gram-negative bacilli including *Pspeudomonas aeruginosa* and *Actinimyces baumannii*. Cefepime also has greater in vitro activity than the third-generation cephalosporins against *Enterobacter* species and *P aeruginosa*. Vancomycin will cover potential MRSA.

9. **C.** CSF requires 2 to 4 days to become sterile, so the best time to recheck it is on day 5, and the patient should be treated for no less than 21 days. Choice A is incorrect because there is no need to check CSF daily knowing that it needs 2 to 4 days to sterilize, and the treatment for ventriculitis should be for 21 days. The same applies for choice B.

10. **A.** No randomized controlled trials of the efficacy of intraventricular antibiotics in CNS device infections have been performed. This treatment modality is potentially toxic and requires careful preparation and delivery to avoid contamination. It should therefore be reserved for circumstances in which conventional intravenous therapy has failed. It may be useful in the following settings:

- Failure of parenteral therapy to sterilize the CSF by day 5 to 7

- Presence of highly resistant organisms sensitive only to antibiotics with poor CSF penetration
- Circumstances in which shunt devices cannot be removed

11. **A.** Echinococcal disease is caused by infection with the metacestode stage of the tapeworm *Echinococcus*. Dogs and other canines are the definitive hosts. However, sheep, goats, camels, horses, cattle, and swine are the intermediate hosts, and humans are accidental hosts. The highest rates of cystic echinococcal endemic disease tend to occur in areas where sheep are raised. Transmission frequently occurs in settings where dogs eat the viscera of slaughtered animals. The dogs then excrete infectious eggs in their stool, which are passed on to other animals or humans via fecal-oral transmission. This may occur via environmental contamination of water and cultivated vegetables or contact between infected domestic dogs and humans. CNS involvement can lead to seizures or signs of raised intracranial pressure; infection of the spinal cord can result in spinal cord compression. On imaging, the hydatid cyst can present in different forms, including the mother-daughter cyst in a solid matrix.

12. **C.** The World Health Organization classification of cystic echinococcosis and its treatment stratified by cyst stage is shown in Table 6-1.

Table 6-1. World Health Organization (WHO) Classification of Cystic Echinococcosis and Treatment Stratified by Cyst Stage

WHO Stage	Description	Stage	Size	Preferred Treatment	Alternate Treatment
CE1	Unilocular unechoic cystic lesion with double-line sign	Active	<5 cm >5 cm	Albendazole alone Albendazole + PAIR	Puncture, aspiration, injection, reaspiration (PAIR)
CE2	Multiseptated, "rosette-like," "honeycomb" cyst	Active	Any	Albendazole + either modified catheterization or surgery	Modified catheterization
CE3a	Cyst with detached membranes (water lily sign)	Transitional	<5 cm >5 cm	Albendazole alone Albendazole + PAIR	PAIR
CE3b	Cyst with daughter cyst in solid matrix	Transitional	Any	Albendazole + either modified catheterization or surgery	Modified catheterization
CE4	Cyst with heterogenous hypoechoic/hyperechoic contents; no daughter cyst	Inactive	Any	Observation	-
CE5	Solid plus calcified wall	Inactive	Any	Observation	-

Abbreviation: CE, cystic echinococcosis.

Reproduced from Junghanss T, da Silva AM, Horton J, et al. Clinical management of cystic echinococcosis: state of the art, problems, and perspectives. *Am J Trop Med Hyg* 2008; 79:301, with permission of The American Society of Tropical Medicine.

13. C. Parenchymal cysticercosis is one of the leading causes of adult-onset seizures, especially in endemic areas such as India and North America. The lesion appears as a ring lesion on noncontrast head CT scan.

Toxoplasmosis symptoms may include simple bilateral lymphadenopathy of the neck, self-limiting constitutional symptoms, and chorioretinitis. It can also present with a picture of encephalitis, fevers, focal neurologic deficit, or seizure especially in immunocompromised patients. Presenting symptoms may include headaches, blurred vision, motor difficulties, and personality changes. The latter may manifest as depression, apathy, psychosis, confusion, memory impairment, slowness of thought, or visual hallucinations. Only 14% of lymphoma patients have seizures as their presenting symptom. Glioblastoma is mainly a solitary lesion that is visualized better on MRI with contrast rather than enhancing on noncontrast head CT. The incidence of seizures is higher with primary tumors than with metastatic lesions, and among patients with primary tumors, seizures are less common with high-grade as opposed to low-grade gliomas. Seizures in glioma can present as focal or generalized seizures, and the type of seizure depends on the location. Seizures are present preoperatively in approximately 30% of patients who are diagnosed with an intracranial meningioma. The risk of seizure is higher with non–skull base tumors and tumors associated with peritumoral edema.

14. A. The potential risk of treatment with antiparasitic therapy is exacerbation of neurologic symptoms due to increased inflammation around the degenerating cyst, particularly in patients with a large number of lesions. The inflammation can be so severe that it can lead to disability or death. For this reason, corticosteroids should be routinely administered together with antiparasitic therapy. The other answers are incorrect. Although there are case reports of use of mannitol to assist with treatment of cerebral edema, this is not a mainstay of initial therapy.

15. C. The neurologic features of early disseminated Lyme disease may include lymphocytic meningitis, unilateral or bilateral cranial nerve palsies (especially of the facial nerve), radiculopathy (Bannwarth syndrome), peripheral neuropathy, mononeuropathy multiplex, cerebellar ataxia (rarely), and encephalomyelitis (rarely).

The classic triad of acute neurologic abnormalities is meningitis, cranial neuropathy, and motor or sensory radiculoneuropathy, but each of these findings may occur alone.

West Nile virus neuroinvasive disease (encephalitis more than meningitis) presents as fever in conjunction with meningitis, encephalitis, flaccid paralysis, or a mixed pattern of disease. The mortality rate of patients with neuroinvasive disease is close to 10%. Risk factors for demise include encephalitis with severe muscle weakness, changes in the level of consciousness, diabetes, cardiovascular disease, hepatitis C virus infection, and/or immunosuppression. Classic symptoms of Rocky Mountain spotted fever (RMSF) include fever, headache, and rash in a person with a history of a tick bite. However, all of these diagnostic clues are rarely identified on the initial patient encounter, leading to delays in appropriate therapy. Malaria can present as impaired consciousness with a Glasgow coma scale score of less than 11, prostration, and convulsions. Tuberculosis can presents with both cardiac and neurologic symptoms including basilar meningitis, which can have facial diplegia as one finding but would more commonly have additional cranial nerves involved. The most common cardiac finding associated with tuberculosis is pericarditis that can be complicated by pericardial effusion. These findings are manifested on an ECG as low-voltage QRS complexes and potentially ST-segment elevations.

16. D. Cryptococcal meningitis is a rare fungal disease in healthy individual and more common in immunocompromised patients. *Cryptococcus neoformans and Cryptococcus gattii* are 2 fungal species that can result in meningitis. In 60% to 80% of patients, India ink of CSF will usually demonstrate round encapsulated yeast organisms consistent with *Cryptococcus*. The advantage of the India ink preparation is that a diagnosis of cryptococcal infection can be made rapidly while confirmatory testing is being performed (eg, CSF culture or antigen). Congo red is a stain used in the diagnosis of amyloidosis. Giemsa and Wright and Field stains are used in the diagnosis of malaria.

17. B. There are many significant clinical and laboratory predictors of death that could be helpful to identify in the early course of cryptococcal meningitis. These factors are: decline in mental status, CSF cryptococcal antigen titer >1:1024, and CSF WBC count <20 cell/μL. Although it is important to keep blood glucose under control in the setting of acute illness, there is no direct correlation between blood glucose and mortality in cryptococcal meningitis patients. WBC within normal limit and thrombocytopenia are not predictors of death in this cohort.

18. **E.** Endocarditis should be considered as a possible etiology in a patient who has 1 major and 3 minor criteria per modified Duke criteria for diagnosis of infective endocarditis.

   The patient meets the modified Duke criteria for endocarditis (positive blood culture with *S*

aureus, febrile, IV drug use, and vascular phenomenon with acute ischemic stroke). Either ischemic or hemorrhagic stroke complicates 10% of infective endocarditis. Given that there is a predisposition for increased hemorrhage, patients with suspected or known endocarditis were excluded from original tPA trials, and suspected or known endocarditis is considered a relative contraindication. Given the patient has a low NIHSS score and known endocarditis, these 2 relative contraindications would push most to not treat with IV tPA. Administration of tPA in the setting of infective endocarditis should weigh the benefits of averting a major neurologic deficit versus precipitating cerebral hemorrhage. Although there are even more limited data for use of intra-arterial therapy for treatment in endocarditis, case reports indicate successful use of intra-arterial

Modified Duke Criteria for Diagnosis of Infective Endocarditis

Major Criteria	Minor Criteria
Positive blood cultures for infective endocarditis (IE) having 1 of the following:	
–Typical microorganisms consistent with IE from 2 separate blood cultures: *Staphylococcus aureus*, *Viridans* streptococci, *Streptococcus gallolyticus* (formerly *Streptococcus bovis*), including nutritional variant strains (*Granulicatella* species and *Abiotrophia defectiva*)	Predisposition: Intravenous (IV) drug use or presence of a predisposing heart condition (prosthetic heart valve or valve lesion associated with significant regurgitation or turbulence of blood flow)
–HACEK group: *Haemophilus* species, *Aggregatibacter* (formerly *Actinobacillus actinomyces comitans*), *Cardiobacterium hominis*, *Eikenella* species, and *Kingella kingae*	
–Community-acquired enterococci, in the absence of a primary focus	
Persistently positive blood culture:	Fever: Temperature ≥38.0°C (100.4°F)
For organisms that are typical cause of IE: at least 2 positive blood cultures from blood samples drawn >12 hours apart	Vascular phenomena: Major arterial emboli, septic pulmonary infarcts, mycotic aneurysm, intracranial hemorrhage, conjunctival hemorrhages, or Janeway lesions
For organisms that are more commonly skin contaminants: At least three positive blood cultures from separate blood draws (with first and last drawn at least 1 hour apart)	Immunologic phenomena: Glomerulonephritis, Osler nodes, Roth spots, or rheumatoid factor
Single positive blood culture for *Coxiella burnetii* or phase I IgG antibody titer >1:800	
Evidence of endocardial involvement (1 of the following):	Microbiology evidence: positive blood cultures that do not meet major criteria or serologic evidence of active infection with organism consistent with IE
Vegetation	
Abscess	
New partial dehiscence of prosthetic valve	
New valvular regurgitation demonstrated by increase or change in preexisting murmur is not sufficient	

therapy without hemorrhage. These reports involve emboli in major vessels (internal carotid artery, M1, basilar artery), and the patient's low NIHSS is indicative of a smaller, more distal vessel, which is less like to be amenable to intra-arterial therapy. Covering the patient with broad spectrum antibiotics and obtain TTE is the next step of management to this patient.

19. **B.** Patients with acute fungal rhinosinusitis usually present acutely with fever, facial pain, nasal congestion, and epistaxis and can have changes in vision or mentation. Facial numbness and diplopia can occur in the setting of cranial nerve involvement. Many patients already have extension of the infection outside the sinuses at the time of presentation.

    The diagnosis of invasive fungal rhinosinusitis is dependent upon histopathologic demonstration of fungal invasion by biopsy of involved areas. Imaging modalities, such as CT scanning, are suggestive but are not sufficiently sensitive or specific to confirm a diagnosis. Evaluation of patients with suspected fungal rhinosinusitis should include early nasal endoscopy with biopsies of affected tissues. Cultures of the biopsy specimen are usually positive. Isolation of the infecting fungus is necessary to guide therapy.

20. **C.** Epidural abscess can be the result of paraspinal steroid/analgesic injection, hematogneous spread, direct bacterial growth or spontaneous. Other possible risk factors include:

    - Epidural catheter
    - Alcoholism
    - Diabetes mellitus
    - HIV infection
    - Trauma
    - Tattooing over the spine
    - Acupuncture
    - IV drug use
    - Hemodialysis

    The median age of onset of spinal epidural abscess is approximately 50 years, with *Staphylcoccus aureus* causing 63% and gram-negative bacilli causing 16% of the cases. *Mycobacterium tuberculosis* is a more frequent cause of epidural abscesses in parts of the developing world. The importance of infection control measures to prevent epidural abscesses associated with epidural catheters was illustrated by a report in which the infecting organism was subsequently isolated from nasal swabs taken from the physician who placed the catheter. Safe injection practices must be used during spinal injection procedures in order to prevent bacterial contamination of medication vials.

The initial manifestations of spinal epidural abscess are often nonspecific and include such signs and symptoms as fever and malaise. The classical diagnostic triad consists of fever, spinal pain, and neurologic deficits. MRI is the preferred test because it is often positive early in the course of the infection and provides the best visualization of the location and extent of inflammatory changes. It should be performed as soon as possible. Consideration should be given to imaging the entire spinal column even when patients have focal signs or symptoms in one region because multiple skip lesions are common and patients may not have pain or tenderness in all of the affected areas.

Two sets of blood cultures should be drawn in all patients with suspected spinal epidural abscess. The best specimen for culture is fluid or pus of the epidural abscess or inflammatory mass obtained by direct needle aspiration, usually using CT guidance. LP for CSF examination is often not performed because the diagnostic yield is low and because of the risk of introducing infection into the CNS.

Antibiotics should be started as soon as the diagnosis is strongly suspected and immediately following the collection of 2 sets of blood cultures. Appropriate empiric parenteral regimens include those listed below.

Antibiotic	Dose	Organism
Vancomycin	30-60 mg/kg IV in divided dosing (adjustment for renal function)	Methicillin-resistant *Staphylococcus aureus*
AND ONE OF THE FOLLOWING:		
Cefotaxime	2 g IV every 6 hours	
Ceftriaxone	2 g IV every 12 hours	
Ceftazidime	2 g IV every 8 hours	To be used if concern for *Pseudomonas aeruginosa*
Cefepime	2 g IV every 8 hours	To be used if concern for *P aeruginosa*

REFERENCES

American Academy of Pediatrics. Rocky Mountain spotted fever. In: Pickering LK, ed. *Red Book: 2012 Report of the Committee on Infectious Diseases.* 29th ed. Elk Grove Village, IL: American Academy of Pediatrics; 2012.

Barouiche RO, Hamill RJ, Greenberg SB, et al. Bacterial spinal epidural abscess. Review of 43 cases and literature survey. *Medicine (Baltimore).* 1992;71:369-385.

Bayer AS, Bolger AF, Taubert KA, et al. Diagnosis and management of infective endocarditis and its complications. *Circulation.* 1998;98(25):2936-2948.

Brouwer MC, Heckenberg SG, de Gans J, Spanjaard L, Reitsma JB, van de Beek D. Nationwide implementation of adjunctive dexamethasone therapy for pneumococcal meningitis. *Neurology.* 2010;75(17):1533-1539.

Brunetti E, Kern P, Vuitton DA, Writing Panel for the WHO-I-WGE. Expert consensus for the diagnosis and treatment of cystic and alveolar echinococcosis in humans. *Acta Trop.* 2010;114:1.

Cao-Lormeau VM, Blake A, Mons S, et al. Guillain-Barré Syndrome outbreak associated with Zika virus infection in French Polynesia: a case-control study. *Lancet.* 2016;387(10027):1531-1539.

Carpio A, Hauser WA. Prognosis for seizure recurrence in patients with newly diagnosed neurocysticercosis. *Neurology.* 2002;59(11):1730-1734.

Chapman AS, Bakken JS, Folk SM, et al. Diagnosis and management of tickborne rickettsial diseases: Rocky Mountain spotted fever, ehrlichioses, and anaplasmosis–United States: a practical guide for physicians and other healthcare and public health professionals. *MMWR Recomm Rep.* 2006;55(RR-4):1-27.

Darouiche RO. Spinal epidural abscess. *N Engl J Med.* 2006;355:2012.

Del Brutto OH, Santibañez R, Noboa CA, Aguirre R, Díaz E, Alarcón TA. Epilepsy due to neurocysticercosis: analysis of 203 patients. *Neurology.* 1992;42(2):389-392.

DelGaudio JM, Swain RE Jr, Kingdom TT, Muller S, Hudgins PA. Computed tomographic findings in patients with invasive fungal sinusitis. *Arch Otolaryngol Head Neck Surg.* 2003;129(2):236-240.

Dirlikov E, Major CG, Mayshack M, et al. Guillain-Barré syndrome during ongoing Zika virus transmission: Puerto Rico, January 1-July 31, 2016. *MMWR Morb Mortal Wkly Rep.* 2016;65(34):910-914.

Dos Santos T, Rodriguez A, Almiron M, et al. Zika virus and the Guillain-Barré syndrome: case series from seven countries. *N Engl J Med.* 2016;375(16):1598-1601.

Garcia HH, Coyle CM, White AC Jr. Cysticercosis. In: Guerrant RL, Walker DH, Weller PF, eds. *Tropical Infectious Diseases: Principles, Pathogens and Practice.* 3rd ed. Philadelphia, PA: Saunders Elsevier; 2011:815.

Garcia HH, Nash TE, Del Brutto OH. Clinical symptoms, diagnosis, and treatment of neurocysticercosis. *Lancet Neurol.* 2014;13(12):1202-1215.

Garg RK, Potluri N, Kar AM, et al. Short course of prednisolone in patients with solitary cysticercus granuloma: a double blind placebo controlled study. *J Infect.* 2006;53(1):65-69.

Ghadiali MT, Deckard NA, Farooq U, Astor F, Robinson P, Casiano RR. Frozen-section biopsy analysis for acute invasive fungal rhinosinusitis. *Otolaryngol Head Neck Surg.* 2007;136(5):714-719.

Gopal AK, Whitehouse JD, Simel DL, Corey GR. Cranial computed tomography before lumbar puncture: a prospective clinical evaluation. *Arch Intern Med.* 1999;159(22):2681-2685.

Hacohen Y, Wright S, Waters P, et al. Paediatric autoimmune encephalopathies: clinical features, laboratory investigations and outcomes in patients with or without antibodies to known central nervous system autoantigens. *J Neurol Neurosurg Psychiatry.* 2013;84(7):748-755.

Hasbun R, Abrahams J, Jekel J, Quagliarello VJ. Computed tomography of the head before lumbar puncture in adults with suspected meningitis. *N Engl J Med.* 2001;345(24):1727-1733.

Hattwick MA, Retailliau H, O'Brien RJ, Slutzker M, Fontaine RE, Hanson B. Fatal Rocky Mountain spotted fever. *JAMA.* 1978.;240(14):1499-1503.

Heckenberg SG, Brouwer MC, van der Ende A, van de Beek D. Adjunctive dexamethasone in adults with meningococcal meningitis. *Neurology.* 2012;79(15):1563-1569.

Heier JS, Gardner TA, Hawes MJ, McGuire KA, Walton WT, Stock J. Proptosis as the initial presentation of fungal sinusitis in immunocompetent patients. *Ophthalmology.* 1995;102(5):713-717.

Helmick CG, Bernard KW, D'Angelo LJ. Rocky Mountain spotted fever: clinical, laboratory, and epidemiological features of 262 cases. *J Infect Dis.* 1984;150(4):480-488.

Hörstrup P, Ackermann R. [Tick born meningopolyneuritis (Garin-Bujadoux, Bannwarth) (author's transl)]. *Fortschr Neurol Psychiatr Grenzgeb.* 1973;41(11):583-606.

Junghanss T, da Silva AM, Horton J, et al. Clinical management of cystic echinococcosis: state of the art, problems, and perspectives. *Am J Trop Med Hyg.* 2008;79:301.

Kayser MS, Titulaer MJ, Gresa-Arribas N, Dalmau J. Frequency and characteristics of isolated psychiatric episodes in anti–N-methyl-d-aspartate receptor encephalitis. *JAMA Neurol.* 2013;70(9):1133-1139.

Kim JM, Jeon JS, Kin YW, et al. Forced arterial suction thrombectomy of septic embolic middle cerebral artery occlusion due to infective endocarditis: an illustrative case and review of the literature. *Neurointervention.* 2014;9:101-105.

Kirkland KB, Wilkinson WE, Sexton DJ. Therapeutic delay and mortality in cases of Rocky Mountain spotted fever. *Clin Infect Dis.* 1995;20(5):1118-1121.

Medina MT, Durón RM, Martínez L, et al. Prevalence, incidence, and etiology of epilepsies in rural Honduras: the Salamá Study. *Epilepsia.* 2005;46(1):124-131.

Oehler E, Watrin L, Larre P, et al. Zika virus infection complicated by Guillain-Barre syndrome: case report, French Polynesia, December 2013. *Euro Surveill.* 2014;19(9):20720.

Panel on Opportunistic Infections in HIV-Infected Adults and Adolescents. Guidelines for the prevention and treatment of opportunistic infections in HIV-infected adults and adolescents: recommendations from the Centers for Disease Control and Prevention, the National Institutes of

Health, and the HIV Medicine Association of the Infectious Diseases Society of America. http://aidsinfo.nih.gov/contentfiles/lvguidelines/adult_oi.pdf. Accessed on October 20, 2015.

Paploski IA, Prates AP, Cardoso CW, et al. Time lags between exanthematous illness attributed to Zika virus, Guillain-Barré syndrome, and microcephaly, Salvador, Brazil. *Emerg Infect Dis.* 2016;22(8):1438-1444.

Parra B, Lizarazo J, Jiménez-Arango JA, et al. Guillain-Barré syndrome associated with Zika virus infection in Colombia. *N Engl J Med.* 2016;375(16):1513-1523.

Patil HV, Patil VC, Rajmane V, et al. Successful treatment of toxoplasmosis with cotrimoxazole. *Indian J Sex Trasm Dis.* 2011;32:44-46.

Prüss H, Dalmau J, Harms L, et al. Retrospective analysis of NMDA receptor antibodies in encephalitis of unknown origin. *Neurology.* 2010;75(19):1735-1739.

Rock RB, Olin M, Baker CA, et al. Central nervous system tuberculosis: pathogenesis and clinical aspects. *Clin Microbiol Rev.* 2008;21:243-261.

Rohmann S, Erbel R, Görge G, et al. Clinical relevance of vegetation localization by transoesophageal echocardiography in infective endocarditis. *Eur Heart J.* 1992;13(4):446-452.

Roithmann R, Shankar L, Hawke M, Chapnik J, Kassel E, Noyek A. Diagnostic imaging of fungal sinusitis: eleven new cases and literature review. *Rhinology.* 1995;33(2):104-110.

Rupprecht TA, Koedel U, Fingerle V, Pfister HW. The pathogenesis of lyme neuroborreliosis: from infection to inflammation. *Mol Med.* 2008;14(3-4):205-212.

Saag MS, Powderly WG, Cloud GA, et al. Comparison of amphotericin B with fluconazole in the treatment of acute AIDS-associated cryptococcal meningitis. The NIAID Mycoses Study Group and the AIDS Clinical Trials Group. *N Engl J Med.* 1992;326(2):83-89.

Schmitt SE, Pargeon K, Frechette ES, Hirsch LJ, Dalmau J, Friedman D. Extreme delta brush: a unique EEG pattern in adults with anti-NMDA receptor encephalitis. *Neurology.* 2012;79(11):1094-1100.

Sendi P, Bregenzer T, Zimmerli W. Spinal epidural abscess in clinical practice. *QJM.* 2008;101:1-12.

Serpa JA, Graviss EA, Kass JS, White AC Jr. Neurocysticercosis in Houston, Texas: an update. *Medicine (Baltimore).* 2011;90(1):81-86.

Sibtubebu SP, Mooss AN, Andukuri VG, et al. Effectiveness of thrombolytic therapy in acute embolic stroke due to infective endocarditis. *Stroke Res Treat.* 2010;2010:841797.

Singhi P, Ray M, Singhi S, Khandelwal N. Clinical spectrum of 500 children with neurocysticercosis and response to albendazole therapy. *J Child Neurol.* 2000;15(4):207-213.

Smedema JP, Katjitae I, Rueter H, et al. Twelve-lead electrocardiography in tuberculous pericarditis. *Cardiovasc J S Afr.* 2001;12:31-34.

Thuny F, Di Salvo G, Belliard O, et al. Risk of embolism and death in infective endocarditis: prognostic value of echocardiography: a prospective multicenter study. *Circulation.* 2005;112(1):69-75.

Torres-Corzo J, Rodriguez-della Vecchia R, Rangel-Castilla L. Bruns syndrome caused by intraventricular neurocysticercosis treated using flexible endoscopy. *J Neurosurg.* 2006;104(5):746-748.

Tunkel AR, Hartman BJ, Kaplan SL, et al. Practice guidelines for the management of bacterial meningitis. *Clin Infect Dis.* 2004;39:1267-1284.

Usatine RP, Sandy N. Dermatologic emergencies. *Am Fam Physician.* 2010;82(7):773-780.

7

Toxidromes

Kara R. Melmed, MD and Shouri Lahiri, MD

Questions

1. A 36-year-old woman presents to emergency department (ED). Her vitals on arrival are heart rate of 135 bpm, blood pressure of 108/60 mm Hg, respiratory rate of 10 breaths/min, and oxygen saturation of 88%. She is drowsy and oriented to self only, with pupillary dilation, marked dysarthria, myoclonus, 4+ reflexes throughout, and ataxia on neurologic exam. She has dry mucous membranes and axillae and diminished bowel sounds and a full bladder on general exam. She was last seen normal 3 hours prior. During her initial evaluation in the ED, she has a generalized tonic-clonic seizure that lasts 45 seconds. The patient is intubated in the ED; blood is sent for toxicology, and an electrocardiogram (ECG) is obtained. This reveals a heart rate of 135 bpm, right axis deviation (125°) as evidenced by terminal R wave in lead aVR, PR prolongation, and widened QRS interval (>100 milliseconds) with premature ventricular beats. What is the next best step in treatment?

   A. Hemodialysis
   B. Forced diuresis
   C. Sodium bicarbonate
   D. Physostigmine salicylate
   E. Flumazenil

2. A 52-year-old man with a history of schizophrenia and diabetes mellitus is transferred to your hospital for altered mental status. His vitals on presentation are heart rate of 115 bpm, blood pressure of 159/95 mm Hg, respiratory rate of 35 breaths/min, and temperatures of 101.3°F. On exam, he is noted to be diaphoretic and pale. He does not follow commands. His pupils are 4 mm and reactive bilaterally, and his motor exam is significant for increased tone throughout with 1+ reflexes. Bowel sounds are normal. Blood work includes white blood cell (WBC) count of 40,000/microL and creatinine of 5 mg/dL. What is the strongest predictor of mortality in this patient?

   A. Creatine phosphokinase levels
   B. Age
   C. Sepsis
   D. Acute respiratory failure
   E. History of diabetes

3. Which of the following statements is true regarding the patient in Question 2?

  A. Incidence of neuroleptic malignant syndrome (NMS) is about 20% among patients taking neuroleptics.

  B. There is no risk of NMS associated with newer generation neuroleptics.

  C. First-line treatment is dantrolene.

  D. There is a high risk of NMS associated with inhalation anesthetics and skeletal muscle relaxants.

  E. Early treatment is oral bromocriptine.

Questions 4 and 5

4. A patient is dropped off at the ED. He is unresponsive, demonstrates shallow respirations, and has a heart rate in the 30s, respiratory rate of 8 breaths/min, and temperature of 94°F. He has pinpoint pupils. He is intubated in the ED. The respiratory depression in this patient is modulated by which of the following?

  A. Activation of cyclic adenosine monophosphate (cAMP) subtype of mu receptors

  B. Activation of voltage-gated potassium channels of mu receptors

  C. Inhibition of G-coupled transmembrane receptors of kappa receptors

  D. Inhibition of cAMP subtype of delta receptors

  E. Activation of voltage-gated potassium channels of kappa receptors

5. The patient in Question 4 is treated with naloxone and admitted to the neurocritical care unit. He is initially stable, although after about 10 hours, the patient starts to demonstrate rhinorrhea, sweating, piloerection, and lacrimation. His pupils become dilated, and he is noted to have muscle twitching. Thirty-six hours after admission, his temperature increases, and he is over-breathing the ventilator. His blood pressure also rises. He is noted to have emesis and diarrhea. Which of the following is true regarding this patient's course?

  A. Withdrawal can be fatal.

  B. Onset of abstinence symptoms is related to pharmacologic half-life of the agent.

  C. Withdrawal symptoms peak at 24 hours after last use of the agent.

  D. Naloxone is a competitive kappa opioid–receptor antagonist.

  E. The duration of action of naloxone is longer than most opioids, making it a potent opioid antidote.

6. A 19-year-old man presents with stupor and cerebellar ataxia to the ED. On exam, he is noted to have spastic hemiplegia and myoclonus. His family states that there is drug use suspected. For the past 2 weeks, he has been experiencing pseudobulbar speech, restlessness, and difficulty with coordination and balance. He is admitted to the neurocritical care unit where, unfortunately, his symptoms rapidly progress and he demonstrates high fevers, akinetic mutism, and hypotonic areflexic paresis. What is most likely seen on magnetic resonance imaging (MRI)?

  A. White matter changes involving the U-fibers

  B. Diffuse increased T2 signal within the white matter tracts of the cerebellum and the brainstem and the deep gray matter structures

  C. Discrete lesions centered in the globus pallidus bilaterally

  D. Mammillary body atrophy with cortical thinning, sulcal widening, and ventriculomegaly

  E. Cortical intracerebral hemorrhage with abnormal-appearing cerebral blood vessels on angiography

7. A 65-year-old woman with a history of epilepsy presents in a coma. She was found in her bedroom with a half-empty open bottle of medications. Pulse is faint and rapid. Blood pressure is greatly reduced. Her respiration is slow and shallow. She is intubated on arrival, and pulmonary edema is evident on postintubation chest x-ray. On general exam, she appears cyanotic. Neurologic exam reveals small reactive pupils, although corneal and gag reflexes are absent. Extremities are flaccid. Deep tendon reflexes are absent, and there is extensor response to plantar simulation. Which of the following statements regarding the pharmacokinetics of the offending agent is true?

   A. The more lipid soluble the agent, the more potent is the effect to the central nervous system (CNS) but the briefer the action.
   B. Increasing plasma pH can increase the rate of entry of the ionized form across the blood-brain barrier.
   C. This agent acts to enhance neuronal transmission via glutamatergic receptors.
   D. This agent acts on postsynaptic γ-aminobutyric acid (GABA) receptors, which increases excitatory potentials.
   E. Decreasing the plasma pH can decrease the rate of entry of the ionized form across the blood-brain barrier.
   F. The more lipid soluble the agent, the easier it is to dialyze off.

8. A 37-year-old woman presents to the ED with anorexia, nausea and vomiting, and constipation. She also complains of double vision. She reports recent travel to Cancun with diarrheal illness. On exam, there is no accommodation or reaction to light. There is marked bilateral ptosis, strabismus, and ophthalmoplegia. The patient also demonstrates dysarthria and dysphagia on exam. She has generalized weakness in her neck, trunk, and limbs. Her deep tendon reflexes are absent. A lumbar puncture is performed, and the protein is normal in her cerebrospinal fluid. Given concern for impending respiratory failure, the patient is admitted to the intensive care unit. The suspected diagnosis is confirmed with electromyography (EMG). What are the EMG findings?

   A. Reduced amplitude of muscle action potentials, prolonged distal motor latencies, conduction block, prolonged or absent F wave, slowed median with normal sural sensory conduction velocity
   B. Continuous discharges of normal motor units with loss of physiologic silent period that occurs 50 to 100 milliseconds after reflex contraction
   C. Reduced amplitude of evoked muscle potentials and an increase in amplitude with rapid repetitive nerve stimulation
   D. Progressive reduction in amplitude with repetitive motor nerve stimulation
   E. Uniform findings throughout the peripheral nervous system of reduced compound muscle action potential amplitude, severe and widespread nerve conduction slowing, and no conduction block

9. A 29-year-old man presents with unsteady gait, drowsiness, confusion, and impairment of memory. The patient suddenly loses consciousness in the ED. His blood pressure is 110/70 mm Hg, and his respiratory rate is 14 breaths/min. The patient was found with an open and empty bottle of alprazolam. Because overdose is suspected, he is immediately given an antidote. What is the mechanism of action of the antidote?

   A. Binds to GABA inhibitory systems to open chloride ion channels
   B. Binds to GABA inhibitory systems to hyperpolarize postsynaptic neurons
   C. Blocks diazepine receptors via blocking glutamate transmission
   D. Blocks activation of inhibitory GABAergic synapses
   E. Unbinds CNS diazepine receptors from GABAergic synapses

Questions 10 and 11

10. A 29-year-old obtunded woman arrives via emergency medical services. Per the paramedics, she was at a party when she suddenly complained of severe headache and then became acutely encephalopathic. Her blood pressure on arrival is 203/87 mm Hg, and her heart rate is 124 bpm. She is mildly hyperthermic and currently maintaining her airway. She is diaphoretic on exam, with large dilated pupils. What is the mechanism of action of the toxic effect of the suspected agent?

 A. Blockage of voltage-gated sodium channels in the neuronal membrane

 B. Inhibition of the presynaptic reuptake of biogenic amines throughout the body

 C. Inhibition of the postsynaptic receptor binding of biogenic amines

 D. Inhibition of GABA A channels, impeding function of the ligand-gated chloride channel

 E. Stimulation of α-adrenergic receptors in arterial smooth muscle cells

11. What is the gravest complication related to the presentation of use of this illicit drug?

 A. Spontaneous subarachnoid or intracerebral hemorrhage

 B. Abstinence that could lead to delirium tremens and be fatal

 C. Acute rhabdomyolysis leading to liver failure

 D. NMS

 E. Severe and irreversible memory loss

Questions 12 and 13

12. A 24-year-old man presents with neck stiffness and low-grade fever. Per report, he suffered a recent skin penetrating injury when visiting a construction site. He now demonstrates large swings in blood pressure and heart rate. He is profusely diaphoretic. He is rigid in all muscles, with a board-like abdomen, extensor posturing of his legs, and pursed lips. The patient also demonstrates paroxysms of tonic contractions. What is the likely mechanism of action of the toxin responsible for this presentation?

 A. Tetanus toxin; prevents the normal exocytosis of neurotransmitters via cleavage of synaptic vesicle surface proteins

 B. Diphtheria toxin; produces demyelination in the proximal parts of spinal nerves

 C. Botulism toxin; interferes with the release of acetylcholine from peripheral motor nerves at the presynaptic membrane of neuromuscular junction

 D. Amanita toxin; disrupts RNA metabolism, causing hepatic and renal necrosis

 E. Ciguatera toxin; blocks neural sodium channels

13. What will be the most likely cause of death in this patient?

 A. Asphyxiation from laryngospasm

 B. Heart failure

 C. Shock due to action of the toxin on the hypothalamus and sympathetic nervous system

 D. Pneumonia

 E. All of the above

14. A 67-year-old man presents with sudden loss of consciousness. He had been complaining of a headache, nausea, dyspnea, confusion, dizziness, and clumsiness. He then had a witnessed seizure and was brought to the ED. Initial computed tomography (CT) scan was normal. He immediately deteriorated, and carbon monoxide poisoning was suspected. The patient was transferred for hyperbaric oxygen therapy. Which of the following statements regarding carbon monoxide poisoning is true?

 A. Binding of carbon monoxide to hemoglobin causes a rightward shift of the oxyhemoglobin dissociation curve, decreasing the offloading of oxygen from hemoglobin to tissue.

 B. Carbon monoxide concentrations are directly proportional to the degree of cerebral hypoxia.

 C. Discrete lesions centered in the globus pallidus bilaterally are pathognomonic for carbon monoxide poisoning.

 D. Carbon monoxide interferes with cellular respiration by binding to mitochondrial cytochrome oxidase.

 E. Hyperbaric oxygen therapy can worsen outcomes in this patient population.

15. A 19-year-old woman with history of depression was brought to the hospital with a change in mental status. On exam, she appears confused and agitated. Her blood pressure is 179/80 mm Hg, her heart rate is 125 bpm and irregular, and her temperature is 100.4°F. She appears to be shivering but is diaphoretic. Her cheeks appear flushed. There are increased bowel sounds on general exam. On her neurologic exam, she has dilated pupils, with muscle rigidity. Hyperreflexia of the lower extremities and bilateral Babinski sign are noted. While in ED, she has a witnessed seizure and is intubated and admitted to the neurocritical care unit. Which of the following is true regarding the etiology and treatment of her presentation?

    A. Activation of the 5-HT2A receptor is thought to be primarily responsible for development of the syndrome.

    B. The 5-HT1A receptor serves a modulatory function by decreasing intrasynaptic concentrations of serotonin.

    C. Use of a depolarizing paralytic, such as succinylcholine, should be considered to control agitation and excess motor activity.

    D. Antagonizing the 5-HT2A receptors is primarily responsible for development of this syndrome.

    E. Phenytoin is first-line treatment for toxin-induced seizures.

16. A 16-year-old patient presents with seizures. Salicylate poisoning is highly suspected. What is the best treatment for this patient?

    A. *N*-Acetylcysteine

    B. Lipid emulsion therapy

    C. Plasma alkalization

    D. Gastrointestinal decontamination

    E. Whole bowel irrigation

17. A 59-year-old male gardener presents with abdominal pain and difficulty breathing. His heart rate is in the low 40s, and his blood pressure is 101/40 mm Hg. On exam, he is noted to have profuse watery nasal discharge, nasal hyperemia, marked salivation, and bronchorrhea, as well as a cough and wheezing with prolonged expiratory phase. On neurologic exam, he demonstrates miosis and flaccid paralysis. He has a witnessed seizure while in the ED. An acute ingestion is suspected. What is the method of action of the offending agent?

    A. Muscarinic receptor antagonist

    B. Blocks neuroeffector site on smooth muscle, cardiac muscle, secretory gland cells, peripheral ganglia

    C. Binds to and activates nicotinic receptors

    D. Hydrolyzes acetylcholine to choline and acetic acid

    E. Inhibits acetylcholinesterase

18. A 37-year-old patient presents after being found down. He is disoriented on arrival and seems to be suffering from severe anxiety. He also appears to see objects that are not visible to anyone else. His blood pressure is 179/50 mm Hg, and his heart rate is 110 bpm and irregular. His temperature is 100.4°F. He is diaphoretic and tremulous. What is the treatment of choice?

    A. Chloral hydrate

    B. Paraldehyde

    C. Barbiturates

    D. Benzodiazepine

    E. Flumazenil

Questions 19-21

19. A 39-year-old man is brought to the hospital via emergency medical services. He appears inebriated. He complains of blurred vision that progressed to complete blindness. He is normotensive. On fundoscopic exam, he has pallor of the optic disc, papilledema, and an afferent papillary defect. CT is obtained, which reveals bilateral basal ganglia lesions. Na is 145 mEq/L, K 4.5 mEq/L, Cl 99 mEq/L, and HCO$_3$ 18 mEq/L. His arterial blood gas values are 7.21/32/98. What is the acid-base disorder seen in this patient?

    A. Respiratory alkalosis

    B. Respiratory acidosis

    C. Mixed metabolic and respiratory acidosis.

    D. Metabolic acidosis, anion gap

    E. Metabolic acidosis, non–anion gap

20. What is the most likely agent ingested by the patient?

A. Ethylene glycol

B. Isopropyl alcohol

C. Methanol

D. Bath salts

E. Synthetic cannabinoids

21. What is the best treatment for the patient?

A. Hemodialysis

B. Lipid emulsion therapy

C. Plasma alkalization

D. Gastrointestinal decontamination

E. Whole bowel irrigation

Answers and Explanations

1. C. This patient's presentation is consistent with tricyclic antidepressant (TCA) toxicity. TCA-induced cardiotoxicity is the most important factor contributing to patient mortality. TCAs cause inhibition of sodium influx through voltage-gated sodium channels. Inhibition of fast sodium channels in His-Purkinje cells leads to delayed depolarization and conduction abnormalities. This impaired sodium entry induces decreased contractility. Sodium blockade results in prolongation of phase 0 of the action potential, and the effects become more pronounced with rapid heart rate, hyponatremia, and acidosis. ECG changes caused by sodium channel blockade include PR and QRS interval prolongation, and right axis deviation may identify patients at high risk for severe toxicity. A terminal right axis deviation >120° and widened QRS interval >100 milliseconds are indications to pursue either sodium bicarbonate therapy or mechanical ventilation–induced respiratory alkalosis. Sodium channel blockade can be overcome by serum alkalization and/or increased serum sodium concentrations via infusion of intravenous (IV) sodium bicarbonate. The rapid influx of sodium promotes release of intracellular calcium stores and improves myocardial contractility.

TCAs have a large volume of distribution and are highly lipophilic. Half-life ranges from 24 to 48 hours, and elimination occurs by hepatic metabolism. Only 1% to 2% of the total body burden of TCAs is found in the blood. Thus, hemodialysis or forced diuresis is unlikely to work.

TCAs are competitive inhibitors of acetylcholine at both central and peripheral muscarinic receptors. Physostigmine is an acetylcholinesterase inhibitor and can reverse antimuscarinic effects and thus has historically been used to reverse TCA effects. The antimuscarinic clinical manifestations are not directly responsible for TCA-related major toxicity or deaths and do not require specific therapy other than supportive care, and given the life-threatening complications associated with physostigmine, this treatment for TCA toxicity is no longer recommended.

Flumazenil may precipitate generalized seizures and should never be given to patients with suspected TCA toxicity.

2. D. Neuroleptic malignant syndrome is associated with rhabdomyolysis, acute kidney injury, systemic infections, and venous thromboembolism. Although rhabdomyolysis is the most common, it is not associated directly with mortality. Nontraumatic rhabdomyolysis is known to cause myoglobinuric acute kidney injury. Acute renal failure occurs in a third of patients with rhabdomyolysis, and the serum creatinine level is directly correlated with creatine phosphokinase levels.

A recent study reported that increased age, acute kidney injury, acute respiratory failure, sepsis, and comorbid congestive heart failure were independent predictors of mortality. Acute respiratory failure was the strongest predictor of mortality.

3. E. Early treatment for NMS is bromocriptine in oral doses of 5 mg 3 times a day up to 20 mg twice a day. If the patient cannot tolerate oral medications, the next step is dantrolene 0.25 to 3.0 mg intravenously. The incidence of NMS is about 0.2% among patients taking neuroleptics; however, the mortality rate is 15% to 30% if not recognized and treated. Generally, the risk is greatest with older generation antipsychotics such as haloperidol, chlorpromazine, fluphenazine, thioridazine, and occasionally even promethazine; however, there is also an associated risk with newer generation drugs such as olanzapine.

Malignant hyperthermia, although similar in presentation and treatment to NMS, occurs with volatile anesthetics and skeletal muscle relaxants such as succinylcholine. The majority of patients with malignant hyperthermia have a mutation in the ryanodine receptor gene.

4. **A.** Opioids activate G-coupled transmembrane receptors. The intermediate cAMP acts on mu, delta, and kappa receptor subtype. These receptors are found in high concentrations in the thalamus and dorsal root ganglia, amygdala, and brainstem raphe, modulating pain, affect, and alertness. The mu-type brainstem receptors are responsible for modulating respirator responses to hypoxia and hypercarbia.

5. **B.** Onset of abstinence symptoms is related to pharmacologic half-life of the agent. In the initial 8 to 16 hours of abstinence, the patient is without symptoms. Then yawning, rhinorrhea, sweating, piloerection, and lacrimation occur. This is followed by an increase in severity of a period of several hours with insomnia, pupillary dilation, muscle twitching, myalgias, and hot and cold flashes. After 36 hours, the patient will experience restlessness with nausea, vomiting, and diarrhea with an increase in temperature, respiratory rate, and blood pressure. Opioid withdrawal symptoms peak 48 to 72 hours after withdrawal. Withdrawal is rarely fatal.

   Naloxone is a competitive mu opioid–receptor antagonist and reverses all signs of opioid intoxication. The onset of action of naloxone given intravenously is less than 2 minutes, and its apparent duration of action is 20 to 90 minutes, which is significantly shorter than most opioids.

6. **B.** Subacute progressive cerebral leukoencephalopathy occurs after heroin use, specifically from the inhalation of heated heroin vapor. This is known colloquially as "chasing the dragon." There are 3 distinct clinical stages. The initial phase consists of pseudobulbar speech, motor restlessness, and cerebellar ataxia; this is followed by an intermediate stage 2 to 4 hours later with rapid worsening of cerebellar symptoms, hyperactive reflexes, spastic hemiplegia or quadriplegia accompanied by myoclonus, and chorea. A quarter of patients will go on develop the terminal stage, with stretching spasms, hypotonic areflexic paresis, akinetic mutism, central pyrexia, and eventually death.

   White matter changes can be seen in posterior regions of the hemispheres and in the internal capsules or even cerebellar white matter. On autopsy, these have been found to be caused by "vacuolating myelinopathy," which causes spongiform degeneration due to formation of vacuoles in the oligodendroglia. On MRI, there is diffuse increased T2 signal within the white matter tracts of the cerebellum and the brainstem and the deep gray matter structures. The white matter appears vacuolated, sparing U-fibers.

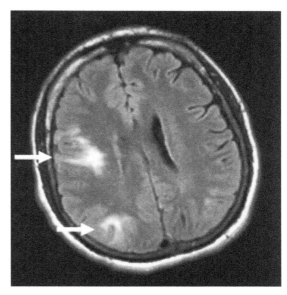

Reproduced with permission from Aminoff MJ, Greenberg DA, Simon RP. *Clinical Neurology*, 9th edition. New York, NY: McGraw-Hill, 2015.

U-fiber involvement can occur with progressive multifocal leukoencephalopathy. Discrete lesions centered in the globus pallidus bilaterally are typically seen in carbon monoxide poisoning. Mammillary body atrophy with cortical thinning, sulcal widening, and ventriculomegaly is seen in chronic alcoholism and Wernicke-Korsakoff syndrome. Intracerebral hemorrhage with abnormal-appearing cerebral blood vessels on angiography is typically associated with amphetamine use.

7. **A.** This patient is suffering from barbiturate toxicity. Barbiturate overdose can result in hypothermia, hypotension, bradycardia, flaccidity, hyporeflexia, coma, and apnea. Severe overdose can mimic brain death.

   The potency of barbiturates is a function of the ionization constant and lipid solubility. The more lipid soluble the agent, the more potent is the effect to the CNS but the briefer the action. The rate of entry of the ionized form of the barbiturate can be increased by lowering the plasma pH.

   Barbiturates suppress neuronal transmission. The mechanism of action is postulated to be enhancement of pre- and postsynaptic GABA inhibition, which reduces excitatory postsynaptic potentials. In particular, inactivation of neurons in the reticular formation of the upper brainstem leads to impaired consciousness or coma. This agent is eliminated via hepatic metabolism and renal excretion.

Pentobarbital acts quickly with quick recovery (3 hours). However, phenobarbital acts more slowly with more prolonged effects. Effects can last 6 or more hours after an average oral dose. The fatal dose of phenobarbital is 6 to 10 g.

Management is supportive care. Supportive measures may also include gastric emptying and activated charcoal. Alkalinization of the urine increases elimination of phenobarbital, but not other barbiturates. This may aggravate pulmonary edema. Long-acting barbiturates may be amenable to hemodialysis or hemofiltration.

Barbiturate withdrawal syndrome is manifested clinically by nervousness, tremor, insomnia, postural hypotension, and weakness. Generalized seizures usually occur between days 2 and 4 and can occur as far out as 7 days. As in delirium tremens seen in alcohol withdrawal syndrome, death can follow a postictal delusional-hallucinatory state.

8. **C.** This patient is suffering from a foodborne illness caused by the exotoxin of *Clostridium botulinum*. The primary site of action of the toxin is at the presynaptic membrane of the neuromuscular junction, where it interferes with the release of acetylcholine from peripheral motor nerves at the neuromuscular synapse. Symptoms first appear within 12 to 36 hours of ingestion. Treatment is antitoxin, which is available from the Centers for Disease Control and Prevention. Early in the course, compound motor action potentials can be normal or have relatively mild reduced amplitude. Repetitive nerve stimulation can either be normal or demonstrate relatively modest increments in amplitude.

Increased distal motor latencies, absent F wave, and decreased median with normal sural sensory conduction velocity are the characteristic EMG findings in Guillain-Barré syndrome. Continuous discharges of normal motor units are characteristic of tetanus toxin. Progressive reduction in amplitude with repetitive motor nerve stimulation is typical for myasthenia gravis. Reduced compound muscle action potential amplitude, severe and widespread nerve conduction slowing, and no evidence

of conduction block are suggestive of Charcot-Marie-Tooth disease type 1 (demyelinating). Diffuse and symmetric findings throughout the peripheral nervous system are characteristic of inherited diseases as opposed to the patchy findings that can occur in acquired peripheral nerve disorders.

9. **D.** Benzodiazepines result in a depressant action on the CNS by binding to specific receptors on GABA inhibitory systems. They act in concert with GABA to open chloride ion channels and hyperpolarize postsynaptic neurons and reduces their firing rate. Primary sites of action are cerebral cortex and limbic system.

Flumazenil rapidly but briefly reverses signs and symptoms of benzodiazepine overdose by binding to CNS diazepine receptors and blocking activation of inhibitory GABAergic synapses. A trial of flumazenil may be diagnostically useful in cases of coma of unknown etiology and hepatic encephalopathy.

10. **B.** Cocaine causes acute coronary syndromes, hypertensive crisis, seizures, rhabdomyolysis, intracranial hemorrhage, pneumomediastinum, and respiratory failure. In general, amphetamines exert their toxicity via CNS stimulation, peripheral release of catecholamines, inhibition of reuptake of catecholamines, or inhibition of monoamine oxidase. In particular, cocaine acts by blocking the presynaptic reuptake of biogenic amines, thus producing vasoconstriction, hypertension, and tachycardia and predisposing to seizure. Cocaine use also causes release of endogenous monoamines. The sympathomimetic effects contribute to the major toxicities of cocaine use. Cocaine has the following effects:

- Inhibition of the presynaptic reuptake of biogenic amines, such as norepinephrine, dopamine, and serotonin, throughout the body
- Analgesic effects due to voltage-gated sodium channel blockage
- Vasoconstrictive effect in most part due to the stimulation of α-adrenergic receptors in arterial smooth muscle cells

First-line therapy for the hypertensive crisis should be benzodiazepines. Refractory patients should receive an α-adrenergic antagonist. β-blocking antihypertensive drugs should be avoided in patients with cocaine-induced hypertensive crisis due to the theoretical risk of unopposed α-adrenergic stimulation that can lead to coronary artery vasoconstriction and exacerbate systemic hypertension.

11. **A.** Spontaneous subarachnoid or intracerebral hemorrhage and cerebral infarction could result from acute hypertension induced by the sympathomimetic actions of cocaine, and the incidence of vascular malformations appears to be high in those with cerebral hemorrhage. Cocaine and amphetamine use is associated with cerebral vasculopathy and an increased risk of stroke. The pathogenesis of amphetamine-associated vasculopathy has been reported as either vasospasm or arteritis, although the exact pathogenesis of the vascular lesions is unknown. Cocaine's major metabolites have been found to be associated with delayed or recurrent coronary or cerebral vasoconstriction. Thrombogenic effects are thought to be related to increase in plasminogen activator inhibitor activity, platelet count, platelet activation, and platelet aggregate, and possibly enhanced by an inflammatory state characterized by elevated C-reactive protein, von Willebrand factor, and fibrinogen concentrations. Cocaine has been associated with acute rhabdomyolysis with acute renal failure, liver dysfunction, and disseminated intravascular coagulation. Abstinence causes insomnia, restlessness, anorexia, and depression.

12. **A.** This patient has tetanus, caused by the anaerobic, spore-forming rod *Clostridium tetani.* Spores can remain dormant for months to years, but when introduced into a wound, they are converted into the vegetative form, which produces the exotoxin tetanospasmin. The toxin is disseminated systemically via blood or lymphatics; however, in local tetanus, the likely mode of spread to the CNS is by retrograde axonal transport. The toxin ascends via the peripheral nerves in the axis cylinders or the perineural sheaths. The tetanus toxin is a zinc-dependent protease that blocks neurotransmitter release. This is done by preventing the normal exocytosis of neurotransmitters via cleavage of synaptic vesicle surface proteins. The toxin thus interferes with the function of the reflex arc by blockade of mainly GABA-inhibitory transmitters at the presynaptic sites. There is a failure of

inhibition with a resulting increase in activation of the neurons that innervate muscles.

13. **E.** Tetanus carries an approximately 50% risk of mortality. Initial treatment includes a single dose of antitoxin with a 10-day course of penicillin, metronidazole, or tetracycline. Survival hinges on supportive care in a critical care setting, which may be necessary for weeks. Most patients with recurrent generalized tonic spasms will require tracheostomy. Support includes judicious use of sedation, preferably benzodiazepines for both sedation and muscle relaxation. Intrathecal baclofen and continuous atropine infusions can also be used in severe cases. Intramuscular botulinum toxin may be used for trismus and local spasm. The patient may even need to be paralyzed to control tetanic paroxysms.

14. **D.** Most carbon monoxide (CO) poisonings are due to smoke exposure, poorly ventilated charcoal or gas heaters, and automobile exhaust. It can present with myocardial infarction, arrhythmias, mental status changes, headache, and generalized weakness. Pulse oximetry overestimates oxyhemoglobin by the amount of carboxyhemoglobin present. Therefore, the oxygen saturation measured by pulse oximetry may be normal despite elevated carboxyhemoglobin. CO has an extreme affinity for hemoglobin—up to 200 to 250 times greater affinity than oxygen. This drastically reduces the oxygen content of blood and subjects the brain to prolonged hypoxia and acidosis. The CO causes a leftward shift of the oxyhemoglobin dissociation curve, decreasing the offloading of oxygen from hemoglobin to tissue. Cardiac toxicity and hypotension generally follow. Delayed neurologic deterioration 1 to 3 weeks after CO exposure occurs more frequently than with other form of cerebral hypoxia. There has been no proven relationship between the amount of CO concentrations and degree of injury. Discrete lesions centered in the globus pallidus bilaterally and occasional in the inner portion of the putamen are characteristic, but similar findings can be seen in other forms of anoxia. The initial treatment is with inspired oxygen as well as hyperbaric oxygen. This greatly reduces the half-life of CO.

15. **A.** This patient has serotonin syndrome. The inhibition of serotine reuptake causes increased cardiovascular and neurologic complications related

to catecholamine excess, such as seizures, hypertension, and various tachydysrhythmias. This is thought to be primarily due to the activation of the 5-HT2A receptor along with the modulatory function of the 5-HT1A receptor, which increases intrasynaptic concentrations of serotonin. Treatment is with cyproheptadine, which has antagonist properties at 5-HT2A receptors.

Supportive care in the intensive care unit is also recommended. The presence of hyperthermia is particularly concerning and is likely attributed to the loss of neuromuscular control. Patients should be sedated, and if this is unsuccessful, neuromuscular blockade should be considered in the intubated patient. Use of a nondepolarizing paralytic is strongly recommended. Use of a depolarizing paralytic, such as succinylcholine, in a patient who already has some amount of rhabdomyolysis could potentially elevate plasma potassium levels to a lethal level. Phenytoin is thought to have limited benefit in toxin-induced seizures as there is no irritable focus causing the seizure, and they are instead related to diffuse neurotransmission problems. Toxin-induced seizures should instead be treated with GABAergic medications.

16. **C.** Salicylate poisoning causes respiratory alkalosis and metabolic acidosis. Urinary alkalinization enhances renal clearance of salicylates. Hypokalemia must first be corrected to succeed in urinary alkalization. Indications for hemodialysis include:

- Seizures
- Coma
- Refractory acidosis
- High serum salicylate levels

Alkalemia should be maintained in mechanically ventilated patients with salicylate poisoning. Therapeutic plasma (or urine) alkalization is achieved by administering sodium bicarbonate, which promotes diffusion of weak nonpolar acids out of the CNS and enhances urinary elimination. This has limited applicability and is generally used in cases such as salicylate poisoning, methotrexate toxicity, or phenobarbital overdose.

N-Acetylcysteine is first-line treatment for acetaminophen toxicity. Lipid emulsion therapy creates an intravascular lipid compartment such that drugs with high lipophilicity will move from the aqueous phase of plasma, where interaction with particular receptors occurs, to the lipid phase, where the drug has relatively limited ability to interact with a particular receptor.

Gastrointestinal decontamination prevents absorption of offending agent. It should consist of single-dose activated charcoal only if patients present within 1 hour after ingestion and if airway is protected.

Whole bowel irrigation with a polyethylene glycol electrolyte solution should be considered for cases involving extended-release preparations to limit prolonged or continued absorption of the drug from the gastrointestinal tract. This is now considered to be less efficacious than originally thought. The routine use of whole bowel irrigation is therefore no longer recommended.

17. **E.** This patient is suffering from cholinergic toxicity (Table 7-1). Cholinergic agents activate muscarinic acetylcholine receptors. Acetylcholine binds to and activates muscarinic and nicotinic receptors. It is regulated by acetylcholinesterase (AChE) within the synaptic cleft via hydrolyzation of the acetylcholine molecule to choline and acetic acid. AChE is inhibited by certain insecticides and results in excessive acetylcholine stimulation. This activates both muscarinic and nicotinic receptors such that the sympathomimetic system is activated and the neuromuscular junction is stimulated.

Table 7-1. Signs and Symptoms of Cholinergic Toxicity

Cholinergic toxicity: Every organ system is effected.
- **Eye:** blurred vision, and miosis.
- **Increase secretions:** lacrimation, profuse watery nasal discharge, nasal hyperemia, marked salivation, and bronchorrhea due to innervation of sweat glands by sympathetic muscarinic receptors.
- **Central nervous system:** effects of excess acetylcholine include seizures, fasciculations, and flaccid paralysis due to stimulation of the nicotinic receptors at the motor end plate.
- **Respiratory system effects (most fatal):** bronchorrhea and bronchoconstriction can lead to prolonged expiratory phase, cough, and wheezing.
- **Cardiac:** bradydysrhythmias and hypotension.
- **Gastrointestinal/urinary:** increase in gastric and intestinal motility with a relaxation of anal sphincter tone causes watery salivation and gastrointestinal hyperactivity with resultant nausea, vomiting, abdominal cramps, tenesmus, and uncontrolled defecation and involuntary urination.

First-line treatment is atropine, which acts as a muscarinic receptor antagonist. Tachycardia is not a contraindication. Pralidoxime chloride is used to treat organophosphate poisoned patients via reactivation of AChE by exerting a nucleophilic attack that splits the organophosphate from the AChE, leaving the regenerated enzyme. Empiric treatment with benzodiazepines is also recommended given high risk of seizures.

18. **D.** This patient is suffering from alcohol withdrawal syndrome (AWS). Benzodiazepines are currently the pharmacologic agents of choice for the treatment of AWS. Benzodiazepines act by binding to specific receptors on GABA inhibitory systems. They act in concert with GABA to open chloride ion channels and hyperpolarize postsynaptic neurons and reduces their firing rate.

  The sedative chloral hydrate was used in the late 1800s to control the agitation and signs and symptoms of AWS. This is rapidly reduced to trichloroethanol, which acts on GABA$_A$ receptors.

Paraldehyde was used starting around the 1890s and was standard of care until the 1970s. Barbiturates act as GABA$_A$ receptor agonists. Flumazenil is the antidote to benzodiazepine overdose and acts by binding to CNS diazepine receptors and blocking activation of inhibitory GABAergic synapses.

19. **D.** The low pH and bicarbonate indicate a metabolic acidosis. The calculated anion gap is 28 (above the normal gap of 8-12); therefore, there is an anion gap acidosis. Metabolic acidosis with an elevated anion gap is a hallmark of toxic alcohol poisoning. The toxic alcohol is metabolized to toxic organic acids that accumulate because there is no natural metabolic pathway of elimination. The differential diagnosis of metabolic acidosis with increase in the anion gap includes:

  - Increase in unmeasured endogenous (eg, lactate) anions
  - Increase in exogenous (eg, salicylate) anions

20. **C.** This patient is suffering from methanol poisoning (Table 7-2).

Table 7-2. Methanol, Ethylene Glycol, and Isopropanol Toxicities

Methanol Poisoning	Ethylene Glycol Poisoning	Isopropanol Poisoning
Known as wood alcohol, this is a commonly used organic solvent	Used primarily in antifreeze	Used in rubbing alcohol
Mechanism:	**Mechanism:**	**Mechanism:**
Methanol → metabolized to formaldehyde (by alcohol dehydrogenase) → then rapidly to formic acid (by formaldehyde dehydrogenase) in the liver.	It forms crystals in the renal tubule. These metabolites might also cause systemic hypocalcemia, resulting in QT prolongation.	It is rapidly absorbed, and approximately 80% is metabolized to acetone by alcohol dehydrogenase. There is no organic acid metabolite and thus no metabolic acidosis. **Ketosis without acidosis is considered diagnostic.**
The metabolite format is a mitochondrial toxin that inhibits cytochrome oxidase, which interferes with oxidative phosphorylation.		Both isopropanol and acetone cause central nervous system (CNS) depression.
Symptoms:	**Symptoms:**	**Symptoms:**
Ocular toxicity	In the CNS can cause cerebral edema and even intracerebral hemorrhage in the globus pallidus and peripheral polyradiculoneuropathy in the peripheral nervous system.	Ingestion can lead to hemorrhagic gastritis. Isopropyl alcohol is metabolized to acetone, and there is no organic acid metabolite and thus no metabolic acidosis. Ketosis without acidosis is considered diagnostic.
Neurons in the basal ganglia are particularly susceptible to methanol toxicity; imaging findings of bilateral basal ganglia lesions in the context of absent hypoxia, hypotension, or carbon monoxide exposure suggest a direct toxic mechanism.	Ethylene glycol can cause a nongap acidosis, often concurrently with anion gap acidosis.	
Renal failure	It also causes nephrotoxicity due to the metabolites.	

Methanol, ethylene glycol, and isopropanol will all induce an osmolar gap. Serum osmolarity (OsmC) can be estimated clinically by equations involving the patient's serum glucose, sodium, and urea nitrogen.

Bath salts are entirely synthetic cathinones, primarily β-ketone amphetamine analogs. Cathinone is a naturally occurring amphetamine analog found in the "khat" plant. Synthetic cannabinoids are also known as spice or K2. These agents bind even more avidly to cannabinoid receptors and have side effects of agitation, delusions, and paranoia. Treatment is with diazepines and haloperidol, often to no avail.

21. **A.** Hemodialysis (HD) is the most effective way to remove methanol from the body. HD is indicated in the setting of severe methanol toxicity, as demonstrated by metabolic acidosis and vision loss. HD works by diffusion taking toxins from high concentration to low concentration and is thus best suited for hydrophilic agents that have a small volume of distribution. Substances with low molecular weight and low protein binding are also more amenable to hemodialysis.

Treatment also includes blocking of metabolism via competitive inhibition of alcohol dehydrogenase (ADH) in order to limit the production of the toxic metabolites. This is done by either ethanol infusion or fomepizole administration. Management in an intensive care unit is recommended. If intubated, hyperventilation should be maintained to mimic the body's compensatory response. Monitoring includes methanol levels (if available), osmolar gap, anion gap, serum creatinine, and ethanol level (if used).

Lipid emulsion therapy creates an intravascular lipid compartment such that drugs with high lipophilicity will move from the aqueous phase of plasma, where interaction with particular receptors occurs, to the lipid phase, where the drug has relatively limited ability to interact with a particular receptor.

Therapeutic plasma (or urine) alkalization involves sodium bicarbonate administration in order to alkalize the serum and obtain ion trapping into the urine in order to enhance elimination of nonpolar weak acids. This has limited applicability and is generally used in cases such as salicylate poisoning, methotrexate toxicity, or phenobarbital overdose.

Gastrointestinal decontamination prevents absorption of the offending agent. It should consist of single-dose activated charcoal only if patients present within 1 hour after ingestion and if the airway is protected.

Whole bowel irrigation with a polyethylene glycol electrolyte solution should be considered for cases involving extended-release preparations to limit prolonged or continued absorption of the drug from the gastrointestinal tract. However, this is now considered to be less efficacious than originally thought.

REFERENCES

Boyer EW. Management of opioid analgesic overdose. *N Engl J Med.* 2012;367:146-155.

Boyer EW, Shannon M. The serotonin syndrome. *N Engl J Med.* 2005;352:1112-1120.

Carlson RW, Kumar NN, Wong-Mckinstry E, et al. Alcohol withdrawal syndrome. *Crit Care Clin.* 2012;28:549-585.

Caroff SN, Rosenberg H, Mann SC, et al. Neuroleptic malignant syndrome in the critical care unit. *Crit Care Med.* 2002;30:2609.

Cassidy S, Henry J. Fatal toxicity of antidepressant drugs in overdose. *Br Med J (Clin Res Ed).* 1987;295:1021-1024.

Choi IS. Delayed neurologic sequelae in carbon monoxide intoxication. *Arch Neurol.* 1983;40:433.

Coburn RF. Endogenous carbon monoxide production. *N Engl J Med.* 1970;282:207-209.

Desai T, Sudhalkar A, Vyas U, Khamar B. Methanol poisoning: predictors of visual outcomes. *JAMA Ophthalmol.* 2013; 131:358-364.

Donofrio PD, Albers JW. AAEM minimonograph #34: polyneuropathy: classification by nerve conduction studies and electromyography. *Muscle Nerve.* 1990;13:889-903.

Farrar JJ, Yen LM, Cook T, et al. Tetanus. *J Neurol Neurosurg Psychiatry.* 2000;69:292-301.

Grossman RA, Hamilton RW, Morse BM, et al. Nontraumatic rhabdomyolysis and acute renal failure. *N Engl J Med.* 1974;291:807-811.

Harrington H, Heller HA, Dawson D, Caplan L, Rumbaugh C. Intracerebral hemorrhage and oral amphetamine. *Arch Neurol.* 1983;40:503-507.

Hedge MW. Miscellaneous central nervous system intoxicants. *Crit Care Clin.* 2012;28:587-600.

Hilberg T, Bugge A, Beylich KM, Ingum J, Bjørneboe A, Mørland J. An animal model of postmortem amitriptyline redistribution. *J Forensic Sci.* 1993;38:81-90.

Hoffman JR, Votey SR, Bayer M, Silver L. Effect of hypertonic sodium bicarbonate in the treatment of moderate-to-severe cyclic antidepressant overdose. *Am J Emerg Med.* 1993;11:336-341.

Holstege CP, Borek HA. Toxidromes. *Crit Care Clin.* 2012;28:479-498.

Ito T, Suzuki T, Wellman SE, Ho IK. Pharmacology of barbiturate tolerance/dependence: GABAA receptors and molecular aspects. *Life Sci.* 1996;59:169-195.

Jammalamadaka D, Raissi S. Ethylene glycol, methanol and isopropyl alcohol intoxication. *Am J Med Sci.* 2010;339: 276-281.

Kass-Hout T, Kass-Hout O, Darkhabani MZ, Mokin M, Mehta B, Radovic V. "Chasing the dragon": heroin-associated spongiform leukoencephalopathy. *J Med Toxicol.* 2011;7:240-242.

Khullar V, Jain A, Sattari M. Emergence of new classes of recreational drugs-synthetic cannabinoids and cathinones. *J Gen Intern Med.* 2014;29:1200-1204.

Krisanda TJ. Flumazenil: an antidote for benzodiazepine toxicity. *Am Fam Physician.* 1993;47:891-895.

Lank PM, Corbridge T, Murray PT. Toxicology in adults. In: Hall JB, Schmidt GA, Kress JP, eds. *Principles of Critical Care.* 4th ed. New York, NY: McGraw-Hill Education; 2015.

Levenson JL. Neuroleptic malignanty syndrome. *Am J Psychiatry.* 1985;142:1137-1145.

Liebelt EL, Francis PD, Woolf AD. ECG lead aVR versus QRS interval in predicting seizures and arrhythmias in acute tricyclic antidepressant toxicity. *Ann Emerg Med.* 1995;26:195-201.

Melli G, Chaudhry V, Cornblath DR. Rhabdomyolosysi: an evaluation of 475 hospitalized patients. *Medicine (Baltimore).* 2005;84:377-385.

Mills KC. Cyclic antidepressants. In: *Critical Care Toxicology: Diagnosis and Management of the Critically Poisoned Patient.* Philadelphia, PA: Elsevier Mosby; 2017:475-484.

Modi S, Dharaiya D, Schultz L, et al. Neuroleptic malignant syndrome: complications, outcomes, and mortality. *Neurocrit Care.* 2016;24:97-103.

Mordel A, Winkler E, Almog S, Tirosh M, Ezra D. Seizures after flumazenil administration in a case of combined benzodiazepine and tricyclic antidepressant overdose. *Crit Care Med.* 1992;20:1733-1734.

Myers RA, Snyder SK, Emhoff TA. Subacute sequelae of carbon monoxide poisoning. *Ann Emerg Med.* 1985;14:1163-1167.

Nelson LS, Lewin NA, Howland MA, Hoffman RS, Goldfrank LR, Flomenbaum NR. Principles of managing the acutely poisoned or overdosed patient. In: Brent J, Burkhart K, Dargan P, et al, eds. *Critical Care Toxicology: Diagnosis and Management of the Critically Poisoned Patient.* Philadelphia, PA: Elsevier Mosby; 2005:37-44.

Okada Y, Tyuma I, Ueda Y, Sugimoto T. Effect of carbon monoxide on equilibrium between oxygen and hemoglobin. *Am J Physiol.* 1976;230:471-475.

Padua L, Aprile I, Monaco ML, et al. Neurophysiological assessment in the diagnosis of botulism: usefulness of single-fiber EMG. *Muscle Nerve.* 1999;22:1388-1392.

Roberts DM, Buckley NA. Enhanced elimination in acute barbiturate poisoning: a systematic review. *Clin Toxicol (Phila).* 2011;49:2-12.

Ropper AH, Samuels MA, Klein JP. *Adam's and Victor's Principles of Neurology.* 10th ed. New York, NY: McGraw-Hill Education; 2014.

Roth D, Alarcón FJ, Fernandez JA, Preston RA, Bourgoignie JJ. Acute rhabdomyolysis associated with cocaine intoxication. *N Engl J Med.* 1988;319:673-677.

Ryan A, Molloy FM, Farrell MA, Hutchinson M. Fatal toxic leukoencephalopathy: clinical, radiological, and necropsy findings in two patients. *J Neurol Neurosurg Psychiatry.* 2005;76:1014-1016.

Schep LJ, Knudsen K, Slaughter RJ, Vale JA, Megarbane B. The clinical toxicology of gamma-hydroxybutyrate, gamma-butyrolactone and 1,4-butanediol. *Clin Toxicol (Phila).* 2012;50:458-470.

Sobel J. Botulism. *Clin Infect Dis.* 2005;41:1167-1173.

Stalberg E. Clinical electrophysiology in myasthenia gravis. *J Neurol Neurosurg Psychiatry.* 1980;43:622-633.

Sullivan EV, Pfefferbaum A. Neuroimaging of the Wernicke-Korsakoff syndrome. *Alcohol Alcohol.* 2009;44:155-165.

Tan TP, Algra PR, Valk J, Wolters EC. Toxic leukoencephalopathy after inhalation of poisoned heroin: MR findings. *AJNR Am J Neuroradiol.* 1994;15:175-178.

Thom SR, Keim LW. Carbon monoxide poisoning: a review epidemiology, pathophysiology, clinical findings, and treatment options including hyperbaric oxygen therapy. *J Toxicol Clin Toxicol.* 1989;27:141-156.

Tomaszewski C. Carbon monoxide. In: Brent J, Burkhart K, Dargan P, et al, eds. *Critical Care Toxicology: Diagnosis and Management of the Critically Poisoned Patient.* Philadelphia, PA: Elsevier Mosby; 2005:1658-1720.

Weaver LK. Clinical practice. Carbon monoxide poisoning. *N Engl J Med.* 2009;360:1217-1225.

Weaver LK. Hyperbaric oxygen in the critically ill. *Crit Care Med.* 2011;39:1784-1791.

Weiner SW. Toxic alcohols. In: Brent J, Burkhart K, Dargan P, et al, eds. *Critical Care Toxicology: Diagnosis and Management of the Critically Poisoned Patient.* Philadelphia, PA: Elsevier Mosby; 2005:1400-1422.

Wolters EC, van Wijngaarden GK, Stam FC, et al. Leucoencephalopathy after inhaling "heroin" pyrolysate. *Lancet.* 1982;2:1233-1237.

Yousry TA, Pelletier D, Cadavid D, et al. Magnetic resonance imaging pattern in natalizumab-associated progressive multifocal leukoencephalopathy. *Ann Neurol.* 2012;72:779-787.

Zimmerman JL. Cocaine intoxication. *Crit Care Clin.* 2012;28:517-526.

Questions

1. A 74-year-old man with no known history has had progressive dysphagia and cognitive decline over the past 8 weeks. He is brought to the emergency department (ED) with acute psychosis after he assaulted his family members and accused them of poisoning him. On examination, his blood pressure is 196/85, heart rate is 120 bpm, respiratory rate is 26 breaths/min, and pulse oximetry of 94%. Limited neurologic examination reveals symmetric/reactive pupils bilaterally, incomprehensible speech, prominent dysarthria, increased tone in all 4 extremities but relatively symmetric strength, brisk reflexes, and upgoing plantar reflex bilaterally.

   During the evaluation, the patient also exhibits frequent involuntarily jerking of his extremities, which is exaggerated when he is startled. A magnetic resonance imaging (MRI) scan is obtained, and diffusion-weighted imaging (DWI) sequence reveals the findings shown in the figure below. Despite extensive lab workup, toxicology, and several lumbar punctures including analysis for cerebrospinal fluid (CSF) 14-3-3 protein, no conclusive diagnosis is found. Unfortunately the patient's symptoms continue to progress and he dies 6 weeks later. What is the most likely diagnosis in this patient?

   A. Intravascular central nervous system (CNS) lymphoma

   B. Anti-Hu encephalomyelitis

   C. Hashimoto encephalopathy

   D. Creutzfeldt-Jacob disease

   E. Acute ischemic stroke

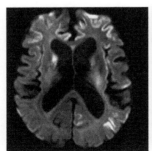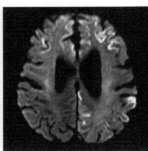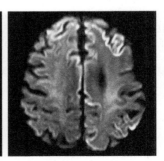

MRI brain, sequential axial diffusion weighted images.

2. A previously healthy 58-year-old man presents with progressive memory loss, intermittent vertigo, and difficulty ambulating at night over the past 3 weeks. He takes no medication and has no prior significant medical issues. On examination, he appears older than stated age. He is alert and oriented to person, place, and year but not month. On memory testing, he has difficulty with recall. Strength and sensory examination are unremarkable. He is diffusely hyperreflexic and is unable to ambulate secondary to ataxia. An MRI of the brain with and without gadolinium contrast is shown below. Despite treatment, the patient continued to progress, and he dies approximately 6 months later. What is the most likely diagnosis?

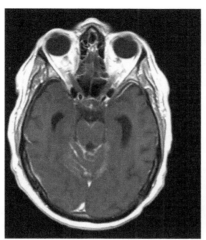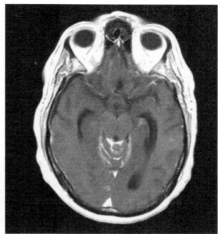

Magnetic resonance imaging of the brain with contrast: T1 postcontrast sequence (axial cross-section).

A. Paraneoplastic syndrome

B. Acute bacterial meningitis

C. Huntington disease

D. Miller Fisher syndrome

E. Wilson disease

3. A 68-year-old man with a past medical history of hypertension and hyperlipidemia presents with rapidly progressive memory changes and headache over the past 6 months. He is admitted to the hospital for further evaluation. Neurologic evaluation reveals a disheveled man oriented to self only with profound inattentiveness who is unable to name the 3 objects presented to him. Cranial nerve, motor, and sensory examinations are normal. Deep tendon reflexes are 3+/4 throughout. A brain MRI (see below) is obtained (A: T2 fluid-attenuated inversion recovery [FLAIR], B: susceptibility weighted imaging [SWI]), whereas T1 postgadolinium scan reveals no enhancement (not shown). Standard CSF testing is unremarkable, and therefore, a brain biopsy is obtained. This reveals reactive gliosis with numerous macrophages in the white matter. Immunohistochemical stain demonstrates amyloid beta in the wall of a small arteriole and multiple capillaries. A special stain is obtained and, when viewed under polarized light, reveals green birefringence. After treatment with high-dose steroids, his memory dramatically improves, corresponding to regression of T2-flair hyperintensities. What is the most likely diagnosis?

A. CNS lymphoma
B. Herpes encephalitis
C. Cerebral amyloid angiopathy–related inflammation
D. Neurosyphilis
E. McLeod syndrome

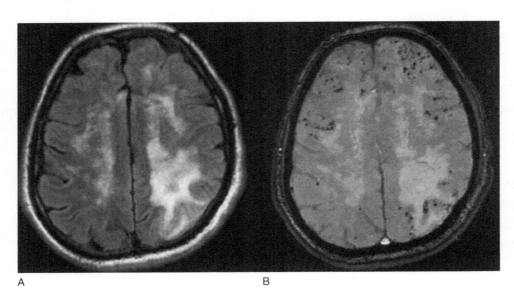

MRI brain, left panel shows axial FLAIR sequence, right panel shows SWI sequence.

4. A 47-year-old man with a past medical history of chronic tobacco use (20 pack-years), hypertension, hyperlipidemia, and chronic obstructive pulmonary disease (COPD) presents with overt functional decline and progressive confusion over the course of 2 weeks. On your examination, he is disoriented and inattentive, with markedly impaired short-term memory, difficulty following complex commands, and poor insight into his condition. Multiple nonblanching skin lesions are observed in his lower extremities. Contrast-enhanced cranial MRI reveals bihemispheric watershed pattern of cerebral infarction (see below). Computed tomography (CT) angiography of the head and neck and digital subtraction angiography (DSA) are unremarkable. Cardiac workup with a transthoracic echocardiogram, transesophageal echocardiogram, and telemetry monitoring is unremarkable. Lab workup, however, is notable for white blood cell (WBC) count of 18,000, with 12% lymphocytes and 57% eosinophils. The patient is treated with high-dose steroids, hydroxyurea, and imatinib with eventual resolution of his symptoms. What is the most likely diagnosis?

A. Hypereosinophilic syndrome
B. Bilateral critical carotid stenosis
C. Acute multiple sclerosis episode
D. Primary CNS angiitis (vasculitis)
E. Reversible cerebral vasoconstriction syndrome (RCVS)

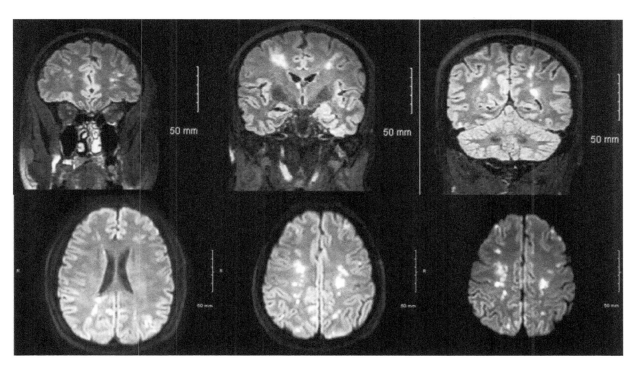

MRI brain, top row shows sequential coronal FLAIR images. Bottom row shows sequential axial FLAIR images.

5. A 75-year-old woman with a long-standing history of rheumatoid arthritis maintained on long-term methotrexate and adalimumab presented with progressive left hemiplegia and global functional decline over the course of 3 months. Brain MRI was obtained on presentation (see below), revealing bilateral, asymmetric (right > left), nonenhancing multifocal areas of periventricular and subcortical white matter confluent lesions with lack of mass effect. Despite extensive workup (including lumbar puncture × 2), the patient's condition continued to progress, and she died 2 months later. A brain autopsy revealed bizarre reactive astrocytes with enlarged nuclei and prominent nucleoli and perivascular cuffing by lymphocytes. Immunohistochemistry using target antibody against SV-40 was positive. What is the most likely diagnosis?

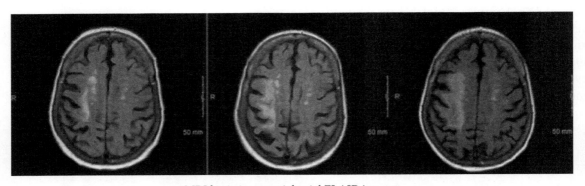

MRI brain, sequential axial FLAIR images.

A. Glioblastoma multiforme

B. Tumefactive-variant multiple sclerosis (MS)

C. Progressive multifocal leukoencephalopathy (PML)

D. Subacute ischemic stroke

E. Brain abscess secondary to immunocompromise

6. A 55-year-old right-handed man with no prior medical history developed new-onset headaches, nausea, and vomiting. Further history reveals that the patient has had subacute memory decline and intermittent agitation over the past few weeks. In the ED, an MRI of the brain with and without contrast was obtained and was unremarkable. A lumbar puncture was obtained and revealed normal opening pressure. CSF analysis revealed 18 WBCs with 98% lymphocytes, normal glucose, normal red blood cells (RBC), and normal protein. CSF cytology and flow cytometry were negative. Additional lab workup revealed positive thyroperoxidase antibody and positive antithyroglobulin antibody but normal thyroid function tests. Paraneoplastic panel was negative. The patient was initially started on 1 specific medication, which led to dramatic improvement of his symptoms and remission at 6, 12, and 18 months of follow-up. What is the most likely medication that was used?

A. Cyclophosphamide

B. Imatinib

C. Rituximab

D. High-dose steroids

E. Temozolomide

7. An 87-year-old man from Connecticut with a past medical history of hypertension presented with 1 week of fatigue, confusion, and anorexia. Following admission to the hospital, his mentation rapidly declined, necessitating intubation. An MRI of the brain with and without contrast was obtained and is shown below (left: T1 postgadolinium; right: T2-FLAIR). A lumbar puncture was obtained and revealed normal opening pressure. CSF analysis revealed protein of 140 mg/dL, glucose of 60 mg/dL, 1 RBC, and 60 nucleated cells with 80% lymphocytes,10% monocytes, and 10% macrophages. CSF herpes simplex virus (HSV) I/II polymerase chain reaction (PCR) and varicella-zoster virus (VZV) PCR were negative. Unfortunately, the patient's condition continued to worsen, and by day 4 of admission, the patient exhibited lack of brainstem reflexes. Care was withdrawn on day 13, and the patient died. What is the most likely diagnosis?

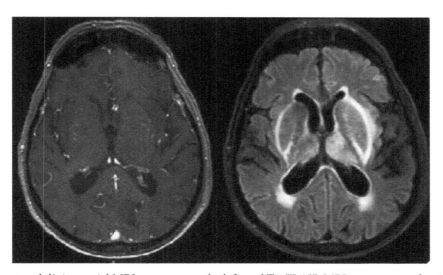

T1 post-gadolinium axial MRI sequence on the left, and T2-FLAIR MRI sequence on the right.

A. Nervous system Lyme disease
B. HSV encephalitis
C. Eastern equine encephalitis (EEE)
D. Human immunodeficiency virus (HIV)-associated dementia
E. Acute CNS lymphoma

8. A 28-year-old African American woman with unremarkable history presents with prominent acute psychiatric manifestation over the course of 3 days, including visual and auditory hallucination, delusions, and insomnia. During the evaluation in the ED, she has numerous seizures. After stabilization, you obtain an MRI brain without contrast, which reveals the findings shown below (T2-FLAIR imaging). After successful treatment, the patient makes a full recovery. What is the most likely diagnosis?

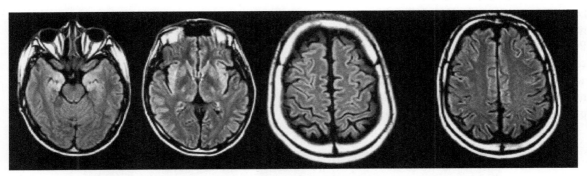

Sequential axial FLAIR brain MRI images.

A. Metastatic CNS disease
B. Anti-NMDA (*N*-methyl-D-aspartate) receptor encephalitis
C. Acute alcohol intoxication
D. Anti-IgLON5 encephalopathy
E. CNS tuberculosis

9. A previously healthy 43-year-old woman is brought emergently to the ED because "she has not been acting right for the past 3 days." Her symptoms started with a high-grade fever, productive cough, and nausea. On examination, she is lethargic and requires constant stimulation to maintain wakefulness. Pupils are sluggish but reactive to light. She has minimal verbal output and intermittently utters unintelligible words. She does not follow any commands. She has 3+/4 deep tendon reflexes. Vitals reveal a respiratory rate of 28 breaths/min, blood pressure of 195/100 mm Hg, heart rate of 47 bpm, temperature of 38.9°C, and pulse oximetry of 90% on 4-L nasal cannula. Viral swab (pulmonary) returns positive with influenza virus PCR (H1N1 strain). A CT of the head without contrast is obtained and is read as unremarkable (not shown here). A chest x-ray reveals diffuse pulmonary infiltrates. The decision is made to intubate given mental status and hypoxia. She is initially sedated for "comfort." You are called approximately 6 hours into her intensive care unit admission. Off-sedation exam (>1 hour) reveals 5-mm pupils that are minimally reactive, negative oculocephalic reflex, negative corneals bilaterally, negative gag/cough reflex, and extensor motor posturing in all 4 extremities. Repeat CT of the head without contrast is obtained (shown below). What is the most likely diagnosis?

A. Status epilepticus

B. Guillain-Barré syndrome

C. Influenza-related acute necrotizing encephalitis with malignant cerebral edema

D. Posterior reversible encephalopathy syndrome (PRES)

E. Anoxic brain injury

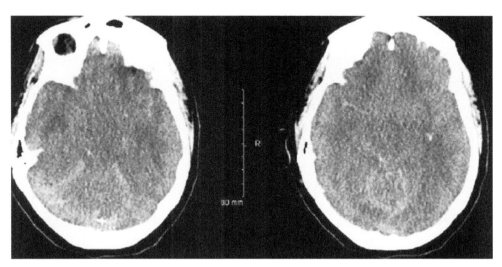

Non-contrast axial head CT.

10. A 51-year-old woman who recently underwent arthroscopic meniscectomy was admitted for a decline in mental status the day after surgery and was intubated for presumed opiate-induced respiratory suppression. Exam off sedation revealed intermittent ability to follow simple commands but not complex commands. She had grossly symmetric strength in all extremities but mildly increased tone. She had brisk reflexes with bilateral upgoing plantar reflexes. An MRI of the brain was obtained 24 hours after her admission and read as normal (not shown). Prolonged electroencephalography (EEG) was obtained and interpreted as mild diffuse slowing. Following stabilization, she was discharged home with near-complete return to preadmission baseline. She was subsequently readmitted approximately 4 weeks after her discharge with failure to thrive, increased tone in all extremities, and confusion. Exam revealed a disheveled woman, inability to follow any commands, unintelligible words, symmetric strength but increased tone in all 4 extremities, brisk reflexes, and upgoing plantar reflexes bilaterally. MRI of the brain with and without contrast was obtained and is shown below. A lumbar puncture was obtained and was nonrevealing. EEG was reported as diffusely slowing. Unfortunately, she continued to decline, and care was withdrawn approximately 3 weeks into her admission. An autopsy was obtained and confirmed her diagnosis. What is the most likely cause of her demise?

A. Delayed post-hypoxic leukoencephalopathy (DPHL)

B. Acute ischemic stroke

C. Alzheimer dementia

D. Acute bacterial meningitis

E. Nonconvulsive status epilepticus

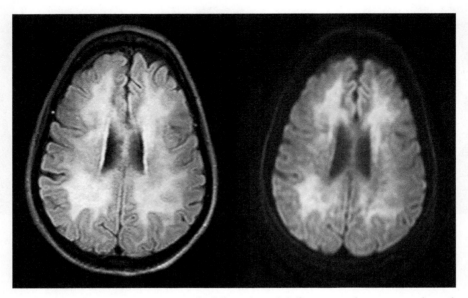

MRI brain, axial FLAIR sequence on the left, and axial diffusion weight image on the right.

11. A 45-year-old man with a long-standing history of alcoholism presents to the ED with acute confusion. On presentation to the ED, his blood pressure is 95/60 mm Hg, heart rate is 120 bpm, respiratory rate is 26 breaths/min, and oxygen saturation is 95%. Ethanol level is <0.1 mg/dL (reference, <0.1 mg/dL), and toxicology is negative. Labs reveal a sodium value of 98 mEq/L. His serum sodium 1 month ago taken at an ED visit for acute alcohol intoxication was 109 mEq/L. A CT of the head without contrast is unremarkable (not shown here). The patient is admitted to the stepdown unit for management of profound hyponatremia. Three days into his admission, you are called to evaluate this patient because he has developed acute-onset quadriparesis and lethargy. Repeat CT of the head without contrast is obtained and unremarkable. Lab workup reveals a serum sodium value of 144 mEq/L, whereas the serum sodium value on the preceding day was 139 mEq/L. What is the next most appropriate step in the management of this patient?

A. Corticosteroids

B. Lowering serum sodium to ~120 mEq/L

C. 1.9% hypertonic saline

D. Plasmapharesis

E. Myoinositol

Answers and Explanations

1. **D.** This patient presents with rapidly progressive neurobehavioral symptoms, a hallmark of Creutzfeldt-Jacob disease (CJD). Rapidly progressive mental deterioration and "startle myoclonus" as exhibited in this patient are 2 cardinal clinical features in CJD. In addition, the MRI reveals restricted cortical diffusion, which, although not specific, is classical for CJD in conjunction with the current clinical picture. CSF 14-3-3 is an adjunctive lab test but is neither specific nor sensitive, with numerous false-positive CSF 14-3-3 results reported in other neurologic disorders. A recent assay (RT-QuIC) has been proposed as a sensitive diagnostic test in CJD, with sensitivity and specificity of 85% to 87% and 99% to 100%, respectively. Unfortunately, there is no treatment for CJD, which is uniformly fatal but with a varied course of weeks to months.

    Choice B is incorrect. Paraneoplastic CNS disorder is an umbrella term for various autoimmune neurologic disorders. Anti-Hu is one of many of the known paraneoplastic orders, which is often multifocal affecting the temporal lobes, brainstem, cerebellum, dorsal roots and autonomic system. See Table 8-1. It is most often found in conjunction with small-cell lung carcinoma. However, even in its most aggressive form, survival is typically months to years. Choice C is incorrect since Hashimoto encephalopathy generally has a more favorable prognosis, and symptoms progress very slowly. Choice A is incorrect as intravascular lymphoma should not present with myoclonus; in addition, the MRI findings and the clinical course (along with CSF findings) in this patient are inconsistent with that diagnosis. There is no evidence of focal neurologic deficits, or MRI findings to suggest acute ischemic stroke which usually is limited to arterial territories. In this case, patient's multifocal T2/fluid-attenuated inversion recovery [FLAIR] hyperintensities not restricted to specific vascular territories.

2. **A.** This patient presents with rapidly progressive neurologic symptoms and an MRI revealing diffuse enhancement throughout the midbrain and brainstem. The most likely diagnosis is a paraneoplastic cerebellar degeneration syndrome. Patients with this disorder typically present with cerebellar signs (such as nausea, vertigo, ataxia, dysarthria, and dysphagia) that typically progress over weeks to months. In roughly two-thirds of patients, no cancer is found at the time of diagnosis. Survival varies but is estimated at a median of 10 to 13 months. Choice B, acute meningitis, is incorrect, as this would present over a much shorter time period (hours to days). Although there is noted pachymeningeal enhancement in the MRI, the clinical hallmarks are incompatible with acute bacterial meningitis, which carries substantial mortality and morbidity if untreated. Choice C is incorrect. Huntington disease is an inherited progressive neurodegenerative disorder characterized by choreiform movement, psychiatric problems, and dementia. Choice D is incorrect, as Miller Fisher syndrome is an acute neuropathy characterized by acute ataxia, diplopia, and muscle weakness and areflexia. Wilson disease (choice E) is incorrect, primarily because Wilson disease presents with structural changes in the basal ganglia (without enhancement). However, Wilson disease does present with some similar clinical manifestations, such as dysarthria, gait abnormalities/ataxia, dystonia, and parkinsonism.

3. **C.** Cerebral amyloid angiopathy–related inflammation is thought to represent a distinct entity from traditional cerebral amyloid angiopathy (CAA). CAA-related inflammation presents with subacute cognitive decline, seizures, headaches, and neurologic deficits. MRI of the brain will typically reveal extensive T2-FLAIR hyperintense lesions, whereas SWI will reveal classical multifocal susceptibility,

Table 8-1. Autoantibodies and Associated Clinical Symptoms

Antibody	Predominant tumor	Comments
Hu (ANNA1)	small-cell lung cancer (SCLC), thymoma	Brainstem encephalitis with bulbar signs and symptoms
Ma2(Ta)	Testicular	Limbic encephalitis, brainstem encephalitis, hypothalamic dysfunction
AMPAR	Lung carcinoma	Memory loss, encephalopathy, seizures, tendency to relapse
NMDAR	Teratoma	Limbic encephalitis, seizures, orafacial dyskinesias, autonomic instability
VGKC	Variety of cancers	Memory loss, encephalopathy, seizures
GluR3		Refractory epilepsy
Ri (ANNA2)	Breast, SCLC	Brainstem syndrome (opsoclonus, myoclonus) cerebellar syndrome, Lambert-Eaton Syndrome
CV2 (CRMP5)	SCLC, thymoma	cerebellar ataxia, movements disorders, myasthenic syndromes
Amphiphysin	Breast, SCLC	Mostly peripheral neuropathy, stiff-person syndrome, myelitis

suggestive of numerous prior microhemorrhages. The clinical course is distinct from CAA, and this entity is typically responsive to steroids, with numerous case series reporting a 66% to 75% response rate to corticosteroids.

CNS lymphoma (choice A) is in the differential diagnosis; however, CNS lymphoma typically reveals contrast enhancement on MRI. Additionally, the time course of CNS lymphoma tends to be more aggressive. Choice B, herpes encephalitis, is incorrect because typically these patients will present with more rapid progressive neurologic deficits. In addition, other common symptoms include alteration in level of consciousness and high-grade fevers. Untreated herpes encephalitis carries a high mortality, and even with treatment, morbidity is

substantial. MRI will typically reveal hemorrhagic temporal lobe lesions. Neurosyphilis, choice D, is incorrect because the imaging and clinical hallmarks are not consistent with that disease entity. Neurosyphilis can be classified into early and late forms. The early form is typically asymptomatic, and the diagnosis is based on CSF abnormalities. Symptomatic meningitis may occur years after the asymptomatic phase and may lead to hydrocephalus and/or arteritis (vasculitis). Late forms may lead to general paresis or tabes dorsalis. McLeod syndrome, choice E, is a rare X-linked disorder caused by *XK* gene mutation. These patients typically present with chorea, restlessness, and small-amplitude involuntarily movements. Brain imaging will typically reveal atrophy of the caudate nuclei.

4. **A.** This patient presents with rapidly progressive encephalopathy and a pattern of watershed infarction on MRI. Vascular imaging ruled out proximal large-vessel occlusion or other vascular lesions. Lab workup was notable for remarkably elevated eosinophils. There is a well-documented watershed pattern of cerebral infarction associated with hypereosinophilia, with a postulated mechanism related to direct endothelial injury from eosinophils due to intravascular release of toxic mediators (ribonuclease, major basic protein, and cationic protein). In hypereosinophilia, there appears to be a predilection for the watershed areas. Treatment of hypereosinophilia depends on the etiology, but in this particular case, the etiology was found to be secondary to BCR-ABL translocation, and hence, treatment with a tyrosine kinase inhibitor (imatinib) was instituted.

Choice B, bilateral carotid stenosis, is incorrect, because although watershed infarcts can be observed with critical vascular stenosis, the normal CT angiography and DSA results essentially rule out this diagnosis. Choice C, multiple sclerosis (MS), is wrong, because neither the clinical picture nor brain imaging (DWI) is suggestive of MS. MS is an autoimmune demyelinating disease of the CNS with an often relapsing-remitting or progressive course. There are no classical clinical findings in MS, but some of the common signs and symptoms include sensory loss, unilateral visual loss, acute or subacute motor weakness, gait disturbance, bladder dysfunction, and vertigo. Brain imaging will typically reveal MS plaques, characterized as hyperintense on T2 and hypointense on T1 and located in the white matter including the corpus collosum, with different degrees of enhancement depending on disease activity. Choice D, primary CNS vasculitis, is in the differential diagnosis; however, the normal DSA makes primary CNS vasculitis less likely. Finally, RCVS (choice E) is incorrect, because the clinical history does not suggest this diagnosis. RCVS is a group of disorders typically associated with severe acute-onset headaches (typically thunderclap in nature) with resultant vasoconstriction. Acute ischemic stroke, intracerebral hemorrhage, and subarachnoid hemorrhage have all been well documented with this disorder.

5. **C.** This patient presented with progressive neurologic deficits along with nonenhancing subcortical white matter changes in the setting of immunocompromised state. The brain MRI revealed typical findings of Progressive Multifocal Leukoencephalopathy (PML), including bilateral, asymmetric, nonenhancing multifocal areas of periventricular and subcortical white matter demyelination that did not conform to the typical cerebral arterial distributions. Lesions in PML lack mass effect and U-fiber involvement. Histopathologic findings as described are classical of PML, along with the SV-40 staining. Unfortunately, there is no treatment for PML. PML is a progressive disease and often fatal.

Choice A, glioblastoma multiforme, is incorrect; lack of enhancement speaks against glioblastoma multiforme. Tumefactive-variant MS, choice B, is incorrect because patients with this disease present with large (often >2 cm) acute lesions associated with cerebral edema, enhancement, and midline shift. Subacute stroke, choice D, is incorrect as neither the clinical history nor the radiographic imaging fits with this diagnosis. Stroke is a clinical diagnosis that results from a vascular occlusion in a particular vascular territory. The progressive nature of symptoms makes this diagnosis unlikely. Finally, brain abscess, choice E, is always a concern in a patient presenting with neurologic symptoms in the setting of an immunocompromised state; however, the lack of ring-enhancing lesions makes cerebral abscess unlikely.

6. **D.** This patient presents with overt nonspecific symptoms with brain imaging revealing no

structural abnormality to explain his symptoms. Lumbar puncture essentially rules out an acute infectious etiology (normal protein, glucose, and RBC). The CSF lymphocytic pleocytosis is a nonspecific finding. Workup reveals positive thyroperoxidase antibody and antithyroglobulin antibody, which are essential features of Hashimoto encephalopathy. The main treatment is high-dose steroids, typically prednisone, with doses ranging from 50 to 150 mg daily. Most patients will achieve remission with this dose. Cyclophosphamide, choice A, may be used in select cases but is not the first-line therapy. Imatinib, choice B, is a BCR-ABL inhibitor that is used in the treatment of chronic myelocytic leukemia. Rituximab, choice C, is a monoclonal antibody and is not used for the treatment of Hashimoto encephalopathy. Temozolomide, choice E, is a chemotherapy agent typically used in the treatment of glioblastoma multiforme.

7. **C.** This patient presents with nonspecific symptoms followed by rapid neurologic decline. MRI of the brain revealed hyperintense signal in the external and internal capsules on FLAIR imaging with minimal enhancement on T1 postgadolinium. CSF revealed mild lymphocytic pleocytosis and elevated protein, which is typically seen with acute viral encephalitis. Eastern equine encephalitis (EEE) is considered to be the most aggressive arthropod-borne encephalitis, with a rapid and often fatal course. Those who survive the initial episodes are often left with severe disability. There is no specific treatment for EEE.

Negative CSF HSV I/II PCR essentially rules out herpes encephalitis (choice B). Nervous system Lyme disease (choice A) is a nonspecific term for a variety of clinical scenarios that may be seen in the setting of *Borrelia burgdorferi* and may include cranial neuropathies, radiculoneuritis, Bannwarth syndrome, meningitis, encephalopathy, and post-Lyme disease, the latter being a controversial entity. However, within the spectrum of neurologic complications of Lyme disease, none is known to manifest with such a rapid and dramatic neurologic picture, along the pictured imaging findings.

HIV-associated dementia (choice D) presents as an indolent progressive memory decline in poorly controlled HIV over months to years. Acute CNS lymphoma (choice E) typically reveals a single or multifocal infiltrative mass or pachymeningeal enhancement, none of which are present here. In addition, CNS lymphoma presents with a more gradual subacute picture rather than hyperacute presentation.

8. **B.** This patient presents with prominent neuropsychiatric symptoms and seizures. Brain imaging reveals T2-FLAIR hyperintensity in bilateral medial temporal lobes, peri-insular region, and bilateral cerebral cortices. While not specific, this imaging pattern is often seen with anti-NMDA receptor encephalitis. The diagnosis of anti-NMDA receptor encephalitis is confirmed by the detection of anti-NMDA antibodies in the serum or CSF. The presence of an ovarian teratoma is common, with appropriately 50% of female patients older than age 18 years having a unilateral or bilateral teratoma. There is an observed predominance in African American women compared to other ethnic or racial groups. Treatment varies by severity of symptoms but may include resection of the tumor if found, glucocorticoids, intravenous immune globulin, and plasma exchange. Prognosis is favorable overall, especially when associated with ovarian teratoma. See Table 8-2.

Metastatic CNS disease, choice A, is in the differential diagnosis, although clinical presentation is highly atypical. A brain metastasis may present with a focal neurologic deficit, corresponding to the neuroanatomic location of the lesion. Seizures are also not uncommon with metastatic brain lesions. Acute alcohol intoxication, choice C, should not present with structural brain imaging abnormalities, and signs and symptoms may vary in severity. These may include nystagmus, slurred speech, disinhibited behavior, ataxia, and memory impairment, and may be severe and include stupor and coma. Anti-IgLON5 encephalopathy, choice D, is an extremely rare newly described paraneoplastic CNS disorder. These patients develop a neurodegenerative rapid eye movement disorder and have abnormal sleep. Choice E is incorrect, because CNS tuberculosis includes 3 distinct clinical categories: tuberculous meningitis, intracranial tuberculomas, and spinal tuberculous arachnoiditis. However, the clinical course of this patient is incompatible with all of the clinical manifestations of CNS tuberculosis.

Autoantibody-Related Encephalitides

Disease Entity	Clinical presentation	Associated Tumor	Laboratory Findings	EEG	Imaging	Treatment and prognosis
Anti-VGKC complex encephalitis	Common presentation: classic limbic encephalitis and brachiofacial dystonic seizures Anti-CSPR2 antibodies are also associated with Morvan's disease Other findings: REM behavior disorder, startle, ataxia, low serum sodium concentration, and intestinal pseudoobstruction	Anti-Lgi1 antibody not associated with tumors Anti-CASPR2 is associated not only with thymoma, but also with other tumors	CSF abnormality in less than half of the patients	EEG shows partial complex seizures and interictal temporal discharges	Hyperintensities on T2 and FLAIR in the temporal areas in over half of the cases, especially when LG-1 is involved	Immunosuppression with steroids, IVIG, and/or PLEX followed by a slow steroid taper. The antibodies usually do not recur after the steroid wean.
Anti-AMPA encephalitis	Limbic encephalitis with prominent psychotic symptoms	Lung, breast, and thymoma in 50% of cases	The patient may have concomitant anti-GAD, TPO, VGCC, and ANA titers CSF is abnormal in a vast majority of cases: protein and pleocytosis	EEG-increased epileptiform activity	Medial temporal hyperintensities or normal	Treatment is similar to NMDA. There are ofter frequent relapses.
Anti-NMDA encephalitis	Common presentation: initially presents with limbic encephalitis In 1 to 2 weeks, may develop akinetic mutism, choreoathetosis, autonomic instability, hypoventilation of consciousness	About half are associated with ovarian teratomas	CSF is almost always abnormal Other findings: presence of ANA and TPO antibodies	Epileptiform activity and slowing	In the majority of cases, there are no abnormalities on MRI. When there are changes, they are in the mesial temporal and limbic cortices, the basal ganglia, and the cerebellum on T2 and FLAIR. There is occasional contrast enhancement of the basal ganglia and the meninges.	Aggressive immuno-suression can slowly improve the symptoms over many months but there is 1/5 chance of recurrence
Anti-GABA$_B$R	Common presentation: limbic encephalitis with prominent seizures Other findings: Up to 50% are associated with N-type VGCC. There are also associations with GAD, TPO, and ANA antibodies.	Mostly thymus and lung		Mesial temporal derivations show increased epileptiform activity	Imaging; Two third has typical changes in the mesial temporal area	Treatment: responds well to treatment without relapses

Reproduced with permission from Salardini A, Biller J. The Hospital Neurology Book. New York, NY: McGraw-Hill, 2016.

9. **C.** This patient presents with altered level of consciousness in the setting of upper respiratory tract infection symptoms. Virology swab testing confirmed H1N1 influenza infection. Influenza-related necrotizing encephalitis with malignant cerebral edema is now recognized as the most severe neurologic complication of seasonal influenza. The pathophysiologic cascade that leads to the development of malignant cerebral edema is poorly understood but is postulated to reflect a severe systemic inflammatory response syndrome (SIRS)-related mechanism. Direct neural invasion by influenza has also been demonstrated, as was reflected in the autopsy in this case. Treatment options are limited, and the course is malignant with almost always a fatal course. There are a few case reports of children who survived such severe illness but were left with a devastated neurologic picture.

Choice A, status epilepticus, is incorrect, because there is no report of convulsions. Nonconvulsive status epilepticus does not present with malignant cerebral edema (although it can be associated from other disease processes that lead to cerebral edema). Choice B is incorrect, because Guillain-Barré syndrome is an acute polyradiculoneuropathy and, in some severe cases, can be mistaken for brain death. Choice D, posterior reverisble encephalopathy syndrome (PRES), is incorrect because although the patient presented with hypertension, it is likely that hypertension was a result of the ongoing intracranial process rather than a cause of it. In addition, the clinical course is too malignant for PRES (although both irreversibility and mortality have been described with PRES). Choice E, anoxic brain injury, is incorrect because although cerebral edema is a feared complication after cardiac arrest and usually reflective of cytotoxic cerebral edema, there is no clinical history to suggest cardiac arrest or anoxia in the first place.

10. **A.** This patient presented following presumed hypoxia from opiate overdose. After initial stabilization, she seemingly recovered but subsequently developed progressive neurologic decline over the course of several weeks. However, she had progressive decline approximately 1 month following her presentation, with repeat brain imaging revealing T2-FLAIR hyperintensities in the deep white matter. Delayed post-hypoxic leukoencephalopathy

(DPHL) is a rare syndrome, in which patients experience an initial inciting hypoxic episode without necessarily anoxia, followed by an initial period of neurologic recovery. The syndrome typically manifests 2 to 40 days after the initial insult and apparent recovery, but then manifests a secondary decline with a progressive course. MRI findings typically reveal diffuse white matter FLAIR hyperintensities matched by restricted diffusion correlates with the timing of the delayed neurologic deficits. Several mechanisms have been postulated to explain the delayed nature of this syndrome including glutamate-induced cytotoxicity and delayed oligodendrocyte apoptosis (hence progressive demyelination in the deep white matter). Unfortunately, there are no treatment options, and supportive care is the mainstay of therapy, with often a severely disabling course.

Choice B, acute ischemic stroke, is an incorrect diagnosis, because brain MRI on initial presentation essentially ruled out a structural cause. Additionally, repeat imaging following readmission revealed multifocal changes that did not reflect any particular vascular territory. Alzheimer dementia, choice C, is incorrect because the time course of Alzheimer disease is much slower. Choice D, acute bacterial meningitis, is incorrect because there was no evidence of bacterial infection on the lumber puncture. Choice E, nonconvulsive status epilepticus (NCSE), is incorrect. NCSE is defined as a condition of ongoing or intermittent seizure activity without convulsions and without recovery of consciousness in between attacks. NCSE symptomology may range from mild confusion to coma, depending on the spatial extent and etiology.

11. **B.** This patient presents with acute confusion in the setting of acute on chronic hyponatremia related to chronic alcoholism. His hyponatremia was unfortunately rapidly corrected, and this patient developed osmotic demyelination syndrome (ODS; previously known as central pontine demyelination). The exact pathogenesis of this syndrome is not clearly understood but has typically been observed in patients who have chronic hyponatremia (typically serum sodium <120 mEq/L) that is rapidly corrected (at rates faster than 8 mEq per 24-hour period). The clinical manifestations, which may rarely be partially reversible, include confusion, lethargy, dysarthria, paraparesis, or quadriparesis. Numerous

cases of "locked-in syndrome" have also been described. The treatment strategy for patients who develop ODS in the setting of rapid sodium correction include relowering serum sodium. There are no randomized controlled trials in humans to affirm the efficacy of such a strategy, but numerous case series have suggested this approach. This strategy is now accepted for patients who develop acute neurologic deficits in the setting of rapid correction of sodium and development of ODS.

Choice A is incorrect because there are no data to support the role of corticosteroids in ODS. Administration of hypertonic saline (choice C) is incorrect, because this will likely increase the sodium level and thus worsen symptoms. Although there are few case reports regarding plasmapheresis in ODS, this is an experimental therapy and is not considered a first-line therapy. Myoinositol (choice E) is incorrect; myoinositol is an agent involved in cellular signaling, and although there are data on using this medication in rat models, none exist in human models, and thus it should not be used beyond research models.

REFERENCES

Akins PT, Belko J, Uyeki TM, et al. H1N1 encephalitis with malignant edema and review of neurologic complications from influenza. *Neurocrit Care.* 2010;13:396-406.

al-Deeb SM, Yaqub BA, Sharif HS, Motaery KR. Neurotuberculosis: a review. *Clin Neurol Neurosurg.* 1992;94(Suppl):S30.

Babi MA, Al Jerdi S, Gorman M. Bilateral border zone infarcts in hypereosinophilic leukemia without proximal vessel stenosis. *J Neurol Neurophysiol.* 2016;7:349.

Babi MA, Pendlebury W, Braff S, et al. JC virus PCR detection is not infallible: a fulminant case of progressive multifocal leukoencephalopathy with false-negative cerebrospinal fluid studies despite progressive clinical course and radiological findings. *Case Rep Neurol Med.* 2015;2015:643216.

Babi MA, Raleigh T, Shapiro RE, et al. MRI and encephalography in fatal eastern equine encephalitis. *Neurology.* 2014;83;1483.

Bahemuka M, Murungi JH. Tuberculosis of the nervous system. A clinical, radiological and pathological study of 39 consecutive cases in Riyadh, Saudi Arabia. *J Neurol Sci.* 1989;90:67-76.

Bharat A, Xie F, Baddley JW, et al. Incidence and risk factors for progressive multifocal leukoencephalopathy among patients with selected rheumatic diseases. *Arthritis Care Res (Hoboken).* 2012;64:612-615.

Bibl D, Lampl C, Gabriel C, et al. Treatment of central pontine myelinolysis with therapeutic plasmapheresis. *Lancet.* 1999;353:1155.

Boba A. Management of acute alcoholic intoxication. *Am J Emerg Med.* 1999;17:431.

Boyd J, Babi MA, Allen G, et al. Fulminant necrotizing encephalitis associated with malignant cerebral edema and transtentorial herniation in the setting of acute seasonal influenza pneumonia. American Academy of Neurology (AAN 2015 Annual meeting). *Neurology.* 2015;84:P6.315.

Calabrese LH, Dodick DW, Schwedt TJ, et al. Narrative review: reversible cerebral vasoconstriction syndromes. *Ann Intern Med.* 2007;146:34-44.

Calisher CH. Medically important arboviruses of the United States and Canada. *Clin Microbiol Rev.* 1994;7:89-116.

Castillo P, Woodruff B, Caselli R, et al. Steroid-responsive encephalopathy associated with autoimmune thyroiditis. *Arch Neurol.* 2006;63:197-202.

Cavuşoglu H, Kaya RA, Türkmenoglu ON, et al. Brain abscess: analysis of results in a series of 51 patients with a combined surgical and medical approach during an 11-year period. *Neurosurg Focus.* 2008;24:E9.

Chong JY, Rowland LP, Utiger RD. Hashimoto encephalopathy: syndrome or myth? *Arch Neurol.* 2003;60:164-171.

Custodio CM, Basford JR. Delayed postanoxic encephalopathy: a case report and literature review. *Arch Phys Med Rehabil.* 2004;85:502-505.

Dalmau J, Gultekin HS, Posner JB. Paraneoplastic neurologic syndromes: pathogenesis and physiopathology. *Brain Pathol.* 1999;9:275-284.

Dalmau J, Rosenfeld MR. Paraneoplastic syndromes of the CNS. *Lancet Neurol.* 2008;7:327-340.

Danek A, Rubio JP, Rampoldi L, et al. McLeod neuroacanthocytosis: genotype and phenotype. *Ann Neurol.* 2001;50:755-764.

Danve A, Grafe M, Deodhar A. Amyloid beta-related angiitis: a case report and comprehensive review of literature of 94 cases. *Semin Arthritis Rheum.* 2014;44:86-92.

Deresiewicz RL, Thaler SJ, Hsu L, et al. Clinical and neuroradiographic manifestations of eastern equine encephalitis. *N Engl J Med.* 1997;336:1867-1874.

Eng JA, Frosch MP, Choi K, et al. Clinical manifestations of cerebral amyloid angiopathy-related inflammation. *Ann Neurol.* 2004;55:250-256.

Ferracci F, Bertiato G, Moretto G. Hashimoto's encephalopathy: epidemiologic data and pathogenetic considerations. *J Neurol Sci.* 2004;217:165-168.

Gable MS, Gavali S, Radner A, et al. Anti-NMDA receptor encephalitis: report of ten cases and comparison with viral encephalitis. *Eur J Clin Microbiol Infect Dis.* 2009;28:1421-1429.

Graus F, Keime-Guibert F, Reñe R, et al. Anti-Hu-associated paraneoplastic encephalomyelitis: analysis of 200 patients. *Brain.* 2001;124:1138-1148.

Halperin JJ, Pass HL, Anand AK, et al. Nervous system abnormalities in Lyme disease. *Ann N Y Acad Sci.* 1988;539:24.

Hardy TA, Chataway J. Tumefactive demyelination: an approach to diagnosis and management. *J Neurol Neurosurg Psychiatry.* 2013;84:1047-1053.

Haywood AM. Transmissible spongiform encephalopathies. *N Engl J Med.* 1997;337:1821-1828.

Kahle KT, Walcott BP, Nahed BV, et al. Cerebral edema and a transtentorial brain herniation syndrome associated with pandemic swine influenza A (H1N1) virus infection. *J Clin Neurosci*. 2011;18:1245-1248.

Hinchey J, Chaves C, Appignani B, et al. A reversible posterior leukoencephalopathy syndrome. *N Engl J Med*. 1996;334:494-500.

Katz Sand IB, Lublin FD. Diagnosis and differential diagnosis of multiple sclerosis. *Continuum (Minneap Minn)*. 2013;19:922-943.

Kinnecom C, Lev MH, Wendell L, et al. Course of cerebral amyloid angiopathy-related inflammation. *Neurology*. 2007;68:1411-1416.

Lee HB, Lyketsos CG. Delated post-hypoxic leukoencephaloathy. *Psychosomatics*. 2001;42:530-533.

Lo YL. Clinical and immunological spectrum of the Miller Fisher syndrome. *Muscle Nerve*. 2007;36:615-627.

Lorincz MT. Neurologic Wilson's disease. *Ann N Y Acad Sci*. 2010;1184:173-187.

Lublin FD, Reingold SC, Cohen JA, et al. Defining the clinical course of multiple sclerosis: the 2013 revisions. *Neurology*. 2014;83:278-286.

Lucchinetti CF, Gavrilova RH, Metz I, et al. Clinical and radiographic spectrum of pathologically confirmed tumefactive multiple sclerosis. *Brain*. 2008;131:1759-1775.

Luft BJ, Steinman CR, Neimark HC, et al. Invasion of the central nervous system by Borrelia burgdorferi in acute disseminated infection. *JAMA*. 1992;267:1364-1367.

Lukehart SA, Hook EW 3rd, Baker-Zander SA, et al. Invasion of the central nervous system by *Treponema pallidum*: implications for diagnosis and treatment. *Ann Intern Med*. 1988;109:855-862.

Manto M, Goldman S, Bodur H. Cerebellar syndrome associated with Hashimoto's encephalopathy. *Rev Neurol (Paris)*. 1996;152:202.

Marques A. Chronic Lyme disease: a review. *Infect Dis Clin North Am*. 2008;22:341-360.

McGuire LI, Poleggi A, Poggiolini I, et al. Cerebrospinal fluid real-time quaking-induced conversion is a robust and reliable test for sporadic Creutzfeldt-Jakob disease: an international study. *Ann Neurol*. 2016;80:160-165.

McMillan HJ, Johnston DL, Doja A. Watershed infarction due to acute hypereosinophilia. *Neurology*. 2008;70:80-82.

Miller DC, Hochberg FH, Harris NL, et al. Pathology with clinical correlations of primary central nervous system non-Hodgkin's lymphoma. The Massachusetts General Hospital experience 1958-1989. *Cancer*. 1994;74:1383-1397.

Oya S, Tsutsumi K, Ueki K, et al. Reinduction of hyponatremia to treat central pontine myelinolysis. *Neurology*. 2001;57:1931-1932.

Peterson K, Rosenblum MK, Kotanides H, Posner JB. Paraneoplastic cerebellar degeneration. I. A clinical analysis of 55 anti-Yo antibody-positive patients. *Neurology*. 1992;42:1931-1937.

Pringsheim T, Wiltshire K, Day L, et al. The incidence and prevalence of Huntington's disease: a systematic review and meta-analysis. *Mov Disord*. 2012;27:1083-1091.

Prusiner SB. Shattuck lecture: neurodegenerative diseases and prions. *N Engl J Med*. 2001;344:1516-1526.

Raschilas F, Wolff M, Delatour F, et al. Outcome of and prognostic factors for herpes simplex encephalitis in adult patients: results of a multicenter study. *Clin Infect Dis*. 2002;35:254-260.

Sabater L, Gaig C, Gelpi E, et al. A novel non-rapid-eye movement and rapid-eye-movement parasomnia with sleep breathing disorder associated with antibodies to IgLON5: a case series, characterisation of the antigen, and post-mortem study. *Lancet Neurol*. 2014;13:575-586.

Salvarani C, Brown RD Jr, Calamia KT, et al. Primary central nervous system vasculitis: analysis of 101 patients. *Ann Neurol*. 2007;62:442-451.

Schabet M. Epidemiology of primary CNS lymphoma. *J Neurooncol*. 1999;43:199-201.

Shapshak P, Kangueane P, Fujimura RK, et al. Editorial neuroAIDS review. *AIDS*. 2011;25:123-141.

Shimada K, Murase T, Matsue K, et al. Central nervous system involvement in intravascular large B-cell lymphoma: a retrospective analysis of 109 patients. *Cancer Sci*. 2010;101:1480-1486.

Shorvon S. What is nonconvulsive status epilepticus, and what are its subtypes? *Epilepsia*. 2007;48:35-38.

Shprecher D, Mehta L. The syndrome of delayed post-hypoxic leukoencephalopathy. *Neuro Rehabilitation*. 2010;26:65-72.

Silver SM, Schroeder BM, Sterns RH, et al. Myoinositol administration improves survival and reduces myelinolysis after rapid correction of chronic hyponatremia in rats. *J Neuropathol Exp Neurol*. 2006;65:37-44.

Sterns RH. Disorders of plasma sodium: causes, consequences, and correction. *N Engl J Med*. 2015;372:55-65.

Sterns RH, Hix JK, Silver S. Treating profound hyponatremia: a strategy for controlled correction. *Am J Kidney Dis*. 2010;56:774-779.

van de Beek D, de Gans J, Spanjaard L, et al. Clinical features and prognostic factors in adults with bacterial meningitis. *N Engl J Med*. 2004;351:1849-1859.

Titulaer MJ, McCracken L, Gabilondo I, et al. Late-onset anti-NMDA receptor encephalitis. *Neurology*. 2013;81:1058-1063.

Trinka E, Cock H, Hesdorffer D, et al. A definition and classification of status epilepticus: report of the ILAE Task Force on Classification of Status Epilepticus. *Epilepsia*. 2015;56:1515-1523.

Wallace IR, Dynan C, Esmonde T. One confused patient, many confused physicians: a case of delayed post-hypoxic leucoencephalopathy. *QJM*. 2010;103:193-194.

Yuki N, Hartung HP. Guillain-Barré syndrome. *N Engl J Med*. 2012;366:2294-2304.

Questions

Questions 1 and 2

An 88-year-old woman with a history of hypertension, osteoporosis, and rheumatoid arthritis on daily aspirin presented to the emergency department (ED) after a mechanical fall, hitting her head on concrete. A head computed tomography (CT) showed a 2-cm subdural hematoma extending along the anterior falx, with no midline shift. Admission vital signs were normal except arterial blood pressure (ABP) of 201/88 mm Hg. Given her elevated ABP, she was given intravenous hydralazine, along with her home antihypertensive medications: carvedilol, clonidine, and prazosin.

Overnight, the patient became hypotensive with ABP of 80/50 mm Hg, and she was treated with 1 L of intravenous normal saline bolus.

Pertinent lab values

Admission:

Sodium (Na) 138 mmol/L, potassium (K) 3.8 mmol/L, chloride (Cl) 104 mmol/L, bicarbonate (HCO$_3$) 23 mmol/L, blood urea nitrogen (BUN) 16 mg/dL, creatinine (Cr) 0.84 mg/dL

Hospital day 1:

Na 138 mmol/L, K 3.7 mmol/L, Cl 105 mmol/L, HCO$_3$ 27 mmol/L, BUN 29 mg/dL, Cr 1.40 mg/dL

Urine chemistry

Urine Cr 60 mg/dL

Urine osmolality 550 mOsm/kg

Urine Na 15 mmol/L

Urea nitrogen 211 mg/dL

1. Based on the available data, what is the etiology of this patient's acute kidney injury (AKI)?

   A. Acute tubular necrosis

   B. Prerenal azotemia

   C. Obstructive acute renal failure

   D. Acute interstitial nephritis

   E. Radiocontrast agent–induced nephropathy

2. In this patient, which of the following autoregulation mechanisms maintain renal perfusion?

   A. Afferent arteriolar vasodilatation and efferent arteriolar vasoconstriction

   B. Afferent arteriolar vasoconstriction and efferent arteriolar vasodilatation

C. Afferent arteriolar vasoconstriction and efferent arteriolar vasoconstriction

D. Afferent arteriolar vasodilatation and efferent arteriolar vasodilatation

E. There is no autoregulatory mechanism in renal perfusion

3. An 87-year-old woman with a past medical history significant for chronic kidney disease, diabetes mellitus, arterial hypertension, congestive heart failure, and atrial fibrillation, status post pacemaker, is admitted to a community hospital for failure to thrive. The patient has not been taking any of her medications for the past 3 months. On hospital day 2, the patient was found to have an acute onset of right gaze preference, left hemiplegia, and left hemisensory deficit. National Institutes of Health Stroke Scale (NIHSS) score was 20. A stat CT of the head was done. The patient received intravenous tissue plasminogen activator. A CT angiogram was performed and showed a right M1 occlusion. The patient was transferred to a comprehensive stroke center for mechanical thrombectomy. She had complete recanalization with a stent retriever with Thrombolysis in Cerebral Infarction (TICI) grade 3 results. Unfortunately, her clinical exam remained poor.

After thrombectomy, the patient was admitted to the neurocritical care unit (NCCU). On arrival to the NCCU, her vital signs were BP 150/70 mm Hg and heart rate 80 bpm. Electrocardiogram (ECG) was obtained and was unremarkable. Troponin was 0.1 ng/mL.

The following day, the patient had a transthoracic echocardiogram that showed ejection fraction of 35% to 40%, hypokinesis of the inferior wall, and mid to distal inferoseptal and anteroseptal walls. A repeat troponin was 196 ng/mL. ECG now reveals ST elevation in leads V_2 to V_4. The heart attack team recommended against coronary angiography as the patient had significant contraindication to

anticoagulation and dual antiplatelet therapy. Medical management was continued, and she maintained a normal BP. She was noted to have decreased urine output, which worsened by day 4.

Repeat vital signs were BP 146/70 mm Hg and heart rate 80 bpm.

Pertinent lab values

Admission:

Na 142 mmol/L, K 4.4 mmol/L, Cl 106 mmol/L, HCO_3 25 mmol/L, BUN 23 mg/dL, Cr 1.7 mg/dL, glucose 190 mg/dL

Hospital day 4:

Na 143 mmol/L, K 4.5 mmol/L, Cl 107 mmol/L, HCO_3 26 mmol/L, BUN 45 mg/dL, Cr 2.5 mg/dL, glucose 224 mg/dL

Urine chemistry

Urine Cr 40 mg/dL

Urine osmolality 300 mOsm/kg

Urine Na 18 mmol/L

Urea nitrogen 211 mg/dL

Based on the available data, what is the cause of this patient's worsening renal function?

A. Postrenal obstruction

B. Radiocontrast agent–induced nephropathy

C. Acute interstitial nephritis

D. Prerenal azotemia

E. Acute tubular necrosis

4. Which of the following is *not* a transport mechanism during renal replacement therapy?

A. Adsorption

B. Convection

C. Diffusion

D. Ultrafiltration

E. Conduction

Questions 5 and 6

An 80-year-old man with history of congestive heart failure is admitted to the neuroscience intensive care unit (ICU) with acute right hemisphere subdural hematoma of 3-cm thickness and 8-mm midline shift. The family refused neurosurgery but agreed to continue medical management. The patient's blood pressure has been low during the ICU stay, and his most recent ABP was 105/70 mm Hg. The patient developed acute kidney failure after being treated aggressively with intravenous furosemide for his heart failure and became anuric. The decision was made to initiate renal replacement therapy.

5. Which of the following renal replacement therapy (RRT) modalities is most appropriate for management of his acute kidney failure?
   A. Intermittent hemodialysis
   B. Peritoneal dialysis
   C. Slow continuous ultrafiltration
   D. Continuous venovenous hemofiltration
   E. All of the above

6. In this patient, which of the following catheter sites is associated with the least risk for catheter dysfunction and least risk for bacteremia?
   A. Right internal jugular vein
   B. Left internal jugular vein
   C. Right subclavian vein
   D. Left subclavian vein
   E. Femoral vein

7. Match the following terms to their definitions:

I. Diffusion	A. Movement of small solute by concentration gradient
II. Convection	B. Movement of solutes by pressure gradient
III. Ultrafiltration	C. Movement of middle and larger solutes by force of water flow, also called solvent drag
IV. Absorption	D. Removal of solutes by adherence of the solute to the membrane

8. A 46-year-old man is admitted to the neuroscience ICU with Guillain-Barré syndrome. On hospital day 3, the bedside nurse calls you stating that his urine output has dropped to less than 5 mL/h over the past 3 hours. What is the next step in management?
   A. Send urine studies
   B. Fluid challenge
   C. Flush or change the urinary catheter to rule out an obstruction
   D. Give a trial of furosemide
   E. Do nothing for the next hour and reassess whether the urinary output spontaneously improves

9. A 25-year-old man was admitted to the neuroscience ICU after severe traumatic brain injury. Glasgow coma scale score was 8 on arrival. The patient developed cerebral edema and was initiated on 3% hypertonic saline with goal to maintain his serum Na between 140 and 150 mEq/L. On hospital day 4, the nurse noted that his urine output, which was previously adequate, had increased to 750 mL/h for the past 3 hours. His serum Na, which was previously 145 mmol/L, is now 155 mmol/L. What is your next step in management?
   A. Give a stat dose of vasopressin
   B. Start patient on fluid replacement with dextrose 5% in water (D5W)
   C. Check urine specific gravity, osmolality, and plasma osmolality
   D. Stat nephrology consult
   E. Given the patient has cerebral edema, change the Na goal from 145 to 155 mEq/L

Questions 10 and 11

A 60-year-old woman presented to the ED with the worst headache of her life. CT head showed diffuse subarachnoid hemorrhage. CT angiogram revealed a posterior communicating aneurysm which was later successfully coiled. During her stay in the neuroscience ICU, she developed worsening hydrocephalus managed by an external ventricular drain and severe vasospasm requiring intra-arterial verapamil. Despite an attempt to maintain euvolemia, on hospital day 6, the nurse reported that the patient's urine output increased to 500 mL/h for the past 3 hour. A stat set of labs revealed Na of 130 mmol/L, which previously was 141 mmol/L. Serum osmolality was 272 mOsm/kg. Stat urine studies were sent and showed urine Na of 42 mmol/L and urine osmolality of 201 mOsm/kg.

10. What is the next step in management of this patient?

    A. Determine the volume status of the patient and start fluid restriction

    B. Determine the fractional excretion of urate

    C. Determine the fractional excretion of urea

    D. Determine the fractional excretion of sodium

    E. Administer 23.4% hypertonic saline

11. In this patient, the fractional excretion of urate was calculated to be 13%. After correcting hyponatremia, the fractional excretion of urate is now 14%. What is the most likely diagnosis?

    A. Cerebral salt wasting (CSW)

    B. Syndrome of inappropriate antidiuretic hormone (SIADH)

    C. Thyroid disease

    D. Verapamil-induced hyponatremia

    E. Adrenal insufficiency

Questions 12-16

A 30-year-old man with history of polysubstance abuse, who was recently diagnosed with human immunodeficiency virus (HIV), was admitted to the ICU after a high-speed motor vehicle collision. The patient was intubated at the scene. On ICU day 2, you received a call from his nurse that his urine output was tea colored.

Pertinent lab values

Urinalysis: reddish-brown color, with large blood, 2+ proteinuria, and muddy-brown casts

Urine toxicology: cocaine

Serum: Na 135 mmol/L, K 3.0 mmol/L, Cl 102 mmol/L, HCO_3 16 mmol/L, BUN 60 mg/dL, Cr: 4 mg/dL, Ca 6.8 mg/dL, phosphate 2.1 mg/dL, albumin 3.2 g/dL

12. Which of the following tests is the next *most* appropriate to order?

    A. Lactate dehydrogenase

    B. Serum myoglobin

    C. Creatine kinase

    D. Aldolase

    E. Hepatic transaminases

13. In this patient, urine myoglobin was 35 mg/dL (normal <1.5 mg/dL) and creatine kinase (CK) level was 150,000U/L (normal male CK <300 U/L). What is the most likely cause of his rhabdomyolysis?

    A. Trauma from the motor vehicle crash

    B. Cocaine

    C. Hypokalemia

    D. Hypocalcemia

    E. All of the above

14. Which of the following is/are the pathophysiologic mechanism(s) of how rhabdomyolysis induces AKI?

    A. Renal vasoconstriction

    B. Formation of intratubular cast

    C. Direct toxicity of myoglobin to kidney tubular cells

    D. Renal vasoconstriction and direct toxicity of myoglobin to the kidney tubular cells

    E. Renal vasoconstriction, formation of intratubular casts, and direct toxicity of myoglobin to the kidney tubular cells

15. After correcting electrolyte abnormalities, a repeat chemistry showed the following: Na 140 mmol/L, K 4 mmol/L, phosphate 4.2 mg/dL, HCO_3 14 mmol/L, BUN 56 mg/dL, and Cr 3.4 mg/dL. His urine output is 25 mL/h. What is the next step in management of this patient?

    A. Initiate renal replacement therapy

    B. Initiate volume repletion with normal saline at 300 mL/h with target urine output of 3 mL/kg of body weight per hour

    C. Mannitol 1 g/kg infusion every 8 hours

    D. Start sodium bicarbonate 100 mmol/L in D5W at 200 mL/h

    E. D5W at 250 mL/h

16. Which of the following electrolyte abnormalities is associated with recovery of renal function in rhabdomyolysis-induced AKI?

    A. Hypercalcemia

    B. Hyperkalemia

    C. Hyperphosphatemia

    D. Hypernatremia

    E. Hyperuricemia

17. A 45-year-old woman with history of diabetes mellitus, hypertension, and end-stage renal disease, who was last seen normal by family 2 days ago, was brought to the ED by family for acting strange. She missed her last 2 sessions of hemodialysis. In the ED, the patient was noted to have a left facial droop and left hemiparesis. Her labs were remarkable for Na 130 mmol/L and K 8.1 mmol/L. ECG showed PR and QRS prolongation. Which of the following is the most appropriate first step in management of this patient?

    A. Hypertonic (3%) saline
    B. Intravenous tissue plasminogen activator (tPA)
    C. Kayexalate dose via nasogastric tube
    D. Continuous venovenous hemodiafiltration
    E. Intravenous calcium gluconate

18. A 50-year-old woman admitted to the ICU for hospital-acquired pneumonia is now intubated, and recent chest x-ray showed evidence of acute respiratory distress syndrome. For the past 5 days, she has had severe diarrhea. She is intubated, alert, and nodding appropriately to orientation questions. Her BP is 115/70 mm Hg with a heart rate of 90 bpm. What acid-base disorder is she suffering from?

    Lab values

    Arterial blood gas (ABG): pH 7.30, Pco_2 60 mm Hg, Po_2 80 mm Hg, HCO_3 30 mmol/L

    Serum: Na 140 mmol/L, K 3.5 mmol/L, Cl 100 mmol/L, HCO_3 31 mmol/L, BUN 25 mg/dL, Cr 1.0 mg/dL, glucose 90 mg/dL

    A. Metabolic acidosis and respiratory alkalosis
    B. Respiratory acidosis and metabolic acidosis
    C. Metabolic acidosis and metabolic alkalosis
    D. Respiratory acidosis and metabolic alkalosis
    E. Respiratory acidosis, metabolic acidosis, and metabolic alkalosis

19. A 55-year-old man with history of diabetes mellitus, congestive heart failure, and chronic kidney disease is admitted for nausea, vomiting, and shortness of breath. Home medications include insulin and furosemide. Which of the following BEST describes his acid-base status?

    Laboratory values

    Serum: Na 140 mmol/L, K 3.9 mmol/L, Cl 99 mmol/L, HCO_3 23 mmol/L, BUN 45 mg/dL, Cr 2.5 mg/dL, glucose 140 mg/dL, albumin 2.0 g/dL

    ABG: pH 7.40, Pco_2 40 mm Hg, Po_2 80 mm Hg, HCO_3 23 mmol/L

    A. Metabolic acidosis and respiratory acidosis
    B. Metabolic acidosis, respiratory alkalosis, and metabolic alkalosis
    C. Metabolic acidosis and metabolic alkalosis
    D. Respiratory acidosis and metabolic alkalosis
    E. Respiratory alkalosis and metabolic alkalosis

20. A 40-year-old man with history of uncontrolled diabetes mellitus and hypertension, who is noncompliant with his medications, is admitted to the neuroscience ICU with left basal ganglia intracerebral hemorrhage. While in the ICU, he developed worsening headache and several episodes of vomiting. A repeat head CT revealed expanding hemorrhage. He required intubation. Which of the following BEST describes his acid-base status?

    Laboratory values

    ABG: pH 7.58, Pco_2 23 mm Hg, Po_2 90 mm Hg, HCO_3 20 mmol/L

    Serum: Na 140 mmol/L, K 4.0 mmol/L, Cl 90 mmol/L, HCO_3 21 mmol/L, BUN 20 mg/dL, Cr 1.5 mg/dL, glucose 600 mg/dL

    Urinalysis: + ketones

    A. Metabolic acidosis and respiratory acidosis
    B. Metabolic acidosis, respiratory alkalosis, and metabolic alkalosis
    C. Metabolic acidosis and metabolic alkalosis
    D. Respiratory acidosis and metabolic alkalosis
    E. Respiratory alkalosis, metabolic acidosis, and metabolic alkalosis

21. A 25-year-old previously healthy African American man presents to the ED with blurry vision and is found to have a blood pressure of 210/138 mm Hg and heart rate of 90 bpm. His blood pressure at his last clinic check-up was normal. Which of the following BEST describes his acid-base status?

Laboratory values

ABG: pH 7.49, P_{CO_2} 47 mm Hg, P_{O_2} 90 mm Hg, HCO_3 34 mmol/L

Serum: Na 140 mmol/L, K 2.7 mmol/L, Cl 85 mmol/L, HCO_3 34 mmol/L, BUN 20 mg/dL, Cr 1.5 mg/dL, glucose 600 mg/dL

Urine: Chloride 50 mmol/L

A. Respiratory alkalosis
B. Metabolic alkalosis, fully compensated, chloride responsive
C. Metabolic alkalosis and respiratory alkalosis
D. Metabolic alkalosis and respiratory acidosis
E. Metabolic alkalosis, fully compensated, chloride resistant

22. A 45-year-old woman is diagnosed with non–anion gap metabolic acidosis. You suspect a type of renal tubular acidosis (RTA) as the etiology because she has polyuria, polydipsia, nephrocalcinosis, unexplained nephrolithiasis, and hypertension. Match the following causes with the type of RTA.

I. Classic distal RTA (type I)	A. Spironolactone
II. Hyperkalemic distal RTA	B. Hypoaldosteronism
III. Proximal RTA (type 2)	C. Obstructive uropathy
IV. Combined RTA (type 3)	D. Systemic lupus erythematosus, amphotericin
V. Hyperkalemic RTA (type 4)	E. Acetazolamide
	F. Valproic acid

23. Which of the following is a possible preventive measure for drug nephrotoxicity?
   A. Urine alkalinization
   B. Sodium administration
   C. Urine acidification
   D. Hydration
   E. All of the above

24. A 55-year-old man with a history of AIDS was brought to the ED by family with 3 days of confusion. He had been complaining of headache for 3 days per family. On arrival to the ED, the patient was confused and holding his head. His vital signs were BP 135/80 mm Hg, heart rate 80 bpm, and temperature 39.6°C. He had a lumbar puncture with opening pressure of 45 mm Hg and was treated for *Cryptococcus* meningitis given positive *Cryptococcus* antigen in cerebrospinal fluid. During his hospital stay on the floor, his BP was low, with systolic BP ranging from 85 to 100 mm Hg.

On hospital day 3, a rapid response was called because the patient was profoundly altered. Vital signs revealed BP 60/35 mm Hg and heart rate 115 bpm. He was given 2 L of normal saline, but he continued to be hypotensive. He was started on norepinephrine to maintain a mean arterial pressure of 65 mm Hg and was transferred to the ICU. While in the ICU, the patient became oliguric on hospital day 6.

Pertinent lab values

Admission:

Na 135 mmol/L, K 3.9 mmol/L, Cl 98 mmol/L, HCO_3 25 mmol/L, BUN 13 mg/dL, Cr 1.2 mg/dL

Hospital day 6:

Na 140 mmol/L, K 3.6 mmol/L, Cl 103 mmol/L, HCO_3 21 mmol/L, BUN 39 mg/dL, Cr 4 mg/dL

Urine chemistry

Urine creatinine 40 mg/dL

Urine osmolality 330 mOsm/kg

Urine sodium 50 mmol/L

Urea nitrogen 211 mg/dL

Microscopic urine analysis: muddy brown granular cast

Based on the available data, what is the etiology of this patient's AKI?
A. Acute tubular necrosis
B. Prerenal azotemia
C. Obstructive acute renal failure
D. Acute interstitial nephritis
E. Radiocontrast agent-induced nephropathy

Answers and Explanations

1. B. This patient had acute kidney injury (AKI) secondary to prerenal azotemia, which is the most common cause of AKI in hospitalized patients. It is due to either a reduction in effective circulating volume or hypotension, leading to renal hypoperfusion. If the hypoperfusion is severe and prolonged, prerenal azotemia can lead to acute tubular necrosis. This patient had a hypotensive episode after being given her home antihypertensive medications. Both prerenal azotemia and acute tubular necrosis exist as a spectrum, and there is a set of biochemical indices that might help differentiate the 2 disorders.

In patients with prerenal azotemia, we typically expect the following:

1. Urinary osmolality is >500 mOsm/kg
2. Urinary sodium concentration <20 mmol/L
3. Urine-to-serum creatinine ratio >40
4. Serum urea-to-creatinine ratio >0.1
5. The fractional excretion of sodium (FE_{Na}), which is based on the fact that sodium reabsorption is enhanced in setting of hypovolemia, is low: <1%

$$FE_{Na} = [(\text{urinary Na/serum Na})/(\text{urinary Cr}/\text{serum Cr})] \times 100.$$

An FE_{Na} <1% suggests prerenal azotemia as cause of AKI.

For patient on diuretics, FE_{Na} is not accurate, and one must calculate the fractional excretion of urea (FE_{Urea}), with a value <35% suggesting prerenal azotemia.

This patient has a urinary osmolality of 550 mOsm/kg, urine sodium of 15 mmol/L, urine-to-serum creatinine concentration (60/1.40) of 43, and FE_{Na} of 0.3%. All of these factors point toward prerenal azotemia as the cause of her AKI.

Causes of Acute Kidney Injury

- Prerenal
  - Absolute volume depletion
  - Decreased effective circulating volume
  - Congestive heart failure
  - Cirrhosis
  - Renal autoregulatory failure
- Postrenal
  - Ureteral obstruction
  - Stones
  - Tumor
  - Fibrosis
  - Bladder outlet obstruction
- Intrinsic renal disease
  - Acute tubular necrosis (ATN)
  - Toxic
  - Ischemic
- Mixed
  - Acute glomerulonephritis (AGN)
  - Acute interstitial nephritis (AIN)
  - Acute renal vasculitis
  - Acute intratubular obstruction
  - Tumor lysis syndrome
  - Drug induced

Reproduced with permission from Lee K. *The NeuroICU Book*. New York, NY: McGraw-Hill; 2012.

2. A. The renal system is controlled by an autoregulatory mechanism. When renal perfusion is compromised because of moderate hypovolemia and hypotension, there are autoregulatory mechanisms in place to maintain a constant glomerular filtration, until the mean arterial pressure falls below 60 to 70 mm Hg. This autoregulation is achieved by afferent arteriolar vasodilatation with a decrease in myogenic tone within the vessel wall and by synthesis and release of intrarenal vasodilators such us prostaglandins and nitric oxide. At the same time, the efferent artery vasoconstricts via angiotensin II, with the goal to keep the glomerular filtration rate constant.

3. B. Radiocontrast agent–induced nephropathy (RCN) is the third leading cause of hospital-acquired AKI. The most important risk factor for RCN is a preexisting renal impairment with a glomerular filtration rate (GFR) <60 mL/min. Other risk factors are divided into nonmodifiable and modifiable.

Nonmodifiable risk factors are older age, history of diabetes mellitus, congestive heart failure, acute myocardial infarction, and depressed left ventricular ejection fraction. Modifiable risk factors include hypovolemia and type of contrast agent used, diuretics, anemia, and angiotensin-converting enzyme inhibitors.

This patient had a preexisting renal impairment, history of diabetes mellitus and systolic heart failure (ejection fraction 35%), and had received 2 loads of contrast: first for the CT angiogram at the community hospital and the second load with the conventional angiogram. All of these factors put her at risk for RCN. In addition, urine osmolality tends to be <350 mOsm/kg. FENa is <1% in the early stages, despite no clinical evidence of hypovolemia or hypotension.

There was no evidence of hypotension or hypovolemia to suggest hypoperfusion to the kidney, essentially ruling out prerenal azotemia and acute tubular necrosis. The absence of any nephrotoxic drug rules out acute interstitial nephritis.

4. E. Renal replacement therapy can involve any of the following 4 major transport mechanisms: convection, diffusion, ultrafiltration, and adsorption. Convection is the movement of solute by pressure gradient. The force of water movement drags solutes across membrane. Diffusion is the movement of solutes across a membrane by concentration gradient. Small molecules easily pass through a membrane by diffusion and convection. Middle and larger sized molecules are cleared primarily by convection. Ultrafiltration, which is a type of convection mechanism, is the passage of water through a membrane under a pressure gradient. Adsorption is the process by which solutes are removed from the blood by clinging to the membrane, which ultimately needs to be changed.

Conduction is the flow of energy from one place to another through a media and has nothing to do with renal replacement therapy.

5. D. There are 3 available modalities of renal replacement therapy (RRT): peritoneal dialysis (PD), intermittent hemodialysis (IHD), and continuous renal replacement therapies (CRRT). Which modality to choose depends on patient's hemodynamics, fluid status, solute removal, and electrolyte abnormalities. PD is a chronic modality of RRT and is a slow process. In critical illness, PD has been shown to be less efficacious and cannot be recommended. IHD can be used in ICU patients who are hemodynamically stable but is not ideal in this patient. The aforementioned patient is hypotensive and has cerebral mass effect, making IHD not an ideal modality. Given this patient's hemodynamics and mass effect from the subdural hematoma, CRRT will be the preferred RRT modality. Slow continuous ultrafiltration (SCUF) and continuous venovenous hemofiltration (CVVH) are examples of CRRT. SCUF only removes fluid and therefore will not improve this patient's electrolyte abnormalities and urea. CVVH, however, will remove fluid and improve electrolytes.

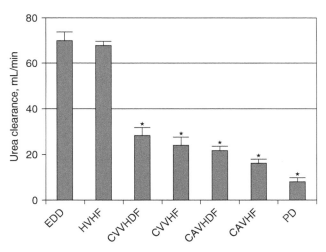

Reproduced with permission from Lee K. *The NeuroICU Book.* New York, NY: McGraw-Hill, 2012.

6. A. According to Kidney Disease: Improving Global Outcomes (KDIGO) guidelines, the following are the preference sites for catheter placement. The first choice is the right jugular vein; catheters in the right internal jugular vein have a straight course into the right brachiocephalic vein and superior vena cava. The second choice is the femoral vein, which is associated with the highest risk of infection. The third choice is left jugular vein; because of more angulation and erratic blood flow, studies have shown catheter dysfunction when compared to the right internal jugular vein. The last choice is the subclavian vein with preference to the dominant side. It is the last choice because of risk of central vein stenosis, which may significantly complicate venous access if chronic hemodialysis is required. It is also associated with erratic blood flow.

7. **I = A; II = C; III = B; IV = D**

8. **C.** This patient is oliguric, which by definition is a urine output less than 0.3 mL/kg/h for at least 24 hours according to the Acute Dialysis Quality Initiative (ADQI). The initial step in management of a patient with oliguria is to rule out urinary obstruction.

    In the ICU, most patients have a urinary catheter; therefore, the first step in a patient with new-onset oliguria is to flush or change the urinary catheter to rule out an obstruction. Fluid challenge and urine studies will help determine if the oliguria is from a prerenal or intrarenal cause.

    Furosemide is not the answer because it does not convert oliguric to nonoliguric renal failure. Doing nothing will only make the oliguria worse, which is associated with worse outcomes.

9. **C.** Polyuria is defined as urine output >30 mL/kg body weight or >200 mL/h for 2 hours. Based on the data in the question, this patient has polyuria. The question now becomes what is the cause of this polyuria. The next step in management of polyuria is to determine the urinary specific gravity (SG), urinary osmolality, serum Na, and serum osmolality.

If SG is <1.005 or urine osmolality is <300 mOsm/kg, this points toward a diagnosis of diabetes insipidus (DI). There are 2 types of DI: central and nephrogenic.

In central DI, there is a decrease in secretion of antidiuretic hormone (ADH), leading to polyuria and polydipsia. In nephrogenic DI, there is an inability to concentrate urine because of resistance to ADH action in the kidney.

This patient likely has central DI from traumatic brain injury. After confirming the diagnosis of central DI, given this patient's poor Glasgow coma scale score, the management will consist of parental fluid replacement and administration of vasopressin.

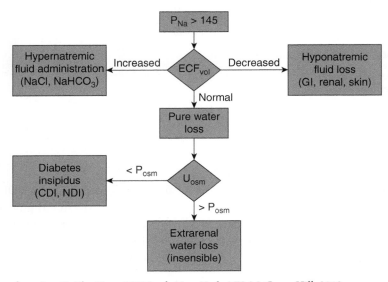

Reproduced with permission from Lee K. *The NeuroICU Book*. New York, NY: McGraw-Hill, 2012.

Pharmacologic Treatment of Central Diabetes Insipidus

Agent	Total daily dose	Frequency administration	Onset of action (h)	Duration of action (h)	Comments
Arginine vasopressin, 20 units/ml	5-10 units subcutaneously	q2-4h	1-2	2-6	Intravenous route may cause vasoconstriction and coronary spasm
Desmopressin acetate (DDAVP)					
10 g/0.1 mL intranasally	10-40 g intranasally	Daily or bid	1-2	8-12	
4 g/mL injection	2-4 intravenously or subcutaneously	Daily or bid	1-2	8-12	

(Adapted from Singer I, Oster JR, Fishman LM. The management of diabetes insipidus in adults. Arch Intern Med. 1997;157(12):1293-1301.)

10 B; 11 A. SIADH and CSW as causes of hyponatremia have significant overlapping clinical findings, making it difficult to differentiate them. Both syndromes happen in the setting of acute intracranial injury, and both have the following features:

1. Concentrated urine with high urinary sodium over 40 mEq/L
2. Nonedematous state
3. Hypouricemia with high fractional excretion of urate

The only difference between SIADH and CSW is the volume status, which is normal/high in SIADH but low in CSW. However, according to several studies, one cannot accurately determine the extracellular volume status in any patient by usual clinical criteria. Falsely determining volume status might lead to erroneous diagnosis, ultimately increasing mortality and morbidity. After determining that the patient is hyponatremic, the **fractional excretion of urate (FE_{urate})** should be calculated:

(Ratio of urine to plasma urate/ Ratio of urine to plasma creatinine) × 100

If the FE_{urate} is >11%, it is consistent with either SIADH or CSW, but repeating FE_{urate} after correction of hyponatremia by any method, such as water

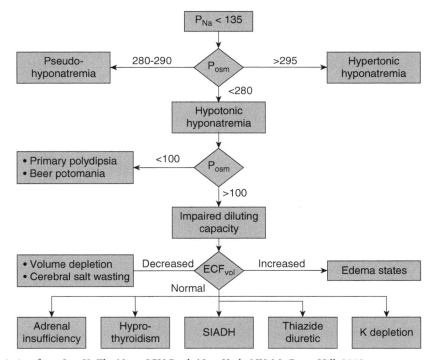

Reproduced with permission from Lee K. *The NeuroICU Book*. New York, NY: McGraw-Hill, 2012.

restriction in the case of SIADH or administration of saline in the case of CSW, will differentiate SIADH from CSW; FE_{urate} will normalize from 11% to 4% in SIADH and remain >11% in CSW.

If FE_{urate} is normal (ie, between 4% and 11%), hyponatremia is due to psychogenic polydipsia.

If FE_{urate} is <4%, hyponatremia is likely secondary to prerenal conditions including volume-depleted states or inadequate perfusion with normal renal function as in true volume depletion, edematous states such as congestive heart failure, cirrhosis, nephrosis, and pre-eclampsia.

12 C. Rhabdomyolysis is a clinical syndrome characterized by muscle injury with release of intracellular content, such as electrolytes, myoglobin, and other sarcoplasmic proteins into circulation. It can lead to AKI. Clinical presentation includes myalgia, weakness, oliguria, or anuria.

Patients with rhabdomyolysis present acutely with pigmented granular casts (muddy brown) and reddish-brown urine (tea colored). The most important test is measurement of serum creatine kinase (CK). CK is elevated within 12 hours after skeletal muscle injury, and persistent elevation is seen for up to 3 to 4 days. The risk of AKI in rhabdomyolysis is low when CK levels are less than 15,000 to 20,000 U/L. Myoglobin is the first enzyme that increases in rhabdomyolysis, but it has a very short half-life (2-3 hours), and its level returns to normal in the first 24 hours after symptoms onset (choice B is incorrect). Aldolase, lactate dehydrogenase, and hepatic transaminases are elevated in rhabdomyolysis, but they lack sensitivity and specificity because there are several other conditions that are associated with elevation of these enzymes (choices A, D, and E are incorrect).

13 E. There are several commonly reported causes of rhabdomyolysis: trauma leading to a crush injury; exertion from strenuous exercise or seizure; muscle hypoxia from a limb compression by head or torso during prolonged immobilization; genetic defects involving disorders of glycolysis, glycogenolysis, or lipid metabolism; infections (Epstein-Barr virus, HIV, influenza A and B); metabolic and electrolyte disorders (hypokalemia, hypophosphatemia, hypocalcemia); drugs and toxins (statins, fibrate, alcohol, cocaine, heroin); and body temperature change (heat stroke, malignant hyperthermia).

14 E. Three mechanisms have been implicated in AKI caused by rhabdomyolysis: renal vasoconstriction, formation of tubular casts, and direct toxicity of myoglobin to kidney tubular cells.

In renal vasoconstriction, there is a decrease in circulatory volume as fluid moves from the intravascular space into the interstitial space of injured muscle. This leads to activation of the sympathetic nervous system, antidiuretic hormone, and renin-angiotensin system, all of which favor vasoconstriction and renal salt and water conservation, with net effect manifested clinically as oliguria with low urine sodium concentration prior to progression to acute tubular injury.

Myoglobin itself is directly toxic to tubular cells. The release of free iron by myoglobin may lead to the formation of oxygen free radicals, as ferrous iron is converted to ferric iron, leading to oxidative injury. Myoglobin can also cause lipid peroxidation of tubular cellular membranes.

The increase in myoglobin levels in the tubules exceeds the absorptive capacity of the proximal tubules. In the distal tubule, myoglobin may complex with Tamm-Horsfall protein, causing formation of casts that lead to intratubular obstruction. An acidic environment (urine pH <6.5) favors the formation of these complexes.

15 B. The treatment of rhabdomyolysis begins with volume repletion with normal saline at a rate of approximately 400 mL/h while monitoring the clinical response or central venous pressure, with target urine output of 3 mL/kg/h. Check serum potassium level frequently and treat hyperkalemia. Correct hypocalcemia only if patient is symptomatic (ie, tetany or seizure) or if severe hyperkalemia occurs.

Check urine pH. If pH <6.5, alternate each liter of normal saline with 1 L of 5% dextrose or 0.45% saline plus 100 mmol of bicarbonate.

Consider treatment with mannitol (up to 200 g/d and cumulative dose up to 800 g). Check for plasma osmolality and plasma osmolal gap, and discontinue mannitol if diuresis (>20 mL/h) is not established.

Maintain euvolemia until myoglobinuria is cleared. Consider renal replacement therapy if there is persistent hyperkalemia of more than 6.5 mmol/L that is symptomatic, rapidly rising potassium, oliguria (<0.5 mL of urine/kg/h for 12 hours), anuria, volume overload, or metabolic acidosis (pH <7.1).

16 A. In a patient with rhabdomyolysis, hypocalcemia is a common complication due to (1) calcium entering the ischemic and damaged muscle cells; (2) hyperphosphatemia inhibiting 1α-hydroxylase in the kidney with less formation of calcitriol, in addition to the renal failure causing low production of 1α-hydroxylase and low calcitriol synthesis; and (3) the formation and deposition of calcium phosphate crystals in necrotic muscles. The recovery of renal function leads to reversal of these mechanisms, and hypercalcemia occurs. This process is unique to rhabdomyolysis-induced AKI.

17 E. This patient likely had a stroke, but she is outside the window for tPA administration given that her last known well time was 2 days prior to presentation. She has life-threatening hyperkalemia. The treatment of hyperkalemia is guided by the following 3 major principles:

- **Membrane stabilization:** Calcium, given either as calcium gluconate or calcium chloride, antagonizes the membrane effects of hyperkalemia by reducing the threshold of potential of cardiac myocytes. Hypertonic (3%) saline administration as a bolus in a patient with hyperkalemia with concurrent hyponatremia has been shown to reverse ECG changes, likely by changing the electrical properties of cardiac myocytes. Neither calcium nor hypertonic saline lowers potassium level.
- **Intracellular shifting:** Shifting of potassium from the extracellular to the intracellular space is accomplished by insulin and dextrose, β-adrenoceptor agonist (albuterol nebulizer), and sodium bicarbonate (better evidence with severe metabolic academia: pH <7.1).
- **Elimination of potassium from the body:** Loop diuretics, cation exchange resin, and emergency dialysis can eliminate potassium from the body. Dialysis is the method of choice for removal of potassium from the body. Peritoneal dialysis (PD), intermittent hemodialysis (IHD), and continuous therapies (continuous venovenous hemofiltration, continuous venovenous hemodiafiltration) may be considered. IHD is the most effective way to remove potassium. PD yields variable results in control of emergent hyperkalemia. It has been used in patients on maintenance PD with moderate hyperkalemia; however, it has a very limited role in the treatment of acute

renal failure associated with severe hyperkalemia with ECG changes in the ICU. Since this patient has an acute stroke, continuous venovenous hemodiafiltration will be the appropriate treatment, but it is not the first step in management, as noted earlier.

18 B. The low pH and high P_{CO_2} indicate a primary respiratory disorder. Since the pH is acidic, the disorder is then a primary respiratory acidosis.

Now let's evaluate acute versus chronic. For acute respiratory acidosis, for every point increase in P_{CO_2} (in mmHg) from normal there is a corresponding increase in HCO_3 (in mmol/L) from normal by 0.1. In our case the P_{CO_2} has changed from 40 (normal) to 60, which should result a HCO_3 change of 2 (expected 26), (60 − 40) = 2. Expected HCO_3 would have been 24 + ΔHCO_3 (2) = 26.

For typical chronic respiratory acidosis, or every point increase in P_{CO_2} (in mmHg) there is a corresponding increase in HCO_3 (in mmol/L) from normal by 0.4. Expected HCO_3 would be 24 + ΔHCO_3 (8) = 32. This is a chronic respiratory acidosis.

Since this is a primary chronic respiratory acidosis, the compensation should be metabolic. Let's calculate the expected pH = 7.4 − [0.003(60 − 40)] = 7.34. Since the measured pH (7.3) is lower than the expected pH, there is a superimposed metabolic acidosis.

Since this patient has diarrhea, she developed a non–anion gap metabolic acidosis, which lowered the HCO_3 and pH. Therefore, this patient has a chronic respiratory acidosis with superimposed non–anion gap metabolic acidosis.

19 C. Since the pH and/or ABG are normal, this is likely a mixed disorder.

First calculate the anion gap (AG): AG = 140 − (99 + 23) = 18. However, we must correct for the low albumin: Adjusted AG = AG + [2.5 (4 − measured albumin)] = 18 + [2.5(2)] = 23.

Gap-gap = (measured AG − 12)/
(24 − measured HCO_3) = (18 − 12)/(24 − 23) = 6

Since gap-gap >1, there is a coexistent metabolic alkalosis. The key to this question is the high anion gap. The coexistence of both metabolic acidosis and metabolic alkalosis normalizes the ABG.

This patient has a mixed anion gap metabolic acidosis and metabolic alkalosis.

20 E. The pH and P_{CO_2} change in opposite direction, indicating a respiratory disorder, and since the pH is alkaline, this is primary respiratory alkalosis.

A decrease of 10 in P_{CO_2} causes a decrease of 2 in HCO_3, which is consistent in acute respiratory alkalosis.

Let's calculate the AG: 140 − (90 + 19) = 31.

Gap-gap = (measured AG − 12)/(24 − measured HCO_3) = (31 − 12)/(24 − 20) = 4.75

Since gap-gap >1, there is a coexistent metabolic alkalosis.

So this patient has acute respiratory alkalosis (likely due to the intracerebral hemorrhage), has anion gap metabolic acidosis (from diabetic ketoacidosis), and has metabolic alkalosis (from vomiting).

21 E. Both pH and P_{CO_2} changes are in the same direction; therefore, this is a primary metabolic disorder. Since the pH is high, indicating an alkalosis, the primary disorder here is metabolic alkalosis.

For compensation, the expected P_{CO_2} = 40 + [0.7(34 − 24)] = 40 + 7 = 47. Expected P_{CO_2} equals the measured P_{CO_2}; therefore, this is a fully compensated metabolic alkalosis.

Since the urine chloride is more than 25 mmol/L, this is likely a chloride-resistant fully compensated metabolic alkalosis. There are 2 causes of metabolic alkalosis: chloride-responsive alkalosis and chloride-resistant alkalosis.

Chloride-responsive metabolic alkalosis is characterized by low urinary chloride concentration (urine chloride concentration <15 mmol/L). The principal causes of this type of metabolic alkalosis include loss of gastric secretions via vomiting, therapy with chloruretic diuretics (thiazides or furosemide), and volume depletion. Patients with chloride-responsive alkalosis improve with infusion of isotonic saline because of volume depletion.

Chloride-resistant metabolic alkalosis is characterized by a urinary chloride concentration >25 mmol/L. Causes of this type of metabolic acidosis include primary aldosteronism, licorice ingestion, and severe hypokalemia. Patients with chloride-resistant metabolic alkalosis have volume expansion and therefore do not improve with infusion with isotonic saline.

22. I = D; II = C; III = F; IV = E; V = A, B

23 E. Preventive measures for drug nephrotoxicity include choosing the appropriate drug dosing for altered kinetics, choosing alternative therapies for drugs with potential nephrotoxicity, and avoiding drug combinations that may result in synergistic nephrotoxicity. Besides those measures, other strategies have been employed to reduce nephrotoxicity, including hydration for drugs such as amphotericin and others that cause crystal-induced nephropathy. In addition, urine alkalinization may reduce crystal precipitation of drugs such as sulfadiazine, whereas urine acidification reduces indinavir precipitation. Sodium administration has been used to prevent amphotericin B nephrotoxicity.

24 A. This patient developed an acute tubular necrosis (ATN) as a result of the profound hypotension. In these patients, the urinary osmolality is <400 mOsm/kg, urinary sodium concentration is >40 mmol/L, and urine-to-serum creatinine ratio is <20. The fractional excretion of sodium (FE_{Na}), which is based on the fact that sodium reabsorption is enhanced in setting of hypovolemia, is >2%.

$$FE_{Na} = [(\text{urinary Na/serum Na})/(\text{urinary Cr/serum Cr})] \times 100$$

An FE_{Na} >2% suggests ATN as the cause of AKI. For patients on diuretics, FE_{Na} is not accurate, and one must calculate the fractional excretion of urea, with a value >35% suggesting ATN.

This patient has urinary osmolality of 350 mOsm/kg, urine sodium of 50 mmol/L, and a urine-to-serum creatinine concentration (40/4) of 10; FE_{Na} is 3.6%. All of these factors point toward ATN as the cause of his AKI.

In addition, the muddy brown granular casts are characteristic of ATN.

REFERENCES

Abuelo JG. Normotensive ischemic acute renal failure. *N Engl J Med.* 2007;357:797-798.

Albright RC. Water and electrolyte disturbances in acute renal failure. In: *Critical Care Nephrology.* 2nd ed. New York NY: Saunders/Elsevier; 2009:399-403.

Bagshaw SM, Berthiaume LR, Delaney A, et al. Continuous versus intermittent therapy for critically ill patients with acute kidney injury: a meta-analysis. *Crit Care Med.* 2008;36:610-617.

Bieber SD, Jefferson JA. Rhabdomyolysis. In: *Nephrology Secrets.* 3rd ed. New York, NY: Mosby; 2012:90-95.

Bitew S, Imbriano L, Miyawaki N, et al. More on renal salt wasting without cerebral disease, response to saline infusion. *Clin J Am Soc Nephol.* 2009;4:309-315.

Bosch X, Poch E, Grau JM. Rhabdomyolysis and acute kidney injury. *N Engl J Med.* 2009;361:62-72.

Capatina C, Paluzzi A, Mitchell R, et al. Diabetes insipidus after traumatic brain injury. *J Clin Med.* 2015;4:1448-1462.

Coppo R, Peruzzi L, Amore A. Antibiotics and antiviral drugs in the intensive care unit. In: *Critical Care Nephrology.* 2nd ed. New York, NY: Saunders; 2009:1687-1692.

Kidney Disease: Improving Global Outcomes (KDIGO) Acute Kidney Injury Work Group. KDIGO clinical practice guideline for acute kidney injury. *Kidney Int (Suppl).* 2012;2:1-138.

Maesaka JK, Abriano L, Mattana J, et al. Differentiating SIADH from cerebral/renal salt wasting: failure of the volume approach and need for a new approach to hyponatremia. *J Clin Med.* 2014;3:1373-1385.

Maesaka JK, Miyawaki N, Palaia T, et al. Renal salt wasting without cerebral disease: value of determining urate in hyponatremia. *Kidney Int.* 2007;71:822-826.

Marino P. Acid-base analysis. In: *The ICU Book.* 4th ed. Philadelphia, PA: Lippincott; 2014:587-599.

Marquis F, Ahern SP, Leblanc M. Etiology of acute renal failure in the intensive care unit. In: *Critical Care Nephrology.* 2nd ed. New York, NY: Saunders; 2009:96-100.

Pannu N, Gibney RTN. Renal replacement therapy in the intensive care unit. *Ther Clin Risk Manag.* 2005;1:141-150.

Petejova N, Martinek A. Acute kidney injury due to rhabdomyolysis and renal replacement therapy: a critical review. *Crit Care.* 2014;18:224.

Reddi AS. Mixed acid-base disorders. In: *Fluid, Electrolyte, and Acid-Base Disorders. Clinical Evaluation and Management.* New York, NY: Springer; 2014:429-442.

Reddi AS. Respiratory acidosis. In: *Fluid, Electrolyte, and Acid-Base Disorders. Clinical Evaluation and Management.* New York, NY: Springer; 2014:407-419.

Ring T. Renal tubular acidosis. In: *Critical Care Nephrology.* 2nd ed. New York, NY: Saunders; 2009:655-662.

Subramanian S, Kellum JA, Ronco C Oliguria. In: *Critical Care Nephrology.* 2nd ed. New York, NY: Saunders; 2009:341-345.

Weisberg LS. Management of severe hyperkalemia. *Crit Care Med.* 2008;36:3246-3251.

Wiederkehr M, Moe O. Core concepts and treatments of metabolic acidosis. In: *Core Concepts in the Disorders of Fluid, Electrolytes and Acid-Base Balance.* New York, NY: Springer; 2013:258-260.

10

Neuro-oncology

Fernando Santos Pinheiro, MD and David Cachia, MD

Questions

1. What molecular mutation is a predictor of improved overall survival in glioblastoma (World Health Organization [WHO] grade IV astrocytoma)?

   A. *PTEN* mutation

   B. *EGFR* mutation

   C. *IDH* mutation

   D. Ki-67

   E. 1p/19q codeletion

2. What is the most common primary malignant brain tumor of childhood?

   A. Glioblastoma

   B. Pilocytic astrocytoma

   C. Meningioma (WHO grade I)

   D. Ganglioglioma

   E. Medulloblastoma

3. A 55-year-old woman with no past medical history presents to the emergency department (ED) with progressive headaches for 2 months prior to presentation. Her neurologic exam is otherwise unremarkable. Brain magnetic resonance imaging (MRI) with contrast reveals an irregularly enhancing 4-cm infiltrating lesion with central necrosis on the right parietal lobe with surrounding vasogenic edema (see figure below). Computed tomography (CT) of the chest, abdomen, and pelvis is unremarkable. Also, blood cultures and transthoracic echocardiography (TTE) were obtained at admission and are also unremarkable. Based on the most likely diagnosis, what is the treatment of choice?

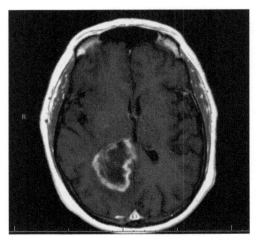

Magnetic resonance imaging of the brain, axial T1 with contrast: right frontoparietal enhancing lesion with central necrosis.

A. Radiation → maximal resection → chemotherapy

B. Neoadjuvant chemotherapy and radiation → maximum resection

C. Maximum safe resection → concurrent chemotherapy and radiation → adjuvant chemotherapy

D. Biopsy → concurrent chemotherapy and radiation → adjuvant chemotherapy

E. Chemotherapy alone for 1 year

4. A 65-year-old woman with history of glioblastoma treated with radiation and temozolomide presents for routine visit 14 months after diagnosis. A brain MRI reveals 2 new enhancing lesions on the same hemisphere of the initial lesion, with mild surrounding vasogenic edema and mass effect (see figure below). Positron emission tomography (PET)-CT revealed hypermetabolism of the new lesions, whereas magnetic resonance spectroscopy revealed an elevated choline-to-creatinine ratio >3, both indicative of tumor recurrence. On exam, the patient has a Karnofsky performance score (KPS) of 90 with some fatigue. What is the next best step in treatment for this patient?

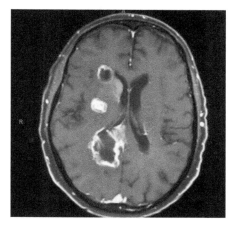

Magnetic resonance imaging of the brain, axial T1 with contrast: multifocal enhancing lesions within the right hemisphere deep white matter.

A. Start bevacizumab

B. Continue observation

C. Start intravenous (IV) dexamethasone 10 mg every 6 hours

D. Arrange hospice consult

E. Start IV vincristine

Questions 5 and 6

A 39-year-old man developed a simple partial seizure involving shaking of the right arm that evolved into a generalized tonic-clonic convulsion while playing golf. After administation of 2 mg of intravenous lorazepam by emergency medical services, the clinical seizure activity stops. He is brought to the ED for additional evaluation. He is seen by you in the ED. Although the patient is not convulsing any longer, he is still confused and unable to follow commands or protect airway 2 hours after the seizure onset. He is afebrile. Review of his medication list shows that the patient is not on any anticonvulsant therapy. He is eventually intubated. A contrasted MRI of the brain is obtained and shown below.

6. Shortly after initiation of the phenytoin infusion the patient became bradycardic (heart rate into 30's) and hypotensive (blood pressure 60's/30's). The infusion was stopped with improvement in his hemodynamics. Rather than continuing with phenytoin infusion, valproic acid was started with a bolus of 40 mg/kg. What is true about use of valproic acid?

A. The potential coagulopathy caused by valproic acid can be reversed by use of desmopressin (DDAVP).

B. Commonly used neuro-oncologic chemotherapeutics are not affected by valproic acid.

C. The use of valproic acid can improve disease-free survival in patients with glioblastoma multiforme (WHO grade IV).

D. Patients on valproic acid need routine ammonia screening.

E. A total level of valproic acid can be checked to guide dosing of the medication after the load.

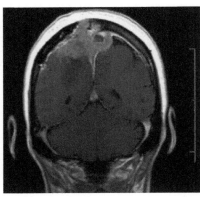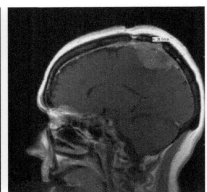

Magnetic resonance imaging of the brain (coronal and sagittal T1 with contrast): right > left parafalcine lesion with destruction of the falx and crossing midline with surrounding edema. There is involvement of the superior sagittal sinus.

5. Which of the following would be the most appropriate next step?

A. Start thiamine load with 100 mg IV then 50 mL dextrose 50% in water (D50W) IV

B. Get a stat electroencephalogram (EEG) study

C. Start empiric antibiotics and perform a diagnostic lumbar puncture (LP)

D. Start intravenous phenytoin with a loading dose of 20 mg/kg

E. Request neuro-oncology consult

7. Which of the following chemotherapeutic agents is most commonly associated with the adverse reaction of peripheral neuropathy?

A. Lomustine

B. Etoposide

C. Vincristine

D. Temozolomide

E. Bevacizumab

Questions 8-10

A 58-year-old women with breast cancer diagnosed 10 years ago, status post bilateral mastectomy and chemotherapy, who is currently on tamoxifen as maintenance therapy, presented to her primary oncologist due to facial numbness and diplopia. Over the past 3 months, the patient has developed numbness of the lower left lip and double vision when looking to the far left. She has also noticed trouble with balance when walking on uneven surfaces, and her right hand is clumsy to the point that she spills coffee when holding a coffee mug. A CT of the head is done and is unremarkable. Brain MRI is shown below.

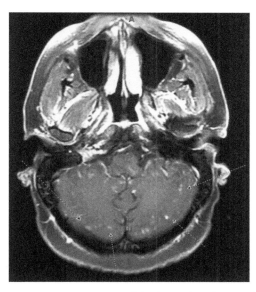

Magnetic resonance imaging of the brain (axial T1 with contrast) with signs of increased hyperintensities in the surface of the cerebellar region.

8. What is the most likely diagnosis?

   A. Leptomeningeal metastasis from primary breast cancer

   B. Intra-axial metastatic disease from primary breast cancer

   C. Cardioembolic strokes

   D. Paraneoplastic cerebellar degeneration

   E. Chemical meningitis from tamoxifen

9. What is the best next step in the workup of the condition described?

   A. LP with opening pressure, cell count and differential, protein, glucose, and cytopathology

   B. Magnetic resonance spectroscopy followed by PET-CT

   C. Esophageal echocardiogram

   D. Biopsy of the lateral ventricle lesion

   E. Discontinue tamoxifen

10. You successfully perform an LP and the results are as follows: opening pressure 9 cm H_2O; glucose 55 mg/dL; protein 255 mg/dL; white blood cells (WBC) 11 cells/microL; red blood cells (RBC) 1 cell/microL; and cytopathology: negative for malignant cells. Despite these results, you continue to have high suspicion for the presumed diagnosis. Two weeks later, the patient continues to deteriorate neurologically. What is the best next step?

    A. Repeat LP with opening pressure, glucose, protein, WBC, and cytopathology

    B. Start stereotactic radiation to the suspected foci

    C. Start empiric systemic chemotherapy

    D. Perform biopsy of 1 of the cerebellar lesions

    E. Obtain whole-body PET

11. An 18-year-old patient arrives in the ED following a 12-minute generalized tonic-clonic seizure witnessed by his mother. The seizure eventually subsided after administration of lorazepam and fosphenytoin IV. He is admitted to the neurologic intensive care unit (ICU) because his mental status is not yet back to baseline and staff is concerned that he may require endotracheal intubation for airway protection. Further investigation reveals that he had just been diagnosed with a testicular mass and is scheduled to have a biopsy tomorrow. According to his mother, he has been very agitated and anxious lately, sometimes paranoid and aggressive toward her over the last 2 weeks. Toxicology screen is negative. CT of the head is also unremarkable. Brain MRI is shown below. You request a bedside EEG. What EEG finding is best correlated to the most likely diagnosis in this case?

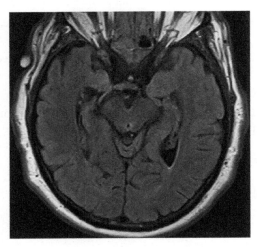

Magnetic resonance imaging of the brain (axial T2 fluid-attenuated inversion recovery): hyperintensity in the bilateral mesial temporal lobes and uncus.

A. Alpha coma
B. Burst suppression
C. Extreme delta brush
D. Phantom spike-and-wave
E. Wicket rhythm

12. Which of the following is a known severe neurologic adverse reaction attributed to the use of the chemotherapeutic agent bevacizumab?
A. Cerebral edema
B. Status epilepticus (convulsive and nonconvulsive)
C. Cerebral infarct (ischemic and hemorrhagic)
D. Malignant hydrocephalus
E. Central pontine myelinolysis

13. What is the most common primary intramedullary spinal tumor in adults?
A. Meningioma
B. Ependymoma
C. Ganglioglioma
D. Schwannoma
E. Oligodendroglioma

14. A 34-year-old woman presented to the ED with altered mental status. She has a history of IV drug use, human immunodeficiency virus (HIV), and hepatitis C for which she takes no medications. Other than the confusion, she seems to have no other systemic involvement. MRI of the brain is shown below. Which organism could be associated with the underlying diagnosis in this woman?

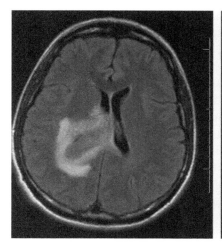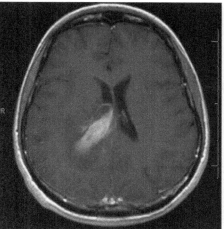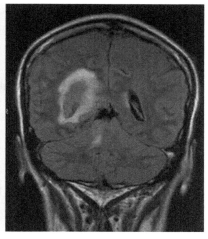

Magnetic resonance imaging of the brain (axial T2/fluid-attenuated inversion recovery [FLAIR] axial T1 with contrast, coronal T2/FLAIR): large right periventricular homogeneously enhancing lesion and surrounding vasogenic edema.

A. Cytomegalovirus (CMV)
B. Epstein-Barr virus (EBV)
C. *Toxoplasma*
D. Syphilis
E. Adenovirus

15. A 24-year-old man presents to the neurology clinic with a 6-month history of progressive headaches, urine incontinence, and ataxic gait. He also has history of bilateral hypoacusis, similar to other members of his family. You request a brain MRI, which reveals obstructive hydrocephalus, secondary to a homogeneously enhancing infratentorial mass compressing the cerebral aqueduct with minimal surrounding edema. Also seen are bilateral enhancing lesions involving cranial nerve VIII. Based on the suspected genetic syndrome, what is the pathology of the mass compressing the cerebral aqueduct?

A. Schwannoma
B. Meningioma
C. Glioblastoma
D. Oligodendroglioma
E. Pilocytic xanthoastrocytoma

16. A 58-year-old man presents to the ED after a witnessed generalized tonic-clonic seizure while gardening in the back yard. The seizure lasted 2 minutes. He arrives to the ED and is already back to his baseline, but complains of significant pounding headache. An MRI of the brain is obtained and is shown below. Neurosurgery is on their way to evaluate the patient. They recommend a single dose of dexamethasone 10 mg IV followed by 4 mg IV every 6 hours. Why is dexamethasone favored over other steroids for treatment of vasogenic edema?

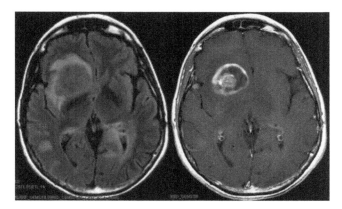

Magnetic resonance imaging of the brain (axial T2/fluid-attenuated inversion recovery [FLAIR] and axial T1 with contrast): 5.5 cm × 6.1 cm × 4.4 cm irregular mass with a necrotic center on the right frontal region with prominent surrounding vasogenic edema and mass effect causing a 6-mm midline shift.

A. Lower mineralocorticoid activity
B. Better penetration across the blood-brain barrier
C. Shorter half-life
D. Decreased risk of hyperglycemia
E. Only steroid available in IV formulation

17. What is the lifetime rate of recurrence of diffuse astrocytoma (WHO grade II) that underwent gross total resection?

    A. 0% to 20%

    B. 20% to 40%

    C. 40% to 60%

    D. 60% to 80%

    E. 80% to 100%

18. Which of the following primary cancers have the potential to both metastasize to the brain and cause intraparenchymal hemorrhage?

    A. Melanoma and renal cancer

    B. Thymoma and prostate cancer

    C. Esophageal and liver cancer

    D. Pharyngeal and pancreatic cancer

    E. Bladder and gastric cancer

19. A 68-year-old man presents to the neurology clinic with progressive fatigue and weakness of the proximal upper and lower extremities that is worse in the morning and tends to improve once he starts to work as a farmer on his ranch in Armadillo, Texas. He has an 80-pack-year smoking history. Lately, he has lost a significant amount of weight, and over the past month, he endorses productive cough with red-stained sputum. He brings a chest x-ray done by his local physician, which reveals a nodular lesion of the right upper lobe along with bibasilar opacities of the lungs. The electromyogram reveals low compound muscle action potential (CMAP) amplitude and an incremental response pattern of motor activation during repetitive nerve stimulation on high-rate frequencies (20-50 Hz). What antibody is associated with his disease process?

    A. GQ1-b

    B. Muscle-specific kinase (MUSK) antibodies

    C. Voltage-gated calcium channel (VGCC) antibodies

    D. N-Methyl-D-aspartate (NMDA) receptor antibodies

    E. Glutamic acid decarboxylase (GAD-65) antibodies

20. A 45-year-old woman presents with progressively worsening headaches and anger outbursts, which is not typical behavior for her. MRI of the brain is shown below (left panel). Pathology is consistent with *IDH1*-mutated glioblastoma. Her KPS 1 week after surgery is 100. She completes radiation therapy along with temozolomide for 6 weeks, after which she starts temozolomide alone. After completing the first cycle of adjuvant chemotherapy, brain MRI with contrast is shown (right panel). The patient is neurologically stable. What is the next most appropriate step?

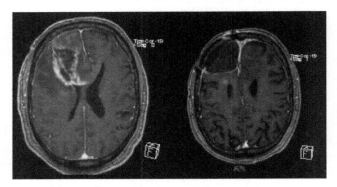

Magnetic resonance imaging of the brain (axial T1 with contrast): left panel shows presence of an enhancing necrotic lesion of the right frontal lobe with surrounding edema; right panel shows repeat scan following surgical resection, radiation, and temozolomide with nodular posterior surgical cavity enhancement.

    A. Increase dose of temozolomide

    B. Request brain fluorodeoxyglucose (FDG)-PET

    C. Add bevacizumab to temozolomide

    D. Perform LP

    E. Repeat brain MRI in 6 months

21. Which of the following meningioma categories is known to cause prominent peritumoral edema?

    A. Meningothelial meningioma

    B. Psammomatous meningioma

    C. Fibrous meningioma

    D. Secretory meningioma

    E. Microcystic meningioma

22. Which of the following primary CNS tumors has the highest risk of metastasizing outside of the CNS?

   A. Glioblastoma

   B. Dysembryoplastic neuroepithelial tumor (DNET)

   C. Ganglioglioma

   D. Oligodendroglioma

   E. Anaplastic meningiomas

23. A 34-year-old man with hypertrophic obstructive cardiomyopathy (HOCM) presented to the ED at the urging of his wife. He was in his usual state of health while at home and had a loss of consciousness that lasted for only a few seconds. On arousal, he was somewhat confused and had a diffuse holocephalic headache. On initial evaluation in the ED, he had a normal neurologic examination and normal vital signs, but on cardiac examination, he had a systolic murmur heard best at the left upper sternal border that increased with Valsalva. Basic laboratory testing was unrevealing. The patient was discharged with tele-monitoring. Given his loss of consciousness at home and ongoing headache an MRI brain was obtained. What is the most likely cause of his syncope?

   A. HOCM due to valvular disease

   B. Atonic seizure

   C. Rupture of a cerebral aneurysm with resulting subarachnoid hemorrhage

   D. Obstructive hydrocephalus from colloid cyst

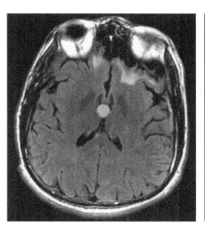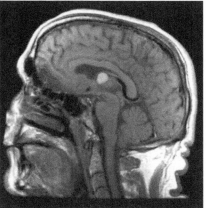

Non-contrast axial (left) and mid-saggital (right) FLAIR sequence of MRI brain. Reproduced with permission from Ropper AH, Samuels MA, Klein JP. *Adams and Victor's Principles of Neurology*, 10e. New York, NY: McGraw-Hill, 2014.

Answers and Explanations

1. **C.** Isocitrate dehydrogenase (*IDH*) gene mutation is thought to occur as one of the early steps in gliomagenesis and is typically present in both lineages of glial tumors—astrocytomas and oligodendrogliomas. It is postulated that WHO grade IV astrocytomas (glioblastoma) expressing *IDH* mutation have arisen from a low-grade glioma. The disease course tends to be more favorable than *IDH* wild-type glioblastomas. *P53* mutation is seen in most low-grade astrocytomas but is not a prognostic marker. 1p/19q codeletion is commonly seen in oligodendrogliomas, but not astrocytomas. Ki-67 is a mitosis marker also unrelated to outcome. *EGFR* and *PTEN* mutations tend to occur more frequently in primary glioblastomas versus secondary glioblastomas.

2. **E.** Primary brain tumors are the most common solid tumors affecting children under age 10. Medulloblastomas are the most common primary malignant brain tumor of childhood, accounting for 15% to 20% of them. All medulloblastomas are considered high-grade tumors, and they are always located in the infratentorial region and are commonly midline. Medulloblastomas can be stratified into average-risk and high-risk subgroups based on age, disease dissemination, and extent of residual disease after surgical resection. More recently, molecular characterization has also stratified medulloblastomas into 4 groups with different biologic behavior and outcomes. The 5-year overall survival rate is 70% for standard-risk patients who undergo surgical resection, radiotherapy, and chemotherapy. Pilocytic astrocytomas, gangliogliomas, and meningiomas are not malignant brain tumors. Glioblastoma is the most common primary malignant brain tumor in adults.

3. **C.** The imaging findings and presentation are concerning for a malignant brain tumor, specifically glioblastoma. Imaging characteristics are heterogenous enhancement with central areas of necrosis and surrounding T2/fluid-attenuated inversion recovery (FLAIR) signal abnormality surrounding the mass. The fact that she is systemically stable and afebrile with normal TTE and negative blood cultures, together with the imaging findings, makes a brain abscess less likely.

   The standard-of-care treatment for glioblastoma is maximal safe resection followed by a 6-week course of radiation with concurrent chemotherapy (temozolomide) followed by adjuvant chemotherapy (temozolomide).

4. **A.** Bevacizumab is approved by the US Food and Drug Administration (FDA) for recurrent glioblastomas monotherapy based on phase II trials that showed improvement in radiographic response and progression-free survival. Bevacizumab is a vascular endothelial growth factor (VEGF) inhibitor that is thought to decrease the blood supply to these very vascular tumors. More recent phase III trials using bevacizumab in newly diagnosed glioblastomas have not shown any survival benefit in adding bevacizumab, so while it is approved treatment for recurrent glioblastomas as described in this case, there is no role for it in the treatment of newly diagnosed glioblastoma cases. Since the patient has not received any treatment for recurrent tumor and has a good functional status, hospice care should be deferred for now. Although dexamethasone is certainly reasonable, it does not have any antineoplastic properties and will only help for symptomatic improvement of the vasogenic edema, of which there is only limited findings. There is no evidence to support the use of vincristine in recurrent glioblastoma.

5. **D.** The suspicion of nonconvulsive status epilepticus should be high in any patient presenting with persistent altered mental status in the setting of a past medical history of epilepsy, brain tumors, and genetic neurologic syndromes. Performing an EEG would be paramount to rule out nonconvulsive status, but should not delay treatment for status epileptics. There are several medications approved for treatment of status epilepticus: phenytoin, valproic acid, and phenobarbital.

6. **E.** The findings of bradycardia and hypotension are commonly seen adverse side-effects of pheyntoin. The bradycardia is due to direct blockade of sodium channels with the myocardium and the hypotension is due to the dilutent (propylene glycol). Valproic acid is approved for treatment of status epilepticus, but it is not without complication. Valproic acid is a CYP450 inhibitor and can interact with a number of medications, including those that are commonly used in neuro-oncology such as bevacizumab and temozolomide. The use of these medications combined can result in increased hematologic complications.

   Valproic acid is also known to cause coagulopathy through varying mechanisms including thrombocytopenia, acquired von Willebrand disease, and depletion of procoagulant proteins. Although rarely an issue for surgical intervention, screening is recommended for surgical interventions where large blood loss is anticipate and treatment with platelets, DDAVP, and fresh frozen plasma may be required. Although valproic acid can commonly (~50% of those taking the medication) cause hyperammonemia, regular screening is not required unless there is an alteration in mental status. There were early data in retrospective reviews that valproic acid was associated with progression-free survival in patients with glioblastoma, but in a large review of multiple trials, there was no improvement in progression-free or overall survival time with use of valproic acid. Although a free level can be checked, only a total level is typically required for medication titration.

7. **C.** Peripheral neuropathy is one of the most common side effects associated with the use of vincristine. The onset is fairly quick after the medication has been started. Both onset and symptom progression are dose dependent. The prevalence of peripheral neuropathy ranges from 35% to 95%. The neuropathy is axonal in pattern and is commonly sensory, although motor and autonomic fibers may also be involved. It may improve after the chemotherapy is discontinued.

8. **A.** Leptomeningeal carcinomatosis (LMC) should be considered in cancer patients presenting with neurologic symptoms that are hard to localize to a single parenchymal region. LMC is most commonly related to solid tumors such as breast and lung cancer and is rarely seen in leukemia and non-Hodgkin lymphoma. The condition may appear anywhere along the gyri/sulci of the brain, ventricular lining, and spinal cord surface. Therefore, the diagnostic workup for LMC should include contrast MRI of the brain and whole spine, along with cerebrospinal fluid (CSF) studies for cytopathology revision. LMC predicts poor prognosis.

9. **A.** If leptomeningeal disease is caught in early stages, the MRI and cytopathologic studies may be negative, although this does not necessarily rule out the condition, and further CSF analysis and imaging should be pursued. In fact, sensitivity after one LP is only 70%, increasing to 95% after 3 high-volume LPs.

10. **A.** Although the first LP was without malignancy, the sensitivity of first LP is only 70%, increasing to 95% after 3 high-volume LPs. Although biopsy of the cerebellar lesions is possible, repeating an LP prior to biopsy is appropriate. Treatment options are very limited, with radiation and intrathecal chemotherapy being therapeutic options. Despite aggressive therapy, the overall survival is still weeks to months in the majority of cases.

11. **C.** Anti-NMDA (*N*-methyl-D-aspartate) receptor encephalitis is seen in young adults presenting with germ cell tumors such as ovarian teratoma or testicular carcinoma. Symptomatic onset is usually acute, with behavioral changes and epileptic seizures being the most common presentation. Extreme delta brush is an EEG pattern characterized by

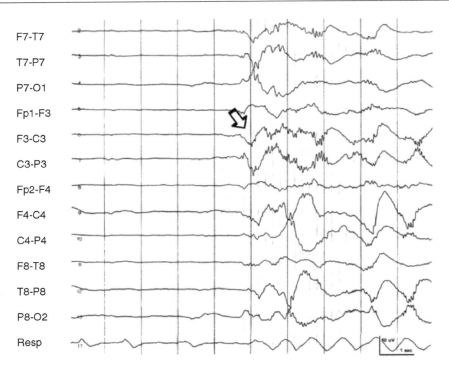

F7-T7

T7-P7

P7-O1

Fp1-F3

F3-C3

C3-P3

Fp2-F4

F4-C4

C4-P4

F8-T8

T8-P8

P8-O2

Resp

Limited EEG with findings of extreme delta brush shown at the arrow. Reproduced with permission from Laoprasert P. *Atlas of Pediatric EEG*. New York, NY: McGraw-Hill, 2011.

slow (delta) waves superimposed with fast (beta) activity, in a continuous and generalized pattern. The pathophysiology of this unique EEG finding is not well stablished. Extreme delta brush is a very specific although not pathognomonic sign of anti-NMDA receptor encephalitis. It is also seen in premature neonates.

12. **C.** Bevacizumab is an antiangiogenesis agent (VEGF inhibitor) with FDA approval for the treatment of recurrent glioblastoma. It significantly decreases vasogenic edema attributed to brain tumors or treatment effect such as radiation, rather than cause edema. Hypertension is the most common adverse reaction seen in up to 25% of patients on bevacizumab. Rare but potentially life-threatening side effects include cerebral infarcts, ischemic or hemorrhagic, that are arterial or venous in origin.

13. **B.** Ependymomas are uncommon central nervous system (CNS) tumors that may occur both in the brain and in the spinal cord. Nevertheless, they are the most common primary intramedullary spinal tumor in adults, accounting of up to 50% of all cases. Such tumors are classified according to the 2016 WHO classification as WHO grade I, II, or III, with some lower grade tumors being

associated with excellent prognosis—even cure—if amenable for gross total resection (eg, myxopapillary ependymomas of the cord). Besides surgery, adjuvant radiation is another therapeutic option, especially for tumors that are incompletely resected or with higher grade histology. Currently there is no role for chemotherapy in the treatment of ependymomas.

14. **B.** The imaging findings are highly suggestive of CNS lymphoma. Typically, this occurs in the periventricular region, with homogenous contrast enhancement. However, immunosuppressed patients can present with atypical imaging patterns. Since systemic workup has been negative, the diagnosis of primary CNS lymphoma is likely. In immunosuppressed patients with primary CNS lymphoma, there is a very frequent association with EBV. Outcomes in immunosuppressed patients with primary CNS lymphoma are typically worse than those in immunocompetent patients.

15. **B.** Neurofibromatosis type 2 (NF2) is an autosomal dominant disease associated with a loss of function of merlin, a protein encoded by the tumor-suppression gene *NF2* located on 22q12.2. NF2 is characterized by bilateral vestibular schwannomas and the propensity to develop other benign tumors such

as meningiomas and ependymoma. The imaging characteristics described are more typical of a meningioma than an ependymoma. The management of NF2 patients is complex and requires a multidisciplinary team and long-term follow-up.

16. **A.** The use of corticosteroids for the acute management of brain edema secondary to a neoplasm has been well established in the setting of symptomatic control, preoperative setup, and postoperative management. Dexamethasone is the steroid of choice in the setting of brain tumor–related vasogenic edema in light of its relative lower mineralocorticoid activity when compared to other steroids as well as longer half-life, which facilitates administration scheduling to once or twice daily. Dexamethasone, methylprednisolone, and hydrocortisone are a few examples of steroids with IV formulation.

17. **E.** Unfortunately brain tumors classified as WHO grade II, III, or IV are invariably incurable. Such tumors exhibit an infiltrative growth pattern that goes beyond the boundaries predicted by MRI scans. Therefore, a surgery is never curative for these tumors. Hence, the goal of surgery is safe maximal resection.

18. **A.** Metastatic (or secondary) brain tumors are 10 times more common than primary brain tumors. Brain metastases occur in approximately 15% of cancer patients as a result of hematogenous dissemination of systemic cancer. The most common tumors to metastasize to the brain are lung, breast, colon, and kidney cancer and melanoma. The most common types of metastatic brain tumors associated with hemorrhagic conversion are melanoma, renal cell carcinoma, choriocarcinoma, thyroid carcinoma, bronchogenic carcinoma, and breast carcinoma.

19. **C.** Paraneoplastic syndromes (PNS) are a relatively rare complication of cancer, affecting less than 1% of patients overall. Nevertheless, certain neoplasms have higher predisposition for developing PNS, including lung, germ cell, and lymphoid cancer.

Lambert-Eaton myasthenic syndrome (LEMS) is a rare autoimmune disorder in the level of the neuromuscular junction, with autoantibodies targeting the voltage-gated calcium channels (VGCC) anchored on the presynaptic membrane. It is characterized by proximal muscle weakness, dysautonomia, and hypoactive reflexes. LEMS presents as a paraneoplastic form in approximately 50% of small-cell lung cancer cases. Early recognition is crucial, and it sometimes precedes the diagnosis of the primary malignancy. As usual, definitive treatment of any paraneoplastic syndrome relies mostly on the management of the primary malignancy, although immunoglobulin therapy and plasmapheresis may be necessary for provisional management.

20. **B.** This case illustrates a common dilemma seen in patients with brain tumors who undergo surgical and radiotherapeutic treatment and then present with a new enhancing lesion on the MRI scan. The clarification of whether such a finding represents a true tumor progression versus treatment effect (also known as pseudoprogression) is of extreme importance so as to not delay effective and time-sensitive management of a recurring tumor. For this purpose, FDG-PET, which measures the degree of FDG metabolism by the tissue, is a good alternative, as it would show hypermetabolic activity in case of a tumor progression or hypometabolic activity in case of treatment effect. The confirmatory diagnosis is, nevertheless, only possible with tissue analysis. Another imaging tool available for this purpose is magnetic resonance spectroscopy, which measures biochemical changes in the area of interest.

21. **D.** Meningiomas are the most common primary brain neoplasms, representing roughly a third of all primary intracranial tumors. Secretory meningiomas are a rare variant, classified as WHO grade I. Yet, despite being considered low grade, they may cause significant morbidity secondary to significant, and sometimes disproportionate, peritumoral edema. Histologically, secretory meningiomas contain glandular lamina with periodic acid-Schiff (PAS)–positive material and eosinophilic secretory globules, also known as pseudopsammoma bodies. Contrast brain MRI scan reveals a vivid homogeneous enhancement of the mass, which tends to protrude outward from the leptomeninges, and it is usually accompanied by a dural tail.

22. **E.** Primary brain tumors are almost exclusively confined to the intracranial space. Nevertheless, meningiomas may rarely metastasize to extracranial locations including liver, bone, soft tissues, and lung. It is assumed that the risk of metastasis of meningiomas is less than 1%, although the risk

increases to approximately 40% among the WHO grade III meningioma subgroup.

23. D. The patient presents with a transient loss of consciousness due to transient obstructive hydrocephalus from his colloid cyst. A colloid cyst is typically located at the roof of the third ventricle, hyperdense, and unilocular and, rarely, can be calcified. Although more commonly found incidentally, the cyst can result in sudden obstructive hydrocephalus.

Atonic, sometimes called "drop," seizures consist of a brief loss of muscle tone and falls that begin in childhood and are part of Lennox-Gasteaut syndrome. Although approximately 40% of subarachnoid hemorrhages can result in a transient loss of consciousness, which is thought to be transient elevation in intracranial pressure, the imaging is not consistent with subarachnoid hemorrhage given the encapsulated and localized hyperdensity on brain MRI. Hypertrophic cardiomyopathy can have syncope as a symptom. The common causes of syncope are inappropriate drop in systolic blood pressure from outflow obstruction/abnormal vascular control or arrhythmia.

REFERENCES

Abdallah C. Considerations in perioperative assessment of valpric acid coagulopathy. *Anaesthesiol Clin Pharmacol.* 2014;30:7-9.

Aghi MK, Nahed BV, Sloan AE, et al. The role of surgery in the management of patients with diffuse low grade glioma: a systematic review and evidence-based clinical practice guideline. *J Neurooncol.* 2015;125:503-530.

Bashir R, McManus B, Cunningham C, et al. Detection of Eber-1 RNA in primary brain lymphomas in immunocompetent and immunocompromised patients. *J Neurooncol.* 1994;20:47-53.

Benit CP, Vecht CJ. Seizures and cancer: drug interactions of anticonvulsants with chemotherapeutic agents, tyrosine kinase inhibitors and glucocorticoids. *Neurooncol Pract.* 2016;3:245-260.

Berg SL, Parsons DW. The pharmacogenomics of vincristine-induced neuropathy: on pins and needles. *JAMA Oncol.* 2015;1:975-976.

Blakeley JO, Plotkin SR. Therapeutic advances for the tumors associated with neurofibromatosis type 1, type 2, and schwannomatosis. *Neuro-Oncol.* 2016;18:624-638.

Bradley WG, Lassman LP, Pearce GW, et al. The neuromyopathy of vincristine in man. Clinical, electrophysiological and pathological studies. *J Neurol Sci.* 1970;10:107-131.

Buhl R, Hugo HH, Mihajlovic Z, et al. Secretory meningiomas: clinical and immunohistochemical observations. *Neurosurgery.* 2001;48:297-301.

Caroline I, Rosenthal MA. Imaging modalities in high-grade gliomas: pseudoprogression, recurrence, or necrosis? *J Clin Neurosci.* 2012;19:633-637.

Casey EB, Jellife AM, Le Quesne PM, et al. Vincristine neuropathy. Clinical and electrophysiological observations. *Brain.* 1973;96:69-86.

Chinot OL, Wick W, Mason W, et al. Bevacizumab plus radiotherapy-temozolomide for newly diagnosed glioblastoma. *N Engl J Med.* 2014;370:709-722.

Chua FH, Low SY, Tham CK, et al. Disseminated extracranial metastatic meningioma. *J Clin Neurosci.* 2016;33:214-216.

Clarke JL. Leptomeningeal metastasis from systemic cancer. *Continuum (Minneap Minn).* 2012;18:328-342.

Czock D, Keller F, Rasche FM, et al. Pharmacokinetics and pharmacodynamics of systemically administered glucocorticoids. *Clin Pharmacokinet.* 2005;44:61-98.

Dalmau J, Gleichman AJ, Hughes EG, et al. Anti-NMDA-receptor encephalitis: case series and analysis of the effects of antibodies. *Lancet Neurol.* 2008;7:1091-1098.

Duffau H. Resecting diffuse low-grade gliomas to the boundaries of brain functions: a new concept in surgical neuro-oncology. *J Neurosurg Sci.* 2015;59:361-371.

Enam SA, Abdulrauf S, Mehta B, et al. Metastasis in meningioma. *Acta Neurochir (Wien).* 1996;138:1172-1177.

Friedman HS, Prados MD, Wen PY, et al. Bevacizumab alone and in combination with irinotecan in recurrent glioblastoma. *J Clin Oncol.* 2009;27:4733-4740.

Fulkerson DH, Horner TG, Hattab EM. Histologically benign intraventricular meningioma with concurrent pulmonary metastasis: case report and review of the literature. *Clin Neurol Neurosurg.* 2008;110:416-419.

Galicich JH, French LA, Melby JC. Use of dexamethasone in treatment of cerebral edema associated with brain tumors. *Lancet.* 1961;81:46-53.

Gatta G, Zigon G, Capocaccia R, et al. Survival of European children and young adults with cancer diagnosed 1995-2002. *Eur J Cancer.* 2009;45:992-1005.

Gilbert MR, Dignam JJ, Armstrong TS, et al. A randomized trial of bevacizumab for newly diagnosed glioblastoma. *N Engl J Med.* 2014;370:699-708.

Gilbert MR, Ruda R, Soffietti R. Ependymomas in adults. *Curr Neurol Neurosci Rep.* 2010;10:240-247.

Glantz MJ, Cole BF, Glantz LK, et al. Cerebrospinal fluid cytology in patients with cancer: minimizing false-negative results. *Cancer.* 1998;82:733-739.

Glauser T, Shinnar S, Gloss D, et al. Evidence-based guideline: treatment of convulsive status epilepticus in children and adults: report of the Guideline Committee of the American Epilepsy Society. *Epilepsy Curr.* 2016;16:48-61.

Graus F, Rogers LR, Posner JB. Cerebrovascular complications in patients with cancer. *Medicine (Baltimore).* 1985;64:16-35.

Grewal J, Saria MG, Kesari S. Novel approaches to treating leptomeningeal metastases. *J Neurooncol.* 2012;106:225-234.

Grossman R, Shimony N, Hadelsberg U, et al. Impact of resecting radiation necrosis and pseudoprogression on survival of patients with glioblastoma. *World Neurosurg.* 2016;89:37-41.

Hang XF, Xu WS, Wang JX, et al. Risk of high-grade bleeding in patients with cancer treated with bevacizumab: a meta-analysis of randomized controlled trials. *Eur J Clin Pharmacol.* 2011;67:613-623.

Happold C, Gorlia T, Chinot O, et al. Does valproic acid or levetiracetam improve survival in glioblastoma? A pooled analysis of prospective clinical trials in newly diagnosed glioblastoma. *J Clin Oncol.* 2016;34:731-739.

Hart MG, Garside R, Rogers G, et al. Temozolomide for high grade glioma. *Cochrane Database Syst Rev.* 2013;4:CD007415.

Hoftberger R, Rosenfeld MR, Dalmau J. Update on neurological paraneoplastic syndromes. *Curr Opin Oncol.* 2015;27:489-495.

Hulsbrink R, Hashemolhosseini S. Lambert-Eaton myasthenic syndrome: diagnosis, pathogenesis and therapy. *Clin Neurophysiol.* 2014;125:2328-2336.

Jaggi AS, Singh N. Mechanisms in cancer-chemotherapeutic drugs-induced peripheral neuropathy. *Toxicology.* 2012;291:1-9.

Kak M, Nanda R, Ramsdale EE, et al. Treatment of leptomeningeal carcinomatosis: current challenges and future opportunities. *J Clin Neurosci.* 2015;22:632-637.

Korf BR. Neurofibromatosis. *Handb Clin Neurol.* 2013;111:333-340.

Kreisl TN, Kim L, Moore K, et al. Phase II trial of single-agent bevacizumab followed by bevacizumab plus irinotecan at tumor progression in recurrent glioblastoma. *J Clin Oncol.* 2009;27:740-745.

Leone MA, Brainin M, Boon P, et al. Guidance for the preparation of neurological management guidelines by EFNS scientific task forces: revised recommendations 2012. *Eur J Neurol.* 2013;20:410-419.

Lu-Emerson C, Plotkin SR. The neurofibromatoses. Part 2: NF2 and schwannomatosis. *Rev Neurol Dis.* 2009;6:E81-E86.

Macdonald RL. Subarachnoid hemorrhage and loss of consciousness. *JAMA Neurol.* 2016;73:17-18.

Mack F, Baumert BG, Schafer N, et al. Therapy of leptomeningeal metastasis in solid tumors. *Cancer Treat Rev.* 2016;43:83-91.

Markand ON. Lennox-Gastaut syndrome (childhood epileptic encephalopathy). *J Clin Neurophys.* 2000;20:426-441.

Massimino M, Biassoni V, Gandola L, et al. Childhood medulloblastoma. *Crit Rev Oncol Hematol.* 2016;105:35-51.

Mohme M, Emami P, Matschke J, et al. Secretory meningiomas: characteristic features and clinical management of a unique subgroup. *Neurosurg Clin N Am.* 2016;27:181-187.

Nuckols JD, Liu K, Burchette JL, et al. Primary central nervous system lymphomas: a 30-year experience at a single institution. *Mod Pathol.* 1999;12:1167-1173.

Parsons DW, Jones S, Zhang X, et al. An integrated genomic analysis of human glioblastoma multiforme. *Science.* 2008;321:1807-1812.

Pavlidis ET, Pavlidis TE. Role of bevacizumab in colorectal cancer growth and its adverse effects: a review. *World J Gastroenterol.* 2013;19:5051-5060.

Ravnik J, Bunc G, Grcar A, et al. Colloid cysts of the third ventricle exhibit various clinical presentations: review of three cases. *Bosn J Basic Med Sci.* 2014;14:132-135.

Regelsberger J, Hagel C, Emami P, et al. Secretory meningiomas: a benign subgroup causing life-threatening complications. *Neuro-Oncol.* 2009;11:819-824.

Reifenberger G, Weber RG, Riehmer V, et al. Molecular characterization of long-term survivors of glioblastoma using genome- and transcriptome-wide profiling. *Int J Cancer.* 2014;135:1822-1831.

Roelz R, Strohmaier D, Jabbarli R, et al. Residual tumor volume as best outcome predictor in low grade glioma: a nine-years near-randomized survey of surgery vs. biopsy. *Sci Rep.* 2016;6:32286.

Rosen LS. VEGF-targeted therapy: therapeutic potential and recent advances. *Oncologist.* 2005;10:382-391.

Ruda R, Gilbert M, Soffietti R. Ependymomas of the adult: molecular biology and treatment. *Curr Opin Neurol.* 2008;21:754-761.

Schmitt SE, Pargeon K, Frechette ES, et al. Extreme delta brush: a unique EEG pattern in adults with anti-NMDA receptor encephalitis. *Neurology.* 2012;79:1094-1100.

Schwarzrock C. Collaboration in the presence of cerebral edema: the complications of steroids. *Surg Neurol Int.* 2016;7(Suppl 7):S185-S189.

Seretny M, Currie GL, Sena ES, et al. Incidence, prevalence, and predictors of chemotherapy-induced peripheral neuropathy: a systematic review and meta-analysis. *Pain.* 2014;155:2461-2470.

Shah R, Vattoth S, Jacob R, et al. Radiation necrosis in the brain: imaging features and differentiation from tumor recurrence. *Radiographics.* 2012;32:1343-1359.

Stupp R, Mason WP, van den Bent MJ, et al. Radiotherapy plus concomitant and adjuvant temozolomide for glioblastoma. *N Engl J Med.* 2005;352:987-996.

Tarapore PE, Modera P, Naujokas A, et al. Pathology of spinal ependymomas: an institutional experience over 25 years in 134 patients. *Neurosurgery.* 2013;73:247-255.

Taylor MD, Northcott PA, Korshunov A, et al. Molecular subgroups of medulloblastoma: the current consensus. *Acta Neuropathol.* 2012;123:465-472.

Titulaer MJ, Lang B, Verschuuren JJ. Lambert-Eaton myasthenic syndrome: from clinical characteristics to therapeutic strategies. *Lancet Neurol.* 2011;10:1098-1107.

Wadzinski J, Franks R, Roane D, et al. Valproate-associated hyperammonemic encephalopathy. *J Am Board Fam Med.* 2007;20:499-502.

Waggenspack GA, Guinto FC. MR and CT of masses of the anterior superior third ventricle. *AJR Am J Roentgenol.* 1989;152:609-614.

Williams L, Frenneaxu M. Syncope in hypertropic cardiomyopathy: mechanisms and consequences for treatment. *Europace.* 2007;9:817-822.

Wu J, Armstrong TS, Gilbert MR. Biology and management of ependymomas. *Neuro-Oncol.* 2016;18:902-913.

Yan H, Parsons DW, Jin G, et al. IDH1 and IDH2 mutations in gliomas. *N Engl J Med.* 2009;360:765-773.

Yoo H, Jung E, Gwak HS, et al. Surgical outcomes of hemorrhagic metastatic brain tumors. *Cancer Res Treat.* 2011;43:102-107.

11

Neuro-hematology

Sanam Baghshomali, MD, Swarna Rajagopalan, MD, and Monisha Kumar, MD

Questions

1. Which of these target-specific oral anticoagulants, when compared to warfarin, is associated with a lower rate of stroke recurrence, lower rate of major bleeding complications, and lower rate of central nervous system (CNS) bleeding?
   A. Dabigatran 150 mg twice daily
   B. Rivaroxaban 20 mg daily
   C. Rivaroxaban 15 mg daily
   D. Apixaban 5 mg twice daily
   E. Aspirin 325 mg daily

2. What is the recommended dose of protamine sulfate 90 minutes after heparin drip has been discontinued?
   A. 1 mg protamine/100 U unfractionated heparin
   B. 0.5 mg protamine/100 U unfractionated heparin
   C. 20 mg of protamine
   D. The dose of protamine depends on patient's weight
   E. There is no need for reversal at 60 to 120 minutes since the half-life of IV heparin is 30 to 45 minutes

3. In patients with ischemic stroke, why is pharmacoprophylaxis of venous thromboembolism (VTE) with low-molecular-weight heparin (LMWH) is preferred to unfractionated heparin (UFH)?
   A. LMWH has proven to be more effective in preventing deep vein thrombosis.
   B. LMWH has lower bleeding complications compared to UFH.
   C. LMWH has higher bioavailability and more predictable pharmacokinetics.
   D. LMWH requires less frequent administration than UFH.
   E. All of the above

4. An 80-year-old woman with known history of atrial fibrillation on apixaban (Eliquis) is brought to the emergency department (ED) unresponsive with new-onset seizure. She was intubated in the field for airway protection. Per her husband, she was last known normal half an hour prior to presentation when he made sure that she took all of her morning medications. Head computed tomography (CT) performed in ED shows a large right frontoparietal hemorrhage. Which of the options below is not an appropriate treatment in reversal of anticoagulation in this patient?

A. Administration of 4-factor prothrombin complex concentrate

B. Administration of activated charcoal

C. Discontinuation of apixaban (Eliquis)

D. Urgent hemodialysis

E. Administration of andexanet alfa

5. Antiphospholipid (aPL) antibodies include which of the following?

A. Anticardiolipin antibody, prothrombin, anti–β_2-glycoprotein

B. Anticardiolipin antibody, phosphatidylserine, prothrombin

C. Lupus anticoagulant, anti–β_2-glycoprotein, prothrombin

D. Lupus anticoagulant, anti–β_2-glycoprotein, anticardiolipin antibody

E. Phosphatidylserine, anticardiolipin antibody, lupus anticoagulant

6. Which of the following statements is true regarding the testing for antiphospholipid syndrome (APLS)?

A. Based on the revised Sapporo APLS Classification Criteria (also known as the Sydney Criteria), aPL antibodies should remain positive after 6 weeks to meet diagnostic criteria.

B. The dilute Russell viper venom time (dRVVT) is the least sensitive but most specific assay for the lupus anticoagulant antibody.

C. Patients at high risk for APS and with a positive rapid plasma reagin (RPR) should be immediately treated with benzathine penicillin G.

D. Antiphospholipid antibody elevations are seen exclusively in APLS.

E. In patients on anticoagulation, anticardiolipin antibody is the only test that can reliably confirm diagnosis of APLS.

7. What are the 4Ts in the 4T score for assessing the likelihood of heparin-induced thrombocytopenia (HIT) type II?

A. Thrombocytopenia, timing, thrombosis, treatment

B. Timing, thrombosis, thrombocytopenia, temperature

C. Thrombosis, thrombocytopenia, timing, testing

D. Thrombocytopenia, temperature, treatment, thrombosis

E. Timing, thrombocytopenia, thrombosis, other cause

8. A patient with active gastric carcinoma is admitted to the hospital with an acute ischemic stroke. While in the hospital, he develops a pulmonary embolism. Which medication best prevents VTE recurrence in this patient?

A. LMWH

B. Argatroban

C. Dabigatran

D. Warfarin

E. Rivaroxaban

9. Regarding the administration of ε-aminocaproic acid (Amicar) to patients with aneurysmal subarachnoid hemorrhage (SAH) who cannot undergo immediate coiling or clipping of aneurysm, which of the following statements is true?

A. ε-Aminocaproic acid increases the incidence of deep venous thrombosis (DVT).

B. ε-Aminocaproic acid decreases the possibility of rebleed from the aneurysm.

C. ε-Aminocaproic acid should be used only for 72 hours or until the aneurysm is secured, whichever comes first.

D. ε-Aminocaproic acid should be discontinued 2 hours prior to surgical or interventional procedure.

E. All of the above

Questions 10-12

A 28-year-old woman with no past medical history presents to the ED with a generalized tonic-clonic seizure. Her family denies any history of seizures but states that she has been confused for the past 3 days and has been complaining of headaches. Head CT does not demonstrate any acute intracranial abnormalities. Laboratory values are significant for hemoglobin of 7.2 g/dL, platelets of 6500/uL, and elevated lactate dehydrogenase. Due to concern for a thrombotic microangiopathy (TMA), a peripheral blood smear and ADAMTS13 level are obtained, which demonstrate schistocytes and absent activity of ADAMTS13.

10. What is the most likely diagnosis?
    A. HELLP (hemolysis, elevated liver enzymes, low platelet count)
    B. Hemolytic-uremic syndrome (HUS)
    C. Disseminated intravascular coagulopathy (DIC)
    D. Thrombotic thrombocytopenic purpura (TTP)
    E. Evans syndrome

11. What is the best treatment for this condition?
    A. Intravenous immunoglobulin (IVIG)
    B. Plasmapheresis
    C. Fresh frozen plasma and steroids
    D. IVIG, fresh frozen plasma, and steroids
    E. Plasmapharesis, fresh frozen plasma, and steroids

12. On day 3 of admission, the patient was receiving plasma exchange, but she becomes comatose and her platelet count remains consistently low. What is the next best step in the treatment of this patient?
    A. Increase steroid dose
    B. Transfuse platelets
    C. Start cryosupernatant
    D. Add IVIG
    E. Start dialysis

13. A 35-year-old woman with no significant medical history except uncomplicated delivery 2 weeks prior was brought in by family for a 3-day history of waxing and waning drowsiness. Her family stated she complained of a headache for 4 days, and she took ibuprofen without relief prior to the onset of her drowsiness. In the ED, she had a witnessed generalized tonic-clonic seizure. Physical examination was significant for decreased alertness, papilledema, and mild left hemiparesis. A noncontrast head CT was unremarkable, but magnetic resonance imaging (MRI)/magnetic resonance venography (MRV) of the head showed a lack of flow void in the superior sagittal sinus, as well as a right superior frontal infarct with mild mass effect and edema. What is the best initial step in management of this patient?
    A. Initiate thrombolytic therapy
    B. Initiate heparin
    C. Initiate high-dose corticosteroid therapy
    D. Initiate antiplatelet therapy
    E. Perform direct cerebral angiography for diagnosis

14. A 20-year-old man with antithrombin (formerly antithrombin III) deficiency and acute lymphoblastic leukemia on L-asparaginase therapy presents with a 5-day history of double vision and new-onset, gradually progressive headache. In the ED, he complains of nausea and has several episodes of emesis. He has a witnessed episode of transient right facial twitching for 2 minutes that resolves without intervention. Within the hour, he becomes acutely comatose. You are consulted by the ED physician. In addition to a stat noncontrast head CT and continuous electroencephalogram, what is the best initial test you recommend?
    A. CT venography (CTV) of head
    B. CT angiography of head
    C. Positron emission tomography (PET) scan
    D. Lumbar Puncture
    E. Digital subtraction cerebral angiography

15. A 58-year-old man with a history of hypertension, diabetes mellitus, coronary artery disease, mitral valve prolapse status post mechanical mitral valve replacement 2 years prior, and lumbar spine spondylosis was admitted to the neurology intensive care unit status post lumbar 2-4 laminectomy and fusion. Warfarin therapy was discontinued 2 days prior to surgery. The surgery was uneventful, estimated blood loss was minimal, and there was good

procedural and postprocedural hemostasis. What is the most reasonable anticoagulation management plan in this patient?

A. Discuss anticipated bleeding risk with neuro-surgeon and start anticoagulation as soon as feasible

B. Delay anticoagulation for 4 weeks after surgery

C. Delay anticoagulation for 3 months after surgery

D. Start novel oral anticoagulant (NOAC)

E. Start antiplatelet agent now

16. A 62-year-old man with a history of a large right parietal glioblastoma multiforme (GBM) tumor was admitted to the neurology intensive care unit for close monitoring status post resection of mass. His surgery was prolonged, complicated by difficulty obtaining hemostasis. The nurse was concerned that he was still bleeding from his incision site, but the neurologic examination was improving, and postoperative imaging was unremarkable. He was extubated without difficulty. Four hours later, he develops sudden-onset dyspnea associated with hypoxemia, requiring oxygen via nasal cannula. He remains hemodynamically stable. A chest CT confirms diagnosis of bilateral segmental pulmonary emboli (PE). Lower extremity Doppler ultrasound confirms thrombosis of the proximal right common femoral vein. What is the best next step in management of this patient?

A. Start anticoagulation

B. Consider for catheter-assisted thrombectomy

C. Start thrombolytic therapy

D. Start antiplatelet therapy

E. Place inferior vena cava filter (IVCF)

17. A 23-year-old woman with no past medical history presented to the hospital with headache and neck stiffness. She was febrile to 102°F and had meningismus and an otherwise unremarkable neurologic examination. She was noted to have the following laboratory abnormalities: white blood cells (WBCs) 16000/microL with 4% bands, platelet count 102,000/µL, fibrinogen 220 mg/dL, prolonged prothrombin time (PT) and partial thromboplastin time (PTT), elevated fibrin degradation products, positive D-dimer, azotemia, metabolic acidosis, and elevated

transaminases. The rest of the basic lab work and noncontrast head CT were unremarkable. Lumbar puncture was performed, and cerebrospinal fluid (CSF) analysis showed 215 WBCs/µL (89% neutrophils), 4 red blood cells/µL, protein 235 mg/dL, and glucose 28 mg/dL versus serum blood glucose 122 mg/dL. Empiric broad-spectrum intravenous antibiotics were administered. Three hours later, she developed acute left hemiparesis. A noncontrast head CT was repeated and showed a 2 cm × 1.2 cm focus of intraparenchymal hemorrhage centered in the right superior frontal white matter. What is the best next step in management of this patient?

A. Administer protamine sulfate

B. Treat underlying cause and provide supportive care

C. Start anticoagulation with UFH

D. Administer recombinant factor VIIa (rFVIIa)

E. Obtain MRI of brain

18. In patients with sickle cell disease (SCD), what is the best strategy for secondary stroke prevention?

A. Start hydroxyurea treatment

B. Start antihypertensive medications

C. Encourage hydration

D. Start systemic anticoagulation

E. Monitor transcranial Doppler (TCD) for possible blood transfusions

19. A 38-year-old man with sickle cell disease was brought in by family after being found down and not able to move his left side. Examination demonstrates normal mental status and language with left hemispatial neglect and left hemiparesis. A noncontrast head CT showed hypodensity in the right parietal area, obscuration of the right lentiform nucleus, and no midline shift. Lab work was significant for hemoglobin of 8.6 g/dL. CTA showed mild right M1 stenosis with good distal flow. He is deemed not to be a candidate for intravenous thrombolysis or mechanical thrombectomy. What is the next best step?

A. Start hydroxyurea therapy

B. Start hyperosmolar therapy

C. Start anticoagulation

D. Start emergent packed red blood cells (pRBCs) or exchange transfusion

E. Start antiplatelet therapy

20. Which of the following would be reversed by the administration of andaxenet alfa?

   A. Argatroban

   B. Edoxaban

   C. Bivalirudin

   D. Dabigatran

   E. Lepirudin

21. Compared to a person with atrial fibrillation (AF) and an international normalized ratio (INR) of 2.0, a person with an INR of 1.8 has a:

   A. Lower risk of stroke and lower risk of excessive bleeding

   B. Lower risk of stroke and higher risk of excessive bleeding

   C. Higher risk of stroke and lower risk of excessive bleeding

   D. Higher risk of stroke and the same risk of bleeding

   E. There is no difference between INR of 1.8 and 2.0

Answers and Explanations

1. **D.** In the ARISTOTLE trial, a total of 18,201 patients with atrial fibrillation (AF) were randomized to apixaban 5 mg twice daily versus warfarin (goal international normalized ratio [INR] between 2 and 3). The results demonstrated a significant decrease in the primary outcome, which was stroke or systemic embolism, and in the number of strokes (hazard ratio [HR], 0.79; 95% CI, 0.66-0.95; $P = .01$). Major bleeding complications (HR, 0.89; 95% CI, 0.35-0.75), including a noticeable reduction in intracranial hemorrhage (HR, 0.42; 95% CI, 0.30-0.58), were also significantly reduced. WASID trial results, which looked at warfarin versus aspirin for treatment of symptomatic intracranial arterial stenosis, showed that warfarin did not have any benefits over aspirin in lowering stroke/vascular death risk while increasing the adverse events. In this trial, patients who were on aspirin had lower rates of major bleeding, myocardial infarction, and sudden death. In the RE-LY trial of 18,234 patients with AF, dabigatran at the twice-daily dose of 150 mg was associated with lower rates of stroke but similar rates of major bleeding compared to warfarin. The rate of stroke prevention in the dabigatran 110-mg arm was equivalent to that in the warfarin arm, but this dose had lower rates of bleeding complications. In the ROCKET-AF trial, 142,64 patients were randomized to either rivaroxaban 20 mg daily (15 mg/d if Cr clearance was 30-49 mm/mL) or warfarin (INR goal 2-3). Results demonstrated an equivalent rate of stroke and major bleeding, with a lower rate of intracranial hemorrhage.

2. **A.** Per the 2015 Neurocritical Care Society (NCS) guidelines for the reversal of antithrombotics after intracranial hemorrhage (ICH), the dose of protamine is 1 mg/100 U unfractionated heparin if heparin was administered during the preceding 2 to 3 hours. It should not be administered faster than 20 mg/min because this can result in significant hypotension, and a single dose should not exceed 50 mg. Subsequent dosing of protamine sulfate may be considered if a posttreatment partial thromboplastin time (PTT) remains significantly prolonged.

3. **E.** The PREVAIL trial demonstrated a 43% reduction of VTE with LMWH compared to UFH. Two other studies established lower rates of hemorrhagic complications with LMWH compared to UFH, making it a safer medication to use in patients with acute ischemic stroke at risk of hemorrhagic conversion. LMWHs have higher bioavailability and more predictable pharmacokinetics.

4. **D.** In all patients on anticoagulation who present with ICH, the anticoagulant should be immediately discontinued and reversal should be considered. Oral factor Xa inhibitors are highly protein bound and do not clear with dialysis; hence, it is an ineffective method of reversal for these agents. Activated charcoal decreases the absorption of apixaban within 6 hours of ingestion with highest efficacy within the first 2 hours of ingestion. However its use is limited in patients who are intubated or who are at high risk of aspiration. Caution should be exercised with its use because emesis may be associated with increased intracranial pressure and brain herniation. Although data regarding prothrombin complex concentrates, activated prothrombin complex concentrates, fresh frozen plasma, and recombinant activated factor VII are insufficient to guide definitive recommendations, the 2015 NCS guidelines for reversal of antithrombotics in ICH suggest administration of these agents, based on animal studies and healthy human studies showing restoration of coagulation factors, decrease in hematoma expansion, decrease in bleeding time, and improvement in coagulation parameters, and offer a conditional recommendation in favor of 4-factor nonactivated prothrombin complex concentrate (PCC) over either activated PCC or recombinant factor VIIa. Andexanet alfa (ANNEXA-A study)

has been studied in healthy elderly individuals and appears to reverse the effects of anticoagulation with apixaban; however, it is not yet approved by the US Food and Drug Administration (FDA).

Mechanism of Action	Medications	Reversal
Direct factor Xa inhibitors	Rivaroxaban	Activated charcoal (50 g) within 2 h of ingestion
	Apixaban	Activated PCC (FEIBA) 50 U/kg IV OR 4-factor PCC 50 U/kg IV
	Edoxaban	Andexanet alfa (pending FDA approval)
Direct thrombin inhibitors	Dabigatran	Activated charcoal (50 g) within 2 h of ingestion, AND idarucizumab 5 g IV (in two 2.5-g/50-mL vials). Consider hemodialysis or idarucizumab redosing for refractory bleeding after initial administration.
	Argatroban	Activated PCC (FEIBA) 50 U/kg IV OR 4-factor
	Bivalirudin	PCC 50 U/kg IV
	Desirudin	
	Lepirudin	

Abbreviations: IV, intravenous; PCC, prothrombin complex concentrate.

Source: Frontera JA, Lewin JJ 3rd, Rabinstein AA, et al. Guideline for reversal of antithrombotics in intracranial hemorrhage: a statement for healthcare professionals from the Neurocritical Care Society and Society of Critical Care Medicine. *Neurocrit Care.* 2016;24:6-46.

Mechanism of Action	Medications	Reversal
Antiplatelets	Aspirin[a,b]	Desmopressin 0.4 μg/kg intravenously × 1
	Dipyridamole[c]	If neurosurgical intervention needed, consider platelet transfusion
	Clopidogrel[d]	
	Prasugrel	
	Ticagrelor	
	Ticlopidine	
	Cilostazol[e]	
	Anagrelide	
	Ibuprofen[f]	
	Naproxen	
	Abixicimab[g]	
	Eptifibatide[b]	
	Tirofiban[b]	
	Vorapaxar[h]	

[a]Irreversible cyclooxygenase-1 and -2 (COX-1 and -2) enzyme inhibitor (inhibits thromboxane A_2).

[b]Aspirin, eptifibatide, and tirofiban are dialyzable.

[c]Reversible adenosine reuptake inhibitor.

[d]Inhibition of P2Y12 adenosine diphosphate receptor.

[e]Phosphodiesterase (PDE) inhibitor.

[f]Reversible COX-1 and COX-2 enzyme inhibitor.

[g]Glycoprotein IIb/IIIa antagonist.

[h]Reversible protease-activated receptor-1 (PAR-1) thrombin receptor antagonist.

Source: Frontera JA, Lewin JJ 3rd, Rabinstein AA, et al. Guideline for reversal of antithrombotics in intracranial hemorrhage: a statement for healthcare professionals from the Neurocritical Care Society and Society of Critical Care Medicine. *Neurocrit Care.* 2016;24:6-46.

Mechanism of Action	Medications	Reversal
Thrombolytics	Alteplase	Cryoprecipitate 10 U IV OR
Catalyze conversion of fibrin-bound plasminogen to plasmin. Plasmin exerts additional proteolytic effects, including cleavage of platelet GPIIIa and GPIb causing inhibition of platelet function	Reteplase Tenecteplase	Antifibrinolytics (tranexamic acid 10-15 mg/kg IV over 20 min or ε-aminocaproic acid 4-5 g IV) if cryoprecipitate is contraindicated
Pentasaccharides Binds with antithrombin and potentiates inhibition of free factor Xa, preventing formation of the prothrombinase complex	Fondaparinux	Activated PCC (FEIBA) 20 U/kg IV or recombinant factor VIIa 90 μg/kg IV

Abbreviations: GP, glycoprotein; IV, intravenous; PCC, prothrombin complex concentrate.

Source: Frontera JA, Lewin JJ 3rd, Rabinstein AA, et al. Guideline for reversal of antithrombotics in intracranial hemorrhage: a statement for healthcare professionals from the Neurocritical Care Society and Society of Critical Care Medicine. *Neurocrit Care.* 2016;24:6-46.

5. **C.** aPL antibodies are a heterogeneous group of antibodies directed against phospholipid-binding proteins. The aPL antibodies included in the international classification criteria are anticardiolipin (aCL) antibody (immunoglobulin [Ig] G or IgM, anti–β_2-glycoprotein 1 (β_2-GP1) antibody [IgG or IgM], and lupus anticoagulant [LA]). Although cardiolipin is a phospholipid, most of the clinically relevant antibodies detected in the assay are actually binding to the phospholipid binding proteins, frequently β_2-GP1, that bind to the cardiolipin in the assay.

6. **B.** APLS is a systemic autoimmune disorder characterized by venous or arterial thrombosis and/or pregnancy morbidity in the presence of persistent laboratory evidence of antiphospholipid antibodies (aPLAs). The dRVVT assay, which is commonly used in laboratories, works via addition of snake venom to dilute rabbit brain phospholipids, activating factor X and subsequently forming fibrin clot. The presence of a lupus anticoagulant will prolong the dRVVT. This test is very specific for LA but is

not sensitive. Testing for LAs should be performed at a minimum of 12 weeks apart based on Sydney investigational criteria.

A history of a false-positive serologic tests for syphilis may also be a clue to the presence of aPLAs. Both the Venereal Disease Research Laboratory (VDRL) and the rapid plasma reagin (RPR) may be positive as both of these assays contain cardiolipin.

Immunoassays for anticardiolipin (aCL) and β_2-glycoprotein (β_2-GP) can and should be done shortly after the acute event and are not affected by thrombotic event or anticoagulation that has been initiated on these patients for treatment of the aforementioned thrombotic event.

7. **E.** The 4T scoring system is used to calculate the pretest probability in patients suspected of having HIT.

	2	1	0
Thrombocytopenia (acute)	50% drop in platelet (PLT) count to nadir of ≥20,000	30%-50% drop in PLT count or nadir of 10,000-19,000	<30% drop in PLT count or nadir of <10,000
Timing of decrease in platelet count or thrombosis	Onset day 5-10 or day 1 if heparin exposure within the past 5-30 days	Onset after day 10 or unclear or day 1 if exposure to heparin within past 30-100 days	Onset ≤4 days with no recent heparin exposure
Thrombosis or other sequelae of HIT	New proven thrombosis, or skin necrosis, or acute systemic reaction after heparin bolus	Suspected thrombosis or recurrent/progressive thrombosis, or erythematous skin lesions	None
Other causes of thrombocytopenia	No other explanation	Possible other causes	Definite other causes

Pretest probability score: 6-8 = high; 4-5 = intermediate; 0-3 = low.

8. **A.** For patients with VTE and no cancer, the 2016 American College of Chest Physicians guidelines recommend dabigatran, rivaroxaban, apixaban, or edoxaban over vitamin K antagonist (VKA) therapy, and suggest VKA therapy over LMWH. However, for patients with **VTE and cancer**, the guidelines suggest LMWH over VKA (grade 2B), dabigatran (grade 2C), rivaroxaban (grade 2C), apixaban (grade 2C), or edoxaban (grade 2C). These recommendations are based on a 2003 study performed by Lee and colleagues. The CLOT trial concluded that LMWH is superior to warfarin for long-term secondary VTE prophylaxis in cancer patients.

9. **E.** Recent studies have demonstrated that in patients who cannot undergo immediate stabilization of ruptured cerebral aneurysm secondary to other medical issues, administration of antifibrinolytic medication for a short period of time can decrease the incidence of early rebleed in these patients. Based on the 2011 NCS guidelines for management of aneurysmal SAH, antifibrinolytic therapy can be continued for 72 hours or until the aneurysm has been secured, whichever comes first. It should be discontinued 2 hours prior to endovascular coil placement or surgical clip placement. It should not be initiated in patients >48 hours after the onset of hemorrhage as it may increase the risk of delayed cerebral ischemia. Two studies have demonstrated that patients who receive antifibrinolytic therapy have higher rates of DVT. Therefore, patients who receive this therapy should be monitored closely for development of DVT.

10. **D.** Thrombocytopenia, hemolysis, and schistocytes (with different degrees and severity) are common features in all TMAs, which make it difficult to differentiate between different syndromes in patients presenting with these abnormalities. However, ADAMTS13 activity levels have been found to vary in these diseases. In DIC, ADAMTS13 levels are decreased, whereas in TTP, the levels are severely decreased to absent, and in HUS, they are within normal range.

11. **E.** Patients who are diagnosed with acquired TTP should be started on plasma exchange upon admission to help remove the autoantibodies against ADAMTS13 and ultra-large von Willebrand factor–platelet strings. Plasma exchange should be accompanied by fresh frozen plasma (FFP) or cryosupernatant as replacement fluid, which helps restore ADAMTS13 levels in plasma. If plasma exchange is not readily available, FFP should be administered until plasma exchange can be initiated. In addition, patients should be started on high doses of steroid (methylprednisolone) to decrease autoantibody production. Other treatments that can be used include rituximab and cyclophosphamide.

12. **C.** Approximately 80% to 90% of patients with acquired TTP can survive 1 episode of TTP with the treatment combination of plasma exchange with FFP or cryosupernatant. If patients do not show any improvement (increase in platelet count) in the first few days of treatment or have deterioration in their exam by, for example, becoming comatose, replacement fluid during plasma exchange can be changed from FFP to cryosupernatant.

13. **B.** This patient has cerebral venous thrombosis (CVT) of the superior sagittal sinus. This is the most common location for CVT. Pregnancy induces changes in the coagulation system that persist into the puerperium and result in a hypercoagulable state, which increases the risk of CVT. The diagnosis of CVT is based on clinical suspicion and imaging confirmation. The diagnostic test of choice is noninvasive venous sinus imaging such as MRV or CT venography (CTV). Invasive catheter angiography, also known as digital subtraction angiography, involves the direct injection of contrast material into a dural sinus or cerebral vein from microcatheter insertion via the internal jugular vein. It is reserved for situations in which an endovascular procedure is being considered. Prompt and adequate treatment with therapeutic anticoagulation is essential in the management of CVT. Most patients have good clinical recovery. There is no role for antiplatelet therapy in acute management of CVT. In a prospective observational study that included 624 patients, treatment with various types, dosages, and durations of steroids did not improve outcome and was detrimental in a subgroup of patients with parenchymal lesions. Therefore, steroids are not recommended in treatment of CVT.

14. **A.** The most likely diagnosis is CVT. The diagnosis of CVT is based on clinical suspicion and imaging

confirmation. Clinical findings are either attributable to increased intracranial pressure (ICP) due to impaired venous drainage or focal symptoms attributable to the location of venous ischemia, infarction, or hemorrhage. Headache, usually due to raised ICP, is the most common symptom in CVT. Other signs and symptoms include papilledema, diplopia due to sixth nerve palsy, seizures, and focal neurologic deficits based on its location. The most widely studied risk factors for CVT include acquired risks (eg, surgery, trauma, pregnancy, puerperium, antiphospholipid syndrome, cancer, exogenous hormones) and genetic risks (inherited thrombophilias). In ISCVT, a large multicenter prospective observational study with 624 patients, 34% of CVT patients had an inherited or acquired prothrombotic condition and 7% had cancer. In addition to cancer itself, certain chemotherapeutic agents, such as L-asparaginase, can contribute to hypercoagulability. The diagnostic test of choice is noninvasive venous sinus imaging such as MRV or CTV. Invasive cerebral angiography is less commonly needed to establish the diagnosis of CVT given the availability of MRV and CTV and, therefore, is reserved for situations in which an endovascular procedure is being considered or if the MRV or CTV results are inconclusive. Although there is limited anecdotal evidence of PET scans in CVT showing reduction in cerebral blood flow and increased blood volume, perfusion imaging in acute CVT is controversial. Unless there is clinical suspicion of meningitis, examination of the cerebrospinal fluid (CSF) is typically not helpful in establishing diagnosis of CVT. There are no specific CSF abnormalities, but frequent findings include elevated opening pressure, elevated cell counts, and elevated protein levels.

15. **A.** The decision to resume full-dose anticoagulant therapy may be influenced by the anticipated risk of bleeding associated with the specific surgery as well as the level of hemostasis achieved perioperatively, weighed against the thromboembolic risk of the individual patient. This merits a multidisciplinary discussion with the operating neurosurgeon to make an individually formulated decision. There is no standard recommended timing for restarting anticoagulation, such as 4 weeks or 3 months, and the individual thromboembolic risk of the patient must be taken into consideration. The risk

of a thromboembolic event varies depending on the clinical indication for anticoagulant therapy as well as presence of comorbid conditions, such as AF. Patients with mitral valve prosthesis are classified as a high-risk group for thrombosis, which is defined as a greater than 10% annual risk for thromboembolism. Other high-risk groups include patients with a caged-ball or tilting-disk aortic valve prosthesis, valve prosthesis with stroke within 6 months, $CHADS_2$ score of 5 or 6, or VTE within 3 months or in the setting of a severe thrombophilia. In a high-risk group, once risk of bleeding has been established, the recommendation is to start anticoagulation as soon as possible. If unfractionated heparin (UFH) is used, it can usually be resumed 24 hours after surgery when there is evidence of adequate hemostasis. To minimize bleeding risk, UFH is recommended to be started without a bolus, at no more than the expected maintenance infusion rate. In a randomized controlled trial comparing dabigatran (NOAC) to warfarin, dabigatran was found to be less effective in preventing thromboembolic complications in patients with mechanical heart valves and was associated with a higher bleeding risk. Anticoagulation is superior to antiplatelet therapy alone for total thromboembolic risk in prosthetic heart valves; thus, starting with an antiplatelet agent is not the best management strategy.

16. **E.** It is established that the perioperative incidence of VTE in patients undergoing surgery for high-grade brain tumors is high, ranging from 3% to 20%. In addition, there is continuing long-term risk of thrombosis throughout the course of disease. In a meta-analysis of 4 studies, UFH or LMWH initiated 24 hours after surgery, compared with mechanical compression devices, had a 38% relative risk reduction in VTE in neurosurgical patients. The optimal treatment in this patient given his history of GBM and a PE is anticoagulation. However, given his recent surgery and difficulty obtaining hemostasis perioperatively, starting anticoagulation at this time could lead to devastating intracranial hemorrhage. IVCF placement should be considered for patients who are at extremely high risk of recurrent venous thromboembolic disease, such as patients who have had an acute episode of PE in whom anticoagulant therapy is contraindicated. Recent neurosurgery is a major contraindication to thrombolysis. There is no role for antiplatelet therapy in management of

acute PE. Guidelines recommend against systemically administered thrombolytic therapy in patients with acute PE not associated with hypotension. Catheter-assisted thrombectomy is reserved for patients with acute PE associated with hemodynamic instability and who have a high bleeding risk, failed systemic thrombolysis, or imminent death (eg, within hours) before systemic thrombolysis can take effect. The patient in this vignette had a high bleeding risk but remained hemodynamically stable, so thrombectomy would not be the best management strategy for him.

17. **B.** The most common clinical manifestations of disseminated intravascular coagulation (DIC) are thrombosis, bleeding, or both, often with resultant multiorgan dysfunction. Common etiologies include malignancies, obstetric complications, infections, trauma, burns, and transfusion reactions. Laboratory abnormalities include prolonged PT, PTT, and thrombin time (TT) due to consumption of coagulation factors, as well as decreased platelet count and increased fibrin degradation products and D-dimer. The cornerstone of DIC management is the treatment of the underlying condition to remove the stimulus for ongoing coagulation and thrombosis, while providing supportive care. Supportive care includes hemodynamic and ventilator support, as well as transfusion of blood products that are tailored individually to each DIC patient. Transfusion strategy should be based on the severity of bleeding, risk of fluid overload, prognosis of the underlying condition, and laboratory tests. The use of protamine sulfate is generally not indicated for the prolonged PTT of DIC. In a patient who is bleeding with a fibrinogen concentration of less than 50 to 60 mg/dL, fibrinogen may be infused in the form of FFP or cryoprecipitate. Usually 10 U of cryoprecipitate (each containing about 200 mg of fibrinogen) will be adequate in adult patients. Although limited preliminary data suggest that rFVIIa could have a potential role in this clinical setting, this has not been studied in a large trial. In addition, thrombosis is a feared complication, and in the absence of large randomized controlled trials that assess safety, rFVIIa transfusion is not currently recommended. Anticoagulation with UFH is contraindicated in the setting of active intracerebral hemorrhage in the setting of DIC. Additional imaging studies, such as MRI, should be reserved for when the patient has unexplained neurologic symptoms despite negative preliminary imaging.

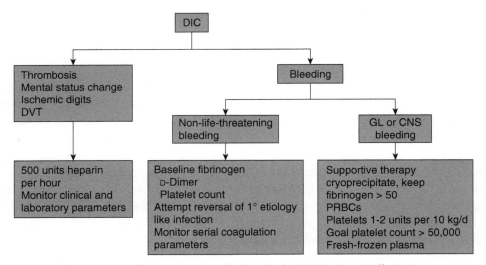

Reproduced with permission from Lee K. *The NeuroICU Book*. New York, NY: McGraw-Hill, 2012.

18. E. Randomized controlled trials (RCTs), such as the Stroke Prevention Trial in Sickle Cell Anemia (STOP) and STOP II demonstrated that prophylactic (typically monthly) red blood cell (RBC) transfusions in children 2 to 16 years of age with SCD, who were at high risk for an initial stroke based on TCD, reduced incidence of strokes. TCD was demonstrated to be a useful tool in monitoring these patients. A long-term follow-up of the STOP trial patients suggested that persistent TCD elevation signals ongoing stroke risk. An RCT failed to demonstrate benefit of switching to hydroxyurea for secondary stroke prevention. Antihypertensive therapy has limited utility in a patient with normal blood pressure. There is no role for systemic anticoagulation in stroke caused by SCD. While SCD patients should remain well hydrated, this is not a sufficient strategy for secondary stroke prevention. TCDs for monitoring stroke risk have only been studied in the pediatric population. In adults with SCD, CNS complications continue to be a major cause of morbidity and mortality, with no current evidence-based strategy for prevention.

19. D. In adults with SCD presenting with an acute stroke, after initial stabilization, the recommended management is emergent transfusion therapy. The goal is to lower the percentage of sickle hemoglobin (Hb S) to ≤30% of total hemoglobin and to aim for a total hemoglobin level of approximately, but not greater than, 10 g/dL. This is best achieved using exchange transfusion, but if it cannot be initiated in a timely fashion, pRBC transfusion should be given. Randomized trials comparing exchange transfusion with simple transfusion for acute stroke in SCD are lacking, but some experts feel that pRBC transfusion does not lower the percentage of Hb S sufficiently without causing hyperviscosity or transfusion-associated circulatory overload. In addition, oxygen therapy should be initiated to keep oxygen saturation at 95%. There is no role for starting hydroxyurea therapy acutely, but it may be a consideration for secondary stroke prevention. There is a possibility of the patient developing malignant edema in the future; however, in the absence of clinical or radiographic findings that suggest it now, there is no role for hyperosmolar therapy. There is no role for antiplatelet therapy in SCD as stroke is presumed to be due to sickling-induced vaso-occlusion, unless stroke workup reveals alternate etiology for stroke. Anticoagulation is not used in the acute management of stroke secondary to SCD.

20. B. Edoxaban is the only direct factor Xa inhibitor. Andexanet alfa is a potential antidote for factor Xa inhibitors which include rivaroxaban, apixaban and edoxaban that acts as a decoy receptor that has a higher affinity for drug than natural Xa. The remaining drugs are all direct thrombin inhibitors. Idarucizumab is a monoclonal antibody for dabigatran.

21. D. The most effective INR for stroke prevention in patients with AF is 2 to 3. As the INR drops below 1.9, the risk of stroke increases, and any benefit in stroke prevention is lost as the INR drops below 1.5. However, the risk of excessive bleeding remains high until the INR is lower than 1.5.

REFERENCES

Bell WR, Braine HG, Ness PM, Kickler TS. Improved survival in thrombotic thrombocytopenic purpura-hemolytic uremic syndrome. Clinical experience in 108 patients. *N Engl J Med*. 1991;325:398-403.

Bertolaccini ML, Amengual O, Andreoli L, et al. 14th International Congress on Antiphospholipid Antibodies Task Force. Report on antiphospholipid syndrome laboratory diagnostics and trends. *Autoimmun Rev*. 2014;13:917-930.

Bockmeyer CL, Claus RA, Budde U, et al. Inflammation-associated ADAMTS13 deficiency promotes formation of ultra-large von Willebrand factor. *Haematologica*. 2008;93:137-140.

Bousser MG. Cerebral venous thrombosis: diagnosis and management. *J Neurol*. 2000;247:252-258.

Buller HR, Agnelli G, Hull RD, et al. Antithrombotic therapy for venous thromboembolic disease: the Seventh ACCP Conference on Antithrombotic and Thrombolytic Therapy. *Chest*. 2004;126(Suppl 3):401S-428S.

Byrnes JJ, Khurana M. Treatment of thrombotic thrombocytopenic purpura with plasma. *N Engl J Med*. 1977;297:1386-1389.

Byrnes JJ, Moake JL, Klug P, Periman P. Effectiveness of the cryosupernatant fraction of plasma in the treatment of refractory thrombotic thrombocytopenic purpura. *Am J Hematol*. 1990;34:169-174.

Canhao P, Cortesao A, Cabral M, et al. Are steroids useful to treat cerebral venous thrombosis? *Stroke*. 2008;39:105-110.

Cannegieter SC, Rosendaal FR, Briët E. Thromboembolic and bleeding complications in patients with mechanical heart valve prostheses. *Circulation*. 1994;89:635-641.

Chemnitz J, Draube A, Scheid C, et al. Successful treatment of severe thrombotic thrombocytopenic purpura with the monoclonal antibody rituximab. *Am J Hematol*. 2002;71:105-108.

Chimowitz MI, Lynn MJ, Howlett-Smith H, et al. Comparison of warfarin and aspirin for symptomatic intracranial arterial stenosis. *N Engl J Med.* 2005;352:1305-1316.

Connolly SJ, Ezekowitz MD, Yusuf S, et al. Dabigatran versus warfarin in patients with atrial fibrillation. *N Engl J Med.* 2009;361:1139-1151.

De Freitas GR, Bogousslavsky J. Risk factors of cerebral vein and sinus thrombosis. *Front Neurol Neurosci.* 2008;23:23-54.

Diringer MN, Bleck TP, Claude Hemphill J 3rd, et al. Critical care management of patients following aneurysmal subarachnoid hemorrhage: recommendations from the Neurocritical Care Society's Multidisciplinary Consensus Conference. *Neurocrit Care.* 2011;15:211-240.

Douketis JD. The perioperative management of antithrombotic therapy: American College of Chest Physicians Evidence-Based Clinical Practice Guidelines (8th Edition). *Chest J.* 2008;133:299S.

Eerenberg ES, Kamphuisen PW, Sijpkens MK, et al. Reversal of rivaroxaban and dabigatran by prothrombin complex concentrate: a randomized, placebo-controlled, crossover study in healthy subjects. *Circulation.* 2011;124:1573-1579.

Eikelboom JW, Connolly SJ, Brueckmann M, et al. Dabigatran versus warfarin in patients with mechanical heart valves. *N Engl J Med.* 2013;369:1206-1214.

Einhäupl KM, Villringer A, Meister W, et al. Heparin treatment in sinus venous thrombosis. *Lancet.* 1991;338:597-600.

Ferro JM. Prognosis of cerebral vein and dural sinus thrombosis: results of the international study on cerebral vein and dural sinus thrombosis (ISCVT). *Stroke.* 2004;34:664-670.

Foreman PM, Chua M, Harrigan MR, et al. Antifibrinolytic therapy in aneurysmal subarachnoid hemorrhage increases the risk for deep venous thrombosis: a case-control study. *Clin Neurol Neurosurg.* 2015;139:66-69.

Freitas GRD, Bogousslavsky J. Risk factors of cerebral vein and sinus thrombosis. *Front Neurol Neurosci.* 2008;8:23-54.

Frontera JA, Lewin JJ 3rd, Rabinstein AA, et al. Guideline for reversal of antithrombotics in intracranial hemorrhage: a statement for healthcare professionals from the Neurocritical Care Society and Society of Critical Care Medicine. *Neurocrit Care.* 2016;24:6-46.

Furlan M, Galbusera M, Noris M, et al. von Willebrand factor-cleaving protease in thrombotic thrombocytopenic purpura and the hemolytic-uremic syndrome. *N Engl J Med.* 1998;339:1578-1584.

Gallagher AM, Setakis E, Plumb JM, et al. Risks of stroke and mortality associated with suboptimal anticoagulation in atrial fibrillation patients. *Thromb Haemost.* 2011;106:968-977.

Galli M, Finazzi G, Bevers EM, Barbui T. Kaolin clotting time and dilute Russell's viper venom time distinguish between prothrombin-dependent and beta 2-glycoprotein I-dependent antiphospholipid antibodies. *Blood.* 1995;86:617-623.

Giannakopoulos B, Passam F, Ioannou Y, Krilis SA. How we diagnose the antiphospholipid syndrome. *Blood.* 2009;113:985-994.

Go AS, Hylek EM, Chang Y, et al. Anticoagulation therapy for stroke prevention in atrial fibrillation: how well do randomized trials translate into clinical practice? *JAMA.* 2003;290:2685-2692.

Granger CB, Alexander JH, McMurray JJ, et al. Apixaban versus warfarin in patients with atrial fibrillation. *N Engl J Med.* 2011.365:981-992.

Gugliotta L, Mazzucconi MG, Leone G, et al. Incidence of thrombotic complications in adult patients with acute lymphoblastic leukaemia receiving L-asparaginase during induction therapy: a retrospective study. The GIMEMA Group. *Eur J Haematol.* 1992;49:63-66.

Gutterman LA, Kloster B, Tsai HM. Rituximab therapy for refractory thrombotic thrombocytopenic purpura. *Blood Cells Mol Dis.* 2002;28:385-391.

Harrigan MR, Rajneesh KF, Ardelt AA, Fisher WS 3rd. Short-term antifibrinolytic therapy before early aneurysm treatment in subarachnoid hemorrhage: effects on rehemorrhage, cerebral ischemia, and hydrocephalus. *Neurosurgery.* 2010;67:935-939.

Herrmann R, Thom J, Wood A, et al. Thrombin generation using the calibrated automated thrombinoscope to assess reversibility of dabigatran and rivaroxaban. *Thromb Haemost.* 2014;111:989-995.

Hillman J, Fridriksson S, Nilsson O, et al. Immediate administration of tranexamic acid and reduced incidence of early rebleeding after aneurysmal subarachnoid hemorrhage: a prospective randomized study. *J Neurosurg.* 2002;97:771-778.

Iorio A, Agnelli G. Low-molecular-weight and unfractionated heparin for prevention of venous thromboembolism in neurosurgery: a meta-analysis. *Arch Intern Med.* 2000;160:2327-2332.

Jones M, McEwan P, Morgan CL, et al. Evaluation of the pattern of treatment, level of anticoagulation control, and outcome of treatment with warfarin in patients with non-valvar atrial fibrillation: a record linkage study in a large British population. *Heart.* 2005;91:472-477.

Kahn SR, Lim W, Dunn AS, et al. Prevention of VTE in non-surgical patients: antithrombotic therapy and prevention of thrombosis, 9th ed: American College of Chest Physicians Evidence-Based Clinical Practice Guidelines. *Chest.* 2012;141(Suppl 2):e195S-e226S.

Kamphuisen PW, Agnelli G, Sebastianelli M. Prevention of venous thromboembolism after acute ischemic stroke. *J Thromb Haemost.* 2005;3:1187-1194.

Kawai N, Shindou A, Masada T, et al. Hemodynamic and metabolic changes in a patient with cerebral venous sinus thrombosis: evaluation using O-15 positron emission tomography. *Clin Nucl Med.* 2005;30:391-394.

Kearon C, Hirsh J. Management of anticoagulation before and after elective surgery. *N Engl J Med.* 1997;336:1506-1511.

Kearon C, Akl EA, Ornelas J, et al. Antithrombotic therapy for VTE disease. *Chest.* 2016;149:315-352.

Lee MT. Stroke Prevention Trial in Sickle Cell Anemia (STOP): extended follow-up and final results. *Blood.* 2006;108:847-852.

Lee AY, Levine MN, Baker RI, et al. Low-molecular-weight heparin versus a coumarin for the prevention of recurrent venous thromboembolism in patients with cancer. *N Engl J Med.* 2003;349:146-153.

Mant MJ, King EG. Severe, acute disseminated intravascular coagulation. A reappraisal of its pathophysiology, clinical significance and therapy based on 47 patients. *Am J Med.* 1979;67:557-563.

Marlu R, Hodaj E, Paris A, et al. Effect of non-specific reversal agents on anticoagulant activity of dabigatran and rivaroxaban: a randomised crossover ex vivo study in healthy volunteers. *Thromb Haemost.* 2012;108:217-224.

Moake JL. Thrombotic microangiopathies. *N Engl J Med.* 2002;347:589-600.

Ono T, Mimuro J, Madoiwa S, et al. Severe secondary deficiency of von Willebrand factor-cleaving protease (ADAMTS13) in patients with sepsis-induced disseminated intravascular coagulation: its correlation with development of renal failure. *Blood.* 2006;107:528-534.

Patel MR, Mahaffey KW, Garg J, et al. Rivaroxaban versus warfarin in nonvalvular atrial fibrillation. *N Engl J Med.* 2011;365:883-891.

Pengo V, Cucchini U, Denas G, et al. Standardized low-molecular-weight heparin bridging regimen in outpatients on oral anticoagulants undergoing invasive procedure or surgery: an Inception Cohort management study. *Circulation.* 2009;119:2920-2927.

Pengo V, Tripodi A, Reber G, et al. Update of the guidelines for lupus anticoagulant detection. Subcommittee on Lupus Anticoagulant/Antiphospholipid Antibody of the Scientific and Standardisation Committee of the International Society on Thrombosis and Haemostasis. *J Thromb Haemost.* 2009;7:1737-1740.

Perry JR. Thromboembolic disease in patients with high-grade glioma. *Neuro-Oncol.* 2012;14(Suppl 4):iv73-iv80.

Perzborn E, Gruber A, Tinel H, et al. Reversal of rivaroxaban anticoagulation by haemostatic agents in rats and primates. *Thromb Haemost.* 2013;110:162-172.

Reynolds MW, Fahrbach K, Hauch O, et al. Warfarin anticoagulation and outcomes in patients with atrial fibrillation: a systematic review and metaanalysis. *Chest.* 2004;126:1938-1945.

Rock GA, Shumak KH, Buskard NA, et al. Comparison of plasma exchange with plasma infusion in the treatment of thrombotic thrombocytopenic purpura. Canadian Apheresis Study Group. *N Engl J Med.* 1991;325:393-397.

Sadler JE, Moake JL, Miyata T, George JN. Recent advances in thrombotic thrombocytopenic purpura. *Hematology Am Soc Hematol Educ Program.* 2004:407-423.

Saposnik, G, Barinagarrementeria F, Brown RD, et al. Diagnosis and management of cerebral venous thrombosis: a statement for healthcare professionals from the American Heart Association/American Stroke Association. *Stroke.* 2011;42:1158-1192.

Sherman DG, Albers GW, Bladin C, et al. The efficacy and safety of enoxaparin versus unfractionated heparin for the prevention of venous thromboembolism after acute ischaemic stroke (PREVAIL Study): an open-label randomised comparison. *Lancet.* 2007;369:1347-1355.

Siegal DM, Curnutte JT, Connolly SJ, et al. Andexanet alfa for the reversal of factor Xa inhibitor activity. *N Engl J Med.* 2015;373:2413-2424.

Squizzato A, Hunt BJ, Kinasewitz GT, et al. Supportive management strategies for disseminated intravascular coagulation: an international consensus. *Thromb Haemost.* 2015;115:896-904.

Starke RM, Kim GH, Fernandez A, et al. Impact of a protocol for acute antifibrinolytic therapy on aneurysm rebleeding after subarachnoid hemorrhage. *Stroke.* 2008;39:2617-2621.

The Optimizing Primary Stroke Prevention in Sickle Cell Anemia (STOP 2) Trial Investigators. Discontinuing prophylactic transfusions used to prevent stroke in sickle cell disease. *N Engl J Med.* 2005;353:2769-2778.

Tsai FY, Nguyen B, Lin WC, et al. Endovascular procedures for cerebrovenous disorders. In: Chiu WT, Chiang YH, Kao MC, et al, eds. *Reconstructive Neurosurgery.* Vienna, Austria: Springer Vienna; 2008:83-86.

Tsai HM, Chandler WL, Sarode R, et al. von Willebrand factor and von Willebrand factor-cleaving metalloprotease activity in *Escherichia coli* O157:H7-associated hemolytic uremic syndrome. *Pediatr Res.* 2001;49:653-659.

Vesely SK, George JN, Lämmle B, et al. ADAMTS13 activity in thrombotic thrombocytopenic purpura-hemolytic uremic syndrome: relation to presenting features and clinical outcomes in a prospective cohort of 142 patients. *Blood.* 2003;102:60-68.

Wang X, Mondal S, Wang J, et al. Effect of activated charcoal on apixaban pharmacokinetics in healthy subjects. *Am J Cardiovasc Drugs.* 2014;14:147-154.

Ware RE, Helms RW, SWiTCH Investigators. Stroke With Transfusions Changing to Hydroxyurea (SWiTCH). *Blood.* 2012;119:3925-3932.

Zheng X, Pallera AM, Goodnough LT, et al. Remission of chronic thrombotic thrombocytopenic purpura after treatment with cyclophosphamide and rituximab. *Ann Intern Med.* 2003;138:105-108.

Zhou W, Zorn M, Nawroth P, et al. Hemostatic therapy in experimental intracerebral hemorrhage associated with rivaroxaban. *Stroke.* 2013;44:771-778.

12

Encephalopathy

David W. Van Wyck, DO and Christa Swisher, MD

Questions

1. A 66-year-old woman with hypertension and diabetes and stage III chronic kidney disease from diabetic nephropathy has been treated in the neurologic intensive care unit (ICU) for a Fisher grade 3, Hunt and Hess grade 3 subarachnoid hemorrhage due to a ruptured left middle cerebral artery (MCA) aneurysm. She required intubation on presentation for markedly diminished mental status and subsequently developed a ventilator-associated pneumonia that was treated with cefepime. Three days into therapy, the patient became intermittently confused and agitated and experienced visual hallucinations and occasional myoclonus. It was subsequently recognized that the cefepime dose was not adjusted for the patient's renal failure, and she was suspected of having a cefepime-induced neurotoxicity. Symptoms resolved within 3 days of changing antibiotic therapy to piperacillin-tazobactam. Which of the following pathophysiologic mechanisms most likely underlies cephalosporin-induced neurotoxicity?

   A. Altered D_2 dopamine and N-methyl-D-aspartate (NMDA) glutamate receptors

   B. Activation of the γ-aminobutyric acid class A receptors (GABA$_A$R), resulting in inhibitory postsynaptic potentials and central excitotoxicity

   C. Free radical formation and altered thiamine metabolism

   D. Increased release of dopamine and inhibition of neuronal Na^+-K^+-ATPase

   E. Blockade of central nervous system muscarinic receptors

2. A 26-year-old woman is admitted for close observation after experiencing multiple witnessed seizures without a return to her baseline neurocognitive status. Her coworker states that she had been experiencing constant holocephalic headaches for several days that had responded poorly to over-the-counter analgesics. Earlier this morning, she complained to coworkers that her headache had worsened and she was seeing zigzag lines in both eyes. In the early afternoon, she became irritable and sleepy for approximately 2 hours prior to her first seizure. Her initial exam was notable for a temperature of 37.3°C, a heart rate of 105 bpm, and a blood pressure of 213/104 mm Hg. She is sleepy but arouses to voice and is confused when attempting to answer questions. Cranial nerves are intact, and she is moving all 4 limbs spontaneously and semi-purposefully. A chemistry panel, complete blood count, and urine drug screen are unremarkable.

Magnetic resonance imaging (MRI) of the brain was obtained as part of her evaluation and is shown below. Which of the following is most frequently associated with condition described in this scenario?

A. Preeclampsia

B. Organ transplantation

C. Guillain-Barré syndrome

D. Chemotherapy

E. Systemic lupus erythematosus

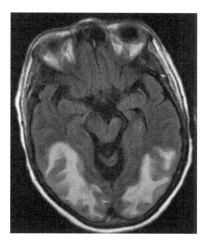

Axial FLAIR brain MRI.

3. Which of the following patients with hepatic encephalopathy is at the highest risk for herniation from intracranial hypertension?

A. A 33-year-old woman with acute liver failure and a plasma ammonia level of 223 μmol/L, who requires a norepinephrine infusion and continuous renal replacement therapy (CRRT).

B. A 68-year-old patient with chronic cirrhosis, a plasma ammonia level of 78 μmol/L, and borderline mild chronic renal failure.

C. A 53-year-old patient with acute chronic hepatic failure and a plasma ammonia level of 135 μmol/L, who is receiving large volumes of crystalloid for underlying pancreatitis and mild acute on chronic renal failure.

D. An 18-year-old patient with acute liver failure who presented over 72 hours after ingestion of large doses of acetaminophen, with a plasma ammonia level of 175 μmol/L, and who is receiving N-acetylcysteine therapy.

E. A 77-year-old patient with alcoholic cirrhosis who develops hepatorenal syndrome after a gastrointestinal bleed with a plasma ammonia level of 112 μmol/L and who requires midodrine and hemodialysis treatments.

4. A 47-year-old woman is admitted for a Fischer grade 3, Hunt and Hess grade 2 subarachnoid hemorrhage (SAH) following the rupture of a right MCA aneurysm. She has a headache, but is otherwise neurologically intact on admission. She successfully undergoes surgical clipping the following day and returns to the neuro-ICU for postoperative monitoring. Four days later, she is noted to have developed acute confusion and intermittent agitation during evening neurochecks. Her vital signs are unremarkable except for a mild sinus tachycardia up to 105 bpm. Additionally, she is now febrile to 38.7°C, and her sodium has decreased from normal range to 131 mEq/L. A review of screening transcranial Doppler ultrasounds reveals steadily increasing right MCA cerebral blood flow velocities with moderate vasospasm noted on the most recent exam. As you arrive at the bedside, she is noted to be markedly more difficult to arouse than earlier in the day. Which of the following is the next most appropriate step in the management of this patient?

A. Start broad-spectrum antibiotics for a suspected infection.

B. Begin hemodynamic augmentation with norepinephrine.

C. Start 1.8% hypertonic saline to correct the sodium deficit.

D. Contact the neurosurgeon on call to request a stat cerebral angiogram and transluminal angioplasty in the setting of previously identified vasospasm.

E. Order a stat computed tomography (CT) angiogram and CT perfusion scan to evaluate for delayed cerebral ischemia from vasospasm.

5. A 46-year-old man was admitted for a embolic strokes following a right carotid dissection that occurred after a bicycle crash. He has a history of migraines, bipolar disorder, and depression, and takes citalopram 40 mg daily and aripiprazole 20 mg daily as an outpatient. He had also reportedly been taking trazadone 50 mg at night for sleep, sumatriptan 50 mg as needed for migraines, and ondansetron 8 mg as needed for nausea and vomiting associated with his migraines; he reportedly has 2 to 3 migraines a week on average. During his hospitalization, he developed a vancomycin-resistant *Staphylococcus aureus* pneumonia and was started on linezolid. Two days later, he was noted on morning rounds to be febrile, diaphoretic, hypertensive, agitated, tremulous, rigid, and with clonus in the hands and feet. Which of the following exam findings is most helpful in establishing the diagnosis of serotonin syndrome over neuroleptic malignant syndrome?

A. Hypertension

B. Rigidity

C. Fever

D. Clonus

E. Tremors

6. A 35-year-old homeless man with no known prior medical history was brought to the emergency department (ED) after being found down and unresponsive on the sidewalk by police. His exam is notable for intact brainstem reflexes and flexion to pain in all 4 extremities. ED evaluation includes a head CT that shows a small left basal ganglia hemorrhage. His exam remains unchanged despite resuscitation in the ED, and respiratory rate is 6 breaths per minute. An arterial blood gas shows a PaO_2 of 52 mm Hg and a $PaCO_2$ of 57 mm Hg. He is intubated for apparent hypoxic and hypercapnic respiratory failure before being transferred to the neuroscience ICU. On arrival, additional evaluation reveals a rectal temperature of 35.1°C, a heart rate of 48 bpm, and nonpitting edema of the hands and feet. Admission labs are notable for a serum sodium of 134 mEq/L, a serum glucose of 54 mg/dL, and a negative urine drug screen. A repeat CT performed 6 hours after presentation shows a stable left basal ganglia hematoma, and an electroencephalogram (EEG) obtained at bedside shows only diffuse, low-amplitude waveforms. On evening rounds, mounding of the biceps muscle tissue to light pressure stimuli is noted. What test would be most beneficial in confirming the diagnosis causing this patient's persistent unresponsiveness?

A. Serum blood cultures

B. MRI of the brain with and without contrast

C. Thyroid-stimulating hormone (TSH), free thyroxine (T_4), and free triiodothyronine (T_3)

D. Carboxyhemoglobin level

E. Plasma ammonia level

7. Which of the following critical care patients receiving opioids is *least likely* to experience delirium as a complication of therapy?

A. A 69-year-old hemorrhagic stroke patient with a history of mild cognitive impairment who receives oxycodone at night to treat agitated confusion

B. A 25-year-old patient with moderate traumatic brain injury and right tibia fracture receiving scheduled, high-dose oxycodone for pain and quetiapine for sedation

C. A 74-year-old woman with a chronic obstructive pulmonary disease (COPD) exacerbation who is intubated and receiving a fentanyl infusion for vent comfort

D. A 34-year-old man involved in a motor vehicle accident who suffered a cervical spinal cord injury, multiple rib fractures, and a ruptured spleen on a hydromorphone infusion

E. A 52-year-old man with status epilepticus with a large head laceration from a fall who is intubated and is receiving continuous fentanyl and midazolam infusions

8. For patients with agitated delirium who have or who are at risk for prolonged QT intervals, which of the following medications has no known association with prolonged QTc intervals?

A. Risperidone

B. Quetiapine

C. Ziprasidone

D. Haloperidol

E. Aripiprazole

9. A 43-year-old woman admitted for severe traumatic brain injury developed toxic acute renal failure. What is the most likely pathogenic mechanism underlying dialysis disequilibrium syndrome?

A. Diencephalic and mesencephalic dysfunction of gray matter surrounding the third and fourth ventricles

B. A combination of microcirculatory abnormalities, altered blood-brain barrier permeability, and a reduction in monoamine neurotransmitters

C. The creation of an osmotic gradient that promotes water movement into the brain

D. Abnormal fatty acid metabolism, free radical damage, and increased ammonia concentrations

E. Formation of new osmoles that increase osmolality and cerebral edema

10. Which of the following statements is true regarding delirium in critically ill patients?

A. Delirium has been associated with long-term cognitive dysfunction in ICU survivors.

B. Limiting sedation increases the risk of self-extubation and self-harm.

C. Dexmedetomidine is just as likely as lorazepam to induce or worsen delirium.

D. Effective pain management has a minimal impact on the control of delirium in an ICU setting.

E. Nicotine replacement therapy is safe and effective and should be prescribed to any patient suspected of agitation and delirium associated with nicotine withdrawal.

11. A 24-year-old woman who is 15 weeks pregnant is admitted after becoming acutely confused during dinner. Her family members state that she has no prior medical history and that, except for a hyperolfactive nausea and vomiting that is sometimes severe and that began 6 weeks ago, her pregnancy has been uncomplicated. She was prescribed antiemetics, but they provided little benefit. On exam, she is sleepy but arousable to voice. She is oriented to person only. When she responds to questions, her answers are often nonsensical and dysarthric. She is afebrile, and vital signs show a blood pressure of 117/73 mm Hg, a heart rate of 102 bpm, a respiratory rate of 17 breaths/min, and an oxygen saturation (SaO_2) of 98% on room air. A chemistry panel and complete blood cell count are within normal limits, and a CT scan of the head is unremarkable. MRI of the brain is shown below. An EEG is notable only for mild diffuse slowing. Which of the following is the most likely diagnosis in this patient?

A. Posterior reversible encephalopathy syndrome

B. Eclampsia

C. Cerebral venous sinus thrombosis

D. Wernicke encephalopathy

E. Idiopathic intracranial hypertension

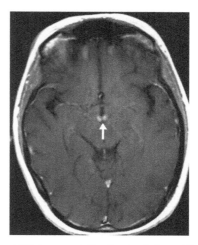

Axial contrast T1 image at the level of the midbrain. There is abnormal hyperintense signal just anterior to the midbrain marked with an arrow. Reproduced with permission from Berkowitz AL. *Clinical Neurology and Neuroanatomy: A Localization-Based Approach.* New York: NY, McGraw-Hill, 2016.

12. Which of the following antibiotic therapies is the most appropriate and effective treatment to combine with lactulose in patients with hepatic encephalopathy?

A. Neomycin

B. Rifaximin

C. Vancomycin

D. Metronidazole

E. Ribavirin

13. An 84-year-old man was found down in his retirement home after suffering a cardiac arrest. Advanced cardiac life support (ACLS) was initiated by emergency medical services, and return of spontaneous circulation was obtained after 10 minutes. He was down for an unknown period of time prior to ACLS initiation. He has a Glasgow coma scale score (GCS) of 6 on presentation (E1, V1, M4). CT of brain shows no acute intracranial process. Therapeutic hypothermia is initiated. Which of the following EEG patterns is most likely to be associated with a poor outcome in a cardiac arrest patient who remains comatose after rewarming?

A. Generalized triphasic waves

B. Diffuse theta slowing

C. Alpha-theta coma pattern

D. Frontal intermittent rhythmic delta (FIRDA)

E. Suppressed background (amplitude <10 μV) with superimposed continuous periodic discharges

14. Which of the following statements is true regarding hypertensive encephalopathy?

    A. Lowering diastolic pressure is more important than lowering systolic pressure.

    B. Sodium nitroprusside is the drug of choice for the treatment of hypertensive encephalopathy.

    C. Hypertensive emergencies are twice as common in women as in men.

    D. Blood pressure should be lowered as quickly as possible to prevent further end-organ damage and to allow transition to oral antihypertensive therapy.

    E. Labetalol provides more consistent and predictable blood pressure control than nicardipine.

15. Which of the following MRI findings is most likely to be associated with acute uremic encephalopathy in a patient with chronic renal failure?

    A. Posterior leukoencephalopathy

    B. T2 hyperintensities of the dorsomedial thalamus, mammillary bodies, and/or periaqueductal gray matter

    C. Bilateral basal ganglia T2 hyperintensities with a brightly hyperintense rim delineating the lateral and medial boundaries of the putamen

    D. Diffusion restriction and fluid-attenuated inversion recovery (FLAIR) hyperintensities involving the central pons

    E. T2/FLAIR hyperintensities involving the dentate nuclei of the cerebellum

16. A 19-year-old female college student with no known prior medical history is admitted to the ICU after being involved in a motor vehicle collision. Her friend, a passenger in the vehicle, stated that the patient had been complaining of abdominal pain for almost a week following an alcoholic drinking binge and seemed to develop increasing confusion and lethargy leading up to the accident. The passenger also stated that the patient "passed out and shook all over" right before crashing the car. During the trauma survey in the ED, the patient had a GCS of 12 (E3, V4, M5); was confused, agitated, and experiencing hallucinations; and had 2 witnessed, generalized tonic-clonic seizures. She was given 8 mg of intravenous lorazepam and 1500 mg of intravenous levetiracetam, which appeared to stop the seizures. She was intubated and placed on a continuous propofol infusion. The patient was then noted to be diaphoretic, tremulous, hypertensive with a blood pressure of 205/101 mm Hg, and tachycardic with a heart rate of 115 bpm. Incidentally, a number of blistering skin lesions over most of her body were noted. Blood tests demonstrated a hyponatremia of 117 mEq/L, a creatinine of 2.3 mg/dL, a neutrophilic leukocytosis of $23.2 \times 10^3/\mu L$, an elevated C-reactive protein of 18.4 mg/L, and an elevated creatinine kinase of 3512 IU/L. CT scans of the head, neck, chest, abdomen, and pelvis were unremarkable. Continuous EEG monitoring was started in the ICU and showed only diffuse, generalized slowing with some frontal beta activity. Which of the following is the most appropriate next step in the treatment of this patient's underlying condition?

    A. Give heme arginate 3 mg/kg and start a 0.9% saline infusion titrated to raise serum sodium by 4 to 6 mEq/L in the first 24 hours

    B. Hydrate at 5 to 10 mL/kg/h with lactated Ringer's solution, start an intravenous fentanyl infusion, and nothing by mouth until pain subsides

    C. Give a conivaptan 20 mg loading dose and continue with a 40-mg/d infusion for 4 days

    D. Start D-penicillamine 500 mg/d and start a 0.9% saline infusion titrated to raise serum sodium by 4 to 6 mEq/L in the first 24 hours

    E. Manage acute seizures and hyponatremia, start a gluten-free diet, and send for IgA endomysial assay, anti-tissue transglutaminase antibodies, and antigliadin antibodies

Answers and Explanations

1. **B.** Antibiotic-associated encephalopathy is felt to be an underrecognized cause of delirium in critically ill patients and has been identified with a number of antibiotic classes. Cefepime in particular has been known to result in neurotoxicity in patients with impaired renal function and may occur in as many as 15% of critically ill patients treated with the drug and should be considered when other causes of encephalopathy have been excluded and the patient's presentation is consistent with an antibiotic-associated encephalopathy. Since cefepime undergoes renal excretion, toxic levels of the drug have been known to accumulate in the blood and cerebrospinal fluid of patients with renal failure, placing them at higher risk for neurologic adverse reactions. A recent review by Bhattacharyya and colleagues evaluated a range of different antibiotics associated with encephalopathy and divided them into 3 phenotype categories. Cephalosporins and penicillins are characterized as causing type 1 antibiotic-associated encephalopathy (AAE), which is characterized by onset within days of initiation, commonly myoclonus, electroencephalogram (EEG) abnormalities (usually severe diffuse slowing, atypical triphasic waves, and multifocal sharp waves), normal magnetic resonance imaging (MRI), and spontaneous resolution within days of cessation of therapy. It is believed to be due to GABA receptor activation, leading to inhibition of postsynaptic potentials and excitotoxicity. Antibiotics associated with this category include penicillin and cephalosporins.

Type 2 AAE involves changes to dopamine and NMDA receptors and is associated with macrolides, procaine penicillin, fluoroquinolones, and sulfonamides.

Type 3 AAE is described solely with metronidazole use and involves free radical formation and altered thiamine metabolism primarily in the cerebellum.

Increased dopamine release and dysfunction of neuronal Na^+-K^+-ATPase are thought to be the underlying mechanisms causing encephalopathy with morphine use. Blockade of central nervous system (CNS) muscarinic receptors is associated with anticholinergic toxicity but is also a component of encephalopathy associated with other medications, such as digoxin.

2. **A.** The patient is manifesting signs and symptoms, as well as imaging findings, that are consistent with posterior reversible encephalopathy syndrome (PRES). PRES is a neurologic syndrome that typically manifests with headaches, confusion, visual disturbances, and seizures. Imaging typically shows evidence of vasogenic edema in the posterior cortical and/or subcortical white matter on T2/fluid-attenuated inversion recovery (FLAIR) sequences, although the anterior circulation can be affected as well. Diffusion-weighted imaging can be positive or negative, and when positive, the underlying structural pathology is often, but not always, reversible. With this in mind, PRES is often considered to be a misleading name for this condition. It is believed to be related to autoregulatory failure that occurs when elevated blood pressures forcibly dilates cerebral arterioles leading to hyperperfusion of the brain and blood-brain barrier breakdown. This results in the entry of fluid and blood products into brain tissue, which leads to cerebral edema. Alternatively, it has been postulated to be due to endothelial dysfunction when it occurs in preeclampsia, autoimmune disorders, and cases involving cytotoxic drugs. In preeclampsia, markers of endothelial dysfunction, such as lactate dehydrogenase, abnormal red cell morphology, fibronectin, tissue plasminogen activator, thrombomodulin, endothelin-1, and von Willebrand factor have all been reported to be elevated. PRES has been reported in numerous other conditions but

remains classically associated with severe hypertension and preeclampsia/eclampsia. Interestingly, there is some suggestion that PRES may be more severe and may be more likely to be nonreversible in cases associated with autoimmunity and/or using cytotoxic drugs.

3. **A.** Hepatic encephalopathy (HE) can occur in both acute and chronic cases of liver failure. In acute liver failure (ALF), it may herald the development of intracranial hypertension and result in transtentorial herniation and death. A plasma ammonia level >200 μmol/L is a well-known risk factor associated with intracranial hypertension. Still, there have been cases of HE with associated intracranial hypertension in the setting of lower plasma ammonia levels, with some authors reporting as many as 25% of ALF cases developing intracranial hypertension in the setting of lower plasma ammonia levels. Intracranial hypertension is most common in ALF and rarely occurs in acute on chronic liver failure (ACLF). Intracranial hypertension does not occur in decompensated cirrhosis. Other risk factors associated with increased risk intracranial hypertension in ALF include patients who meet Kings College Criteria, which are as follows:

- Have a sustained elevation in plasma ammonia levels
- Require continuous renal replacement therapy for acute renal failure
- Are <35 years of age
- Require the use of vasopressors
- Have multiple organ system dysfunction
- Have higher sequential organ failure assessment (SOFA) scores

Patient A is therefore at the highest risk for intracranial hypertension. Patients B, C, and E are older, have chronic liver failure or ACLF, and have lower overall ammonia levels. Patient E is also receiving hemodialysis, which is less likely to result in intracranial hypertension. Patient D is young and experiencing acute liver failure from an acetaminophen overdose, but treatment with *N*-acetylcysteine has been associated with improved mortality and lower incidences of cerebral edema in these patients. It is most beneficial when given up to 24 hours after ingestion, but has also proven to benefit patients with established ALF even when given beyond this window.

4. **E.** Fever is common in aneurysmal subarachnoid hemorrhage (aSAH) and develops in up to 75% of patients at some point during their hospital stay. Furthermore, fever in aSAH may have a number of etiologies, which makes it important to quickly and correctly identify the source. The 2 most common and concerning sources of fever in SAH patients are neurogenic fever and infection. Prior studies have indicated that as many as 50% of aSAH patients have fevers related to an infectious etiology. On the other hand, fever of central origin is common and may be associated with developing vasospasm. Vasospasm occurs in as many as 70% of patients with aSAH, but only 40% will develop signs and symptoms of delayed cerebral ischemia (DCI).

In this patient, there are a number of indicators that are worrisome of the development of DCI, including the Fisher grade assigned to her SAH, her sudden change in mental status in the setting of fever, hyponatremia, and increasing arterial vasospasm on screening transcranial Doppler ultrasounds. The best way to evaluate these concerns is to order a CT angiogram and perfusion scan. The CT angiogram can demonstrate vessel narrowing, whereas the CT perfusion scan can show evidence of developing ischemia with high sensitivity and specificity.

Requesting a stat angiogram or starting hemodynamic augmentation can be considered, but with febrile encephalopathy from infection being a significant consideration, it would be more appropriate to confirm the ischemia before sending the patient for an invasive procedure or starting vasopressor therapy. Likewise, starting broad-spectrum antibiotics should be reserved until DCI can be excluded. Hyponatremia in the setting of SAH may be related to the syndrome of inappropriate antidiuretic hormone or cerebral salt wasting and should be addressed, but it would be unusual for encephalopathy to develop unless the serum sodium concentration acutely fell below 115 to 120 mEq/L. It is recommended that this patient's hyponatremia be evaluated and treated, but identification and treatment of DCI and vasospasm is of upmost importance, since DCI is the leading cause of morbidity and mortality in SAH.

5. **D.** Serotonin syndrome (SS) is believed to be an underdiagnosed cause of encephalopathy. It generally occurs in patients who have been taking a

serotonergic agent, such as a selective serotonin reuptake inhibitor (SSRI) or tricyclic antidepressant (TCA), who are then given another medication with serotonergic activity (additional SSRIs or TCAs, opiates, cough medications, antibiotics, antiemetics, and/or migraine medications). SS and a similar condition, neuroleptic malignant syndrome (NMS), can have overlapping features but can be distinguished on the basis of clinical history and exam (Table 12-1). Both are important to recognize and both can be life threatening in severe cases. Therapies for SS and NMS differ, and treatments for each can potentially worsen the other in the setting of misdiagnosis.

Table 12-1. Comparison Between Serotonin Syndrome and Neuroleptic Malignant Syndrome

Serotonin Syndrome (SS)	Neuroleptic Malignant Syndrome (NMS)
Serotonin agonist use	Antipsychotics
Occurs over hours to days	Occurs over days to weeks
Both can present with mental status changes, autonomic instability, hyperthermia, rigidity, agitation, tremors, incontinence, and diarrhea	
Differs by the presence of clonus and/or hyperreflexia	NMS more often manifests with hyporeflexia
Tachycardia is more characteristic of SS	NMS manifests with bradycardia
	NMS is associated with low serum iron levels
Both can have lab abnormalities such as elevated creatinine kinase levels, myoglobinuria, metabolic acidosis, elevated creatinine from rhabdomyolysis, and leukocytosis	

Both are treated with hydration, control of autonomic symptoms, and treatment of rigidity, hyperthermia, and agitation. SS may also be treated with serotonin antagonists, such as cyproheptadine, although evidence of their efficacy is weak.

NMS is treated with dopamine agonists such as bromocriptine as well as dantrolene, which blocks calcium release in muscles. Electroconvulsive therapy has also been used in medication-refractory cases of NMS.

6. **C.** The patient manifests with signs and symptoms classically associated with myxedema coma.

Myxedema coma is a rare but serious manifestation of severe, untreated hypothyroidism with a mortality rate of up to 60%. It is rarely seen in modern clinical practice because of the ease with which screening thyroid assays can be performed. Patients with poorly treated hypothyroidism often decompensate into myxedema coma following a precipitating event, which may include trauma, infection, or acute neurologic injuries such as seizures or cerebrovascular insults (hemorrhagic or ischemic). Coma is rare, despite the name, and most patients present with varying degrees of altered mental status and consciousness. Additional signs and symptoms that have classically been associated with myxedema coma include hypothermia, bradycardia, hyponatremia, hypoglycemia, and hypotension. The mounding of muscle tissue in the biceps is an uncommon finding known as myoedema. While it is classically associated with hypothyroid myopathy and serves as a clue to the underlying diagnosis in this case, it has also been associated with other conditions such as anorexia nervosa and has even been noted in normal individuals. The condition can be easily identified by a high TSH and low or undetectable free T_4 and T_3 levels. Since TSH can be lowered by concomitant critical illness, a free T_4 and T_3 should always be checked when this condition is suspected because a TSH alone may not be sufficient to identify the thyroid dysfunction. Because of the high mortality associated with myxedema coma, treatment with thyroid hormone and glucocorticoids should not be delayed while awaiting laboratory confirmation in suspected cases. While carboxyhemoglobin and plasma ammonia levels and blood cultures are reasonable tests to evaluate coma, they are not as likely to help with the diagnosis, considering the patient's clinical history and evaluation. An MRI of the brain is likewise unlikely to yield any additional diagnostic information in this case.

7. **D.** Pain is a well-known and modifiable risk factor for delirium in ICU patients. However, opioids have also been shown to increase the risk for developing delirium. In a review on delirium in the ICU, it was noted that opioid-induced delirium is related to the analgesic and sedative effects of opioids. When opioids are used to address pain, as in trauma and burn patients, it has been noted that opioids reduce the risk of delirium. Alternatively, opioids

used primarily for sedation in general medical and surgical ICU patients or in conjunction with other sedatives, especially benzodiazepines, resulted in an increased risk of delirium. Care should also be used in patients with primary neurologic conditions, as encephalopathy may result from these injuries and be exacerbated by delirium developing secondary to oversedation. Patient D, who is younger and receiving opioids primarily for pain control, is therefore the least likely to develop delirium as a result of opioid use.

8. **E.** Agitated delirium may require treatment with antipsychotic medications in order to prevent a patient from harming himself or herself or others. One of the more concerning and serious adverse effects associated with antipsychotic mediations is prolonged QT intervals, which increase the risk for torsade de pointes, a polymorphic ventricular tachycardia that can degenerate into ventricular fibrillation and sudden cardiac death. Critically ill patients may have medical comorbidities or require other medications that increase the risk for prolongation of the QT interval. Lurasidone, clozapine, and aripiprazole have been found not to cause a prolonged QT interval. Aripiprazole also has an intramuscular formulation that may be administered to patients unable or unwilling to take an oral formulation. Haloperidol is a first-generation antipsychotic and has a higher association with prolonged QT intervals than second-generation medications. The remaining options are all second-generation antipsychotics. Risperidone and quetiapine have a lower overall risk for prolonged QT intervals compared with typical antipsychotics and can be considered in patients who are at risk for prolonged QT intervals but have a prolonged QTc that measures less than 500 milliseconds. For patients with a QTc longer than 500 milliseconds, however, these drugs should be avoided in favor of aripiprazole or other medications with some antipsychotic effects such as trazadone, valproate, or benzodiazepines. Ziprasidone has the highest association with prolonged QT intervals among the second-generation antipsychotics and should be avoided in any patient with or at risk for prolonged QT intervals.

9. **C.** Dialysis disequilibrium syndrome (DDS) is a rare complication associated with the initiation of hemodialysis treatment. It is identified by the development of neurologic symptoms, most commonly encephalopathy, during dialysis, although no diagnostic test or criteria exist, making it a diagnosis of exclusion. Symptoms that develop during or immediately following the dialysis session include headache, nausea, restlessness, blurry vision, disorientation, nausea, muscle cramps, and dizziness. Symptoms often resolve within several hours, although in rare cases, confusion, seizures, and coma may occur. It must be differentiated from other, more common causes of encephalopathy in critically ill patients, including uremia, systemic infection, meningitis, cerebral ischemia, intracerebral hemorrhage, other forms of metabolic disturbances such as hyponatremia, hypoglycemia, and/or drug-induced encephalopathy. The mechanism underlying DDS is unclear, but it is believed to be due to a reverse osmotic shift that occurs when blood urea nitrogen (BUN) is rapidly removed, thereby promoting the shift of water into cells. Slower reduction in BUN via lower blood flow rates and/or the use of ultrafiltration may help prevent DDS. Dialysis should be stopped in any patient who develops severe manifestations such as seizures or coma. Intracerebral acidosis resulting in increased osmolality and cerebral edema from osmoles formed during dialysis has been proposed as an alternative hypothesis to explain DDS. However, subsequent experiments have not demonstrated any significant formation of organic osmolytes after rapid dialysis. Diencephalic and mesencephalic dysfunction of gray matter around the third and fourth ventricles occurs with thiamine deficiency and Wernicke encephalopathy. Microcirculatory abnormalities, altered blood-brain barrier permeability, and a reduction in monoamine neurotransmitters are some of the mechanisms underlying septic encephalopathy. Abnormal fatty acid metabolism, free radical damage, and increased ammonia concentrations are some of the mechanisms believed to lead to hepatic encephalopathy.

10. **A.** Delirium is a common complication in hospitalized critical care patients and occurs in as many as 70% to 80% of patients according to some studies. Delirium is specifically characterized as fluctuating levels of attention that occur over hours to days that are caused by an underlying medical condition, substance intoxication, or as a side effect of therapy.

Structural disruptions involving any number of the brain's arousal or attention centers (eg, ascending reticular activating center, thalamus, hypothalamus) or abnormalities in various neurotransmitters are involved in the complex underlying pathophysiology of delirium. It is also important to recognize that delirium has been linked to increased morbidity, mortality, prolonged hospitalization, and other medical complications such as fever, tachycardia, and hypertension.

The Awakening and Breathing Controlled (ABC) trial was a randomized trial (daily sedation awakening plus spontaneous breathing trial vs daily spontaneous breathing trials alone) and demonstrated decreased ICU length of stay and 90-day mortality in the intervention group. Of the survivors, delirium in ICU patients was associated with long-term cognitive dysfunction. It should be noted, however, that this trial did not include patients with primary neurologic disease and did not assess for secondary neurologic complications that may have occurred as a result of the patients' ICU hospitalization. Nevertheless, additional studies in stroke patients have shown worsened Mini-Mental State Exam scores were worse at 3 and 6 months in patients who were determined to have had delirium during their hospitalization.

Based on the MENDS and SEDCOM trials, dexmedetomidine is believed to be less likely than benzodiazepines and neuroleptics to induce or worsen delirium, although these trials also excluded primary neurologic pathologies. Effective pain management has a clear impact on reducing the risk of delirium and may also reduce the risk of other conditions such as posttraumatic stress disorder. Nicotine withdrawal has been associated with agitated delirium in critical care patients. Nicotine replacement therapy is controversial, however, with several studies showing increased delirium and seizures, providing conflicting data on the possibility of increased mortality in the nicotine replacement arms.

11. **D.** The patient is presenting with history, signs, and symptoms of Wernicke encephalopathy (WE) associated with hyperemesis gravidarum. WE is the result of thiamine deficiency (vitamin B_1) and is characterized by the classic triad of encephalopathy, gait ataxia, and oculomotor dysfunctions, although rarely are all 3 features present. Nystagmus is the most common ocular abnormality, although lateral and vertical gaze palsies can occur as well. Thiamine is important in energy utilization pathways, particularly as a cofactor for α-ketoglutarate dehydrogenase, transketolase, and pyruvate dehydrogenase. Thiamine is therefore important in highly metabolic regions of the brain. While it is classically associated with alcoholism, it can occur in systemic malignancy, prolonged fasting or starvation, dialysis patients, acquired immunodeficiency syndrome, anorexia nervosa, after gastrectomy, and with hyperemesis in pregnancy. The diagnosis is usually clinical, but an MRI of the brain may demonstrate T2 hyperintensities involving the dorsomedial thalami, periaqueductal gray area, mammillary bodies, or other structures previously mentioned to be affected by thiamine deficiency. Patients often respond favorably and rather quickly to parenteral doses of thiamine, and pregnant women, particularly those with nausea and vomiting, should be prescribed daily oral thiamine supplementation to reduce the risk of WE.

Posterior reversible encephalopathy syndrome and eclampsia can both present with encephalopathy, but the absence of seizures, hypertension, and visual disturbances makes this less likely. Furthermore, eclampsia is rare in pregnant women before 20 weeks of gestation. The absence of headaches, seizure, focal neurologic deficits, and/or a CT with findings such as absent venous flow, an intraluminal thrombus, or hemorrhages and signs of edema or infarcts that do not correspond with arterial territories make Cerebral venous sinus thrombosis less likely. Idiopathic intracranial hypertension (IIH) most often affects overweight women of childbearing age. It can be associated with nausea and vomiting and can worsen with pregnancy, but a history of headache, visual disturbances (diplopia, transient visual obscurations, photopsias), and/or vertigo would be expected. Encephalopathy is also not associated with IIH.

12. **B.** The mainstay of therapy for hepatic encephalopathy (HE) is lactulose, which works by lowering colonic pH. When the colonic pH is lowered to approximately 5, this favors the formation of nonabsorbable NH_4^+ over NH_3 and traps it in the colon, allowing for a reduction in plasma ammonia levels. Oral antibiotics, however, are commonly added when there is an insufficient response to

lactulose monotherapy or when lactulose is not tolerated due to excessive diarrhea, abdominal pain, or other common adverse effects. Broad-spectrum antibiotics, such as rifaximin, are believed to work by reducing the amount of ammonia-producing bacteria in the gut. While rifaximin has not been clearly shown to be superior to lactulose, it has been shown to be better tolerated, with some evidence that it may reduce mortality as well. Furthermore, although it has not clearly been shown to reduce hospital length of stay, it has been shown in several studies to reduce the number of hospital readmissions. Other antibiotics may be helpful in HE but have more side effects associated with their use or are understudied in HE. Although neomycin has historically be used successfully to treat HE by reducing gut bacteria, it has a significant side effect profile including ototoxicity, nephrotoxicity, and enterocolitis. Vancomycin and metronidazole have been used in HE, but there are limited data supporting their use, and side effects such as neurotoxicity associated with metronidazole and nephrotoxicity associated with vancomycin limit their appeal. Ribavirin is an antiviral used to treat hepatitis C; it has no role in the treatment of HE.

13. **E.** EEG has been used to monitor patients with hypoxic ischemic encephalopathy (HIE) for seizures after undergoing therapeutic hypothermia. EEG has also been used to help generate a neurologic prognosis in patients after cardiac arrest. Despite some debate as to the clinical value of EEG in making a prognosis in patients with HIE, this modality remains the most commonly used prognostic tool. Several patterns have been identified as being associated with a poor prognosis in both hypothermic and normothermic HIE patients. Westhall and colleagues prospectively evaluated EEG patterns in previously recorded EEGs from patients in the Targeted Temperature Management Trial and determined that "highly malignant" patterns, or those with suppression, suppression with periodic discharges, or burst-suppression, predicted a poor outcome (a cerebral performance category score of 3-5 after 180 days) in half of the patients without false predictions. Using the American Clinical Neurophysiology Society terminology to define "highly malignant" patterns, they reported a specificity for predicting poor outcome of 100%, although sensitivity was reported at 50%.

Other malignant patterns, such as periodic or rhythmic patterns, patterns with pathologic or nonreactive backgrounds, or patterns with a reversed anterior-posterior gradient, did not predict a poor outcome when occurring in isolation (specificity of 48% and sensitivity of 99%), but the identification of at least 2 malignant features significantly increased the specificity for predicting a poor neurologic outcome (96%), although sensitivity decreased to 76%.

Other types of EEG patterns or "benign EEG" patterns that did not contain any of the pathologic features listed above were highly associated with good outcomes (a cerebral performance category score of 1-2 after 180 days). Numerous other studies have identified similar "malignant" patterns that are generally indicative of a poor outcomes, but many have been plagued by lack of consensus on pattern definitions and interrater variability.

Choices A, B, C, and D are malignant or benign patterns, as defined earlier, and are therefore less likely to have a poor outcome than pattern E, which has a suppressed background.

14. **A.** Hypertensive encephalopathy (HE) occurs in the setting of rapid changes in blood pressure that exceed the brain's autoregulatory capacity and result in cerebral edema and nonspecific neurologic symptoms such as headache, blurry vision, dizziness, nausea, vomiting, and confusion. HE is a form of hypertensive crisis. It is often the result of poorly controlled hypertension and/or patient noncompliance. However, HE is a diagnosis of exclusion, and alternative sources for blood pressure elevation should be sought, such as acute ischemic or hemorrhagic stroke, acute myocardial infarction, head injury, pregnancy, or medication/toxin, such as cocaine, amphetamines, or monoamine oxidase inhibitors. Once the diagnosis of HE is made, the goals should be to lower mean arterial pressure (MAP) by 10% to 15% in the first hour and 25% in the first 24 hours using titratable intravenous (IV) antihypertensive medications such as clevidipine 1 to 32 mg/h, nicardipine 5 to 15 mg/h, and labetalol as a 10- to 20-mg bolus followed by an infusion at 0.5 to 2 mg/min. Lowering blood pressure more aggressively increases the risk of cerebral hypoperfusion and stroke. Targeting the diastolic pressure with initial therapies will more effectively lower MAP than targeting the systolic pressure since diastole counts for twice as much when calculating

the MAP because two-thirds of the cardiac cycle is spent in diastole.

Sodium nitroprusside was previously recommended as the agent of choice in acute hypertensive crisis; however, the risk of cyanide toxicity in the setting of agents with fewer side effects has relegated this agent to second- or third-line use in most institutions. There is literature to suggest that sodium nitroprusside increases intracranial pressure, which should typically be avoided in the acute setting.

Hypertensive emergencies are more common in men than in women and in African Americans more often than other ethnic groups. Nicardipine and labetalol appear to be equally efficacious and safe; however, nicardipine was noted to provide a more predictable and consistent blood pressure–lowering effect than labetalol. Furthermore, labetalol should not be used in patients who are hypertensive from cocaine ingestion without an additional agent to provide α-receptor blockade.

15. **C.** Uremic encephalopathy can occur in both chronic and acute renal failure and is typically a sign of severe renal dysfunction. It most often manifests when the glomerular filtration rate falls below 15 mL/min and as various toxins accumulate in the kidneys. The underlying pathophysiology is complex and not completely understood. Metabolic acidosis is a common complication of worsening renal failure as the kidneys become unable to clear daily dietary acid loads. It is this acidosis that is believed to result in what is called the "lentiform fork sign" in which bilateral basal ganglia hyperintensities are accompanied by a bright rim demarcating the medial and lateral boundaries of the putamen forming a fork-like appearance. Although rare, this has been described in a number of cases of uremic encephalopathy and may help explain some of the movement disorders (tremors, myoclonus, asterixis) that often accompany uremic encephalopathy. Posterior leukoencephalopathy occurs more commonly in hypertensive encephalopathy and, in particular, with posterior reversible encephalopathy syndrome.

T2 hyperintensities of the dorsomedial thalamus, mammillary bodies, and/or periaqueductal gray matter are findings classically associated with Wernicke encephalopathy. Diffusion restriction involving the central pons is the classic finding in osmotic demyelination that can occur with overly rapid correction of sodium in hyponatremia. T2/FLAIR hyperintensities involving the dentate nuclei are a common finding that occurs with metronidazole toxicity.

16. **A.** This patient is suffering from an acute porphyria. Porphyrias are rare disorders of heme biosynthesis that can present with acute neurovisceral and/or cutaneous attacks. A number of enzyme deficiencies are involved in the various porphyrias and are categorized as either hepatic or erythropoietic, although most forms are hepatic in nature. There are 4 types of acute porphyrias (Table 12-2).

Table 12-2. Types of Acute Porphyrias and Their Presentations

Type of Acute Porphyria	Symptoms	Cutaneous Lesions
Acute intermittent porphyria (AIDP)	The acute attacks are indistinguishable from one another and they share the following symptoms: <ul><li>The major symptom is severe abdominal pain of neuropathic origin</li><li>Neuropsychiatric symptoms</li><li>Neuropathy (motor > sensory)</li><li>Electrolyte disturbances; hyponatremia develops in as many as 40% of acute porphyric episodes</li></ul>	No
δ-Aminolevulinic acid dehydratase porphyria (ADP)		No
Hereditary coproporphyria (HCP)		Yes
Variegate porphyria (VP)		Yes

Attacks can last several days to weeks and can be triggered by alcohol intake, as in this case. Hyponatremia is believed to play a prominent role in the development of seizures in these patients. An acute porphyria can be quickly confirmed by a clinical history and an elevated urine porphobilinogen. Porphyrin biochemistry on urine, stool, or plasma will differentiate the specific porphyria subtype. Acute attacks are treated with intravenous heme arginate 3 mg/kg, which reduces the production of heme precursors by suppressing δ-aminolevulinic acid synthases (ALAS), the rate-limiting enzyme in the heme biosynthesis pathway. Intravenous carbohydrate loads have also been used to treat acute porphyria, but care must be taken to avoid worsening hyponatremia through the administration of dextrose solutions. A high index of suspicion must be present to diagnose this condition, but it should be considered in any patient with acute abdominal pain of unclear origin and neuropsychiatric symptoms.

Aggressive hydration with lactated Ringer's solution, bowel rest, and pain control with opioids compose the initial therapy for acute pancreatitis. Although pancreatitis is a consideration given the patient's alcohol use, it would not be expected to manifest with cutaneous symptoms or neuropsychiatric features.

Conivaptan is a vasopressin analog that is sometimes used in severe syndrome of inappropriate antidiuretic hormone (SIADH). While addressing SIADH in this patient may be necessary, conivaptan should not be the initial treatment and can potentially raise the sodium too quickly and place the patient at risk for osmotic demyelination. D-Penicillamine is the treatment for Wilson disease and is not appropriate in this patient.

A gluten-free diet and testing for IgA endomysial antibodies, anti-tissue transglutaminase antibodies, and antigliadin antibodies compose the initial management for celiac disease. Celiac disease can manifest with abdominal pain and epilepsy, but blistering and severe electrolyte disorders are unlikely.

REFERENCES

Ahuja CK, Yadav MK, Khandelwal N. Mystery case: syndrome of bilateral basal ganglia lesions in uremic encephalopathy. *Neurology.* 2016;86:e182-e183.

Alagiakrishnan K, Wien C. An approach to drug induced delirium in the elderly. *Postgrad Med J.* 2004;80:388-393.

Bass NM, Mullen K, Sanyal A, et al. Rifaximin treatment in hepatic encephalopathy. *N Engl J Med.* 2010;362:1071-1081.

Besur S, Schmeltzer P, Bonkovsky HL. Acute porphyrias. *J Emerg Med.* 2015;49:305-312.

Bhattacharyya S, Darby RR, Raibagkar P, et al. Antibiotic-associated encephalopathy. *Neurology.* 2016;86:963-971.

Bhavsar AS, Verma S. Abdominal manifestations of neurologic disorders. *Radiographics.* 2013;33:135-153.

Brouns R, De Deyn PP. Neurological complications in renal failure: a review. *Clin Neurol Neurosurg.* 2004;107:1-16.

Brummel NE, Girard TD. Preventing delirium in the intensive care unit. *Crit Care Clin.* 2013;29:51-65.

Chun LJ, Tong MJ, Busuttil RW, Hiatt JR. Acetaminophen hepatotoxicity and acute liver failure. *J Clin Gastroenterol.* 2009;43:342-349.

Commichau C, Scarmeas N, Mayer SA. Risk factors for fever in the neurologic intensive care unit. *Neurology.* 2003;60:837-841.

Crepeau AZ, Rabinstein AA. Continuous EEG in therapeutic hypothermia after cardiac arrest: prognostic and clinical value. *Neurology.* 2013;80:339-344.

Dority JS, Oldham JS. Subarachnoid hemorrhage: an update. *Anesthesiol Clin.* 2016;34:577-600.

Ferreira TS, Reis F, Appenzeller S. Posterior reversible encephalopathy syndrome and association with systemic lupus erythematosus. *Lupus.* 2016;25:1369-1376.

Frontera, JA. Delirium and sedation in the ICU. *Neurocrit Care.* 2011;14:463-474.

Fugate JE, Kalimullah EA, Hocker SE, et al. Cefepime neurotoxicity in the intensive care unit: a cause of severe, underappreciated encephalopathy. *Crit Care.* 2013;17:R264.

Fugate JE, Wijdicks EF, Mandrekar J, et al. Predictors of neurologic outcome in hypothermia after cardiac arrest. *Ann Neurol.* 2010;68:907-914.

Girard TD, Kress JP, Fuchs BD, et al. Efficacy and safety of a paired sedation and ventilator weaning protocol for mechanically ventilated patients in intensive care (Awakening and Breathing Controlled trial): a randomised controlled trial. *Lancet.* 2008;371:126-134.

Gish DS, Loynd RT, Melnick S, Nazir S. Myxoedema coma: a forgotten presentation of extreme hypothyroidism. *BMJ Case Rep.* 2016;2016:bcr2016216225.

Gyanendra K, Munish KG. Lentiform fork sign: a unique MRI picture. Is metabolic acidosis responsible? *Clin Neurol Neurosurg.* 2010;112:805-812.

Hinchey J, Chaves C, Appignani B, et al. A reversible posterior leukoencephalopathy syndrome. *N Engl J Med.* 1996;334:494-500.

Hornung K, Nix WA. Myoedema. A clinical and electrophysiological evaluation. *Eur Neurol.* 1992;32:130-133.

Hwang JJ, Hwang DY. Treatment of endocrine disorders in the neuroscience intensive care unit. *Curr Treat Options Neurol.* 2014;16:271.

Jawaro T, Yang A. Management of hepatic encephalopathy: a primer. *Ann Pharmacother.* 2016;50:569-577.

Jiang Q, Jiang XH. Rifaximin versus nonabsorbable disaccharides in the management of hepatic encephalopathy: a meta-analysis. *Eur J Gastroenterol Hepatol.* 2008;20:1064-1070.

Kandiah PA, Kumar G. Hepatic encephalopathy: the old and the new. *Crit Care Clin.* 2016;32:311-329.

Kastrup O, Schlamann M, Moenninghoff C, et al. Posterior reversible encephalopathy syndrome: the spectrum of MR imaging patterns. *Clin Neuroradiol.* 2015;25:161-171.

Katus LE, Frucht SJ. Management of serotonin syndrome and neuroleptic malignant syndrome. *Curr Treat Options Neurol.* 2016;18:39.

Kimer N, Krag A. Systematic review with meta-analysis: the effects of rifaximin in hepatic encephalopathy. *Aliment Pharmacol Ther.* 2014;40:123-132.

Kramer CL, Pegoli M, Mandrekar J, et al. Refining the association of fever with functional outcome in aneurysmal subarachnoid hemorrhage. *Neurocrit Care.* 2017;26(1):41-47.

Lucidarme O, Seguin A, Daubin C, et al. Nicotine withdrawal and agitation in ventilated critically ill patients. *Crit Care.* 2010;14:R58.

Morgan HG, Barry R, Morgan MH. Myoedema in anorexia nervosa: a useful clinical sign. *Eur Eat Disord Rev.* 2008;16:352-354.

Norton J, Hymers C, Stein P, et al. Acute porphyria presenting as major trauma: case report and literature review. *J Emerg Med.* 2016;51(5):e115-e122.

O'Hara-McCoy H. Posterior reversible encephalopathy syndrome: an emerging clinical entity in adult, pediatric and obstetrical care. *J Am Acad Nurse Pract.* 2008;20:100-106.

Oliveira-Filho J, Ezzeddine MA, Segal AZ, et al. Fever in subarachnoid hemorrhage: relationship to vasospasm and outcome. *Neurology.* 2001;56:1299-1304.

Patel N, Dalal P, Panesar M. Dialysis disequilibrium syndrome: a narrative review. *Semin Dial.* 2008;21:493-498.

Peacock WF, Hilleman DE, Levy PD, et al. A systematic review of nicardipine vs labetalol for the management of hypertensive crises. *Am J Emerg Med.* 2012;30:981-993.

Phillips SJ, Whisnant JP. Hypertension and the brain. The National High Blood Pressure Education Program. *Arch Intern Med.* 1992;152:938-945.

Rabinstein AA, Wijdicks EF. The value of EEG monitoring after cardiac arrest treated with hypothermia. *Neurology.* 2012;78:774-775.

Rehman T, Deboisblanc BP. Persistent fever in the ICU. *Chest.* 2014;145:158-165.

Ries R, Sayadipour A. Management of psychosis and agitation in medical-surgical patients who have or are at risk for prolonged QT interval. *J Psychiatr Pract.* 2014;20:338-344.

Rodgers GM, Taylor RN, Roberts JM. Preeclampsia is associated with a serum factor cytotoxic to human endothelial cells. *Am J Obstet Gynecol.* 1988;159:908-914.

Sharma P, Eesa M, Scott JN. Toxic and acquired metabolic encephalopathies: MRI appearance. *AJR Am J Roentgenol.* 2009;193:879-886.

Sheng AZ, Shen Q, Cordato D, et al. Delirium within three days of stroke in a cohort of elderly patients. *J Am Geriatr Soc.* 2006;54:1192-1198.

Silver SM. Cerebral edema after rapid dialysis is not caused by an increase in brain organic osmolytes. *J Am Soc Nephrol.* 1995;6:1600-1606.

Westhall E, Rossetti AO, van Rootselaar AF, et al. Standardized EEG interpretation accurately predicts prognosis after cardiac arrest. *Neurology.* 2016;86:1482-1490.

Wilson CD, Shankar JJ. Diagnosing vasospasm after subarachnoid hemorrhage: CTA and CTP. *Can J Neurol Sci.* 2014;41:314-319.

Woytowish MR, Maynor LM. Clinical relevance of linezolid-associated serotonin toxicity. *Ann Pharmacother.* 2013;47:388-397.

Yahia M, Najeh H, Zied H, et al. Wernicke's encephalopathy: a rare complication of hyperemesis gravidarum. *Anaesth Crit Care Pain Med.* 2015;34:173-177.

13

Neuropharmacology

Ali Daneshmand MD, MPH, Arnavaz Hajizadeh Barfejani, PharmD, and Xuemei Cai, MD

Questions

1. A 35-year-old right-handed man presents to the emergency department (ED) with a 2-day history of a severe headache, confusion, and slurred speech. On arrival, his temperature is 37.5°C, blood pressure is 132/68 mm Hg, heart rate is 96 bpm, and respiratory rate is 19 breaths/min. His neurologic examination is notable for lethargy and inattention. He underwent a lumbar puncture, which revealed glucose of 50 mg/dL and protein of 150 mg/dL and a white blood cell count of 170 cells/μL with a lymphocytic predominance. His magnetic resonance imaging (MRI) scan is shown below. Which statement is true regarding treatment for his condition?

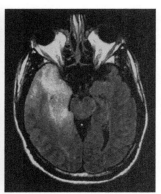

Sequential images of axial FLAIR MRI at the level of the upper pons and lower midbrain.

A. Dexamethasone 40 mg daily for 4 days is a useful adjunctive treatment for improved functional outcome in this condition.

B. Acyclovir should be administered intravenously at a dose of 2 mg/kg of actual body weight and administered every 8 hours for one week.

C. Acute tubular necrosis is a common renal side effect of treatment.

D. If antivirals are begun within 4 days of onset of the illness in an awake patient, survival is greater than 90%.

E. Quantitative polymerase chain reaction (PCR) testing should guide antiviral treatment duration.

2. A 26-year-old man is admitted to the hospital with rapidly ascending weakness after a gastrointestinal illness. He is started on plasma exchange. On hospital day 7, he develops worsening bifacial weakness and shortness of breath with difficulty clearing secretions. Which of the following medications is contraindicated at induction for endotracheal intubation?

A. Rocuronium

B. Fentanyl

C. Atropine

D. Etomidate

E. Succinylcholine

3. A 67-year-old right-handed woman presents to the ED with 3 days of productive cough, shortness of breath, and fever. She is on amlodipine for hypertension, aspirin, and metoprolol for coronary artery disease, methotrexate and prednisone for rheumatoid arthritis, and paroxetine for depression. A chest x-ray shows consolidation of the left lower lung. She is started empirically on levofloxacin but continues to decline. She becomes hypotensive on day 3 and was started on norepinephrine as well as linezolid and cefepime given a significant history of previous vancomycin-resistant enterococcal infections. On day 4, she becomes agitated and tachycardic, with a new temperature of 39.4°C. On neurologic examination, she has new myoclonus in all limbs with stimulation. Which of the following medications may have contributed to her new symptoms?

A. Levofloxacin

B. Prednisone

C. Cefepime

D. Linezolid

E. Norepinephrine

4. A 45-year-old man with history of hepatitis C presents to the ED with headache and altered mental status. A head computed tomography (CT) scan is obtained and shown below. In the preceding weeks, he had developed fever and shortness of breath. A bronchoscopy reveals septated, acute angle branching hyphae. What would be the best treatment agent?

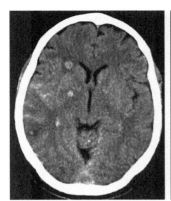 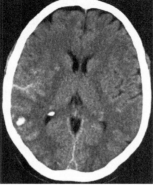

Sequential axial non-contrast head CT at the level of the upper midbrain and thalami.

A. Voriconazole

B. Amphotericin B

C. Caspofungin

D. Fluconazole

E. Micafungin

5. A 47-year-old woman with history of obesity undergoes an emergent cholecystectomy due to gallbladder perforation. One week after surgery, she develops symmetrical paresthesias in the feet, which then ascend to the trunk, chest, and both arms. Her general physical examination reveals livedo reticularis and fissures in the angles of the mouth. Her abdomen is swollen and sensitive to palpation. On further examination, there is weakness in all limbs with a distal preponderance. Proprioception is impaired, and Lhermitte sign is present. Deep tendon reflexes are absent in upper extremities and decreased in lower extremities. What is the most likely cause of her symptoms?

A. Subacute combined degeneration due to B_{12} deficiency

B. Peripheral neuropathy due to nitrous oxide inhalation

C. Peripheral neuropathy due to B_{12} deficiency

D. Cervical myelopathy due to hypoxic ischemic insult

E. Subacute combined degeneration due to hypoxic ischemic insult

6. A 31-year-old woman at 30 weeks of gestation presents to the ED with a moderate headache and nuchal rigidity. A noncontrast head CT shows subarachnoid hemorrhage predominantly in the right Sylvian fissure and interhemispheric fissure. Conventional angiogram shows a 1.5-cm right middle cerebral artery (MCA) bifurcation aneurysm with a broad neck. She undergoes surgical clipping. Which of the following agents has the least potential of affecting the fetus?

A. Fentanyl

B. Thiopental

C. Etomidate

D. Succinylcholine

E. Propofol

7. A 72-year-old right-handed man with a history of hypertension is brought to the ED after being struck by a car while crossing the street. On arrival, he is normothermic, hypertensive with a blood pressure of 188/112 mm Hg, and tachycardic with a heart rate of 116 bpm. A head CT demonstrates small punctate subcortical hemorrhages in bilateral temporal and frontal lobes. The patient is admitted to the neurocritical care unit. He becomes restless and agitated overnight. Which of the following sedatives would be preferred in this patient?

A. Dexmedetomidine

B. Midazolam

C. Propofol

D. Fentanyl

E. Ketamine

8. A 58-year-old right-handed man with history of atrial fibrillation is found in his apartment with right-sided hemiparesis and aphasia. A head CT reveals a full territory left MCA infarction with significant midline shift. The patient undergoes emergent decompressive craniectomy. He remains comatose on postoperative day 8 (3 days after cession of all sedative medications). Which of the following agents is least likely to contribute to his depressed mental status?

A. Diazepam

B. Midazolam

C. Fentanyl

D. Propofol

E. Flurazepam

9. A 48-year-old right-handed man with a history of seizure disorder is admitted for refractory status epilepticus. He was loaded with intravenous (IV) levetiracetam and IV phenytoin. He continues to have subclinical seizure activity on electroencephalogram (EEG) and is started on a propofol infusion. On day of 4 of hospitalization, he develops sudden onset of severe metabolic acidosis, bradycardia, and hypotension, which requires vasopressor treatment. Which biochemical marker could have been used for early diagnosis and prevention of hemodynamic instability in this patient?

A. Potassium

B. Creatinine

C. Triglycerides

D. Bilirubin

E. Bicarbonate

10. A 28-year-old man with history of alcohol abuse is brought to the ED after a motorcycle crash. His initial vital signs are significant for blood pressure of 140/90 mm Hg, heart rate of 50 bpm, and respiratory rate of 26 breaths/min. A head CT shows a small left frontal and temporal subdural hemorrhage with scattered subarachnoid hemorrhage. He becomes agitated on hospital day 2, requiring multiple doses of haloperidol and lorazepam for management of his agitation. On hospital day 7, the patient becomes hypertensive to 184/118 mm Hg and hyperthermic to 39.4°C, with worsening mental status and hypertonicity throughout. A repeat head CT does not show any significant changes. What would be the next step in the management of his symptoms?

A. Lumbar puncture

B. Discontinuation of haloperidol

C. Discontinuation of lorazepam

D. Initiation of IV midazolam infusion

E. Initiation of bromocriptine

11. A 31-year-old obese woman with history of myasthenia gravis undergoes transsternal thymectomy. She receives her usual dose of pyridostigmine prior to surgery. After induction with IV propofol and fentanyl, neuromuscular monitoring is applied. A single bolus of rocuronium is administered to facilitate tracheal intubation. At the end of the surgical procedure, she is given neostigmine and glycopyrrolate. Which of the following statements is correct regarding management of this patient?

A. Acetylcholinesterase inhibitors cause tachycardia via modulation of muscarinic receptors.

B. Glycopyrrolate is a sympathomimetic agent that blocks muscarinic side effects of neostigmine.

C. Glycopyrrolate is an anticholinergic agent that blocks muscarinic side effects of neostigmine.

D. Neostigmine reduces the sweating capacity, which can lead to hyperthermia.

E. Atropine is associated with less tachycardia than glycopyrrolate.

12. A 69-year-old woman with a history of diabetes mellitus, end-stage renal disease, alcoholic cirrhosis, and coronary artery disease presents after cardiac arrest and return of spontaneous circulation. During induced hypothermia, which of the following neuromuscular blockade agents would be most appropriate to reduce shivering for rapid induction of targeted temperature management?

   A. Vecuronium

   B. Pancuronium

   C. Rocuronium

   D. Cisatracurium

   E. Succinylcholine

13. A 66-year-old woman of East Asian descent with a recent diagnosis of hypertension starts an herbal medication for blood pressure management. One week later, she is found unconscious in her apartment. In the ED, her blood pressure is 60/30 mm Hg, heart rate is 40 bpm, and respiration rate is 20 breaths/min. Her pupils are small, and bowel sounds are present. Which of the following would be the most effective cardiovascular stimulant in the management of her symptoms?

   A. Amphetamine

   B. Clonidine

   C. Isoproterenol

   D. Norepinephrine

   E. Tyramine

14. A 67-year-old man with history of hypertension and atrial fibrillation is found mute with right-sided weakness in his apartment. A head CT shows a left frontal intraparenchymal hemorrhage. The patient's wife states that he is taking a blood-thinning medication. Which of the following anticoagulants has a direct antidote for reversal?

   A. Dabigatran

   B. Rivaroxaban

   C. Enoxaparin

   D. Warfarin

   E. Apixaban

15. A 51-year-old woman with metastatic breast cancer is found drowsy in her home and brought to the ED. On arrival, she is comatose with a blood pressure of 104/64 mm Hg, heart rate of 61 bpm,

respiratory rate 7 breaths/min, and temperature of 36.7°C. Her pupils are miotic and sluggishly reactive to light. What would be the next step in the management of this patient?

   A. Head CT

   B. Arterial blood gas

   C. Intubation

   D. IV naloxone 0.4 mg, repeat every 2 to 3 minutes, maximum dose: 10 mg

   E. IV naloxone 0.4 mg, repeat every 2 to 3 minutes, maximum dose: 2 mg

16. A 71-year-old man with a history of hypertension has a witnessed cardiac arrest at home. The patient's wife performs cardiopulmonary resuscitation. On paramedic arrival, the patient is found to be in ventricular fibrillation. Return of spontaneous circulation is achieved after defibrillation. The patient remains comatose on arrival to the hospital and is started on therapeutic hypothermia. Which of the following statements is correct regarding therapeutic hypothermia?

   A. Patients may develop hyperkalemia and hypermagnesemia.

   B. Therapeutic hypothermia reduces urine output.

   C. Therapeutic hypothermia enhances the immune response and apoptosis.

   D. Hypothermia can lead to hypoglycemia by decreasing the secretion of glucagon and cortisol.

   E. Plasma levels of propofol and fentanyl increase during hypothermia.

17. A 45-year-old man with a history of pheochromocytoma, mitral stenosis, and chronic kidney disease is admitted to the intensive care unit for hypertensive emergency. He is started on an IV infusion of nitroprusside. On day 3 of hospitalization, the patient develops delirium, tremor, and hyperreflexia. What is the most likely explanation for his symptoms?

   A. Thiocyanate toxicity

   B. Cyanide toxicity

   C. Arterial vasodilation

   D. Reduced cerebral perfusion

   E. Hypernatremia

18. An 81-year-old woman who presents with severe headache and left visual field cut is found to have a right occipital intraparenchymal hemorrhage with surrounding edema and midline shift. Her blood pressure is elevated at 210/102 mm Hg. Which of the following medications should be used with caution in this patient?

A. Nicardipine
B. Labetalol
C. Hydralazine
D. Enalapril
E. Esmolol

19. A 6-year-old boy with a history of type 3 von Willebrand disease is brought to the ED with nausea, vomiting, and somnolence. A head CT demonstrates a cerebellar hemorrhage. What would be the first step in the management of the patient after life support measures?

A. Emergent posterior craniotomy
B. Fresh frozen plasma administration
C. Desmopressin administration
D. Extraventricular drainage
E. Close monitoring for neurologic deterioration

20. A 67-year-old woman with a history of hypertension, atrial fibrillation on warfarin, diabetes mellitus, and heart failure with reduced ejection fraction presents with acute-onset right-sided weakness and is found to have an ischemic stroke in the left internal capsule. Hospital course is subsequently complicated by monomorphic ventricular tachycardia, which is treated with amiodarone. Which of the following statements is correct regarding this patient?

A. The dose of warfarin should be reduced by one-third to one-half after initiation of amiodarone.
B. The dose of amiodarone should be reduced by one-third to one-half in patients on warfarin.
C. The dose of warfarin should be increased by one-third to one-half after initiation of amiodarone.
D. The dose of amiodarone should be increased by one-third to one-half in patients on warfarin.

E. In patients on amiodarone, international normalized ratio (INR) cannot be used to monitor warfarin efficacy.

21. A 37-year-old woman with aneurysmal subarachnoid hemorrhage status post surgical clipping develops confusion on postoperative day 3. She is noted to have poor skin turgor on exam. Her laboratory workup is remarkable for a serum sodium of 121 mEq/L. After 24-hour treatment with IV normal saline and 3% hypertonic saline, she remains lethargic, with a repeat sodium of 122 mEq/L. What should be the next step in the management of her symptoms?

A. Demeclocycline
B. Fludrocortisone
C. Desmopressin
D. Fluid restriction
E. Midodrine

22. A 67-year-old woman with a history of hypertension, Hashimoto thyroiditis, diabetes mellitus complicated by neuropathy, and end-stage renal disease status post kidney transplant presents with a severe headache and subsequent generalized tonic-clonic seizure. Her MRI is shown below. Which of the following medications is most likely associated with her presentation?

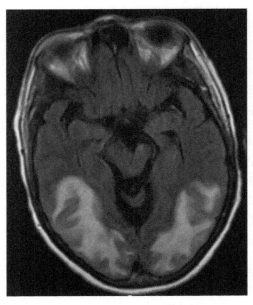

Axial FLAIR sequence of the brain at the level of the midbrain.

A. Prednisone

B. Cyclosporine

C. Levothyroxine

D. Pioglitazone

E. Pregabalin

23. A 53-year-old woman with history of bipolar mood disorder on lithium is admitted to the hospital with diarrhea. On the second day of hospitalization, she develops palpitations. During the episode, her blood pressure is 102/64 mm Hg. Her urine toxicology test is unrevealing, and basic metabolic profile, calcium, magnesium, liver, and thyroid function tests are within normal limits. The electrocardiogram (ECG) strip is shown below. What should be the next step in the management of this patient?

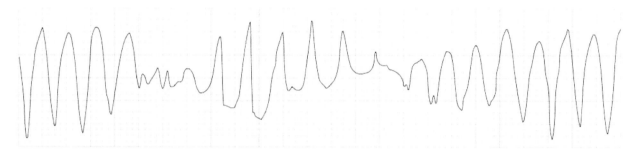

Telemetry strip tracing.

A. Infusion of calcium gluconate

B. Infusion of magnesium sulfate

C. Cardioversion

D. Infusion of lidocaine

E. Infusion of amiodarone

24. A 31-year-old woman with history of asthma and pituitary adenoma undergoes endoscopic transsphenoidal resection of the tumor. Thirty minutes into the procedure, she develops hypotension and hypoxia secondary to bronchoconstriction. Which of the following medications can cause her symptoms?

A. Fentanyl

B. Buprenorphine

C. Morphine

D. Remifentanil

E. Succinylcholine

25. A morbidly obese 44-year-old man is admitted to the intensive care unit due to trauma and grade 3 burns in his bilateral lower extremities. His hospital course is further complicated by acute kidney injury secondary to myoglobinuria and rhabdomyolysis. He is started on enoxaparin 1 mg/kg twice daily for deep venous thrombosis (DVT) prophylaxis. Which of the following statements is correct about this patient?

A. The patient is on appropriate dose of enoxaparin for DVT prophylaxis.

B. The dose of enoxaparin should be decreased in this patient.

C. Enoxaparin cannot be used for DVT prophylaxis in this patient.

D. Anti–factor Xa assays should be used to monitor enoxaparin efficacy.

E. Laboratory monitoring of anticoagulation is not required in this patient.

26. A 37-year-old man with history of seizure disorder is admitted to the neurocritical care unit with status epilepticus and is loaded with IV fosphenytoin and started on oral phenytoin. Twenty-four hours later, EEG monitoring reveals ongoing epileptiform discharges, and IV valproic acid is administered. Which of the following statements is correct?

A. Total phenytoin serum concentration increases following administration of valproic acid.

B. Free phenytoin serum concentration decreases following administration of valproic acid.

C. Volume of distribution of total phenytoin is decreased by valproic acid.

D. The change in phenytoin level after initiation of valproic acid is significant and sustained.

E. Valproic acid induces hepatic metabolism of phenytoin.

27. A 51-year-old man presents to the ED with severe headache, nausea, and vomiting. His initial blood pressure is 174/106 mm Hg. A head CT demonstrates a perimesencephalic subarachnoid hemorrhage. He is given an antihypertensive agent. Subsequently, the patient develops nausea, and his oxygen saturation drops to 88%. Which of the following medications can contribute to his hypoxia?

A. Labetalol

B. Nicardipine

C. Enalapril

D. Nimodipine

E. Metoprolol

28. 77-year-old man with a remote history of ischemic stroke is admitted from a nursing facility with lethargy, disorientation, and confusion. Nursing records indicate that the patient did not have any fever, diarrhea, or fluid loss. Urine output is recorded as 700 mL/d. Physical examination is normal except for orthostatic hypotension and dry mucous membranes. He weighs 70 kg. Laboratory results are as follows:

Serum: Na^+ = 168 mEq/L, K^+ = 4.6 mEq/L, Cl^- = 114 mEq/L, HCO_3^- = 26 mEq/L, creatinine = 1.9 mg/dL, blood urea nitrogen (BUN) = 64 mg/dL, glucose = 110 mg/dL
Urine: Na^+ = 12 mEq/L, osmolality = 600 mOsm/kg H_2O

Calculate his free water deficit assuming a normal serum Na^+ concentration of 140 mEq/L.

A. 3.75 L

B. 4.5 L

C. 5.25 L

D. 7 L

E. 8.4 L

29. A 26-year-old man presents to the ED after an assault. He is unconsciousness with multiple fractures. Head CT reveals a right frontal epidural hematoma with overlying depressed skull fracture. He undergoes emergent evacuation and is admitted to the intensive care unit. On the fourth day of hospitalization, the patient develops acute hypoxic respiratory failure. A chest x-ray shows diffuse infiltrates, and arterial blood gas (ABG) shows Pao_2/Fio_2 ratio of 150. Despite management strategies, which include antimicrobial treatment and prone mechanical ventilation, an ABG on the sixth day of hospitalization shows Pao_2/Fio_2 ratio of 90. Which of the following treatments can improve oxygenation in this patient?

A. IV furosemide

B. Permissive hypercapnia

C. IV methylprednisolone

D. Inhaled epoprostenol

E. Inhaled surfactant

Answers and Explanations

1. **D.** Herpes simplex virus (HSV) is the most common cause of sporadic acute encephalitis and, if left untreated, confers >70% mortality. However, early treatment can improve mortality and morbidity associated with the infection. Appropriate treatment with intravenous acyclovir at a dose of 10 mg/kg of ideal body weight (in cases of significant obesity, adjusted body weight can be used to calculate dose) should be administered every 8 hours for 3 weeks. Hydration should be administered concomitantly with acyclovir treatment in order to prevent crystal nephropathy, the most common cause of renal toxicity, although acute tubular necrosis or acute interstitial nephritis can occur as well. Although HSV PCR is an important diagnostic test and may remain persistently positive for up to 2 weeks after initiation of treatment, the potential correlation of viral load with prognosis or other clinical features of disease remains uncertain. Although there are animal data and limited case report data regarding use of adjunctive corticosteroids, as yet, there are no significant large human data supporting the use of dexamethasone in this setting. The German Trial of Acyclovir and Corticosteroids in HSV Encephalitis (GACHE) is an ongoing large randomized controlled trial testing the hypothesis that adjuvant dexamethasone 40 mg daily for 4 days confers a survival and functional outcome improvement.

2. **E.** Patients with neuromuscular disease may require high doses of neuromuscular blockade agents due to upregulation of acetylcholine receptors. Patients with neuromuscular disease can develop life-threatening hyperkalemia and rhabdomyolysis from depolarizing agents such as succinylcholine due to upregulation of acetylcholine receptors. Dangerous cardiac arrhythmias such as ventricular fibrillation and ventricular tachycardia may result; defibrillation in these cases may be ineffective in the presence of high potassium levels. High levels of calcium and repeated doses of calcium may be required to overcome the effect of hyperkalemia while monitoring the response to electrocardiography. Such depolarizing neuromuscular blockade agents are to be strictly avoided in Guillain-Barré syndrome. In patients who have undergone plasma exchange (PLEX), the half-life of these medications is extended due to removal of metabolizing enzymes.

3. **D.** Linezolid is a weak monoamine oxidase inhibitor (MAOI). Patients who receive concomitant treatment with an adrenergic or serotonergic agent such as the selective serotonin reuptake inhibitors (SSRIs) may develop serotonin syndrome, which is characterized by autonomic instability, increased muscle tone, altered mental status, and hyperthermia. Treatment is focused on removal of the offending medication and supportive care to treat autonomic instability and hyperthermia. Hyperthermia results from muscle contraction, not from change in hypothalamic set point, so antipyretics typically do not have efficacy in fever reduction in this condition; in severe cases of hyperthermia, use of nondepolarizing neuromuscular blockade agents with other external cooling methods may be required. Other therapies may include cyproheptadine, a 5-HT$_{1A}$ antagonist that binds 85% to 95% of serotonin receptors. Patients who are genetically deficient in the cytochrome P450 2D6 enzyme (8% of whites) are more susceptible if they are taking drugs such as paroxetine, venlafaxine, tricyclic antidepressants, dextromethorphan, and methadone. Medications that inhibit cytochrome P450 2D6 and 3A4 may also increase risk of increased serotonergic signaling.

   Similar to serotonin syndrome, neuroleptic malignant syndrome (NMS) is also characterized by hyperthermia, increased muscle tone, autonomic instability, and altered mental status. Typically the onset is slower, within 7 days of introduction of a neuroleptic as opposed to within 24 hours after introduction of serotonin-enhancing agents. The pathogenesis of NMS relates to reduced dopaminergic activity in the central nervous system. Use of neuroleptic agents or abrupt withdrawal of dopamine agonists has been associated with this syndrome.

4. **A.** Fungal infections account for an increasing proportion of central nervous system (CNS) infections, mainly secondary to the widespread use of immunosuppressive therapy and aging population. Common clinical presentations are chronic granulomatous meningitis, brain abscess, or fungal arteritis. Cryptococcosis, blastomycosis, coccidioidomycosis, and histoplasmosis most often present as chronic meningitis.

   The CT scan shows multiple hemorrhagic lesions, both cortical and subcortical, as well as subarachnoid hemorrhage. CNS aspergillosis usually occurs as part of disseminated infection that often originates from the lung. CNS aspergillosis can lead to vascular involvement, leading to thrombosis from fungal hyphae blocking intracerebral blood vessels and causing infarction and hemorrhage. Vascular involvement from aspergillosis can also lead to mycotic aneurysm formation from destruction of internal elastic lamina and inflammation and infiltration of media and adventitia. Other CNS manifestations include meningitis and granuloma formation.

   Voriconazole is the drug of choice for the treatment of invasive aspergillosis. There are reports that voriconazole is up to 20% more effective than amphotericin B. In cases of severe disseminated or CNS disease, amphotericin B is often used in combination. In case series of CNS involvement, mortality is close to 100% despite treatment with amphotericin B; however, up to a 35% response rate has been observed with voriconazole. Voriconazole is available in both intravenous and oral preparations with excellent bioavailability. If the creatinine clearance is less than 50 mL/min, the oral form should be used (due to accumulation of intravenous [IV] vehicle). The most common side effects include reversible visual disturbances and rash.

5. **A.** Nitrous oxide (N_2O) is an inhaled anesthetic agent that irreversibly oxidizes the cobalt ion in vitamin B_{12}. It prevents methylcobalamin from acting as a coenzyme in the production of methionine and subsequently S-adenosyl-methionine, which is necessary for methylation of myelin sheath phospholipids. The end result of nitrous oxide toxicity is subacute combined degeneration of the spinal cord, as described in classic vitamin B_{12} deficiency. The posterior columns are involved, with loss of position and vibration senses, ataxia, broad-based gait, and, occasionally, Lhermitte sign.

6. **D.** Both depolarizing and nondepolarizing muscle relaxants are highly ionized at physiologic pH with very limited placental transfer. Anesthesia induction drugs such as etomidate, thiopental, and propofol are highly lipophilic and not ionized at physiologic pH; thus, placental transfer is quite rapid. The opioids freely traverse the placenta because of their high lipid solubility and low molecular weight.

7. **A.** Dexmedetomidine is an IV selective α_2-agonist that revolutionized the field of critical care and anesthesia due to its specific pharmacokinetic and pharmacodynamic characteristics. Patients on dexmedetomidine can have regular sleep-wakefulness cycles, which in return improves delirium and agitation. In the Maximizing Efficacy of Targeted Sedation and Reducing Neurological Dysfunction trial, it is reported that the use of dexmedetomidine IV infusion for 24 to 120 hours results in an increased number of delirium-free and coma-free days compared to lorazepam. In comparison to propofol, dexmedetomidine has been found to be equally effective for sedation in the intensive care unit with the additional advantage of minimal respiratory depression, suppression of consciousness, and hemodynamic effects.

8. **D.** Propofol is an IV general anesthetic agent that exerts sedative and hypnotic properties at low doses and has amnestic properties similar to benzodiazepines. Its rapid onset and offset of action makes it the sedative agent of choice in patients in whom rapid awakening is important. Many benzodiazepines are converted initially to active metabolites with long half-lives. After several days of therapy with agents such as diazepam and flurazepam, accumulation of active metabolites can lead to excessive sedation. Fentanyl is a highly lipophilic opioid with rapid onset of action.

However, this high lipophilicity can lead to a prolonged duration of effect, especially after repeated dosing or infusion.

9. C. Propofol infusion syndrome (PRIS) is a rare condition associated with long-term (usually >48 hours) infusion of propofol. The clinical features are acute refractory bradycardia with at least 1 of the following findings: metabolic acidosis (base deficit >10 mmol/L), hyperlipidemia, rhabdomyolysis, and enlarged or fatty liver. The syndrome can be caused by either a direct mitochondrial respiratory chain inhibition or impaired mitochondrial fatty acid metabolism mediated by propofol. Young age, exogenous catecholamine or glucocorticoid administration, severe critical illness of central nervous system or respiratory system, inadequate carbohydrate intake, and subclinical mitochondrial disease are predisposing factors for PRIS. Rise in serum levels of creatine kinase and triglycerides attributed to propofol alone occurs in patients at risk of developing PRIS. Treatment options are limited. Hemodialysis or hemoperfusion with cardiorespiratory support has been the most successful treatment.

10. B. Neuroleptic malignant syndrome (NMS) is a life-threatening neurologic complication associated with neuroleptic or antipsychotic drug use. It is often associated with phenothiazine and haloperidol use. However, cases have been reported in the setting of dopaminergic agent withdrawal or use of newer antipsychotic drugs. It can occur days or months after initiation of the offending agent. The symptoms include hyperthermia, autonomic dysfunction, rigidity, stupor, diaphoresis, and other signs of sympathetic overactivity. Serum creatine phosphokinase is elevated, and patients may develop acute kidney injury due to myoglobinuria. The mainstay of treatment is discontinuation of antipsychotic medication and supportive care with IV hydration and diuresis. Oral bromocriptine and IV dantrolene have also proven beneficial, especially if used early in the course of the condition.

11. C. Cholinesterase inhibitors, such as neostigmine and physostigmine, reverse nondepolarizing muscle blockade. These agents are also used to diagnose and treat myasthenia gravis. The effects of neostigmine are usually apparent in 5 minutes, peak at 10 minutes, and last more than 1 hour. Muscarinic side effects, such as bradycardia and bronchospasm, are minimized by prior or concomitant administration of an anticholinergic agent. The onset of action of glycopyrrolate is similar to neostigmine and is associated with less tachycardia compared to atropine.

12. D. Atracurium and cisatracurium convert to less active metabolites by plasma esterases and spontaneous Hofmann elimination. Because of these alternative routes of metabolism, both agents do not exhibit an increased half-life in patients with impaired renal function and, therefore, are good choices in this setting. Of note, the elimination half-life of atracurium and cisatracurium's neurotoxic metabolite laudanosine increases in renal failure but is of unknown clinical significance. Succinylcholine has a brief duration of action due to its rapid hydrolysis by butyrylcholinesterase synthesized by the liver and found in the plasma, but duration of action is relatively short, and repeated dosing is not recommended due to potential for bradyarrhythmias and asystole. Chronic renal failure by itself is not a contraindication to the use of succinylcholine for neuromuscular blockade in the setting of endotracheal intubation provided that the serum potassium is not acutely elevated. In renal failure, the elimination half-life of pancuronium increases by 97%. Rocuronium and vecuronium are both steroid-based neuromuscular blockade agents and undergo both hepatic and renal elimination.

13. D. The patient shows signs of sympathetic autonomic failure: hypotension, bradycardia, and miosis. These signs are compatible with an overdose of a drug that causes marked depletion of stored catecholamine transmitter such as reserpine. Herbal medications often contain potent synthetic drugs in addition to (or instead of) the advertised constituents.

Amphetamine and tyramine are adrenergic agents that act via release of catecholamines from the nerve terminal and would, therefore, be ineffective in this patient. Clonidine works primarily on presynaptic nerve endings, although it can activate α_2-receptors located elsewhere. Isoproterenol would stimulate the heart but has no α-agonist action and might exacerbate the hypotension. Norepinephrine has the necessary combination of direct action and α_1, α_2, and β_1 effects.

14. **A.** With the emergence of non–vitamin K antagonist oral anticoagulants for stroke prevention in patients with nonvalvular atrial fibrillation, the quest for reversal agents also has begun for the inevitable hemorrhagic complications that arise with therapy. Idarucizumab, a monoclonal antibody, is the first medication that is developed to reverse the anticoagulant effects of dabigatran. Vitamin K is necessary for synthesis of certain coagulation factors in liver (factors II, VII, IX, and X), and therapeutic doses of warfarin reduce the total amount of these factors, resulting in diminished biological activity. Thus, vitamin K is considered an indirect antidote of warfarin. Prothrombin complex concentrates (PCCs) are the 3 or 4 vitamin K–dependent factors as well as protein C and protein S and are not a direct antidote to warfarin or non–vitamin K antagonist oral anticoagulants. Protamine is a positively charged polypeptide that binds to heparin forming a salt; protamine is considered 60% effective at neutralizing the anti-Xa effect of enoxaparin.

15. **D.** Opioids are widely used for the management of pain in patients with metastatic cancer. Coma, miosis, and respiratory depression are the classic triad of opioid overdose. Overdose is diagnosed with injection of naloxone, an opioid antagonist, which will lead to prompt recovery of the symptoms. In adults, an initial naloxone dose of 0.4 to 2 mg is recommended. This dose may be repeated every 2 to 3 minutes until the full reversal is achieved or to a maximum of 10 mg.

16. **E.** Therapeutic hypothermia induces diuresis in which patients may develop significant hypokalemia, hypomagnesemia, and/or hypophosphatemia. Close monitoring of serum electrolytes is necessary, and aggressive supplementation might be required. Hypothermia decreases insulin sensitivity and insulin secretion, which can lead to hyperglycemia. Most of the enzymes in the body are highly temperature sensitive; thus, drug metabolism is reduced by hypothermia. This will lead to decreased clearance of various drugs from serum. Plasma levels of propofol increase by approximately 30% and fentanyl by 15% when individuals are hypothermic by 3°C.

17. **A.** Sodium nitroprusside is a short-acting vasodilator that is used to treat severe hypertension and heart failure with reduced ejection fraction. It acts by relaxing vascular (both arterial and venous) smooth muscle as a nitric oxide donor. Nitroprusside is rapidly hydrolyzed and releases free cyanide, which normally is converted quickly to thiocyanate by the liver and blood vessels. Acute cyanide poisoning may occur with short-term high-dose nitroprusside infusions (>10-15 μg/kg/min for ≥1 hour). Thiocyanate toxicity may result from prolonged infusions (>3 μg/kg/min for ≥48 hours), especially in patients with renal insufficiency. This leads to confusion, delirium, tremor, hyperreflexia, and in rare cases, seizures and coma.

18. **C.** After intracerebral hemorrhage (ICH), blood pressure often increases during the first 24 hours and then declines spontaneously. Elevated systolic blood pressure is associated with higher mortality in patients with ICH; thus, blood pressure monitoring and treatment are critical in ICH management, although the optimum target is still under investigation.

Hydralazine is a potent cerebral vasodilator and inhibitor of cerebral blood flow autoregulation, both of which can increase cerebral blood flow and intracranial pressure (ICP). This patient already shows signs and symptoms of increased ICP with headache and midline shift; therefore, the use of hydralazine may be detrimental in this situation.

19. **C.** ICH in children with von Willebrand disease (vWD) is rare, yet does occur, especially in patients with type 3 vWD. Early and effective treatment is important for an optimal outcome, which requires prompt correction of the hemostatic defect.

The vasopressin V2 receptor agonist, 1-deamino-8-d-arginine vasopressin or desmopressin (DDAVP), increases the plasma concentration of von Willebrand factor (vWF) and factor VIII. Factors VIII:C and vWF levels increase to 2 to 5 times baseline with a peak at 60 minutes after the completion of intravenous infusion of DDAVP (90-120 minutes after subcutaneous and intranasal application).

20. **A.** Amiodarone is a potent antiarrhythmic agent and is widely used for both ventricular and supraventricular tachyarrhythmias. It has many important drug interactions, and all medications should be reviewed when the drug is initiated and

when the dose is adjusted. Amiodarone is a substrate for liver cytochrome CYP3A4 and inhibits CYP3A4. Other inhibitors include azithromycin, cimetidine, cyclosporine, metronidazole, fluoxetine, fluconazole, and valproic acid which all can lead to increased levels of amiodarone if given concurrently. Drugs that induce CYP3A4 (including phenytoin, nafcillin, carbamazepine, phenobarbital, and rifampin) decrease amiodarone concentration when coadministered. Amiodarone inhibits several cytochrome P450 enzymes including CYP3A4 and may result in high levels of many drugs including statins, digoxin, and warfarin. The dose of warfarin should be reduced by one-third to one-half following initiation of amiodarone, and the INR should be closely monitored.

21. **B.** Cerebral salt wasting (CSW) syndrome is commonly seen following subarachnoid hemorrhage. Patients develop natriuresis and present with symptoms of hyponatremia, usually with confusion and lethargy. Signs of dehydration, such as poor skin turgor, are common in these patients and can be helpful in differentiating it from the syndrome of inappropriate antidiuretic hormone (SIADH). Patients with CSW are hypovolemic, whereas SIADH patients have normal to elevated plasma volume. Misdiagnosis of CSW as SIADH may be disastrous, as fluid restriction in SIADH will result in rapid worsening of hyponatremia. The treatment for CSW is repletion of salt and fluid, usually by IV administration of normal saline. IV or oral fludrocortisone can be used to help promote retention of sodium in patients who do not seem to respond solely to normal saline treatment. Fludrocortisone has high mineralocorticoid effects on the distal renal tubules, which increases sodium reabsorption, potassium excretion, hydrogen ion secretion, and water retention.

22. **B.** Reversible posterior leukoencephalopathy syndrome (RPLE), also known as posterior reversible encephalopathy syndrome (PRES), is a hypertensive encephalopathy that occurs secondary to the inability of posterior circulation to autoregulate in response to acute changes in blood pressure. Hyperperfusion with resultant disruption of the blood-brain barrier results in vasogenic edema most commonly in the parieto-occipital regions. In severe cases, hemorrhage and infarction can

develop. Patients usually present with a headache, seizures, altered mental status, and visual disturbance. Multiple immunosuppressive drugs have been associated with this condition. Among them, calcineurin inhibitors (cyclosporin, tacrolimus, and sirolimus) and interferons are noteworthy. It has been proposed that cyclosporin causes PRES via changes in the blood-brain barrier permeability, increased fluid overload, and hypertension.

23. **B.** Torsade de pointes (TdP) is a form of ventricular tachycardia that can lead to sudden cardiac death. Prolongation of QT interval increases the risk of TdP development. An increasing list of medications is associated with QT prolongation, among them phenothiazines, fluoroquinolones, lithium, ephedrine, and methylphenidate.

Many episodes of TdP are self-limiting and short in duration. IV magnesium sulfate is effective to prevent recurrent episodes, even in patients with a normal serum magnesium level. Immediate cardioversion is indicated in patients who develop hemodynamic instability.

24. **C.** Morphine causes mast cell activation and histamine release, which can lead to bronchoconstriction and vasodilation. It has the potential to precipitate or exacerbate asthmatic attacks and should be avoided in patients with a history of asthma. Other opioid agonists associated with a lower incidence of histamine release, such as the fentanyl derivatives, may be better choices for these patients.

25. **D.** Several studies have shown that low-molecular-weight heparins (LMWH), such as enoxaparin, dalteparin, and tinzaparin, are as efficacious as heparin in several thromboembolic conditions. Weight-based dosing of LMWH leads to predictable pharmacokinetics and plasma levels in patients with normal renal function. However, LMWH levels are typically measured in the setting of renal insufficiency, obesity, and pregnancy. LMWH levels can be determined by anti-Xa units. For enoxaparin, peak therapeutic levels should be 0.5 to 1 unit/mL for twice-daily dosing (determined 4 hours after administration) and 1.5 units/mL for once-daily dosing.

26. **D.** The pharmacokinetic properties of phenytoin are affected by its binding to serum proteins, by

its dose-dependent elimination, and by its metabolism by the hepatic cytochrome P450 enzymes. Phenytoin is highly bound to plasma proteins (90%), mainly albumin. Small variations in the percentage of phenytoin that is protein bound significantly change the amount of free (active) drug. Some medications can compete with phenytoin for binding sites on plasma proteins and increase free phenytoin. However, the effect on free phenytoin is only short-lived and usually does not cause clinical complications unless inhibition of phenytoin metabolism also occurs. In this example, valproic acid competes for protein binding sites and also inhibits phenytoin hepatic metabolism, resulting in marked and sustained increases in free phenytoin. The displacement of phenytoin from serum proteins by valproic acid exceeds metabolism inhibition capacity. Thus, total phenytoin clearance increases after valproic acid ingestion, whereas, total phenytoin level decreases.

27. **B.** Nicardipine is a dihydropyridine calcium channel blocker that leads to relaxation of smooth muscle, with no effect on the myocardium. Common side effects associated with nicardipine include hypotension/orthostatic hypotension, edema, flushing, tachycardia, palpitations, and nausea. Nicardipine increases pulmonary vascular dilation and pulmonary blood flow, which can lead to hypoxia due to increased intrapulmonary shunting.

28. **E.** The patient's hypernatremia is due to water deficit rather than Na^+ gain, as the patient has orthostatic changes. In general, men and women should have a total body water percentage of 60% and 50%, respectively.

$$\text{Free water deficit} = \% \text{ Body water} \times \text{Mass (kg)} \times$$
$$(\text{Current Na} - \text{Ideal Na})/(\text{Ideal Na})$$
$$\text{Free water deficit} = 0.6 \times 70 \times (168 - 140)/(140)$$
$$= 8.4 \text{ L}$$

29. **D.** Acute respiratory distress syndrome (ARDS) is acute hypoxic respiratory failure not secondary to heart failure and volume overload with radiographic evidence of bilateral lung opacities. In the presence of positive end-expiratory pressure >5 cm H_2O, a Pao_2/Fio_2 <300 is applied to diagnose and grade ARDS.

Epoprostenol is a prostacyclin that binds to endothelial prostacyclin receptors and raises cyclic adenosine monophosphate, which activates protein kinase A. Protein kinas A promotes phosphorylation and inhibition of the myosin light chain kinase, leading to smooth muscle relaxation and vasodilation. Epoprostenol is approved for idiopathic pulmonary hypertension, where it has been shown to improve survival and reduce morbidity. In ARDS, inhaled epoprostenol similarly improves oxygenation and decreases pulmonary artery pressure. However, due to the limited number of randomized controlled trials, current use of epoprostenol is reserved for those refractory to traditional therapies.

Multiple studies confirm the efficacy of surfactant therapy in preventing and treating neonatal respiratory distress syndrome (NRDS) in preterm infants. It has been established that the use of surfactant for treatment of NRDS is associated with a decreased risk of pneumothorax, pulmonary interstitial emphysema, bronchopulmonary dysplasia, and mortality. However, in adults, randomized controlled trials have shown limited success in ARDS.

REFERENCES

Abella BS, Leary M. Therapeutic hypothermia. In: Hall JB, Schmidt GA, Kress JP, eds. *Principles of Critical Care.* 4th ed. New York, NY: McGraw-Hill; 2015.

Armao D, Bouldin T. Pathology of the nervous system. In: Reisner HM, ed. *Pathology: A Modern Case Study.* New York, NY: McGraw-Hill; 2015.

Bajwa SJ, Kulshrestha A. Dexmedetomidine: an adjuvant making large inroads into clinical practice. *Ann Med Health Sci Res.* 2013;3:475-483.

Benowitz NL. Nitroprusside. In: Olson KR, ed. *Poisoning & Drug Overdose.* 6th ed. New York, NY: McGraw-Hill; 2012.

Bhardwaj A, Mirski MA, eds. *Handbook of Neurocritical Care.* New York, NY: Springer Science & Business Media; 2010.

Birmes P, Coppin D, Schmitt L, et al. Serotonin syndrome: a brief review. *CMAJ.* 2003;168:1439-1442.

Blunk JA, Schmelz M, Zeck S, et al. Opioid-induced mast cell activation and vascular responses is not mediated by μ-opioid receptors: an in vivo microdialysis study in human skin. *Anesthes Analg.* 2004;98:364-370.

Butterworth JF IV, Mackey DC, Wasnick JD. Cholinesterase inhibitors & other pharmacologic antagonists to neuromuscular blocking agents. In: Butterworth JF IV, Mackey DC, Wasnick JD, eds. *Morgan & Mikhail's Clinical Anesthesiology.* 5th ed. New York, NY: McGraw-Hill; 2013.

Butterworth JF IV, Mackey DC, Wasnick JD. Hypotensive agents. In: Butterworth JF IV, Mackey DC, Wasnick JD, eds. *Morgan & Mikhail's Clinical Anesthesiology.* 5th ed. New York, NY: McGraw-Hill; 2013.

Devlin JW, Roberts RJ. Pharmacology of commonly used analgesics and sedatives in the ICU: benzodiazepines, propofol, and opioids. *Crit Care Clin.* 2009;25:431-449.

Eerenberg ES, Kamphuisen PW, Sijpkens MK, et al. Reversal of rivaroxaban and dabigatran by prothrombin complex concentrate clinical perspective. *Circulation.* 2011;124:1573-1579.

Flippo TS, Holder WD. Neurologic degeneration associated with nitrous oxide anesthesia in patients with vitamin B12 deficiency. *Arch Surg.* 1993;128:1391-1395.

Fuller BM, Mohr NM, Skrupky L, et al. The use of inhaled prostaglandins in patients with ARDS: a systematic review and meta-analysis. *Chest J.* 2015;147:1510-1522.

Hibbs RE, Zambon AC. Agents acting at the neuromuscular junction and autonomic ganglia. In: Brunton LL, Chabner BA, Knollmann BC, eds. *Goodman & Gilman's: The Pharmacological Basis of Therapeutics.* 12th ed. New York, NY: McGraw-Hill; 2011.

Hjalmarsson A, Blomqvist P, Sköldenberg B. Herpes simplex encephalitis in Sweden, 1990-2001; incidence, morbidity, and mortality. *Clin Infect Dis.* 2007;45:875-880.

Hoffbrand A. Megaloblastic anemias. In: Kasper D, Fauci A, Hauser S, Longo D, Jameson J, Loscalzo J, eds. *Harrison's Principles of Internal Medicine.* 19th ed. New York, NY: McGraw-Hill; 2015.

Hunter JD, Sharma P, Rathi S. Long QT syndrome. *Contin Edu Anaesth Crit Care Pain.* 2008;8:67-70.

Hasan D, Lindsay KW, Wijdicks EF, et al. Effect of fludrocortisone acetate in patients with subarachnoid hemorrhage. *Stroke.* 1989;20:1156-1161.

Hinchey J, Chaves C, Appignani B, et al. A reversible posterior leukoencephalopathy syndrome. *N Engl J Med.* 1996;334:494-500.

Hume JR, Grant AO. Agents used in cardiac arrhythmias. In: Katzung BG, Trevor AJ, eds. *Basic & Clinical Pharmacology.* 13th ed. New York, NY: McGraw-Hill; 2015.

Hypothermia after Cardiac Arrest Study Group. Mild therapeutic hypothermia to improve the neurologic outcome after cardiac arrest. *N Engl J Med.* 2002;346:549-556.

Kam PC, Cardone D. Propofol infusion syndrome. *Anaesthesia.* 2007;62:690-701.

Labarque V, Stain AM, Blanchette V, et al. Intracranial haemorrhage in von Willebrand disease: a report on six cases. *Haemophilia.* 2013;19:602-606.

MacDougall C, Chambers HF. Protein synthesis inhibitors and miscellaneous antibacterial agents. In: Brunton LL, Chabner BA, Knollmann BC, eds. *Goodman & Gilman's: The Pharmacological Basis of Therapeutics.* 12th ed. New York, NY: McGraw-Hill; 2011.

Martinez-Torres F, Menon S, Pristch M, et al. GACHE Investigators: protocol for German trial of acyclovir and corticosteroids in herpes-simplex-virus-encephalitis (GACHE): a multicenter, multinational, randomized, double-blind, placebo-controlled German, Austrian and Dutch trial. *BMC Neurol.* 2008;8:40.

Martyn JA, Richtsfeld M. Succinylcholine-induced hyperkalemia in acquired pathologic states: etiologic factors and molecular mechanisms. *Anesthesiology.* 2006;104:158-169.

McNamara JO. Pharmacotherapy of the epilepsies. In: Brunton LL, Chabner BA, Knollmann BC, eds. *Goodman & Gilman's: The Pharmacological Basis of Therapeutics.* 12th ed. New York, NY: McGraw-Hill; 2011.

Mikkelsen ME, Lanken PN, Christie JD. Acute lung injury and the acute respiratory distress syndrome. In: Hall JB, Schmidt GA, Kress JP, eds. *Principles of Critical Care.* 4th ed. New York, NY: McGraw-Hill; 2015.

Naguib M, Lien CA. Pharmacology of muscle relaxants and their antagonists. In: Miller RD, ed. *Miller's Anesthesia.* 6th ed. Philadelphia, PA: Churchill-Livingstone; 2005:481-572.

Pandharipande PP, Pun BT, Herr DL, et al. Effect of sedation with dexmedetomidine vs lorazepam on acute brain dysfunction in mechanically ventilated patients: the MENDS randomized controlled trial. *JAMA.* 2007;298:2644-2653.

Pasi KJ, Collins PW, Keeling DM, et al. Management of von Willebrand disease: a guideline from the UK Haemophilia Centre Doctors' Organization. *Haemophilia.* 2004;10:218-231.

Pema PJ, Horak HA, Wyatt RH. Myelopathy caused by nitrous oxide toxicity. *AJNR Am J Neuroradiol.* 1998;19:894-896.

Perucca ES, Hebdige S, Frigo GM, et al. Interaction between phenytoin and valproic acid: plasma protein binding and metabolic effects. *Clin Pharm Ther.* 1980;28:779-789.

Polderman KH. Application of therapeutic hypothermia in the intensive care unit. *Intensive Care Med.* 2004;30:757-769.

Pollack Jr CV, Reilly PA, Eikelboom J, et al. Idarucizumab for dabigatran reversal. *N Engl J Med.* 2015;373:511-520.

Porter RJ, Meldrum BS. Antiseizure drugs. In: Katzung BG, Trevor AJ, eds. *Basic & Clinical Pharmacology.* 13th ed. New York, NY: McGraw-Hill; 2015.

Raghunathan K, Connelly NR, Robbins LD, et al. Inhaled epoprostenol during one-lung ventilation. *Ann Thoracic Surg.* 2010;89:981-983.

Reddi AS. *Fluid, Electrolyte and Acid-Base Disorders: Clinical Evaluation and Management.* New York, NY: Springer Science & Business Media; 2013.

Roppolo LP, Walters K. Airway management in neurological emergencies. *Neurocrit Care.* 2004;1:405-414.

Ropper AH, Samuels MA. Disorders of the nervous system caused by drugs, toxins, and chemical agents. In: Ropper AH, Samuels MA, eds. *Adams & Victor's Principles of Neurology.* 10th ed. New York, NY: McGraw-Hill; 2014.

Ruhnke M, Kofla G, Otto K, et al. CNS aspergillosis. *CNS Drugs.* 2007;21:659-676.

Seedat A, Winnett G. Acyclovir-induced acute renal failure and the importance of an expanding waist line. *BMJ Case Rep.* 2012;2012:bcr2012006264.

Sessler DI. Complications and treatment of mild hypothermia. *Anesthesiology.* 2001;95:531-543.

Shields SH, Holland RM, Pippin R, et al. Pharmacology of antiarrhythmics and antihypertensives. In: Tintinalli JE, Stapczynski J, Ma O, et al, eds. *Tintinalli's Emergency Medicine: A Comprehensive Study Guide.* 8th ed. New York, NY: McGraw-Hill; 2016.

Stovell M, Smith S, Udberg M, et al. Pre-PRIS? Prospective monitoring for early markers of propofol infusion syndrome. *Crit Care.* 2013;17:P391.

Suarez JI, eds. *Critical Care Neurology and Neurosurgery*. New York, NY: Springer Science & Business Media; 2004.

Thomas K. Bleeding disorders. In: Hall JB, Schmidt GA, Kress JP, eds. *Principles of Critical Care*. 4th ed. New York, NY: McGraw-Hill; 2015.

Trevor AJ, Katzung BG, Kruidering-Hall M. Antifungal agents. In: Trevor AJ, Katzung BG, Kruidering-Hall M, eds. *Katzung & Trevor's Pharmacology: Examination & Board Review*. 11th ed. New York, NY: McGraw-Hill; 2015.

Trevor AJ, Katzung BG, Kruidering-Hall M. Opioid analgesics and antagonists. In: Trevor AJ, Katzung BG, Kruidering-Hall M, eds. *Katzung & Trevor's Pharmacology: Examination & Board Review*. 11th ed. New York, NY: McGraw-Hill; 2015.

Trevor AJ, Katzung BG, Kruidering-Hall M. Sedative-hypnotic drugs. In: Trevor AJ, Katzung BG, Kruidering-Hall M, eds. *Katzung & Trevor's Pharmacology: Examination & Board Review*. 11th ed. New York, NY: McGraw-Hill; 2015.

Trevor AJ, Katzung BG, Kruidering-Hall M. Sympathomimetics. In: Trevor AJ, Katzung BG, Kruidering-Hall M, eds. *Katzung & Trevor's Pharmacology: Examination & Board Review*. 11th ed. New York, NY: McGraw-Hill; 2015.

Tunkel AR, Glaser CA, Bloch KC, et al. The management of encephalitis: clinical practice guidelines by the Infectious Diseases Society of America. *Clin Infect Dis*. 2008;47:303-327.

Venn RM, Grounds RM. Comparison between dexmedetomidine and propofol for sedation in the intensive care unit: patient and clinician perceptions. *Br J Anaesth*. 2001;87:684-690.

Weitz JI. Blood coagulation and anticoagulant, fibrinolytic, and antiplatelet drugs. In: Brunton LL, Chabner BA, Knollmann BC, eds. *Goodman & Gilman's: The Pharmacological Basis of Therapeutics*. 12th ed. New York, NY: McGraw-Hill; 2011.

Wlody DJ, Weems L. Anesthesia for neurosurgery in the pregnant patient. In: Cottrell JE, Young WL, eds. *Cottrell and Young's Neuroanesthesia*. New York, NY: Elsevier Health Sciences; 2016.

Yaksh TL, Wallace MS. Opioids, analgesia, and pain management. In: Brunton LL, Chabner BA, Knollmann BC, eds. *Goodman & Gilman's: The Pharmacological Basis of Therapeutics*. 12th ed. New York, NY: McGraw-Hill; 2011.

Yandle G, deBoisblanc BP. Persistent fever. In: Hall JB, Schmidt GA, Kress JP, eds. *Principles of Critical Care*. 4th ed. New York, NY: McGraw-Hill; 2015.

Yeh EH, Bickford CL, Ewer MS. The diagnosis and management of cardiovascular disease in patients with cancer. In: Fuster V, Walsh RA, Harrington RA, eds. *Hurst's the Heart*. 13th ed. New York, NY: McGraw-Hill; 2011.

Zehnder JL. Drugs used in disorders of coagulation. In: Katzung BG, Trevor AJ, eds. *Basic & Clinical Pharmacology*. 13th ed. New York, NY: McGraw-Hill; 2015.

14

Neuromonitoring

Michael Reznik, MD, Andrew Martin, MD, Shivani Ghoshal, MD, Alexandra Reynolds, MD, and Jan Claassen, MD, PhD, FNCS

Questions

1. An 82-year-old woman with a history of hypertension and chronic kidney disease is admitted to the hospital with 3 days of increasing confusion of waxing and waning quality. Exam shows occasional asterixis and is otherwise nonfocal. Electroencephalogram (EEG) leads are placed demonstrating the below tracing. Which of the following is essential in the workup and treatment of this patient?

   A. Start an antiepileptic drug (AED), such as levetiracetam
   B. Initiate a load with a benzodiazepine
   C. Complete a thorough investigation for metabolic derangements and/or infection
   D. Obtain an immediate magnetic resonance imaging (MRI) of the brain
   E. All of the above

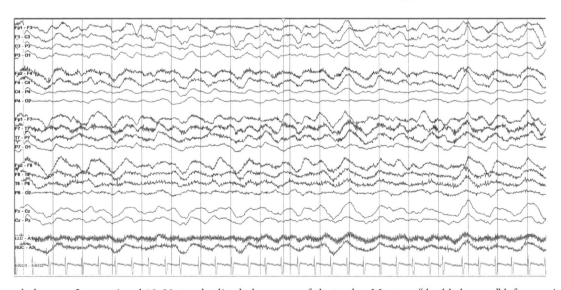

Electroencephalogram: International 10-20 standardized placement of electrodes. Montage "double banana" left over right.

2. A 53-year-old man is admitted with 2 days of fever, worsening confusion, and aphasia. On arrival to the emergency department (ED), he has an episode of speech arrest with automatisms followed by tonic stiffening and generalized convulsions for 1 minute before spontaneously resolving. He is difficult to arouse afterward. His EEG is shown below. What is the best next step in management?

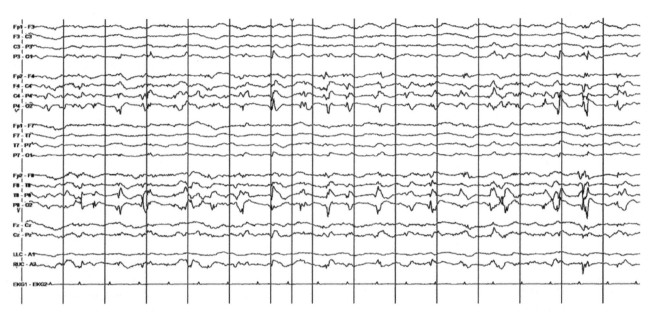

Electroencephalogram: International 10-20 standardized placement of electrodes. Montage "double banana" left over right.

A. Begin empiric antiviral therapy with intravenous acyclovir
B. Perform MRI of the brain with and without contrast
C. Start a standing AED
D. Perform lumbar puncture
E. Give aspirin as the aphasia is likely due to an ischemic stroke

3. A 67-year-old patient suffered a cardiac arrest. Cardiopulmonary resuscitation (CPR) was initiated, and return of spontaneous circulation was obtained after 25 minutes. The patient is subsequently cooled for 24 hours and then rewarmed. It is now 96 hours following the cardiac arrest, and the patient is normothermic. He remains intubated and sedated in the neurologic ICU. The patient is comatose with intact brainstem reflexes. EEG monitoring shows the below pattern. What can be told to the patient's family regarding prognosis?

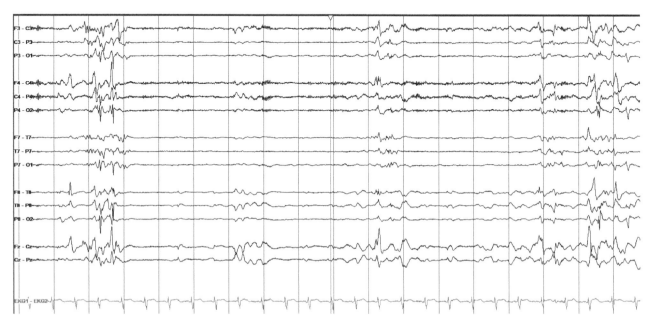

Electroencephalogram: International 10-20 standardized placement of electrodes without FP1 and FP2 placement. Montage "double banana" left over right.

    A. The EEG shows burst suppression, which is an indicator of invariably poor outcome after cardiac arrest.

    B. The EEG shows burst suppression, which is nonspecific and of no prognostic value.

    C. The EEG shows frequent seizures, and the patient should be treated with AEDs.

    D. There is not enough information currently available to accurately prognosticate.

    E. The EEG shows generalized periodic discharges, which indicate a highly epileptogenic cortex.

4. A 54-year-old patient suffered a cardiac arrest. CPR was initiated, and return of spontaneous circulation was obtained after 18 minutes with an initial rhythm of ventricular fibrillation. The patient is subsequently cooled to 36°C for 24 hours and then rewarmed over 24 hours. He remains intubated in the neurologic ICU. The patient is comatose, and generalized jerking of the limbs is noted with every spike on the EEG shown below. What can be told to the patient's family regarding prognosis?

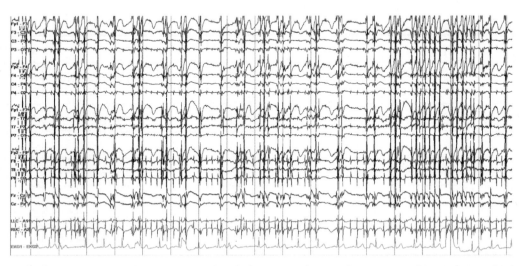

Electroencephalogram: International 10-20 standardized placement of electrodes. Montage "double banana" left over right.

A. This is muscle artifact caused by purposeful motor activity, which portends a favorable prognosis.

B. This is myoclonic status epilepticus, which is highly correlated with poor outcome, although in rare instances, good neurologic recovery has been reported.

C. No prognostic information can be given until the patient has been normothermic for 72 hours.

D. This is myoclonic status epilepticus, which is easily treated, although it has no correlation with a patient's prognosis.

E. No prognostic information can be given without first performing an MRI of the brain.

5. While admitted to the medical ICU for pneumonia and treated with meropenem, a 48-year-old man with a history of epilepsy managed with levetiracetam has a generalized tonic-clonic seizure lasting 7 minutes before he is given 4 mg of intravenous (IV) lorazepam with resolution of the convulsions. Following the seizure, he is difficult to arouse and does not follow commands. What is the most appropriate next step in management?

A. Transfer the patient into the neurointensive care unit for close neurologic monitoring; he is likely oversedated from the lorazepam and will improve once this clears in 12 to 18 hours.

B. The patient has postictal confusion and should be monitored clinically, but no further treatment is necessary because he has a history of known epilepsy and the seizure was likely provoked by his acute illness.

C. Begin continuous EEG monitoring as soon as possible if it is available.

D. Change the patient's antibiotic regimen because meropenem is highly epileptogenic, but do not make any further changes to his antiseizure medications.

E. Administer another 4 mg of IV lorazepam and continue his home levetiracetam.

6. A 47-year-old woman is admitted to the neurointensive care unit after suffering a Hunt and Hess grade 4, modified Fisher grade 4 subarachnoid hemorrhage (SAH). Conventional angiogram reveals a ruptured anterior communicating artery aneurysm that is subsequently secured with coil embolization. Given the high-grade SAH, a thorough neurologic exam is difficult. Continuous video EEG monitoring is initiated. The initial record is notable only for bilateral and symmetric theta range slowing. On post bleed day 4, there is a change in the record (quantitative EEG shown below with alpha/delta ratio [ADR] in top row and total power in bottom row). Which of the following is true, and what is the next appropriate step in treatment?

A. There is a bilateral loss of fast activity and/or increase in delta activity (indicated by a change in total power and decreased ADR); differential includes bi-hemispheric delayed cerebral ischemia (DCI) and intracranial hypertension, among other potential causes (including sedation effects), and the patient should be imaged with a computed tomography (CT) scan and CT angiogram.

B. There is an intermittent and asymmetric increase in total power suggesting seizure activity, and the patient's antiepileptic regimen should be optimized.

C. There is a change in total power and ADR indicative of sleep morphology, which is indicative of good prognosis.

D. There is a change in total power and decreased ADR indicative of a grave prognosis, and further family discussion regarding goals of care should be initiated.

E. There is an increase in total power and decrease in ADR, which is expected on post bleed day 4, and no change in treatment is necessary.

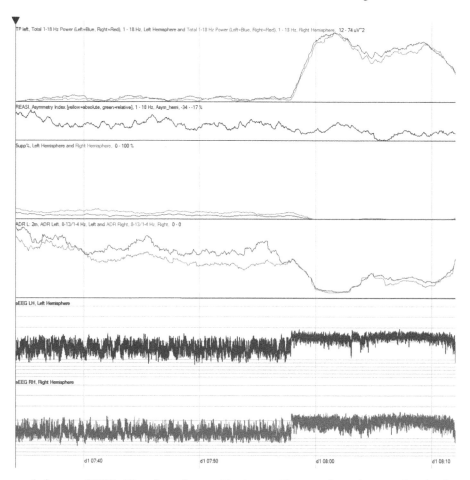

Qualitative electroencephalogram (EEG): Time lapsed over 45 minutes. Top panel: total power (total voltage of EEG). Second panel: asymmetric index right-left balance of power in EEG. Third panel: suppression percentage: amount of time with suppression. Fourth panel: alpha-delta ratio is the ratio time with alpha frequency to delta frequency. Fifth and sixth panels: amplitude-integrated EEG (left and right hemispheres, respectively).

7. For which of the following patients is discontinuation of continuous EEG monitoring most reasonable?

   A. A 55-year-old man admitted with sepsis with deteriorating mental status found to have frequent epileptiform discharges but no seizures over 12 hours of recording

   B. A 55-year-old man admitted with out-of-hospital cardiac arrest, now status post rewarming from targeted temperature management, but who remains comatose

   C. A 55-year-old man admitted with 3 generalized convulsive seizures, now awakened after being initially stuporous, who has had no epileptiform discharges over 12 hours of recording

   D. A 55-year-old man admitted with refractory status epilepticus requiring intubation and midazolam infusion, who has been seizure free for the past 48 hours of recording—for 24 hours after achieving a stable dose of midazolam, for 12 hours as midazolam was weaned off, and for 12 hours afterward

8. A 55-year-old woman with no past medical history presents to the hospital after sudden-onset severe headache. She is diagnosed with an SAH and undergoes coiling of a right internal carotid aneurysm. While being monitored in the ICU, she is noted to be more difficult to arouse. Transcranial Doppler ultrasounds are done, and the report appears below. Which of the following statements is correct?

Transcranial Doppler Ultrasound Mean Velocities Obtained from Standard Temporal Bone Windows

Left (L)		Right (R)	
Mean Velocity (cm/s)		Mean Velocity (cm/s)	
L-MCA	140	R-MCA	147
L-ACA	−40	R-ACA	−90
L-term ICA	100	R-term ICA	103
L-PCA	55	R-PCA	44
L-Ext ICA	−52	R-Ext ICA	−33

Abbreviations: ACA, anterior cerebral artery; ICA, internal carotid artery; MCA, middle cerebral artery; PCA, posterior cerebral artery.

A. These findings may be consistent with vasospasm bilaterally.

B. These findings may be consistent with vasospasm on the right only.

C. These findings may be consistent with vasospasm on the left only.

D. These findings are not consistent with vasospasm.

E. The Lindegaard ratio on the left is consistent with hyperemia.

9. According to Brain Trauma Foundation guidelines, for which of the following patients with traumatic brain injury (TBI) is intracranial pressure (ICP) monitoring most indicated?

   A. Age 35; Glasgow coma scale (GCS) 9; abnormal head CT showing a 5-mm subdural hematoma; blood pressure (BP) 80/50 mm Hg

   B. Age 85; GCS 9; abnormal head CT showing a 5-mm subdural hematoma; BP 100/70 mm Hg

   C. Age 55; GCS 7; normal head CT; BP 80/50; decerebrate posturing

   D. Age 39; GCS 9; normal head CT; BP 80/50

   E. All of the above

10. A 45-year-old man is brought to the hospital after being struck by a vehicle at high speed. On initial exam in the ED, he opens his eyes to pain and moans and does not follow commands or speak, pupils are briskly reactive, he has corneal and cough reflexes, and to painful stimulus, he flexes in the arms and triple flexes in the legs. He is immediately intubated. His head CT reveals diffuse cerebral edema, small amounts of SAH bilaterally, large blossoming right frontal contusion, effaced lateral and third ventricles, and left subdural hematoma. Which of the following is the best choice with regard to intracranial monitoring?

   A. He does not need invasive monitoring of his ICP, as he has an exam to follow.

   B. He should have a right frontal extraventricular drain placed.

   C. He should have a left temporal subarachnoid bolt placed.

D. He should have a right frontal intraparenchymal monitor placed in the area of the lesion.

E. He should have a right frontal intraparenchymal monitor placed near, but not in, the area of the lesion.

11. A 51-year-old man presents with a large right cerebellar hemorrhage with effacement of the fourth ventricle and moderate obstructive hydrocephalus. On exam, he opens his eyes to noxious stimulus, he does not attend or follow commands, his pupils are 1 mm and minimally reactive, he has corneal and cough reflexes, and he extends his arms and triple flexes in the legs bilaterally. He is intubated, and an extraventricular drain (EVD) is immediately placed and opened at 20 cm H_2O. Despite EVD placement, his exam does not improve. His ICP reads at 12 cm H_2O. Which of the following statements is true?

A. His ICP is 12 cm H_2O, so he cannot be herniating.

B. His EVD should be dropped to drain more cerebrospinal fluid (CSF).

C. Medical management should be used, targeting his ICP.

D. He needs surgery despite the ICP measurement.

E. An EVD should not have been placed.

12. A 24-year-old man with TBI has been in the ICU for 2 days. He was intubated on arrival because he had GCS of 3 on exam, with a CT scan that showed evidence of global cerebral edema. An EVD was placed when he arrived in the ICU. Because of excellent medical management, his ICPs have been controlled in the range of 12 to 16 cm H_2O. While bathing the patient, the nurse calls you to come see his ICP waveform. He is lying flat with the EVD clamped, and his waveform appears below. The ICP reads at 19 cm H_2O. Which of the following is most likely?

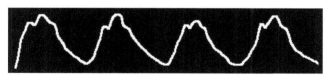

Extraventricular drain (EVD) waveform: Four intracranial pressure waveforms recorded from EVD.

A. The nurse did not re-zero the EVD.

B. The EVD may need to be replaced, as it is no longer working.

C. The ICP is still reading below 20 cm H_2O, so there is nothing to worry about.

D. The waveform suggests reduced compliance, and the patient should not remain flat for very long.

E. The waveform suggests increased compliance as the peaks are blunted.

13. Which of these noninvasive measurements is most specific for elevated intracranial pressure?

A. Ultrasound of the optic nerve sheath yielding a diameter of approximately 5 mm bilaterally

B. EEG recording showing frontal intermittent rhythmic delta activity (FIRDA)

C. EEG recording showing severe diffuse slowing

D. Transcranial Doppler measurements showing an elevated pulsatility index

E. Sluggish pupillary responses to light

14. Which of the following findings on ancillary testing is most consistent with a diagnosis of brain death?

A. Oscillatory flow (reversal of flow during diastole) on transcranial Doppler ultrasounds

B. Present flow on transcranial Doppler ultrasounds with a pulsatility index >1.2

C. Isoelectric EEG for at least 1 hour at a sensitivity of 7 μV/mm

D. ICP waveform with P2 higher than P1

E. A CT angiogram that shows no opacification of any internal or external carotid artery branches

15. A 62-year-old woman is post bleed day 7 from a Hunt and Hess grade 5, modified Fisher grade 4 subarachnoid bleed from a basilar tip aneurysm, now secured. Her exam off sedation is notable for equal and reactive pupils, a right corneal reflex, an intact vestibulo-ocular reflex, and a cough. She has mild flexor posturing to painful stimuli in her upper extremities. Over the past 3 days, her systolic BPs have ranged from 160 to 270 mm Hg. An EVD has been in place since the time of admission with ICPs ranging from 5 to 22 mm Hg and central perfusion pressures ranging from 60 to 140 mm Hg. An MRI of the brain shows new small scattered infarcts between days 4 and 8, and her CT angiogram shows diffuse mild vasospasm of her anterior and posterior circulation. She has been on nimodipine since admission. What is the best next step in management to decrease the risk of delayed cerebral ischemia in this patient with high-grade SAH?

A. Increase nimodipine dose

B. Aggressively lower systolic BP to <160 mm Hg

C. Empirically increase cerebral perfusion pressure range goals

D. Place brain oxygenation and cerebral microdialysis monitors

E. Continue current care

16. A 53-year-old woman is post bleed day 5 from a Hunt and Hess grade 4, modified Fisher grade 4 SAH from a ruptured right MCA aneurysm, now secured. Her cerebral perfusion pressure goals are 80 to 100 mm Hg. She has an EVD ICP monitor, as well as brain tissue oxygenation and cerebral microdialysis monitors in her right frontal lobe. Readings from earlier in the day have consistently shown $PbtO_2$ >25 mm Hg and lactate/pyruvate (L/P) ratio <35, whereas her most recent readings are below these levels. What is the best next step in management to reduce the patient's risk of delayed cerebral ischemia?

Trends of Partial Pressure of Parenchymal Oxygen ($PbtO_2$; mm Hg), Brain Temperature (°C), Cerebral Perfusion Pressure (CPP), and Microdialysis Concentrations of Parenchymal Lactate and Pyruvate (mmol/L) Over Time

	2 p.m.	3 p.m.	4 p.m.	5 p.m.	6 p.m.	7 p.m.
$PbtO_2$	21.1	14.6	15.0	28.3	29.2	32.7
Brain temperature	37.9	38.2	38.2	38.2	37.6	38.2
CPP	86	74	78	101	109	120
Lactate (L)	6.3	7.9	8.1	8.2	7	6.7
Pyruvate (P)	150	172	180	221	199	193
L/P ratio	42.1	46	45	36.9	35.1	34.7

A. Continue current care

B. Increase cerebral perfusion pressure

C. Aggressive temperature management

D. Start continuous EEG monitoring

E. Decrease fraction of inspired oxygen (FiO_2)

17. A 47-year-old man is postoperative day 3 from left carotid stenting. Prior to his procedure, he was noted to have complete occlusion of his right internal carotid artery, 80% stenosis of his left internal carotid artery, and a large arteriovenous malformation (AVM) within his left anterior circulation. Postoperatively, the patient's course was complicated by a 40-mL hemorrhage from his left AVM, and he cannot be placed on antiplatelet agents. The patient is intubated and sedated for ventilator synchrony and has an ICP monitor in place. What is the next best step to monitor this patient's progress?

A. Continuous EEG monitoring to evaluate for seizures

B. Continue current care

C. Place a perilesional $PbtO_2$ monitor

D. Serial CT brain perfusion studies

E. Daily transcranial Doppler ultrasounds

18. A 45-year-old man is post bleed day 8 from a Hunt and Hess grade 5, modified Fisher grade 4 SAH from a posterior cerebral artery (PCA) aneurysm that is now secured. His CPP goals are 80 to 100 mm Hg. He has an EVD ICP monitor, as well as brain tissue oxygenation and cerebral microdialysis monitors. His most recent readings are below. What is the best next step in management to reduce the patient's risk of delayed cerebral ischemia?

Trends of Partial Pressure of Parenchymal Oxygen (PbtO₂; mm Hg), Brain Temperature (°C), Cerebral Perfusion Pressure (CPP), and Microdialysis Concentrations of Parenchymal Lactate and Pyruvate (mmol/L) Over Time

	2 a.m.	3 a.m.	4 a.m.	5 a.m.	6 a.m.
PbtO₂	54	42.4	47.3	40.4	42.9
Brain temperature	38.2	38.5	38.7	39.2	39
CPP	101	104	99	93	90
Lactate (L)	8.3	8.2	8.6	7.5	9.1
Pyruvate (P)	202	192	202	186	167
L/P ratio	44	42.7	42.5	50.8	54.4

A. Decrease cerebral perfusion pressure
B. Increase cerebral perfusion pressure
C. Aggressive temperature management
D. Continue current care
E. Decrease FiO₂

19. A 53-year-old woman is postoperative day 3 from right carotid stenting. Her course was complicated by a 30-mL frontotemporal hemorrhage, and antiplatelet agents were stopped. She has an EVD ICP monitor and right-sided multimodality monitor with brain tissue oxygenation, brain temperature, and microdialysis. Her numbers are below. Her serum hemoglobin is 8.3 mg/dL. What is the immediate next best step in this patient's management?

Trends of Partial Pressure of Parenchymal Oxygen (PbtO₂; mm Hg), Brain Temperature (°C), Cerebral Perfusion Pressure (CPP), Intracranial Pressure (ICP; mm Hg), Fraction of Inspired Oxygen (FiO₂; %), and Microdialysis Concentration of Parenchymal Lactate (L) and Pyruvate (P) Over Time

	3 p.m.	4 p.m.	5 p.m.	6 p.m.	7 p.m.
PbtO₂	35	28.2	19	17.6	14.4
Brain temperature	37.9	38.1	38	37.8	37.8
FiO₂	40	40	40	40	40
ICP	15	15	16	16	17
CPP	55	58	63	67	72
L/P ratio	42.1	46	52.6	58	62.3

A. Increase FiO₂
B. Continue current care
C. Transcranial Doppler
D. Increase CPP
E. CT angiogram of the head and neck

20. A 49-year-old woman is post bleed day 7 from a Hunt and Hess grade 3, modified Fisher grade 4 SAH from a left MCA bifurcation aneurysm that is now secured. She has had steadily increasing transcranial Doppler velocities in her left MCA territory for the past several days, but has remained without focal deficits, with systolic BPs ranging from 120 to 140 mm Hg. Given that she is at high risk of vasospasm and delayed cerebral ischemia, the clinical team has stressed the importance of maintaining euvolemia for adequate cerebral perfusion and have placed a pulse index continuous cardiac output (PiCCO) monitoring device (which measures cardiac output using pulse contour analysis and transpulmonary thermodilution). The patient then suddenly develops weakness in her right side, and her BP is noted to be 90/50 mm Hg. Which of the following management choices is most appropriate given the PiCCO values for stroke volume variation (SVV), cardiac index (CI), global end-diastolic index (GEDI), and extravascular lung water index (ELWI)?

A. SVV 14, CI 2.5, GEDI 550, ELWI 8; hold IV fluids, start inotrope infusion
B. SVV 14, CI 2.5, GEDI 550, ELWI 22; IV fluid bolus only
C. SVV 10, CI 2.5, GEDI 550, ELWI 22; diurese with IV furosemide
D. SVV 10, CI 2.5, GEDI 550, ELWI 14; hold IV fluids, start inotrope infusion
E. SVV 10, CI 2.5, GEDI 550, ELWI 14; IV fluid bolus then start inotrope infusion

Answers and Explanations

1. **C.** Generalized rhythmic delta activity (GRDA), frontally predominant (formerly FIRDA), is a nonspecific EEG pattern that has been associated with a wide variety of pathologies. Most commonly, this pattern is seen in patients with mild to moderate toxic metabolic encephalopathy and/or underlying structural lesions. In this patient, the most likely cause is encephalopathy due to uremia as indicated by the presence of asterixis on exam and the patient's history of chronic kidney disease. The cause for this patient's encephalopathy should be further investigated with a thorough laboratory workup. The absence of focal findings in the neurologic exam make a structural brain lesion less likely, although MRI of the brain could be considered at a later time if no clear cause of encephalopathy is found in the diagnostic workup. There is no indication for AED in this patient as this is not an epileptic pattern and addition of an AED may worsen the patient's confusion.

2. **A.** Lateralized periodic discharges (LPDs; formerly PLEDs) are a nonspecific indicator of an acute brain dysfunction or unilateral (usually destructive) brain lesions. LPDs have classically been associated with herpes simplex virus (HSV) encephalitis, which is high on the differential for this patient. Empiric treatment of HSV encephalitis should be initiated as soon as possible and should not be delayed for diagnostic workup (including brain imaging and cerebrospinal fluid [CSF] HSV polymerase chain reaction [PCR], in addition to routine CSF studies). Treatment with a prophylactic AED would likely be beneficial in this patient, but should not delay administration of antiviral therapy. The patient is likely aphasic due to HSV preferentially affecting the temporal lobes, and aspirin may increase the risk of hemorrhage.

3. **D.** The question stem indicates that the patient is intubated and sedated following cooling protocol after cardiac arrest. The EEG shows burst suppression, which can be seen with high doses of anesthetic medications (such as propofol or midazolam) commonly used for sedation in the intensive care unit setting. These medications should be withheld and allowed to clear before information is gathered and interpreted for prognostication purposes. In the absence of any sedating medications, burst suppression may indicate a poor prognosis (especially "burst suppression with identical bursts"), but consists of heterogeneous EEG activity with diverse probabilities of recovery.

4. **B.** Prior to the advent of therapeutic hypothermia after cardiac arrest, myoclonic status epilepticus was associated with a uniformly poor outcome. In the era of postarrest targeted temperature management, the definitive association of myoclonic status epilepticus with a poor neurologic outcome is less clear. Although this pattern remains a strong predictor of poor outcome, several case reports of good neurologic recovery have been published. Although neurologic exam at 72 hours post rewarming and MRI of the brain may provide additional prognostic information, the EEG can provide some guidance in their absence. Treatment of postanoxic myoclonic status can be highly refractory to treatment with AEDs.

5. **C.** The differential diagnosis for depressed level of consciousness following a seizure includes both drug effect and postictal confusion. However, prior studies have demonstrated the presence of nonconvulsive status epilepticus in 48% of patients after apparent control of convulsive status epilepticus. Accordingly, continuous EEG monitoring should be initiated in patients with a depressed level of consciousness following prolonged seizure activity. Alteration of the treatment plan should be guided by EEG findings.

6. **A.** The hallmark of neurocritical care is to prevent further brain injury after an initial neurologic insult. Treatment of aneurysmal subarachnoid hemorrhage (SAH) is a model example of this goal as patients are at high risk for subsequent brain injury due to vasospasm and delayed cerebral ischemia (DCI). Early detection is crucial to avoid irreversible injury. Although in awake patients, serial neurologic exams provides a reliable method of detecting DCI, this is often not possible in patients with high-grade (Hunt and Hess grades 4 and 5) SAH. Quantitative EEG has been demonstrated to be highly sensitive for detection of DCI. Most sensitive for this is a change in the total power followed closely by a reduction in ADR following stimulation.

7. **C.** Retrospective studies have shown that between 10% and 16% of patients undergoing EEG monitoring for altered mental status in medical and surgical intensive care units (ICUs) were found to have electrographic seizures, whereas a prospective study showed that 11% of all patients admitted to a medical ICU with severe sepsis were found to have electrographic seizures on continuous EEG. The timing of continuous EEG discontinuation is controversial, however. In one study, 12% of ICU patients with recorded seizures did not have their first seizure until after the first 24 hours of monitoring. Another study showed that a lack of epileptiform discharges in the first 2 hours of monitoring was predictive of a <5% risk of seizures by 72 hours; if epileptiform discharges were present, 16 hours of seizure-free monitoring were required to have a similarly low risk of seizures at 72 hours. As for patients with refractory status epilepticus who are on anesthetic infusions, expert guidelines, including those from the Neurocritical Care Society, recommend continuing EEG monitoring for the duration of the anesthetic wean and for at least 24 hours afterward (and potentially much longer depending on the half-life of the anesthetic used). Finally, continuous EEG monitoring is an important part of management and prognostication for patients who remain comatose after cardiac arrest.

8. **B.** After SAH, vasospasm can result in delayed cerebral ischemia. Transcranial Doppler ultrasound allows noninvasive monitoring of blood flow velocity, which can serve as a surrogate for the diameter of cerebral arteries. Mean velocities in the middle cerebral artery (MCA) of >200 cm/s have a positive predictive value of 87% for angiographic spasm, and velocities <120 cm/s have a negative predictive value of 94% for angiographic spasm. However, high velocities may also occur due to hyperemia. To distinguish hyperemia from vasospasm, the velocity can be normalized by calculating the Lindegaard ratio, by dividing the mean velocity in the MCA by the mean velocity in the ipsilateral extracranial internal carotid artery (ICA). A Lindegaard ratio >3 signifies hyperemia, and a ratio <3 signifies vasospasm. In this case, while the left MCA mean velocity is elevated at 120 cm/s, the Lindegaard ratio is 2.7 (140/−52), suggesting hyperemia and not vasospasm. The right MCA mean velocity is also elevated at 147 cm/s, but because the right external ICA velocity is lower (−33), the Lindegaard ratio is 4.5, and these findings may therefore be suggestive of moderate vasospasm.

9. **C.** According to the 2016 Brain Trauma Foundation guidelines, "management of severe TBI patients using information from ICP monitoring is recommended to reduce in-hospital and 2 week post-injury mortality" (Level II B). However, severe TBI is defined as GCS ≤8, meaning that the first 2 patients would normally be classified as moderate TBI if their exam did not worsen any further. Of note, the previous edition of the Brain Trauma Foundation guidelines from 2007 suggested that ICP "should be monitored in all salvageable patients with a severe traumatic brain injury and an abnormal computed tomography (CT) scan [revealing] hematomas, contusions, swelling, herniation, or compressed basal cisterns."

ICP monitoring is indicated in patients with severe TBI with a normal CT scan if 2 or more of the following features are noted at admission:

- Age over 40 years
- Unilateral or bilateral motor posturing
- Systolic BP <90 mm Hg

Overall, monitoring ICP does not change outcomes, only the use of these measurements in addition to clinical assessment for treatment decisions.

10. D. The patient in the question has suffered a severe TBI, with GCS 7 (E2, V2, M3) and multicompartmental brain injury. The Brain Trauma Foundation guidelines recommend ICP monitoring in this scenario. However, subarachnoid bolts are rarely used because of unreliable measurements. The 2 main ICP monitoring devices in current use are the extraventricular drain (EVD) and the intraparenchymal monitor (IPM), and there are no clear guidelines on which to use. The EVD can be therapeutic in the case of hydrocephalus or intraventricular hemorrhage, in addition to being a monitoring device. However, it can be challenging to place when the ventricles are effaced and only transduce readings onto a monitor when clamped. In contrast, an IPM is often easier to place and can be placed along with other monitors to perform simultaneous monitoring of partial brain oxygen saturation, cerebral blood flow, or microdialysis, although it offers no therapeutic potential and cannot be recalibrated once it is inserted. IPMs are best suited for measuring pressures in a region of interest, while EVDs tend to be more representative of global ICP (and may potentially miss focal areas of increased ICP).

The presence of a right frontal contusion makes the location for placement of any potential right-sided IPM crucial, especially if other monitoring modalities besides the ICP monitor are also to be placed. The best option would be to place a right frontal perilesional IPM, which may give important information about local (as well as global) ICP; further, other monitoring modalities would be able to help identify tissue at risk, while an intralesional

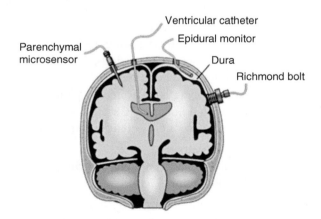

Parenchymal microsensor
Ventricular catheter
Epidural monitor
Dura
Richmond bolt

Redrawn from Mayer SA. *Management of increased intracranial pressure.* In: Wijdicks EFM, Diringer MN, Bolton CF, et al, eds. Continuum: Critical Care Neurology. Minneapolis, MN: American Academy of Neurology; 1997:47-61.

IPM would only indicate ongoing cell death in already damaged brain tissue.

11. D. This patient presented with a large cerebellar hemorrhage, which can be life-threatening due to mass effect, obstructive hydrocephalus, and herniation. Because of the obstructive hydrocephalus, an EVD may be placed to prevent supratentorial complications. However, given that the highest regional ICP exists in the posterior fossa where the lesion is located, EVD placement carries the risk of upward herniation. If one is placed, it should therefore be kept open at a relatively high pressure or clamped with intermittent small amount of CSF drainage at a time until the compartment is decompressed. Indeed, in such a scenario, the ICP as measured supratentorially does not necessarily represent infratentorial ICP and, therefore, does not exclude the possibility of ongoing downward herniation. While medical management, in the form of hypertonic saline or mannitol, can be used as a temporizing measure, emergent surgery is indicated to evacuate the hematoma and decompress the posterior fossa.

12. D. The patient has an EVD, which does need to be re-zeroed when the patient changes position (unlike intraparenchymal monitors, which do not). If it is not re-zeroed, however, only the ICP reading itself will be affected, not the waveform. ICP monitoring waveform has a flow of 3 peaks:

- Peak one (P1), which is also called percussion wave, represents arterial pulsation
- Peak two (P2), which is also called tidal wave, represents intracranial compliance
- Peak three (P3), which is also called dicrotic wave, represents aortic valve closure

In our patient, although his ICP is not >20 cm H_2O, his waveform suggests poor intracranial compliance, with a P2 (ie, second peak) component that is as high or higher than the P1 component (ie, first peak). The ICP likely will continue to rise as the patient lies flat, and he likely cannot tolerate lying flat for long. This patient should have the head of bed placed at 30° or above, and should not be sent for long imaging studies that require remaining supine. The image below depicts different commonly encountered ICP waveforms. The first panel is a normal tracing. There is a progressively higher

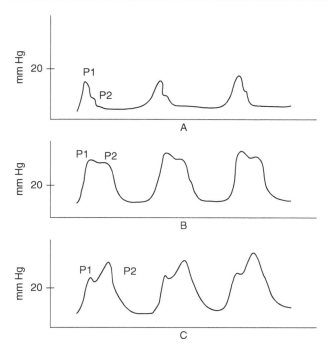

Intracranial pressure tracing: The first panel is a normal tracing. There is a progressively higher P2 wave, which is seen with noncompliant brain even in the setting of normal intracranial pressure.

P2 wave, which is seen with noncompliant brain even in the setting of normal ICP.

13. **A.** Several studies have shown that optic nerve sheath diameter greater than approximately 5 mm has a sensitivity of 88% to 94% and specificity of 76% to 94% in detecting ICP >20 cm H_2O.

   EEG monitoring can identify signs of globally increased ICP—for example, FIRDA and diffuse slowing in cases of diffuse ICP increases—however, these are highly nonspecific as they are more often seen with metabolic or toxic encephalopathies. Elevated pulsatility index on transcranial Doppler can be seen in patients with increased ICP, but also in other states of elevated distal cerebrovascular resistance. Sluggish pupillary responses have many possible causes in addition to increased ICP, including pharmacologic causes and local structural causes (eg, local compression of the oculomotor nerve). However, unilateral pupillary unresponsiveness or sluggishness in a patient with a large focal brain lesion is certainly more concerning.

14. **A.** Transcranial Doppler ultrasounds in a patient with brain death can show reversal of normal

anterograde flow during diastole, also called oscillatory flow, or systolic spikes. The pulsatility index is calculated by subtracting the diastolic flow velocity from the systolic flow velocity and dividing it by the mean flow velocity and reflects distal cerebrovascular resistance. While elevated pulsatility index values are found in severe TBI, an elevated pulsatility index is not specific to a diagnosis of brain death. When using EEG as an ancillary test for brain death, sensitivity must be increased to a maximum of 2 μV/mm for at least 30 minutes. While the normal ICP waveform has 3 components, with P1 (percussion wave) being larger than P2 (tidal wave) and P3 (dichrotic wave), a noncompliant waveform may show a P2 higher than P1. This can be seen in patients with elevated ICP but does not mean the patient is brain dead. Finally, angiographic studies that show opacification of external carotid artery but not internal carotid artery branches are consistent with brain death, but the gold standard is conventional angiography; CT angiograms can yield false-negative results if the contrast bolus is poorly timed, which would be manifested as a lack of any arterial opacification whatsoever.

15. **D.** This patient has a high-grade SAH with a limited exam and MRI evidence of ongoing delayed cerebral ischemia with a wide range of systolic pressures and central perfusion pressures. Finding the most appropriate cerebral perfusion goal is the most important next step in her care. Although there is low-quality evidence in the literature, there is strong recommendation for use of microdialysis in the setting of those at risk for cerebral hypoxia and delayed cerebral ischemia. Multimodality monitoring can give information for early detection of brain ischemia or vulnerability not disclosed by routine ICP and cerebral perfusion pressure (CPP) surveillance. Brain oxygenation (PbtO$_2$) reflects the partial pressure of oxygen at the end of the capillary circuit. It reflects oxygen supply while testing optimal CPP ranges, as well as adequate oxygen extraction. Cerebral microdialysis analyzes substrates within the extracellular fluid of subcortical white matter. Trends in its values can help predict energy crisis.

16. **B.** This patient is at risk of delayed cerebral ischemia after SAH. In this scenario, PbtO$_2$ numbers are initially low and L/P ratios are high. PbtO$_2$ is a

balance between oxygen delivery and oxygen consumption in brain cells. It can be affected by a number of parameters, such as cerebral metabolism, cerebral blood flow, sedation, low inspired oxygen, ICP and CPP changes, and other traumatic changes in the cellular environment. The goal with $PbtO_2$ monitoring is to assess which change will have the greatest effect on $PbtO_2$ trends. In the case of this patient, $PbtO_2$ and brain metabolism improve with increasing CPPs.

17. **C.** ICP and CPP *should not* be used as surrogates for $PbtO_2$ because cerebral oxygenation can vary independently from ICP. Both CPP and ICP may be normal during discrete episodes of cerebral hypoxia. This patient is at high risk for thrombosis of his unprotected carotid stent. Due to his intracerebral hemorrhage, he may also have compartmentalization of ICPs, further complicating local CPPs to the remaining viable left hemisphere. A monitoring device will be able to reflect the patient's local brain physiology and measure oxygen delivery and consumption for the at-risk tissue. Trends in these values help guide further interventions.

18. **C.** The L/P ratio (LPR) reflects the state of cerebral oxidative metabolism, with direct measurement of anaerobic and aerobic metabolites (lactate and pyruvate). LPR is a sensitive marker for cerebral ischemia when coupled with $PbtO_2$ values, but LPR and lactate levels can also be elevated in the setting of increased metabolic need without hypoxia or ischemia. In this patient's case, both the LPR and pyruvate values are high in the setting of normal $PbtO_2$. This indicates increased oxygen consumption or mitochondrial dysfunction, likely in the setting of the patient's worsening fevers. Fever control in this patient will decrease the brain's metabolic need and improve homeostasis.

19. **E.** The values in the table are from a patient with a recent carotid stent, not on antiplatelet agents. The decreasing cerebral oxygenation and increasing LPRs are concerning for progressive stent thrombosis, given that these numbers do not appear to improve with increasing CPPs, which is the first thing that must be excluded in this scenario. (Note, however, that complete thrombosis would likely cause the LPR to rise even more sharply than in this scenario, while the $PbtO_2$ would likely have an even sharper drop.) This can be done with a conventional or CT angiogram or carotid Doppler ultrasound. If this does not show evidence of stent thrombosis, then CPP may actually need to be decreased, as this may represent a case of postrevascularization luxury perfusion; a further increase of the patient's CPP is also undesirable in the setting of the patient's recent hemorrhage (which itself may have been caused by luxury perfusion). Meanwhile, although increasing FiO_2 would indeed increase the $PbtO_2$ reading, it would not address the underlying issue of overall blood flow. Transcranial Doppler ultrasounds may be helpful in diagnosing luxury perfusion but would not help in excluding carotid stent thrombosis.

20. **D.** A PiCCO catheter is an arterial line with an additional thermistor on its tip, which allows for pulse counter analysis (yielding stroke volume variation) and continuous cardiac output, along with intermittent measurements, including global end-diastolic index (GEDI), extravascular lung water index (ELWI), and cardiac index (CI), that are based on transpulmonary thermodilution (requiring the presence of a concurrent central line). This information is of particular value to patients with SAH, whose clinical course often depends on their volume status. A study of PiCCO monitoring in SAH patients showed that patients with poor-grade SAH had significantly higher extravascular lung water index and lower cardiac index than good-grade SAH patients, and those who ended up developing DCI had a significantly lower GEDI than those who did not. This finding of lower GEDI in patients with DCI was confirmed in another multicenter prospective study, suggesting that serial GEDI measurements may prove to be instrumental in the prevention of DCI. Interpretation is relatively straightforward.

CI below 3.0 is considered abnormal, suggesting the need for intervention based on other values. GEDI less than 650 to 700 suggests the need for cardiac support with fluids, inotropes, or both; SVV greater than 10 to 12 suggests fluid responsiveness; and ELWI greater than 10 suggests fluid overload. The scenario for choice A suggests a highly fluid-responsive patient who should first be given IV fluids. In the scenario for choice B, the high ELWI means fluid boluses should be administered with caution, and inotropic support should either be given first or in conjunction. Meanwhile, although diuresis may indeed be eventually indicated in the scenario for choice C, one should be cautious in doing so as a first step in a patient with hypotension, especially when he or she has SAH (since fluid status plays a major role in the development of DCI). Instead, inotropes should probably be started first, with further interventions to follow. The patient in choice E does not appear to be fluid responsive and instead may have fluid overload, suggesting that inotropes should be the first course of action.

REFERENCES

Accolla, EA, Kaplan PW, Maeder-Ingvar M, et al. Clinical correlates of frontal intermittent rhythmic delta activity (FIRDA). *Clin Neurophysiol.* 2011;122:27-31.

Bouzat P, Oddo M, Payen JF. Transcranial Doppler after traumatic brain injury: is there a role? *Curr Opin Crit Care.* 2014;20:153-160.

Bradshaw MJ, Venkatesan A. Herpes simplex virus-1 encephalitis in adults: pathophysiology, diagnosis, and management. *Neurotherapeutics.* 2016;13:493-508.

Brain Trauma Foundation. Guidelines for the management of severe traumatic brain injury. 3rd ed. *J Neurotrauma.* 2007;24(Suppl 1).

Brain Trauma Foundation. Guidelines for the management of severe traumatic brain injury. 4th ed. https://braintrauma .org/guidelines/guidelines-for-the-management-of -severe-tbi-4th-ed#/. Accessed November 1, 2016.

Brophy GM, Bell R, Claassen J, et al. Guidelines for the evaluation and management of status epilepticus. *Neurocrit Care.* 2012;17:3-23.

Carrera E, Schmidt JM, Fernandez L, et al. Spontaneous hyperventilation and brain tissue hypoxia in patients with severe brain injury. *J Neurol Neurosurg Psychiatry.* 2010;81:793-797.

Chou SH, Robertson CS, Participants in the International Multi-Disciplinary Consensus Conference on Multimodality Monitoring. Monitoring biomarkers of cellular injury and death in acute brain injury. *Neurocrit Care.* 2014; 21(Supp 2):S187-S214.

Claassen J, Mayer SA, Kowalski RG, et al. Detection of electrographic seizures with continuous EEG monitoring in critically ill patients. *Neurology.* 2004;62:1743-1748.

Datar S, Rabinstein AA. Cerebellar hemorrhage. *Neurol Clin.* 2014;32:993-1007.

DeLorenzo RJ, Waterhouse EJ, Towne AR, et al. Persistent nonconvulsive status epilepticus after the control of convulsive status epilepticus. *Epilepsia.* 1998;39:833-840.

De Riva N, Budohoski KP, Smielewski, et al. Transcranial Doppler pulsatility index: what it is and what it isn't. *Neurocrit Care.* 2012;17:58-66.

Emilia M, Andraus C. Periodic EEG patterns: importance of their recognition and clinical significance. *Arq Neuropsiquiatr.* 2012;70:145-151.

Foreman B, Claassen J. Quantitative EEG for the detection of brain ischemia. *Crit Care.* 2012;16:216.

Francoeur CL, Mayer SA. Management of delayed cerebral ischemia after subarachnoid hemorrhage. *Crit Care.* 2016;20:277.

Gilmore EJ, Gaspard N, Choi HA, et al. Acute brain failure in severe sepsis: a prospective study in the medical intensive care unit utilizing continuous EEG monitoring. *Intensive Care Med.* 2015;41:686-694.

Greer DM, Wang HH, Robinson JD, et al. Variability of brain death policies in the United States. *JAMA Neurol.* 2016;73:213-218.

Harders AG, Gilsbach JM. Time course of blood velocity changes related to vasospasm in the circle of Willis measured by transcranial Doppler ultrasound. *J Neurosurg.* 1987;66:718-728.

Hawthorne C, Piper I. Monitoring of intracranial pressure in patients with traumatic brain injury. *Front Neurol.* 2014;5:121.

Helbok R, Olson DM, Le Roux PD, et al. Intracranial pressure and cerebral perfusion pressure monitoring in non-TBI patients: special considerations. *Neurocrit Care.* 2014;21(Suppl 2):S85-S94.

Hillered L, Vespa PM, Hovda DA. Translational neurochemical research in acute human brain injury: the current status and potential future for cerebral microdialysis. *J Neurotrauma.* 2005;22:3-41.

Hofmeijer J, van Putten M. EEG in postanoxic coma: prognostic and diagnostic value. *Clin Neurophysiol.* 2016;127:2047-2055.

Kasotakis G, Michailidou M, Bramos A, et al. Intraparenchymal vs extracranial ventricular drain intracranial pressure monitors in traumatic brain injury: less is more? *J Am Coll Surg.* 2012;214:950-957.

Kimberly HH, Shah S, Marill K, et al. Correlation of optic nerve sheath diameter with direct measurement of intracranial pressure. *Acad Emerg Med.* 2008;15:201-204.

Kurtz P, Gaspard N, Wahl AS, et al. Continuous electroencephalography in a surgical intensive care unit. *Intensive Care Med.* 2014;40:228-234.

Lazaridis C, Robertson CS. The role of multimodal invasive monitoring in acute traumatic brain injury. *Neurosurg Clin N Am.* 2016;27:509-517.

Le Roux P, Menon DK, Citerio G, et al. Consensus Summary Statement of the International Multidisciplinary Consensus Conference on Multimodaility Monitoring in Neurocritical Care. *Neurocrit Care.* 2014;21:1-26.

Lindegaard KF, Nornes H, Bakke SJ, et al. Cerebral vasospasm diagnosis by means of angiography and blood velocity measurements. *Acta Neurochir.* 1989;100:12-24.

Lui TN, Fairholm DJ, Shu TF, et al. Surgical treatment of spontaneous cerebellar hemorrhage. *Surg Neurol.* 1985;23: 555-558.

Messerer M, Daniel RT, Oddo M. Neuromonitoring after major neurosurgical procedures. *Minerva Anestesiol.* 2012;78: 810-822.

Moretti R, Pizzi B. Optic nerve sheath ultrasound for detection of intracranial hypertension in intracranial hemorrhage patients: confirmation of previous findings in a different patient population. *J Neurosurg Anesthesiol.* 2009;21:16-20.

Oddo M, Carrera E, Claassen J, et al. Continuous electroencephalography in the medical intensive care unit. *Crit Care Med*. 2009;37:2051-2056.

Oddo M, Villa F, Citerio G. Brain multimodality monitoring: an update. *Curr Opin Crit Care*. 2012;18:111-118.

Purkayastha S, Sorond F. Transcranial Doppler ultrasound: technique and application. *Semin Neurol*. 2012;32:411-420.

Rajajee V, Vanaman M, Fletcher JJ, et al. Optic nerve ultrasound for the detection of raised intracranial pressure. *Neurocrit Care*. 2011;15:506-515.

Roh DJ, Morris NA, Claassen J. Intracranial multimodality monitoring for delayed cerebral ischemia. *J Clin Neurophysiol*. 2016;33:241-249.

Roh D, Park S. Brain multimodality monitoring: updated perspectives. *Curr Neurol Neurosci Rep*. 2016;16:56.

Ropper AH, Kehne SM, Wechsler L. Transcranial Doppler in brain death. *Neurology*. 1987;37:1733.

Rosenthal ES. The utility of EEG, SSEP, and other neurophysiologic tools to guide neurocritical care. *Neurotherapeutics*. 2012;9:24-36.

Rosenthal G, Hemphill JC 3rd, Sorani M, et al. Brain tissue oxygen tension is more indicative of oxygen diffusion than oxygen delivery and metabolism in patients with traumatic brain injury. *Crit Care Med*. 2008;36:1917-1924.

Sandroni C, Caiou A, Cavallaro F, et al. Prognostication in comatose survivors of cardiac arrest: an advisory statement from the European Resuscitation Council and the European Society of Intensive Care Medicine. *Intensive Care Med*. 2014;40:1816-1831.

Schmidt JM, Rincon F, Fernandez A, et al. Cerebral infarction associated with acute subarachnoid hemorrhage. *Neurocrit Care*. 2007;7:10-17.

Stecker MM, Sabau D, Sullivan L, et al. American clinical neurophysiology society guideline 6: minimum technical standards for EEG recording in suspected cerebral death. *J Clin Neurophysiol*. 2016;33:324-327.

Tagami T, Kuwamoto K, Watanabe A, et al. Optimal range of global end-diastolic volume for fluid management after aneurysmal subarachnoid hemorrhage: a multicenter prospective cohort study. *Crit Care Med*. 2014;42:1348-1356.

Vespa P, Bergsneider M, Hattori N, et al. Metabolic crisis without brain ischemia is common after traumatic brain injury: a combined microdialysis and positron emission tomography study. *J Cereb Blood Flow Metab*. 2005;25:763-774.

Vora YY, Suarez-Almazor M, Steinke DE, et al. Role of transcranial Doppler monitoring in the diagnosis of cerebral vasospasm after subarachnoid hemorrhage. *Neurosurgery*. 1999;44:1237-1247.

Westover MB, Shafi MM, Bianchi MT, et al. The probability of seizures during EEG monitoring in critically ill adults. *Clin Neurophysiol*. 2015;126:463-471.

Yoneda H, Nakamura T, Shirao S, et al. Multicenter prospective cohort study on volume management after subarachnoid hemorrhage. *Stroke*. 2013;44:2155-2161.

Yopneda S, Nishimoto A, Nukada T, et al. To-and-fro movement and external escape of carotid arterial blood in brain death cases. A Doppler ultrasonic study. *Stroke*. 1974;5:707-713.

15

Neurointerventional Surgery

Mohammad El-Ghanem, MD, Gaurav Gupta, MD, Sudipta Roychowdhury, MD, and Fawaz Al-Mufti, MD

Questions

1. A 10-day-old neonate with severe hydrocephalus is being evaluated for refractory congestive heart failure. As part of the evaluation, a cranial ultrasound is performed and demonstrates an abnormal vascular structure. Brain magnetic resonance imaging (MRI)/magnetic resonance venography (MRV) and computed tomography (CT) scan are obtained and shown below. Which of the following is the best treatment option?

   A. Start anticoagulation using low-molecular-weight heparin

   B. Continued aggressive medical management with surgical intervention planned at 5 to 6 months of age

   C. Urgent referral for endovascular embolization

   D. Placement of a ventriculoperitoneal shunt

   E. Microsurgical removal of the abnormality

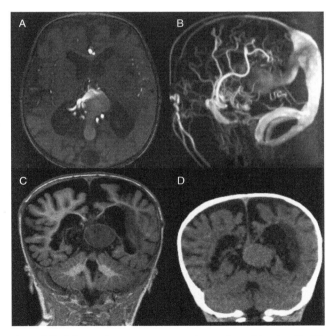

A and B. Magnetic resonance angiography of brain. **C.** T2 fluid-attenuated inversion recovery coronal magnetic resonance imaging of brain. **D.** Noncontrast coronal compute tomography scan.

2. A 42-year-old right-handed woman presented for the evaluation of headaches. Upon evaluation, an unruptured left middle cerebral artery (MCA) bifurcation aneurysm (10 mm in diameter) was found. Which of the following statements regarding management and risk of rupture is correct?

A. Based on the International Study of Unruptured Intracranial Aneurysms (ISUIA), the 5-year risk of aneurysm rupture in this particular patient is 14.5%.

B. Based on the ISUIA study and the Unruptured Cerebral Aneurysm Study (UCAS) Japan, anterior circulation aneurysms have a higher risk of rupture when compared with posterior circulation aneurysms.

C. Patient age and comorbidities are not taken into consideration when planning management.

D. Based on the ISUIA study, the 5-year risk of aneurysm rupture in this particular patient is 2.6%.

E. Uncontrolled hypertension and cigarette smoking are associated with lower risk of aneurysm rupture.

3. A 63-year-old right-handed man with history of smoking, hypertension, and diabetes mellitus presents with acute-onset left-sided hemiparesis and hemineglect, with conjugate eye deviation to the right, with onset of symptoms 3 hours before emergency department (ED) evaluation. Brain CT scan without contrast was unremarkable. CT angiogram showed proximal right MCA filling defect consistent with acute occlusion. Which of the following statements is correct regarding endovascular mechanical thrombectomy (EMT) in this patient?

A. Intravenous (IV) tissue plasminogen activator (tPA) should not be combined with EMT.

B. Based on recent trials, an angiographic reperfusion score of Thrombolysis in Cerebral Infarction (TICI) 2a is associated with highest functional outcome.

C. In this patient, the best evidence supports a therapeutic window of 24 hours from symptom onset.

D. The likelihood of good outcome with a modified Rankin Scale (mRS) score of 0 to 2 at 90 days and a reperfusion score of modified TICI (m-TICI) 2b to 3 is 49%.

E. Patient must receive EMT irrelevant of his prestroke mRS.

Questions 4-7

A 40-year-old right-handed woman with no past medical history and no history of trauma is admitted with abrupt severe headache and rapidly deteriorating mental status. On examination, she is confused and drowsy, moving all 4 extremities to painful stimuli. Her brain CT scan is shown below.

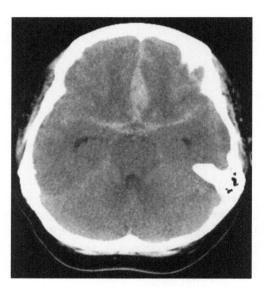

Noncontrast axial computed tomography of the head.

4. Which of the following statements is correct regarding this patient?

A. Giant aneurysms in the anterior circulation have a 60% risk of rupture.

B. Saccular berry aneurysms account for 70% of all aneurysms.

C. Ruptured saccular aneurysm is a rare cause of nontraumatic subarachnoid hemorrhage (SAH).

D. Fusiform aneurysms account for 30% of total aneurysms.

E. The most common location of fusiform aneurysms is the posterior circulation.

5. What is the risk of rebleeding during this hospitalization estimated to be?

    A. Risk of rebleeding in the first 24 hours is 80%.

    B. Daily risk of rebleeding is 2% to 3%.

    C. Rebleeding risk in the first 2 weeks is 5%.

    D. One-month risk of rebleeding is 10%.

    E. After the initial SAH, the 10-year cumulative risk of recurrent SAH after clipping is 9%.

6. After stabilizing the patient and providing proper treatment in the neurointensive care unit (neuro-ICU), a conventional cerebral angiogram was performed and is shown below. Which of the following statements is correct regarding the management of the patient's condition?

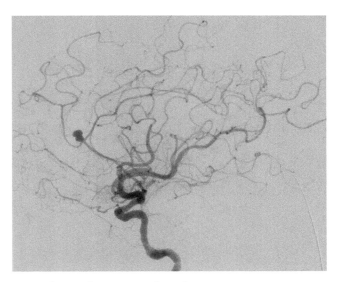

Internal carotid angiogram, lateral view.

    A. No further intervention is needed, and the patient can be managed only medically in the neuro-ICU.

    B. In the presence of impaired cardiovascular status, delayed intervention (surgical/endovascular) beyond 72 hours is highly recommended.

    C. Microsurgical clipping has a lower risk of secondary seizures compared to the endovascular approach.

    D. Based on the International Subarachnoid Aneurysm Trial (ISAT), endovascular coiling has low risk of death or dependency compared to the surgical approach.

    E. Microsurgical clipping has a higher risk of rebleeding compared to the endovascular procedure.

7. Seven days after admission and despite best medical treatment in the neuro-ICU, the patient started to have worsening mental status and left-sided weakness. Transcranial Doppler ultrasound showed progressive increased intracranial cerebral blood flow velocities. Which statement is correct regarding the patient's current condition?

    A. Local (intraventricular) administration of a calcium channel blocker is effective in preventing and treating this condition and is equally as effective as peripheral administration.

    B. Studies support the use of triple-H therapy to treat this condition.

    C. Intra-arterial balloon angioplasty has a long-term effect and targets more proximal arteries.

    D. Evidence supports the use of statins to prevent this condition.

    E. Achieving rapid subarachnoid blood clearance is significantly associated with better outcome.

8. A 35-year-old right-handed man presented with acute-onset right arm weakness, headache, and left anterior neck pain that he noted after he finished working out at the gym. He had no prior significant medical history. General examination was unremarkable. In the neurologic examination, a remarkable right arm drift with mild hemiparesis was noted. Brain and neck MRI scans were obtained followed by cerebral angiogram shown below. Which of the following statements is correct about the best way to manage this patient?

A. Starting both dual antiplatelet therapy and statins is recommended.

B. A high-dose IV steroid is the treatment of choice.

C. Lifelong IV heparin is recommended.

D. Carotid stenting is the mainstay of treatment.

E. Antiplatelet or short-term anticoagulation can be considered in treating this patient.

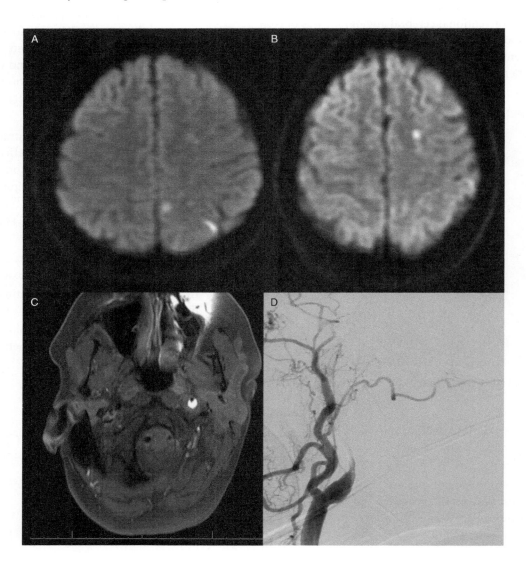

Questions 9 and 10

A 35-year-old woman with no significant past medical history presented with acute-onset right-sided hemiparesis that started 1 day prior. She also describes a history of multiple attacks of transient neurologic symptoms consistent with transient ischemic attacks (TIAs). MRI of the brain and cerebral angiogram are shown below.

9. What is the most likely explanation of this patient's clinical condition?

   A. Bilateral cardioembolic ischemic strokes

   B. Bilateral strokes secondary to hypercoagulable state

   C. Moyamoya disease

   D. Primary cerebral angiitis (vasculitis)

   E. Demyelinating disease

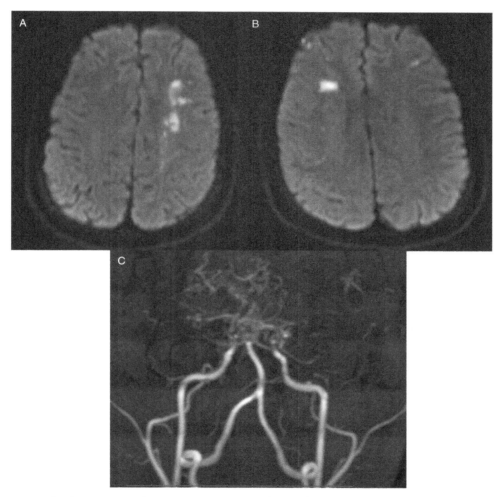

A and B. Diffusion-weighted imaging axial magnetic resonance imaging of the brain. **C.** Magnetic resonance angiography of the brain, anterior view.

10. Cerebral angiogram was performed for further evaluation (shown below). Which of the following is correct regarding the patient's condition?

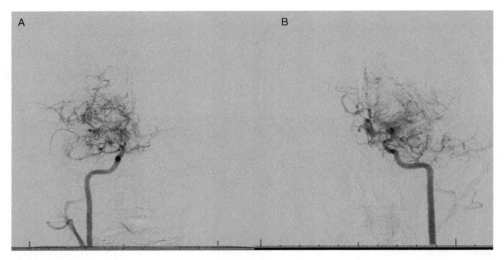

A. Right internal carotid artery angiogram, anterior projection. **B.** Left internal carotid artery angiogram, anterior projection.

    A. This condition can only lead to ischemic type of strokes.

    B. Long-term anticoagulation is recommended.

    C. The prognosis of young pediatric patients (<4 years old) is worse than adult patients.

    D. According to the 2015 revised diagnostic criteria for this disease, a cerebral angiogram is required in all unilateral disease.

    E. Treatment of this patient consists of high-dose IV steroids followed by long-term immunosuppressive therapy.

Questions 11-13

A 26-year-old right-handed woman presents with a history of persistent nonspecific headaches. As part of her diagnostic workup, the primary physician ordered a brain MRI, shown below.

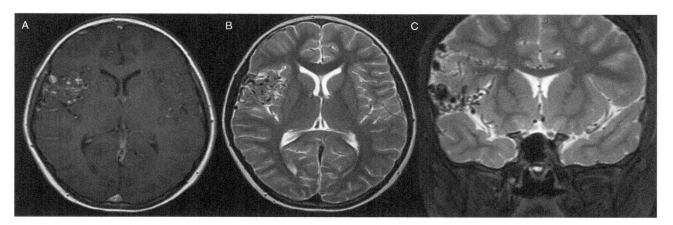

A. Axial brain magnetic resonance imaging (MRI) with contrast. **B.** Axial T2-weighted brain MRI. **C.** Coronal brain MRI.

11. Given the fact that the patient had no prior brain hemorrhage, what is the annual risk of bleeding secondary to this lesion?

A. 1%

B. 3%

C. 7%

D. 10%

E. 17%

12. What is the lifetime risk of hemorrhage in this particular patient?

A. 90%

B. 80%

C. 70%

D. 60%

E. 50%

13. Which of the following statements is correct regarding patient management?

A. Since the lesion was diagnosed incidentally with no signs of hemorrhage, no further treatment is recommended.

B. The effect of radiosurgery is immediate, with significant reduction in risk of bleeding within 1 week.

C. Complete cure following endovascular treatment has been reported in 45% to 50% of cases.

D. A recent randomized controlled trial concluded that medical management with interim follow-up is superior to intervention.

E. Overall permanent morbidity following endovascular treatment is estimated at 1%.

14. A 36-year-old right-handed man presented to the ED for sudden onset of headaches and left hemiplegia. His medical and familial history was noncontributory. Neurologic examination was significant for left hemiparesis. Upon further evaluation, cerebral angiogram was obtained and showed a left deep thalamic arteriovenous malformation (AVM) with a nidus of 4 cm in diameter and associated deep venous drainage. Based on Spetzler-Martin grading, what grade is this AVM?

A. Grade I

B. Grade II

C. Grade III

D. Grade IV

E. Grade V

15. A 70-year-old right-handed man with past medial history of prior ischemic strokes, chronic cigarette smoking, hypertension, and diabetes was referred by his primary physician for evaluation of recurrent spells of slurred speech and right arm numbness consistent with TIAs. The MRI of his brain and a cerebral angiogram showed right deep right MCA watershed ischemic infarcts and 60% right mid-MCA stenosis. In addition to controlling diabetes and recommending that the patient stop smoking, what is the most appropriate treatment for this lesion?

    A. Balloon angioplasty alone

    B. Balloon angioplasty and stenting of the right MCA

    C. Anticoagulant with warfarin and statin therapy

    D. Antiplatelet and statin therapy

    E. Antiplatelet and anticoagulant

16. A 79-year-old right-handed man with history of severe congestive heart failure with an ejection fraction of <20, uncontrolled hypertension end-stage renal failure, coronary artery disease, diabetes, and dyslipidemia presented to the ED after awakening with nonsense speech and right arm and lower face weakness. Initial CT of the brain showed chronic and subacute small lacunar strokes in the left MCA distribution. By the next day, he had improved significantly to the point where he had only mild right arm weakness and few paraphasic errors. Stroke workup was done including carotid ultrasound and CT angiography of the head and neck and both showed 80% to 89% left internal carotid stenosis just distal to the origin with bilateral common carotid bifurcation at the level of C2 spinal vertebrae. Which of the following statements is correct regarding this patient's management?

    A. Based on available evidence, medical treatment, with antithrombotic and risk factors modification, is the treatment of choice.

    B. Urgent carotid endarterectomy is strongly indicated.

    C. Endarterectomy is not indicated.

    D. Based on the patient's characteristics, internal carotid stenting carries lower risk compared to surgical intervention.

    E. Endarterectomy is highly recommended in high carotid bifurcation and is associated with low risk of complications.

17. A 70-year-old right-handed woman with past medical history significant for uncontrolled hypertension, diabetes, and dyslipidemia presented to the hospital with a 1-day history of left arm weakness and slurred speech. MRI of the brain showed acute small right corona radiata ischemic stroke, and CT angiography of the head and neck revealed 70% to 80% right internal carotid stenosis. Carotid endarterectomy (CEA) was considered. When is the recommended timing for this procedure based on current evidence?

    A. Within 2 weeks after stroke

    B. Urgent, as soon as possible

    C. Delayed until 3 to 4 months after stroke

    D. No current evidence available

    E. Within 2 months after stroke

18. A 27-year-old woman with no significant past medical history was admitted at 32 weeks of gestation with severe headaches, nausea, and vomiting. The patient had no previous history of trauma. A CT scan of the head revealed a right frontal lobe intracranial hemorrhage with adjacent subarachnoid hemorrhage. Which of the following statements is correct regarding this patient's condition?

    A. Most cerebral AVM hemorrhages occur between 20 weeks of pregnancy and 6 weeks postpartum.

    B. In pregnant patients with unruptured AVM, vaginal delivery will increase the cerebral AVM bleeding risk.

    C. The radiation dose of stereotactic radiotherapy in the treatment of pregnant women with cerebral AVM is above the safety threshold.

    D. The Spetzler-Martin classification for operative risk does not apply in pregnant patients with AVM.

    E. There is no role of endovascular treatment in pregnant patients with ruptured AVM.

19. A 31-year-old woman from Japan, with a history of headaches and transient right arm and leg weakness consistent with TIAs, presented to the ED with acute-onset right arm, face, and leg weakness of 2 days in duration. She also describes new-onset left arm pain, which is precipitated while combing her hair. Neurologic examination revealed right-sided hemiparesis and right lower face weakness, CT and magnetic resonance angiography of the head and neck are shown below. What is the most likely diagnosis?

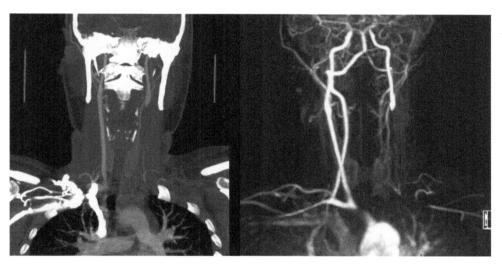

A. Extensive arterial dissection

B. Ischemic stroke with large artery thrombosis secondary to hypercoagulable state

C. Normal vascular variation

D. Takayasu arteritis

E. Cardioembolic stroke; extensive cardiac workup is warranted

20. A 36-year-old woman with no significant past medical history presented complaining of progressive spastic paraparesis and numbness in the lower extremities. Physical examination revealed increased tone in both legs with moderate bilateral symmetric weakness, hyperreflexia, and upgoing toe reflex. Sensory examination showed sensory loss below T10 dermatome. Thoracic spine MRI was consistent with spinal AVM at the level of T10 thoracic vertebrae. Spinal angiogram is recommended for further evaluation. Which of the following statements is correct regarding spinal angiography procedure?

    A. Blood supply to mid-lower thoracic spinal cord is through supreme intercostal artery.

    B. Anterior and posterior spinal arteries are in the midline.

    C. Right and left lower lumbar arteries both arise from the lateral wall of the aorta.

    D. Upper thoracic right-sided intercostal arteries arises from the lateral wall, and left-sided intercostal arteries are more posterior.

    E. Lumbar and lower thoracic region segmental branches usually arise just above the level of the pedicle.

21. A 44-year-old man with no significant past medical history presented with a left cranial nerve III deficit and sudden-onset severe headache. Physical examination showed a dilated right pupil with intact extraocular muscle movements; the rest of the examination was unremarkable. CT angiography of the head revealed a right posterior communicating artery aneurysm. For further evaluation, a diagnostic conventional angiogram was scheduled. Which of the following statements regarding the procedure is correct?

    A. In patients receiving heparin, the heparin infusion should be stopped 3 hours prior to the angiogram.

    B. Minimum platelet count for angiography is 50,000 plt/microL.

C. Contrast-induced nephropathy is usually defined as an increase in serum creatinine of 25% to 50% over baseline.

D. Metformin-associated lactic acidosis is very common and is associated with a 70% mortality rate.

E. Bovine aortic arch is when the innominate artery and right common carotid artery share a common origin.

22. A 55-year-old woman with history of coiled anterior communicating artery aneurysm 3 years ago presented to the same-day surgery unit for a follow-up cerebral angiogram. The procedure was done using the transfemoral artery approach. Which of the following is correct regarding femoral artery access site for a transcatheter procedure?

    A. The femoral artery is grossly located one-third of the distance from the anterior superior iliac spine to the symphysis pubis.

    B. Females have a lower risk of access site complication compared with males.

    C. Several studies found that left groin puncture is associated with an increased risk of femoral pseudoaneurysms and arteriovenous fistula formation.

    D. High stick is one of the risk factors for the development of arteriovenous fistula.

    E. Access site hematoma commonly requires surgical evacuation.

Answers and Explanations

1. **C.** This patient has a vein of Galen malformation (VGM). VGM is a rare congenital vascular malformation that results from maldevelopment of the intracranial embryonic midline venous system at the level of the median prosencephalic vein of Markowski, which is considered as the embryonic precursor of the vein of Galen. VGMs are postulated to arise during the fetal period; they consist of a cerebral arteriovenous malformation draining into the vein of Galen. The age of presentation varies and can be immediately after birth ("neonatal period"; 44% of cases), in infancy (41%), or in the early childhood and adult period (12%). Clinically, patients can have different presentations, including high cardiac output failure secondary to venous shifting phenomena, hydrocephalus (communicating and no-communicating), and cerebral ischemia due to steal phenomena and intracranial hemorrhage.

   Ideally, if the patient's clinical condition is stable and the patient is not in heart failure or does not have signs of cerebral ischemia, treatment should be deferred until 5 to 6 months of age to minimize the risk of affecting brain maturation. Untreated, the mortality rate reaches 100%. Treatment options include surgical, medical, endovascular, and combined. The timing of treatment has always been controversial; the 12-point Bicêtre scoring system is one method used to guide patient selection and timing of intervention in the neonatal period.

   The main goal of medical treatment is to decrease the flow through VGM and hemodynamically stabilize the patient until definite treatment can be done safely.

   Despite advances in microneurosurgical techniques, complete removal of the lesion in newborns is seldom accomplished or advised because of the hemodynamic instability, location of the lesion, poor myelination of the brain parenchyma (in younger patients), and cerebral venous hypertension. As a result, currently, surgical treatment is reserved for the evacuation of intracranial hematomas, management of hydrocephalus, or in cases of embolization failure.

   Congestive heart failure refractory to medical management in a newborn necessitates emergency embolization to relieve the hemodynamic overload. In such cases, staged partial, rather than complete, obliteration is the goal of endovascular embolization to allow for redistribution of blood flow to the heart and brain to permit normal cardiac and neurologic development. The advances of endovascular therapy, together with a comprehensive multidisciplinary approach involving pediatric intensive care units, have considerably enhanced the prognosis of patients with VGM.

2. **D.** Unruptured intracranial aneurysms (UIA) occur in approximately 3% of the population. Most of these lesions are found incidentally, are asymptomatic and typically carry a benign course. The natural history of UIA was evaluated in 7 large observational studies. The ISUIA and the cohort of Japanese patients with UCAS Japan study are 2 examples of large cohort studies exploring the natural history of UIAs. In both studies, data showed strong associations between the size of aneurysm and risk of rupture. In the ISUIA study, data indicated that aneurysm size (especially in patients who were diagnosed with UIAs) and location have a significant role in determining the risk of future rupture.

   In the same study, the risk of aneurysm rupture over 5 years was 0% among aneurysms in the anterior circulation <7 mm in diameter (0.1% per year), 2.6% for aneurysms between 7 and 12 mm in diameter, 14.5% for those 13 to 24 mm in diameter, and 40% for diameters >25 mm (Table 15-1). Across all aneurysm sizes, rupture risks were higher among the posterior circulation aneurysms. The Japanese cohort displayed similar results to ISUIA with clear association between the risk of rupture and aneurysm size; however, the Japanese study did not

Table 15-1. Anterior Circulation Aneurysm and 5-Year Rupture Risk

Anterior Circulation Aneurysm Size (mm)	5-Year Risk of Rupture (%)
<7 mm	0%
7-12 mm	2.6%
13-24 mm	14.5%
>25 mm	40%

show any increased risk of rupture between anterior versus posterior circulations. However, it did show an elevated risk of rupture in aneurysms involving anterior communicating or posterior communicating arteries compared to other aneurysm locations. Other elements that have been reported to be associated with rupture of a UIA include prior history of subarachnoid hemorrhage, presence of daughter sac, multiple aneurysms, hypertension (uncontrolled), cigarette smoking, and heavy alcohol consumption. The main factor in UIA management is balancing the risk of rupture versus risk of intervention (surgical or endovascular), and it should be individualized for each patient. If the UIA is deemed to have low risk for rupture, then conservative management is reasonable. This mainly focuses on optimizing the modifiable factors associated with higher risk of rupture, which include smoking cessation and blood pressure control in conjunction with radiographic imaging to monitor aneurysm growth (may include noninvasive imaging 6-12 months after initial discovery of a UIA). It has been shown that aneurysms that demonstrate growth on follow-up have rupture rates of about 3% per year compared to about 0.1% per year for stable-size aneurysms. Once the risk of rupture becomes higher than intervention risk, the decision to intervene is considered; the type of intervention (endovascular vs craniotomy) depends on several factors, including patient's age, comorbidities, procedural risks, and aneurysmal factors (location, size, and morphology). Options for endovascular therapies include coiling alone or balloon-assisted/stent-assisted coil embolization and flow-diverting stenting.

3. **D.** Approximately one-third of acute ischemic strokes are caused by an occlusion of a large, proximal cerebral vessel. The natural history of an acute ischemic stroke from a large vessel occlusion (LVO) is poor and has challenged stroke therapy. Since its approval, unless contraindicated, IV tPA is still considered the standard of care for patients suffering from acute ischemic stroke within 3 hours of symptoms onset, with an extended time window up to 4.5 hours in certain patient populations. However, <50% of patients with LVO treated with IV thrombolysis recanalize; part of this failure is secondary to the clot burden and the inability of IV tPA to recanalize large-size clots. IV tPA is not contraindicated if EMT is considered, and EMT should not delay IV tPA administration. Multiple randomized controlled trials (RCTs) have assessed the efficacy of EMT compared with medical management for acute ischemic stroke. First-generation trials, such as the SYNTHESIS Expansion and MR RESCUE studies, did not show superiority of endovascular therapy over IV tPA following acute ischemic stroke. However, with the advances in endovascular technology and devices, the recent MR CLEAN, EXTEND-IA, ESCAPE, REVASCAT, and SWIFT PRIME studies have all established improved functional outcomes (efficacy and superiority) via endovascular therapy with no differences in mortality and intracerebral hemorrhage. Table 15-2 provides a summary of recent trials.

The recent trials shown in Table 15-2 have helped clarify some predictors of response to EMT, for example, presence of a LVO, evidence of significant neurologic deficit to justify the risk of intervention, and treatment initiation within time window from onset. The recent trials generally enrolled patients with National Institutes of Health Stroke Scale (NIHSS) scores >6. Although recent trial data suggest that EMT is unlikely to lead to a mRS of 0 to 2 in these patients, EMT doubled the chance of improving these patients' baseline mRS.

The m-TICI score is simple and has good interobserver reliability. It is clear that patients have the best chance at recovery when angiographic reperfusion is m-TICI 2b/3. The angiographic definition of success should therefore be at least m-TICI 2b/3 reperfusion, with a time goal of reperfusion within 30 minutes after starting the procedure. The functional clinical outcome (measured by mRS) reported in the second-generation trials improved with increasing effectiveness of recanalization. Patients with partial recanalization (TICI 2a) did not do as well as those with

Table 15-2. Summary of Acute Ischemic Stroke Thrombectomy Trials

Study	Location	Window/ Eligibility	LVO Determination MCA/ICA	Imaging Other than CTA/ ASPECT	Use of Stent-Retriever (%)	Premature Termination	Outcome	Outcome (%), EMT vs Medical
MR CLEAN, N = 500	16 sites, Netherlands	≤6 hours	Yes	No	82	No	mRS at 90 days	32 vs 19
EXTEND IA, N = 70	14 centers, Australia, New Zealand	≤4.5 hours 6 hours EMT CTP core <70 mL	Yes	Rapid CTP	100	Yes, because of external evidence/efficacy	Reperfusion at 24 hours and early neurologic improvement	71 vs 40
ESCAPE, N = 316	22 sites, United States, Canada, UK, SK	≤12 hours Multiphasic CTA	Yes	Multiphasic CTA	86	Yes, because of external evidence/efficacy	mRS at 90 days	53 vs 29
REVASCAT, N = 206	4 centers, Spain	≤8 hours IVtPA failure or IVtPA contraindicated	Yes	No	100	Yes, because of external evidence/efficacy	mRS (shift analysis) at 90 days; mRS (0-2) at 90 days	44 vs 28
SWIFT PRIME, N = 196	39 sites, United States/ Europe	≤4.5 hours 6 hours EMT CTP small core 50 mL (71 patients) ASPECTS ≥6 (125 patients)	Yes	Rapid CTP	100	Yes, because of external evidence/efficacy	mRS 0-2 at 90 days	60 vs 35

Abbreviations: ASPECT, Alberta Stroke Program Early Computed Tomography score; CTA, computed tomography angiogram; CTP, computed tomography perfusion scan; EMT, endovascular mechanical thrombectomy; ICA, internal carotid artery; IVtPA, intravenous tissue plasminogen activator; MCA, middle cerebral artery; mRS, modified Rankin Score; SK, South Korea; UK, United Kingdom.

near complete/complete recanalization. TICI 2b/3 reflected the highest functional outcome (34% with a TICI grade of 2a had an mRS score of 0 to 2 at 90 days vs 49% with a TICI grade of 2b/3).

Based on recent trials, American Heart Association/American Stroke Association published an update of the 2013 Guidelines for the Early Management of Patients with Acute Ischemic Stroke Regarding Endovascular Treatment, and the following recommendation was added: Patients should receive endovascular therapy with a stent retriever if they meet all the following criteria: prestroke mRS score 0 to 1; acute ischemic stroke receiving IV tPA within the recommended therapeutic window "according to guidelines from professional medical societies"; causative occlusion of the internal carotid artery or proximal MCA (M1); age ≥18 years; NIHSS score of ≥6; Alberta Stroke Program Early Computed Tomography Score (ASPECTS) of ≥6; and treatment can be initiated (groin puncture) within 6 hours of symptom onset.

4. **E; 5 B; 6 D; 7C.** Aneurysmal subarachnoid hemorrhage (SAH) is a health burden with high mortality and permanent disability rates. SAH secondary to aneurysmal rupture accounts for approximately 80% of SAH. The main risk factors for developing cerebral aneurysms are hypertension, smoking, chronic alcohol use, female sex, and family history of intracranial aneurysms in first-degree relatives. Aneurysms are often an incidental finding during investigations for various neurologic symptoms (eg, nonspecific headache, cranial neuropathies, or symptoms of brainstem dysfunction). However, the most common presenting feature of an aneurysm is SAH. Once the diagnosis of nontraumatic SAH is established, noninvasive cerebral vascular imaging is commonly used to establish the etiology. Studies have shown that saccular berry aneurysms account for 90% of the total aneurysm morphology, and their rupture is the most common cause of SAH. Fusiform aneurysms, which are commonly located in the posterior circulation, account for the remaining 10%.

In patients with aneurysmal SAH, the peak rate of rebleeding occurs in the first 24 hours and is reported to range from 4% to 14%. The rebleed rate has been estimated to be approximately 20% within the first 2 weeks of the initial bleeding and 40% at 1 month. The roughly daily rate of rebleeding is 2% to 3% per day. After clipping, the long-term risk (10-year risk) of recurrent SAH is 3.2%.

The leading cause of morbidity and mortality after surviving the rupture of an intracranial aneurysm is delayed cerebral ischemia (DCI), which is strongly linked to the occurrence of vasospasm. DCI is defined as vasospasm including clinical deterioration. Cerebral vasospasm typically occurs between days 4 and 14 after aneurysm rupture and resolves spontaneously after 21 days. Traditionally, "triple-H" therapy, a combination of hypervolemia, induced arterial hypertension, and hemodilution, has been the cornerstone of treatment. However, recent data showed that isolated induced hypertension (tolerated by the cardiac status) and euvolemia are more effective. Dihydropyridine calcium channel blockers (eg, nimodipine) are recommended for all patients with aneurysmal SAH. A dose of 60 mg 6 times daily for 21 days improves the rate of good outcome significantly.

Strong evidence supports that magnesium does not reduce the incidence of clinical vasospasm. Based on current studies, including the Simvastatin in Aneurysmal Subarachnoid Hemorrhage (STASH) trial, statins are not recommended and have no significant effect on preventing or treating vasospasm secondary to aneurysmal SAH. Although, a good result is associated with using calcium channel blockers peripherally, intrathecal (intraventricular) injection of nicardipine did not show any effect on outcome in multiple studies; however, it was able to reduce transcranial Doppler–measured flow velocities. The use of intrathecal thrombolytic drugs is associated with a higher subarachnoid blood clearance rate; however, no consistent benefits on long-term outcome have been shown. Finally, endovascular treatment has become an integral part of the management of patients with medically refractory vasospasm because it can produce angiographic resolution. Two methods have been used: intra-arterial vasodilator and balloon angioplasty. Typically, angioplasty targets proximal arteries with immediate long-term effect; in contrast, the effect of intra-arterial vasodilators is transient and usually targets more distal arteries. Due to limited data, further randomized studies are needed to carefully evaluate the effect of the endovascular approach in such conditions.

The main goal of therapy in aneurysmal SAH is to secure the aneurysm (by complete and permanent occlusion of the aneurysm sac) by either surgical clipping or endovascular intervention. Successful intervention will prevent subsequent complications. Although the data did not provide solid evidence regarding the effect of intervention timing on outcome, most clinicians advocate for early intervention, with the aims of lowering the risk of rebleeding and enabling safe and effective management of vasospasm. An analysis of data from a Nationwide Inpatient Sample that included 32,048 US patients with aneurysmal SAH revealed that patients treated early (within 48 hours of admission) with coiling or surgery are more likely to be discharged with little or no disability.

Microsurgical techniques, endovascular approaches, and a combination of both are all options used to treat aneurysms. The main question is which approach carries lower risk in each particular patient. To answer which approach is better, multiple studies have attempted to compare microsurgical clipping with endovascular coiling. Currently, only 3 randomized, prospective studies compare microsurgical clipping and endovascular coiling. One of the large studies is the International Subarachnoid Aneurysm Trial (ISAT). In this study and the subsequent follow-up reports, the rate of occlusion was higher in clipped aneurysms (82%) compared to coiled aneurysms (66%), and coiling resulted in a significant decrease in the rate of death or dependency compared to clipping (24% vs 31%, respectively). Furthermore, the rebleeding rate was low, and the rate of epilepsy was higher in microsurgical patients. Discussing the details of these trials is beyond the scope of this chapter; please refer to the references for more information. In 2012, in response to multiple criticisms of ISAT, the Barrow Ruptured Aneurysm Trial (BRAT) was conducted. BRAT had similar findings as the ISAT with improved outcomes in the coiled group at 12 months. These finding persisted at the 3-year follow-up published in 2013. Although coiling currently appears to be advantageous, additional long-term studies are needed.

8. **E.** Arterial dissection is one of the potential etiologies of ischemic stroke in young adults (<50 years old); it is the most common lesion of the cervical arteries after atherosclerosis. Dissection has traditionally been described as either spontaneous or secondary to major trauma. A population-based study published in 2006 estimated the incidence as 1.72 per 100,000 per year for internal carotid artery dissections and 0.97 per 100,000 for vertebral artery dissection. As a stroke etiology, arterial dissection was found to account for about 2% of all ischemic strokes. Apart from trauma, dissection is likely multifactorial, and both environmental and genetic risk factors have been implicated. When involving the cervical internal carotid, dissection typically begins 2 to 3 cm distal to the internal carotid origin; distally, the skull base limits the dissection extent. Clinical manifestations of dissections include both local and ischemic-related events (either due to thromboembolic phenomena or flow impairment). For example, locally, carotid artery dissection can cause Horner syndrome, neck pain, facial pain, and cranial neuropathies. Conventional angiography was the diagnostic mainstay for many years; however, it has now been largely replaced by noninvasive imaging, such as CT angiography (CTA) and MR angiography (MRA). MRA can be combined with axial T1-weighted cervical MRI (see part C of figure) with fat suppression to better identify small intramural hematomas and does not require radiation. Treatment with antiplatelet agents is recommended over oral anticoagulants (Level of Evidence IA).

9. **C; 10 D.** Moyamoya disease (MMD) is a chronic, progressive steno-occlusive cerebrovascular disease affecting the terminal portion (intracranial) of the internal carotid artery (ICA) with associated abnormal vascular network at the base of the brain. The term MMD refers to isolated and primary moyamoya angiopathy, which is usually bilateral. In contrast, moyamoya syndrome refers to moyamoya angiopathy pattern associated with other manifestations, with or without a well-known associated inherited or acquired condition; this can be unilateral or bilateral. MMD was described in 1960 by a Japanese neurosurgeon. For an unknown reason, MMD is relatively more common in the East Asian population (Korea and Japan), as compared with those in the Western Hemisphere. Based on Japanese studies, female sex is associated with a higher incidence, and females are affected at a younger age compared to male patients. MMD may present with multiple different clinical symptoms including

ischemic stroke, hemorrhagic stroke, seizures, headache, and cognitive impairment. The main 2 forms are ischemia and hemorrhagic strokes. Most children with MMD develop ischemic complications, such as transient ischemic attack and cerebral infarction, and around half of adult patients have intracranial hemorrhage and half have ischemic stroke. In the past, the proposed diagnostic criteria consisted of 3 principal factors: (1) stenosis or occlusion at the terminal portion of the ICA and/or at the proximal portion of the anterior and/or middle cerebral arteries; (2) abnormal vascular networks in the vicinity of the occlusive or stenotic lesions in the arterial phase; and (3) bilateral involvement. However, the diagnostic criteria were modified in 2015, including patients with unilateral terminal ICA as well. The newer criteria require performing cerebral angiography. Based on various angiographic findings, Suzuki and Takaku proposed an angiographic staging system consisting of 6 stages. This staging system is mainly based on serial angiographic changes over time in the degree of development of MMD. The modified Suzuki grading system was recently introduced, which provides precise grading based on 1 angiographic study with classification of posterior circulation involvement. Traditionally, surgical revascularization has been performed on ischemic MMD patients. It aims to improve cerebral blood flow and restore reserve capacity. Recently, endovascular treatment (using angioplasty with or without stenting) has been proposed; however, evidence is limited to case reports, and it should not be considered as standard therapy. Antiplatelet therapy using aspirin and avoiding dehydration and low blood pressures are used for stroke prevention and hypoperfusion-induced events. Anticoagulation is not indicated. IV steroids are not a treatment option used in this disease. The prognosis in patients with MMD is poor; however, pediatric patients (<4 years old) have a better prognosis than adults.

11. **B; 12 B; 13 D.** Arteriovenous malformations (AVMs) are congenital vascular lesions that may appear throughout the central nervous system. They consist of direct connections between arteries and veins, without an intervening capillary bed or normal brain tissue. AVMs are assumed to appear during fetal life; however, the exact etiology is unknown. The estimated prevalence is as high as 0.5% of the general population based on the Cooperative Study of Intracranial Aneurysms and Subarachnoid Hemorrhage and early autopsy series. AVMs can commonly cause the following clinical presentations: hemorrhage (most common presentation, around 50% of patient with AVM), seizures (second most common), and headaches. Risk of hemorrhage is thought to be around 3% to 4% yearly after diagnosis of an AVM in patients who present without intracranial hemorrhage. Assuming a 3% annual risk, lifetime risk can be calculated using the following simple formula: Lifetime risk (%) = 105 – the patient's age in years. The yearly risk after a clinical hemorrhage was reported to be as high as 7% in the first year.

14. **D.** One of the popular grading systems established to predict outcome (rate of obliteration, morbidity,

Table 15-3. Spetzler-Martin Grading System

Graded Features	Points Assigned
Size of arteriovenous malformation	
Small (<3 cm)	1
Medium (3-6 cm)	2
Large (>6 cm)	3
Eloquence of adjacent brain	
Noneloquent	0
Eloquent	1
Pattern of venous drainage	
Superficial only	0
Deep	1

Arteriovenous malformation grade (1-5) equals total number of points.

and mortality) in surgically treated patient is the Spetzler-Martin grading system (Table 15-3).

Based on this grading system, risk of permanent major neurologic morbidity was negligible in grades I, II, and III AVMs. However, patients with high-grade AVMs had a worse outlook compared to low-grade lesions. For example, in patients with grades IV and V AVMs, the permanent major neurologic morbidity rate was noted to be as high as 22%.

In 2011, a large meta-analysis from 137 studies concluded that although overall case fatalities were low, there was still a considerable risk of significant complications leading to permanent neurologic deficits after AVM resection, radiosurgery, and embolization (up to 7%). The final decision about the most appropriate treatment for any patient with an AVM will take into account many factors, such as age, neurologic status, associated clinical risk factors, and angioarchitectural features of the AVM. All 3 treatment modalities—microsurgery, endovascular embolization, and radiosurgery—have an established role in treatment of patients with AVMs. For ruptured AVM (patient presents with intracranial bleeding), most clinicians treat patients on a semi-elective basis after proper medical management, to allow patient stabilization and recovery from the initial insult; however, others advocate early intervention in most cases, especially for expanding hematoma and/or when the lesion is accessible surgically. In patients with unruptured AVMs, debates have occurred in the past about whether preventive lesion eradication offers a clinical benefit. Recently, in 2014, results from the large Randomized Trial of Unruptured Brain AVMs (ARUBA) were published. ARUBA is the first RCT assessing the outcomes from 2 management strategies (medical management with interventional therapy or medical management alone) in patients diagnosed with unruptured AVMs. ARUBA concluded that in unruptured AVMs with interim follow-up, medical management alone was superior to medical management with interventional therapy. It confirmed a low spontaneous rupture rate of 2% per year. Although the study was halted early and did introduce many controversies in this field, it provided valuable results and raised more questions that need to be answered in future studies.

Radiosurgery as a treatment option can be used alone or with other therapy, the advantages of radiosurgery are that it is minimally invasive, relatively low-risk, and useful for treatment of surgically inaccessible lesions. Disadvantages include a latency period (usually 2-3 years) until AVM obliteration occurs (risk of hemorrhage persists during the latency period) and that it is most effective for smaller lesions. Regarding endovascular treatment alone, complete AVM obliteration has been reported in 5% to 10% of cases. The relatively low cure rate with embolization alone is probably due to few AVMs with several pedicles that can be safely catheterized. Most of the time, endovascular embolization is followed by radiosurgery and/or microsurgery. The overall rate of permanent morbidity following endovascular therapy varies between studies; however, it has been estimated to be between 2% and 14%, with mortality between 1% and 3%.

15. **D.** The most likely cause of this patient's symptoms is the evident stenosis of the right MCA, and the most appropriate treatment, based on available evidence, for this lesion is optimization of risk factors and antiplatelet therapy.

   Intracranial atherosclerosis is a common cause of stroke and is associated with a high risk of recurrent stroke, especially in patients with a recent stroke or TIA and severe arterial stenosis. The SAMMPRIS trial was designed to assess whether percutaneous transluminal angioplasty and stenting plus aggressive medical treatment is more effective than aggressive medical treatment alone in high-risk patients with intracranial atherosclerotic disease. The results showed that at 30 days, the risk of stroke or death using aggressive medical treatment was less than that of stenting of the intracranial vessels (5.8% vs 14.7%). At 1 year, the risk of the primary event was higher among those in the stent group compared to those in the aggressive medical treatment group (20% vs 12%). These results persisted over extended follow-up (2 years of follow-up) in subsequent reports. Given the current evidence, the role of stenting of intracranial arteries is not clear, and therefore, the best option is antiplatelet therapy. The patient will still need strict and aggressive risk factor control including statin therapy. According to SAMMPRIS, aggressive medical management includes aspirin, at a dose of 325 mg/d, or clopidogrel, at a dose of 75 mg/d, for 90 days after enrollment; management of the primary risk factors (elevated systolic blood pressure and elevated low-density lipoprotein [LDL] cholesterol levels); and management of secondary risk factors (diabetes, elevated non–high-density lipoprotein [non-HDL] cholesterol levels, smoking, excess weight, and insufficient exercise) with the help of a lifestyle modification program. With respect to the primary risk factors, target systolic blood pressure was <140 mm Hg (<130 mm Hg in the case of patients with diabetes), and target LDL cholesterol level was <70 mg/dL (1.81 mmol/L).

16. **D.** Carotid stenosis is a major cause of ischemic stroke; therefore, the goal of carotid artery stenosis

treatment is to reduce the risk secondary to this disease process. Carotid endarterectomy (CEA) has been an effective approach to preventing stroke, and recently, carotid artery stenting has provided a less invasive alternative. Numerous studies have demonstrated that carotid artery stenting is inferior to endarterectomy because stenting increases the stroke or death rate within 30 days of treatment. Other studies, including more than 2500 patients from 2002 to 2008, have shown that carotid artery stenting might be equivalent to endarterectomy, especially in patients younger than 70-years old.

CREST (Carotid Revascularization Endarterectomy Versus Stent Trial) is considered one of the largest RCTs to evaluate the efficacy of carotid artery stenting versus CEA in patients with carotid stenosis. CREST concluded that there were no significant advantages for either intervention for primary end points (defined as stroke, myocardial infarction, or death) for symptomatic carotid disease. The rate of stroke or death with carotid stenting among symptomatic patients (6.0%) was lower than the rates achieved in prior trials, whereas the same low rate compared to prior trials was noted among symptomatic patients who underwent endarterectomy (3.2%). However, the periprocedural stroke and death rates were significantly higher in the stenting group up to 10 years postoperatively. The optimal timing of surgical or endovascular treatment of carotid stenosis after a cerebral ischemic event is controversial. Surgery within 7 days of a stroke has been found to be a risk factor for complications with CEA. Meta-analysis has shown that endarterectomy in neurologically stable patients with TIA or minor stroke is not associated with a substantially higher operative risk than delayed endarterectomy, and the same can be concluded regarding the stenting option based on CREST subanalysis.

17. **D.** Most clinicians wait 1 to 2 weeks after stroke to perform CEA and proceed more quickly for TIA or crescendo TIA. The following factors increase the risk of surgical intervention in carotid stenosis, and stenting is an alternative option: (1) a previous history of myocardial infarction, angina, or hypertension; (2) coronary artery disease; (3) congestive heart failure; (4) age >75 years old; (5) high carotid bifurcation; (6) prior endarterectomy; and (7) prior neck radiation.

18. **A.** Commonly, AVMs present at a young age (between 20 and 40 years of age). For women, this age is considered the age of pregnancy, and potentially, AVM can occur during pregnancy. Pregnancy with cerebral AVM is a complex situation, and multiple potential scenarios can happen (preexisting AVM prior to pregnancy, incidentally found during pregnancy, and intracranial bleeding prior to or during pregnancy); in every situation, the management is different and complex. Studies have found that the hemorrhagic risk of cerebral AVM during pregnancy was between 3% and 6%. AVM bleeding in pregnant patients can lead to a maternal mortality rate of 28% and fetal death rate of 14%. Most cerebral AVM hemorrhages occur between 20 weeks of pregnancy and 6 weeks postpartum; during the same period, maternal physiology and hemodynamics take place. Treatment of AVMs in pregnant patients is very challenging, and a careful analysis of each case should be done to decide on the optimum treatment. An emergency operation is necessary for AVM bleeding in pregnant patients if intracranial hematoma causes worsening of neurologic symptoms or cerebral herniation. As in nonpregnant patients, cerebral AVM operation risk should be graded according to the Spetzler-Martin classification. Endovascular intervention is considered a valid treatment option; however, its use is limited to few case reports and definite guidelines are not available. Although there is limited evidence, radiosurgery use has been described during pregnancy; however, this is not recommended and is highly controversial. The radiation dose of stereotactic radiotherapy in the treatment of pregnant patients with cerebral AVM is below the safety threshold. However, it is not considered a first option in treating this group of patients. There is no evidence suggesting that vaginal delivery will increase the cerebral AVM bleeding risk, with no evidence to support that cesarean section can prevent the hemorrhage of AVM.

19. **D.** Takayasu arteritis (TA) is a rare, chronic large-vessel granulomatous arteritis of unknown etiology that affects the aorta and its major branches. TA is commonly seen in Japan, South East Asia, India, and Mexico. TA tends to occur in female patients in the second or third decade of life. The most frequently affected large arteries are ascending/descending aorta and the subclavian

and extracranial arteries such as carotids. According to a Japanese nationwide registry, there were at least 5881 TA patients in Japan in 2011, and the prevalence is thought to be >0.004%. A set of classification criteria for TA was established by the American College of Rheumatology; however, in clinical practice, the use of these criteria is limited to differentiate the disease from other possible causes such as giant cell arteritis or atherosclerotic disease. Treatment choices are limited to observational studies and usually are based on case-by-case clinician decision. Treatment is mainly focused on controlling the activity of inflammation with immunosuppressive therapy. A revascularization approach, either surgical or interventional, can be considered in certain cases, typically after controlling the active phase of the disease.

20. **D.** See Table 15-4 for the blood supply to different spinal regions. The anterior spinal artery is in the midline. The posterolateral spinal arteries are slightly off midline. Upper thoracic right-sided intercostal arteries arise from the lateral wall of the aorta; the left are more posterior. Right and left lower lumbar arteries both arise from the posterior wall of the aorta. Lower lumbar arteries may have a common origin of both the right and left lumbar artery from the aorta. Remember, in lumbar and lower thoracic regions, segmental branches usually arise just below the level of the pedicle.

Table 15-4. Spinal Cord Blood Supply

Level	Feeding Arteries
Upper cervical	Vertebral, ascending pharyngeal, occipital deep cervical
Lower cervical	Vertebral, deep cervical, ascending cervical
Upper thoracic	Supreme intercostal, superior intercostal
Mid-lower thoracic	Intercostal
Upper lumber	Lumber
Lower lumber	Ileolumber
Sacrum	Sacral (anterior and lateral)

21. **D.** Iodinated contrast-induced nephropathy usually appears as an acute worsening in renal function within 3 to 4 days of exposure. It is usually defined as an increase in serum creatinine of 25% to 50% over baseline or an absolute rise in serum creatinine of 0.5 to 1 mg/dL. For patients with dialysis-dependent renal failure, arrangements should be made with the patient's nephrologist to schedule dialysis after the angiogram. In patients receiving heparin, the heparin infusion should be stopped 6 hours prior to the angiogram. If the need is urgent, an angiogram can be done in patients on heparin or who are coagulopathic with minimal risk. The initial puncture should be made with a micropuncture set to minimize potential bleeding. Minimum platelet count for angiography is 75,000 cells/μL. Metformin-associated lactic acidosis is a rare complication and is associated with 50% mortality rate. Bovine aortic arch is when the innominate artery and left common carotid artery share a common origin.

22. **C.** Percutaneous-based vascular procedures continue to increase as endovascular techniques improve and provide a less morbid approach than the open vascular procedures. Femoral access has been and is currently the most frequently used arterial access. The femoral artery is located one-half the distance from the anterior superior iliac spine to the symphysis pubis. Medial to the femoral artery lays the femoral vein, with the femoral nerve found lateral to the femoral artery. In almost all patients, the femoral artery crosses over the femoral head, with 99% of the bifurcation occurring below the midfemoral head. Typically, the femoral access site should be proximal to the bifurcation. The most common complications associated with percutaneous vascular intervention involve the access point of the procedure. Patient-specific factors associated with femoral access site complications include female sex, extremes in body weight, previous access or bypass procedures, and high femoral artery bifurcation, whereas factors linked to procedural technique include left versus right groin, method of puncture, site of arterial entry, size of sheath used, use of anticoagulation during or after the procedure and closure device use.

The reported incidence of access site complications varies in the literature, mainly because of the retrospective nature of these reviews. The most common complications include groin hematoma, pseudoaneursyms, arteriovenous fistula, retroperitoneal hemorrhage, and vessel occlusion. In a recent series, the incidence of pseudoaneurysms was 5.3%, arteriovenous fistula 0.6%, and femoral artery dissection 1.6%. Furthermore, left groin punctures were found to be associated with higher risk of pseudoaneurysm and fistula compared to right femoral artery access. The incidence of hematoma formation following femoral artery catheterization also varies in the literature. However, operative evacuation of hematoma is rarely required. Identifying patients at risk of having access site complication after percutaneous catheterization is primitive to avoid subsequent associated morbidities.

REFERENCES

Akbik F, Hirsch JA, Cougo-Pinto PT, et al. The evolution of mechanical thrombectomy for acute stroke. *Curr Treat Options Cardiovasc Med.* 2016;18(5):32.

Alibaz-Oner F, Direskeneli H. Update on Takayasu's arteritis. *Presse Med.* 2015;44(6 Pt 2):e259-e265.

Berkhemer OA, Fransen PS, Beumer D, et al. A randomized trial of intraarterial treatment for acute ischemic stroke. *N Engl J Med.* 2015;372(1):11-20.

Bonati LH, Bobson J, Algra A, et al. Short-term outcome after stenting versus endarterectomy for symptomatic carotid stenosis: a preplanned meta-analysis of individual patient data. *Lancet.* 2010;376:1062-1073.

Brinjikji W, Zhu YQ, Lanzino G, et al. Risk factors for growth of intracranial aneurysms: a systematic review and meta-analysis. *AJNR Am J Neuroradiol.* 2016;37:615-620.

Brott TG, Halperin JL, Abbara S, et al. 2011 ASA/ACCF/AHA/AANN/AANS/ACR/ASNR/CNS/SAIP/SCAI/SIR/SNIS/SVM/SVS guideline on the management of patients with extracranial carotid and vertebral artery disease: a report of the American College of Cardiology Foundation/American Heart Association Task Force on Practice Guidelines, and the American Stroke Association, American Association of Neuroscience Nurses, American Association of Neurological Surgeons, American College of Radiology, American Society of Neuroradiology, Congress of Neurological Surgeons, Society of Atherosclerosis Imaging and Prevention, Society for Cardiovascular Angiography and Interventions, Society of Interventional Radiology, Society of NeuroInterventional Surgery, Society for Vascular Medicine, and Society for Vascular Surgery Developed in Collaboration with the American Academy of Neurology and Society of Cardiovascular Computed Tomography. *J Am Coll Cardiol.* 2011;57(8):e16-e94.

Campbell BCV, Mitchell PJ, Kleinig TJ, et al. Endovascular therapy for ischemic stroke with perfusion-imaging selection. *N Engl J Med.* 2015;372(11):1009-1018.

Chimowitz MI, Bäzner H, Nelson PK. Stenting versus aggressive medical therapy for intracranial arterial stenosis. *N Engl J Med.* 2011;365(11):993-1003.

Ciccone A, Valvassori L, Nichelatti M, et al. Endovascular treatment for acute ischemic stroke. *N Engl J Med.* 2013; 368(10):904-913.

Drake CG, Peerless SJ. Giant fusiform intracranial aneurysms: review of 120 patients treated surgically from 1965 to 1992. *J Neurosurg.* 1997;87(2):141-162.

D'Souza S. Aneurysmal subarachnoid hemorrhage. *J Neurosurg Anesthesiol.* 2015;27(3):222-240.

Fleetwood IG, Steinberg GK. Arteriovenous malformations. *Lancet.* 2002;359(9309):863-873.

Goyal M, Demchuk AM, Menon BK, et al. Randomized assessment of rapid endovascular treatment of ischemic stroke. *N Engl J Med.* 2015;372(11):1019-1030.

Gupta AK, Varma DR. Vein of Galen malformations: review. *Neurol India.* 2004;52:43-53.

Gupta AK, Rao VR, Varma DR, et al. Evaluation, management, and long-term follow up of vein of Galen malformations. *J Neurosurg.* 2006;105:26-33.

Harrigan MR, Deveikis JP. Arteriovenous malformations. In: *Handbook of Cerebrovascular Disease and Neurointerventional Technique.* Totowa, NJ: Humana Press; 2013: 571-602.

Harrigan MR, Deveikis JP. Diagnostic cerebral angiography. In: *Handbook of Cerebrovascular Disease and Neurointerventional Technique.* Totowa, NJ: Humana Press; 2013:99-131.

Harrigan MR, Deveikis JP. Intracranial aneurysms and subarachnoid haemorrhage. In: *Handbook of Cerebrovascular Disease and Neurointerventional Technique.* Totowa, NJ: Humana Press; 2013:483-569.

Harrigan MR, Deveikis JP. Spinal angiography. In: *Handbook of Cerebrovascular Disease and Neurointerventional Technique.* Totowa, NJ: Humana Press; 2013:133-151.

Hishikawa T, Sugiu K, Date I. Moyamoya disease: a review of clinical research. *Acta Med Okayama.* 2016;70(4):229-236.

Hoang S, Choudhri O, Edwards M, et al. Vein of Galen malformation. *Neurosurg Focus.* 2009;27:E8.

Ishibashi T, Murayama Y, Urashima M, et al. Unruptured intracranial aneurysms: incidence of rupture and risk factors. *Stroke.* 2009;40:313-316.

Jovin TG, Chamorro A, Cobo E, et al. Thrombectomy within 8 hours after symptom onset in ischemic stroke. *N Engl J Med.* 2015;372(24):2296-2306.

Juvela S, Poussa K, Lehto H, Porras M. Natural history of unruptured intracranial aneurysms: a long-term follow-up study. *Stroke.* 2013;44:2414-2421.

Kidwell CS, Jahan R, Gornbein J, et al. A trial of imaging selection and endovascular treatment for ischemic stroke. *N Engl J Med.* 2013;368(10):914-923.

Kim T, Lee H, Bang JS, et al. Epidemiology of moyamoya disease in Korea: based on National Health Insurance Service data. *J Korean Neurosurg Soc.* 2015;57(6):390-395.

Kim T, Oh CW, Bang JS, et al. Moyamoya disease: treatment and outcomes. *J Stroke.* 2016;18(1):21-30.

Lasjaunias PL, Chng SM, Sachet M, et al. The management of vein of Galen aneurysmal malformations. *Neurosurgery.* 2006;59(Suppl 3):S184-S194.

Lal BK, Meschia JF, Howard G, Brott TG. Carotid stenting versus carotid endarterectomy: what did the carotid revascularization endarterectomy versus stenting trial show and where do we go from here? *Angiology.* 2016;pii:0003319716661661.

Lee VH, Brown RD Jr, Mandrekar JN, Mokri B. Incidence and outcome of cervical artery dissection: a population-based study. *Neurology.* 2006;67(10):1809-1812.

Lee EJ, Lee HJ, Hyun MK, et al. Rupture rate for patients with untreated unruptured intracranial aneurysms in South Korea during 2006-2009. *J Neurosurg.* 2012;117:53-59.

Lu X, Li Y. The clinical characteristics and treatment of cerebral AVM in pregnancy. *Neuroradiol J.* 2015;28(4):385-388.

Mackey J. Evaluation and management of stroke in young adults. *Continuum (Minneap Minn).* 2014;20(2 Cerebrovascular Disease):352-369.

McDougall CG, Spetzler RF, Zabramski JM, et al. The barrow ruptured aneurysm trial. *J Neurosurg.* 2012;116(1):135-144.

Mohr JP, Parides MK, Stapf C, et al. Medical management with or without interventional therapy for unruptured brain arteriovenous malformations (ARUBA): a multicentre, non-blinded, randomised trial. *Lancet.* 2014;383(9917):614-621.

Molyneux A, Kerr R, International Subarachnoid Aneurysm Trial (ISAT) Collaborative Group, et al. International Subarachnoid Aneurysm Trial (ISAT) of neurosurgical clipping versus endovascular coiling in 2143 patients with ruptured intracranial aneurysms: a randomized trial. *J Stroke Cerebrovasc Dis.* 2002;11(6):304-314.

Molyneux AJ, Kerr RS, Yu LM, et al. International subarachnoid aneurysm trial (ISAT) of neurosurgical clipping versus endovascular coiling in 2143 patients with ruptured intracranial aneurysms: a randomised comparison of effects on survival, dependency, seizures, rebleeding, subgroups, and aneurysm occlusion. *Lancet.* 2005;366(9488):809-817.

Mugikura S, Takahashi S, Higano S, et al. Predominant involvement of ipsilateral anterior and posterior circulations in moyamoya disease. *Stroke.* 2002;33(6):1497-1500.

Murayama Y, Takao H, Ishibashi T, et al. Risk analysis of unruptured intracranial aneurysms: prospective 10-year cohort study. *Stroke.* 2016;47:365-371.

Nasr DM, Brown RD Jr. Management of unruptured intracranial aneurysms. *Curr Cardiol Rep.* 2016;18:86.

National Institute of Neurological Disorders and Stroke rt-PA Stroke Study Group. Tissue plasminogen activator for acute ischemic stroke. *N Engl J Med.* 1995;333(24):1581-1587.

Perkins WJ, Lanzion G, Brott TG. Carotid stenting vs endarterectomy: new results in perspective. *Mayo Clin Proc.* 2010;85:1101-1108.

Perret G, Nishioka H. Report on the cooperative study of intracranial aneurysms and subarachnoid hemorrhage. Section VI. Arteriovenous malformations. An analysis of 545 cases of cranio-cerebral arteriovenous malformations and fistulae reported to the cooperative study. *J Neurosurg.* 1966;25(4):467-490.

Powers WJ, Derdeyn CP, Biller J, et al. 2015 American Heart Association/American Stroke Association Focused Update of the 2013 guidelines for the early management of patients with acute ischemic stroke regarding endovascular treatment: a guideline for healthcare professionals from the American Heart Association/American Stroke Association. *Stroke.* 2015;46(10):3020-3035.

Priebe HJ. Aneurysmal subarachnoid haemorrhage and the anaesthetist. *Br J Anaesth.* 2007;99(1):102-118.

Saver JL, Goyal M, Bonafe A, et al. Stent-retriever thrombectomy after intravenous t-PA vs. t-PA alone in stroke. *N Engl J Med.* 2015;372(24):2285-2295.

Spetzler RF, McDougall CG, Albuquerque FC, et al. The barrow ruptured aneurysm trial: 3-year results. *J Neurosurg.* 2013;119(1):146-157.

Siddiq F, Adil MM, Qureshi AI. Factors and outcomes associated with early and delayed aneurysm treatment in subarachnoid hemorrhage patients in the United States. *Neurosurgery.* 2012;71(3):670-677; discussion 677-678.

Sonobe M, Yamazaki T, Yonekura M, Kikuchi H. Small unruptured intracranial aneurysm verification study: SUAVe study, Japan. *Stroke.* 2010;41:1969-1977.

UCAS Japan Investigators, Morita A, Kirino T, et al. The natural course of unruptured cerebral aneurysms in a Japanese cohort. *N Engl J Med.* 2012;366:2474-2482.

van Beijnum J, van der Worp HB, Buis DR, et al. Treatment of brain arteriovenous malformations: a systematic review and meta-analysis. *JAMA.* 2011;306(18):2011-2019.

Vanninen R, Koivisto T, Saari T, et al. Ruptured intracranial aneurysms: acute endovascular treatment with electrolytically detachable coils: a prospective randomized study. *Radiology.* 1999;211(2):325-336.

Veldeman M, Höllig A, Clusmann H, et al. Delayed cerebral ischaemia prevention and treatment after aneurysmal subarachnoid haemorrhage: a systematic review. *Br J Anaesth.* 2016;117(1):17-40.

Wiebers DO, Whisnant JP, Huston J 3rd, et al. Unruptured intracranial aneurysms: natural history, clinical outcome, and risks of surgical and endovascular treatment. *Lancet.* 2003;362:103-110.

Yan J, Wen J, Gopaul R, et al. Outcome and complications of endovascular embolization for vein of Galen malformations: a systematic review and meta-analysis. *J Neurosurg.* 2015;123:872-890.

16

Brain Death

Sarah Wahlster, MD, and David M. Greer, MD, MA, FNCS

Questions

A 24-year-old woman suffers a pulseless electrical activity (PEA) arrest following a prolonged asthma attack. Bystanders perform cardiopulmonary resuscitation and call 911; emergency medical services (EMS) arrive at the scene within 15 minutes. Return of spontaneous circulation is achieved after 45 minutes. She is taken to a nearby hospital, and on initial evaluation, she is hemodynamically stable, but her neurologic exam is concerning for brain death. Her condition remains unchanged 48 hours after completing targeted temperature management (TTM). Following further conversations with her family, a clinical examination is repeated.

1. Which of the following parameters is a prerequisite for a brain death evaluation according to the 2010 American Academy of Neurology (AAN) criteria?

   A. Underlying structural etiology confirmed by history and visualized on neuroimaging

   B. Presence of severe electrolyte abnormalities

   C. Systolic blood pressure (SBP) >90 mm Hg in the absence of any vasopressors

   D. Required hypothermia for 24 hours, if there was a cardiac arrest

   E. Family consent to proceed with the exam, or clear and unequivocal documentation of organ donation status (such as a driver's license or other legal paperwork)

2. Which of the following clinical findings is compatible with the diagnosis of brain death?

   A. Presence of pupillary response to a bright light

   B. Inability to complete oculocephalic testing due to cervical spine injury

   C. Presence of spinal reflexes

   D. Unilateral absence corneal reflexes to saline drop

   E. Presence of diabetes insipidus

3. Which of the following statements regarding the clinical brain death exam is true?

    A. Severe hyperammonemia should be corrected before initiating the evaluation.

    B. The AAN criteria mandate a waiting period of at least 24 hours after the completion of therapeutic hypothermia or TTM in cardiac arrest patients.

    C. The oculocephalic reflex should be performed with the head of bed angled at 30°.

    D. The Lazarus sign is a commonly seen phenomenon in brain dead patients, and if observed, ancillary testing is required.

    E. The vestibulo-ocular reflex is tested by irrigating each ear with 50 mL of ice water and confirming the absence of reactive eye movements during 1 minute of observation.

4. A 74-year-old man with a history of hypertension and hyperlipidemia is found down by his grandson a few hours after he had breakfast with his family. EMS is called, and he is minimally responsive (Glasgow coma scale [GCS] score 4); initial blood pressure (BP) is 240/120 mm Hg, heart rate (HR) is 50, oxygen saturation (SO_2) is 85%, and temperature is 34°C. He is intubated at the scene, started on nicardipine, and taken to an emergency department (ED). On arrival, his BP is 200/100 mm Hg, HR is 55 bpm, SO_2 is 96% on 60% fraction of inspired oxygen (FiO_2), and temperature is 35°C. A head computed tomography (CT) scan is shown below. A detailed clinical exam performed by a neurology attending physician is consistent with brain death (as required per hospital protocol). An apnea trial demonstrates no spontaneous respirations during 10 minutes of observation (initial Pco_2 36 mm Hg, final Pco_2 64 mm Hg). What is the appropriate course of action?

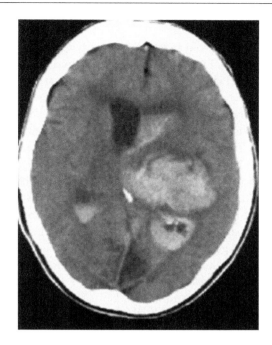

    A. Declare the patient brain dead and notify the family as well as the organ procurement organization.

    B. Repeat the apnea test.

    C. Obtain an electroencephalogram (EEG) to confirm the diagnosis of brain death.

    D. Admit the patient and repeat the brain death evaluation once he is consistently normothermic.

    E. Treat the patient's elevated BP (goal normotension) and repeat the brain death evaluation.

5. What is the highest core temperature allowable for clinical brain death testing?

    A. 38°C

    B. 38.5°C

    C. 39°C

    D. 40°C

    E. None of the above

Questions 6-8

A 45-year-old man presents with a Hunt and Hess grade 5, Fisher grade 4 subarachnoid hemorrhage (SAH) due to a ruptured internal carotid artery (ICA) aneurysm. After the patient is hemodynamically stabilized, his initial neurologic exam in the ED is concerning for brain death. He is admitted to the intensive care unit (ICU). Temperature is 39°C, BP is 150/80 mm Hg, HR is 84 bpm, SO_2 is 98% on 40% FiO_2 on volume assist control ventilation with a tidal volume (TV) of 450 mL, respiratory rate (RR) is 14 breaths/min, positive end-expiratory pressure (PEEP) is 5 cm H_2O, and the last arterial blood gas (ABG) is pH $paCO_2$ 28 mmHg/paO_2 155. His labs are notable for sodium 145 mEq/L, potassium 5.0 mEq/L, creatinine 1.8 mg/dL (baseline 1.0), creatine kinase 8000 Units/L, and white blood cells 9000 cell/L. His electrocardiogram (ECG) shows diffuse nonspecific ST-segment depressions (<1 mm) and T-wave inversions. His clinical exam is consistent with a diagnosis of brain death.

6. Which of the following is the most appropriate next step before proceeding with an apnea test?

   A. Start aminocaproic acid to minimize further bleeding from the aneurysm while the evaluation is ongoing.

   B. Increase the PEEP to 15 cm H_2O to improve oxygenation and repeat an ABG in 30 minutes.

   C. Decrease the RR to 10 breaths/min and repeat an ABG in 30 minutes.

   D. Give a bolus of normal saline to improve his renal function and treat the hyperkalemia.

   E. Request an urgent cardiology consult and obtain a transthoracic echocardiogram.

7. Which of the following values is consistent with a positive apnea test?

   A. PCO_2 >60 mm Hg, or 20-mm Hg increase over baseline value

   B. PCO_2 >80 mm Hg, or 20-mm Hg increase over baseline value

   C. PCO_2 >60 mm Hg, or 30-mm Hg increase over baseline value

   D. PCO_2 >80 mm Hg, or 30-mm Hg increase over baseline value

   E. None of the above

8. Which of the following statements regarding apnea testing is true?

   A. The recommended duration of apnea during apnea testing is 6 to 8 minutes.

   B. Apnea testing should be aborted if the oxygen saturation is <90% for >30 seconds.

   C. Apnea testing should be aborted if the SBP drops below 100 mm Hg.

   D. End-tidal capnography is required during apnea testing.

   E. Hypotension is the most frequently encountered complication during apnea testing.

9. Which of the following statements regarding EEG in brain death testing is true?

   A. In some countries, an EEG is a mandatory part of the brain death evaluation.

   B. A minimum of 8 scalp electrodes are required.

   C. The sensitivity should be increased to at least 2 μV for 30 minutes with appropriate calibrations.

   D. Absent activity of EEG was one of the principal requirements in the definition of brain death by the Harvard Criteria.

   E. All of the above are true.

10. A 29-year-old woman is admitted to the ICU following a motor vehicle accident. Her injuries include severe traumatic brain injury (TBI; GCS 3 in the field) with large bitemporal contusions, diffuse SAH, multiple facial and skull base fractures, an unstable fracture of C3 with spinal cord compression and cord signal change from C2 to C5, a left-sided hemothorax (stabilized after chest tube insertion), and a femoral fracture. Her neurologic examination is consistent with brain death. Her family understands the gravity of the situation, and they state that she is an organ donor and agree to proceed with the "full brain death evaluation." What are the appropriate next steps?

    A. Perform an apnea test, and if consistent with brain death, sign a death certificate. If the patient cannot tolerate the study, order an ancillary test.

    B. Perform an apnea test; also order an EEG given her young age. If either study is consistent with brain death, sign a death certificate.

C. Contact the organ procurement organization (OPO) and ask them to evaluate the patient; forego apnea testing, since the clinical exam and scans are clearly consistent with the diagnosis of brain death.

D. Check a serum and urine toxicology screen because you suspect that the accident might have been related to a drug overdose. Proceed with apnea testing and, if needed, ancillary testing only if the toxicology screen is negative.

E. Obtain an ancillary study (4-vessel angiogram or cerebral scintigraphy) to assess cerebral perfusion and do not attempt apnea testing. Contact the OPO to assess the patient, pending results of the ancillary study.

11. Which statement is true regarding the presence of confounding medications and drugs in brain death testing?

A. EEG is a reliable ancillary test that can help determine brain death when sedating drugs are a potential confounder.

B. It is reasonable to proceed with brain death evaluation if the blood alcohol content is under 0.08%.

C. The train of 4 test is an electrophysiologic study that can be helpful to assess the effect of benzodiazepines and barbiturates.

D. The 2010 AAN guidelines recommend waiting at least 48 hours from ingestion and repeating a toxicology screen for patients who have been given benzodiazepines or barbiturates.

E. If the patient is a long-standing chronic opioid user (taking up to 200 mg/d of oxycodone), it is feasible to proceed with brain death evaluation even after the patient recently received several doses of fentanyl in the ED.

12. In the presence of normal renal and hepatic function, how much time should pass before a confounding drug is thought to be nearly or completely eliminated?

A. 24 hours from administration or ingestion, if documented

B. 2 half-lives

C. 5 half-lives

D. 10 half-lives

E. Typically 2 half-lives, but if circumstances are unclear, emergent dialysis should be considered

13. For brain dead patients, when is the exact time of death that should be documented in the patient's chart?

A. When the patient is disconnected from the ventilator after withdrawal of care or organ removal

B. When asystole has been observed for ≥5 minutes on telemetry (after withdrawal of care or in the operating room after organ procurement)

C. When ABG results from the apnea trial are reported by the laboratory and fulfill criteria

D. When the patient is officially accepted as an organ donor

E. When the nuclear scan, if used for ancillary testing, is completed

14. A 66-year-old woman with a history of hypertension, end-stage renal disease (glomerular filtration rate 30 mL/min), congestive heart failure, hepatitis C, and atrial fibrillation on warfarin collapses while having dinner with her family. Her husband calls 911, and she is intubated with propofol, fentanyl, and succinylcholine. She is taken to a local ED, where CT of head is performed (shown below). After completing a clinical examination, the ED resident suspects that she is brain dead. Which of the following findings should alert him to reconsider his diagnosis?

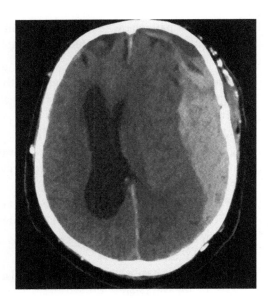

A. Triple flexion
B. Spontaneous facial myokymias
C. An upgoing toe (Babinski sign) on the left side
D. Pupils <1 mm
E. Cyclical constriction and dilation in light-fixed pupils

15. The patient presented in Question 14 is admitted to the ICU and evaluated by the neurology team the following morning. Her exam is now notable for absent pupillary, corneal, oculocephalic, and vestibulo-ocular reflexes; she has no gag but a weak cough is present; and spontaneous respirations are intermittently noted on the ventilator. Her nurse also notices that her urine output has increased to 300 to 500 mL/h over the past few hours. The patient is a registered organ donor, and her family reaffirms that "this is what she would want." What is the most appropriate course of action at this point?

A. Explain to the family that, unfortunately, this patient cannot be an organ donor due to her age and multiple comorbidities. Hold off on contacting the organ procurement organization (OPO) and recommend withdrawal of care.

B. Explain to the family that the patient is not brain dead. Ask the OPO to evaluate whether she is an eligible organ donor. Observe the patient for 24 hours; if her exam does not progress to brain death by then, recommend withdrawal of care to avoid prolonged suffering for the patient and her family.

C. Explain to the family that the patient is not brain dead. Recommend donation after cardiac death (DCD) and contact the OPO to evaluate whether she is an eligible candidate.

D. Ask the OPO to evaluate whether she is an eligible organ donor. Continue to monitor the patient until her exam progresses to brain death, pending further input from the OPO. Start aggressive fluid resuscitation and a vasopressin drip.

E. Start intravenous fluids, place a central line, and initiate a vasopressin drip. Start acetylcysteine for renal protection. Order a transthoracic echocardiogram and full hepatitis serologies and perform a bronchoscopy to help determine whether the patient is an eligible donor. Once these tests are completed, contact the OPO to determine her eligibility as an organ donor.

Answers and Explanations

1. A. Prerequisites for performing a brain death evaluation are listed in Table 16-1. Normotension is also a prerequisite; however, the SBP should be >100 mm Hg, and vasopressors may be used to achieve this goal. Family consent or documentation of organ donation status is not mandatory prior to a brain death evaluation in most states and is not listed as a prerequisite according to the 2010 AAN criteria. In the setting of a cardiac arrest, there is no requirement for prior therapeutic hypothermia to make the diagnosis of brain death because not all patients qualify for cooling.

Table 16-1. Prerequisites for Performing a Brain Death Evaluation (All Criteria must be Fulfilled)

1.1. Coma with a clearly established irreversible and proximate cause (determined by history, exam, neuroimaging)
1.2. Exclude presence of a central nervous system depressant drug
1.3. Normothermia or near-normal core body temperature (>36°C)
1.4. No recent administration or residual presence of paralytic agents (can check train of 4 twitches)
1.5. Absence of a severe electrolyte, acid-base, or endocrine abnormality
1.6. Systolic blood pressure ≥100 mm Hg (vasopressors or vasopressin may be used)
1.7. No spontaneous respirations noted on the ventilator

2. C. The requirements for a neurologic exam consistent with brain death are listed in Table 16-2. Spinal reflexes can be present in the context of brain death. In the event of inability to complete oculocephalic reflex testing, then vestibulo-ocular testing with cold water irrigation should occur. Diabetes insipidus (DI) can be observed in up to 85% of patients who experience brain death as a result of pituitary injury, but the presence of DI is not a mandatory finding for brain death declaration.

Table 16-2. Neurologic Examination (All Criteria must be Fulfilled)

2.1. **Coma:** no eye opening to noxious stimuli, no motor response to noxious stimuli in all 4 limbs other than spinally mediated reflexes.
2.2. Absence of **pupillary response** to a bright light. *Constricted pupils can be suggestive of drug intoxication.*
2.3. **Oculocephalic reflex** absent (tested only if cervical spine integrity ensured).
2.4. Absent **corneal reflex** tested with a cotton swab, piece of tissue paper, or squirt of water.
2.5. **No facial movement** or grimacing to deep pressure at the supraorbital ridge or temporomandibular joint.
2.6. Absence of ocular movement (1 minute of observation) during **vestibulo-ocular reflex** testing, confirm patency of the external auditory canals, then irrigate each ear with ~50 mL of ice cold water with head elevated at 30°.
2.7. Absent **gag reflex**, stimulate posterior pharynx with a tongue blade or suction device.
2.8. Absent **cough reflex** to tracheal suctioning, advance catheter to the level of the carina.

3. E. The 2010 AAN criteria suggest that a longer waiting period may be indicated after cardiac arrest, particularly after the use of therapeutic hypothermia (TH) or targeted temperature management (TTM). Factors that need to be taken into consideration include the presence of sedative agents and paralytics, which may be required during TH or TTM to control shivering. In addition, the metabolism of these drugs may be delayed in the context of lower body temperatures. However, no specific waiting period is defined, and each case needs to be assessed individually. While considered a metabolic abnormality, hyperammonemia is not thought to significantly affect brainstem reflexes and does not have to be corrected.

The oculocephalic reflex is assessed by brisk rotation of the head in the horizontal and vertical plane. The head of bed should be angled at 30° when performing the vestibulo-ocular reflex. Named after Lazarus of Bethany, who was raised from the dead by Jesus in the Gospel of John, the Lazarus sign is a reflexive, stereotypical movement during which the patient raises his or her arms and then crosses them on the chest. A rare phenomenon, it can be encountered in brain dead patients during apnea testing or even after extubation. See Table 16-2.

4. **D.** As highlighted in Table 16-1, normothermia or a near-normal core body temperature is a mandatory prerequisite for a brain death evaluation. In this case, the rise in Pco_2 is adequate; however, both the clinical exam and apnea testing can be confounded by hypothermia and should be repeated in this case; the patient cannot be declared brain dead at this point. It appears that all clinical parameters can be assessed in this patient, and he has tolerated an apnea test. Unless he becomes unstable or does not tolerate a repeat apnea test, there is no indication for an ancillary test according to the AAN guidelines. Normotension is a prerequisite with a minimal SBP target (Table 16-1); however, no upper limit is strictly defined. It may be reasonable to control hypertension to avoid intracerebral hemorrhage expansion while the evaluation is ongoing, but the presence of hypertension does not preclude brain death testing.

5. **E.** Although the AAN criteria define normothermia (>36°C) as a prerequisite, no upper temperature limit is specified, as the presence of fevers is not thought to confound testing of brain death reflexes or the apnea test. See Table 16-3.

6. **C.** See Table 16-3. In this case, the patient is not eucapneic, which is a prerequisite prior to initiating an apnea test. It appears that the patient is oxygenating well, and the PEEP should be decreased to 5 cm H_2O prior to the apnea test. Desaturations after the PEEP is decreased suggest that the patient may not tolerate the test. Use of aminocaproic acid and hydration are reasonable treatment options given the clinical picture, but since his exam is already consistent with brain death, the effort appears futile at this point. Patients presenting with high-grade aneurysmal SAH frequently warrant a cardiac workup and are commonly noted to have ECG changes; however, the patient does not appear

Table 16-3. Apnea Testing (All Criteria must be Fulfilled)

Prerequisites

3.1. Patient is **eupneic** (PaCO₂ 35-45 mm Hg)

3.2. Patient is **normotensive** (systolic blood pressure [SBP] ≥100 mm Hg and hemodynamically stable, even with the use of vasopressors)

3.3 Patient is **normothermic**

3.4. Patient is **euvolemic**

3.5. Patient is **not hypoxic**

3.6. No evidence of **CO₂ retention**

Procedure

Preoxygenate with 100% FiO₂ for ≥10 minutes to PaO₂ >200 mm Hg.

3.7. Decrease **PEEP to 5 cm H₂O** (patient should remain well oxygenated).

3.8. **Disconnect** the patient from the ventilator.

3.9. **Preserve oxygenation** by delivering 100% O₂ via a suction catheter to the level of the carina at 6 L/min.

3.10. Assess carefully for **spontaneous respiratory movements** (gasp, chest rise, abdominal excursions).

3.11. Draw an ABG after **8-10 minutes** and **reconnect** the patient to the ventilator.

3.12. **No respiratory effort and PCO₂ ≥60 mm Hg or > 20 mm Hg from** pretest ABG consistent with brain death.

If the ABG is not conclusive and patient hemodynamically stable, repeat apnea test for 10-15 minutes.

Abort if

3.13. Patient becomes **hemodynamically unstable** (SBP <90 mm Hg)

3.14. Patient **desaturates** with SO₂ <85% for >30 seconds. Retry with T-piece, CPAP 10 cm H₂O, and 100% O₂ at 12 L/min.

Abbreviations: ABG, arterial blood gas; CPAP, continuous positive airway pressure; PEEP, positive end-expiratory pressure.

hemodynamically unstable, and in light of his clinical exam, further investigations are not urgently indicated.

7. **A.** An apnea test that is consistent with brain death is one where the PCO_2 increases to >60 mm Hg or there is an increase of 20 mm Hg over the baseline value.

8. **E.** The recommended duration of apnea testing is 8 to 10 minutes on the first attempt. If the

ABG does not meet criteria and the patient is stable, it can be repeated for a longer time period (10-15 minutes). Apnea testing should be aborted if the patient's SBP falls below 90 mm Hg or if the patient desaturates to an SO_2 <85% for >30 seconds. End-tidal capnography is not required during apnea testing. The most commonly encountered complication is hypotension.

9. E. Absent activity of EEG is one of the major requirements in the original brain death description, and EEG remains a mandatory ancillary test in some countries. A minimum of 8 scalp electrodes are required, and the sensitivity should be increased to at least 2 µV for 30 minutes with appropriate calibrations (Table 16-4).

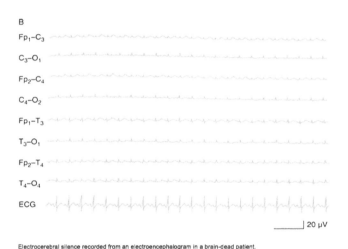

Electrocerebral silence recorded from an electroencephalogram in a brain-dead patient.

Reproduced with permission from Lee K. *The NeuroICU Book.* New York, NY: McGraw-Hill, 2012.

10. E. Ancillary testing is required either when the clinical exam cannot be performed (eg, due to confounding drugs or injuries) or if apnea testing is not possible, not conclusive, or aborted due to instability.

In this particular case, the patient's exam might be confounded by her cervical spine injury; an absent motor response to noxious stimuli might be due to sensory or motor deficits related to the spinal cord injury, and absent chest movements during the apnea test can be a result of diaphragmatic dysfunction due to lack of innervation. Therefore, an ancillary test is necessary to determine brain death. In general, it is advisable to check a urine toxicology

Table 16-4. Ancillary Testing

Cerebral Angiogram

4.1. Inject contrast in the aortic arch under high pressure and reach both anterior and posterior circulation.

4.2. No intracerebral filling should be detected at the level of entry of the carotid or vertebral artery to the skull.

4.3. The external carotid should be patent.

4.4. Filling of the superior sagittal sinus may be delayed (due to extracranial to intracranial late contrast shunting).

Cerebral Scintigraphy

4.5. The isotope should be injected within 30 minutes after its reconstitution.

4.6. Anterior and both lateral image planar image counts (500,000) should be obtained immediately, between 30 and 60 minutes and 2 hours later.

4.7. Can confirm correct intravenous injection by assessing uptake in the liver.

4.8. No tracer in the anterior and middle cerebral artery or basilar artery territory (hollow skull phenomenon); no tracer in the superior sagittal sinus. Minimal tracer can come from the scalp.

Electroencephalogram

4.9. A minimum of 8 scalp electrodes are required.

4.10. Interelectrode impedance should be between 100 and 10,000 Ω.

4.11. The integrity of the entire recording system needs to be tested.

4.12. The distance between electrodes should be at least 10 cm.

4.13. The sensitivity should be increased to at least 2 µV for 30 minutes with appropriate calibrations.

4.14. The high-frequency filter should not be <30 Hz; the low-frequency filter should not be >12 Hz.

4.15. A lack of reactivity to intense somatosensory or audiovisual stimuli should be demonstrated.

Transcranial Doppler

4.16. Only useful if a reliable sign is found (complete absence of flow might be due to inadequate transtemporal windows). Assess either for reverberating flow or small systolic peaks in early systole.

4.17. There should be bilateral as well as anterior and posterior insonation. The probe should be placed at the temporal bone above the zygomatic arch and the vertebrobasilar arteries. Insonation through the orbital window can be considered to obtain a signal.

screen to exonerate exposure to sedating drugs before brain death testing. However, in this case, an ancillary study will be necessary regardless of the toxicology screen results. Neither test is affected by the presence of confounding medications.

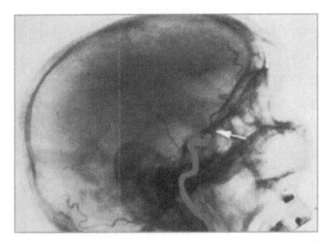

Reproduced with permission from Lee K. *The NeuroICU Book.* New York, NY: McGraw-Hill, 2012.

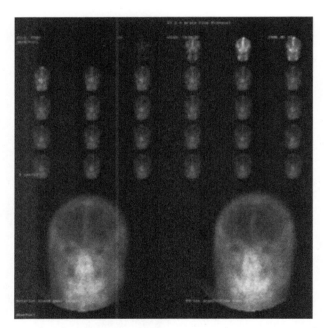

Reproduced with permission from Lee K. *The NeuroICU Book.* New York, NY: McGraw-Hill, 2012.

11. **B.** If the blood alcohol level is below the legal driving limit (0.08%), it is reasonable to proceed with the brain death evaluation. The EEG tends to be affected by sedating drugs, including benzodiazepines, opioids, and barbiturates. The train of

4 test is performed to exonerate the presence of paralytic agents. The AAN criteria do not specify a defined waiting period after receiving benzodiazepines or barbiturates. Even in light of a presumably high tolerance for sedating drugs, the presence of any potentially confounding agent needs to be excluded before proceeding with brain death determination.

12. **C.** The AAN criteria recommend waiting 5 times the drug's half-life, assuming normal renal and hepatic function.

13. **C.** Brain death is considered equal to cardiac death, and the time of death is once the brain death determination is complete, either when the ABG is reported or (if exam or apnea testing are precluded) if single-photon emission CT or 4-vessel angiogram is officially interpreted by an attending physician. The timing of withdrawal of care or organ donation and the time of cardiac arrest are not relevant because the patient has already been declared dead by then.

14. **D.** Constricted pupils may suggest drug intoxication, especially in the context of the patient receiving intravenous fentanyl. Permissive signs include cyclical constriction and dilation in light-fixed pupils (hippus), facial myokymias, triple flexion, plantar flexion with plantar or dorsal stimulation, a prominent Babinski sign (unilateral or bilateral), and reflexive movements (stereotypical and reproducible), such as the Lazarus sign.

15. **D.** This patient still has a cough, and spontaneous respirations are noted; therefore, she is not brain dead at this point. However, the progression of her exam with presence of DI suggests that she will likely become brain dead soon. There is no specific defined maximum waiting period. It appears that donation would be consistent with her wishes. Contacting the OPO and asking them to assess the patient is appropriate in this setting. Her comorbidities may preclude donation, but the determination of donor status and further workup should be led by the OPO. Correcting her volume deficit due to DI with fluids and vasopressin while waiting for the decision by the OPO regarding donation is appropriate, especially if she will indeed qualify as an organ donor.

REFERENCES

A definition of irreversible coma. Report of the Ad Hoc Committee of the Harvard Medical School to Examine the Definition of Brain Death. *JAMA*. 1968;205:337-340.

Darby JM, Stein K, Grenvik A, et al. Approach to management of the heart beating "brain dead" organ donor. *JAMA*. 1989;261:2222-2228.

Wahlster S, Wijdicks EF, Patel PV, et al. Brain death declaration: practices and perceptions worldwide. *Neurology*. 2015;84:1870-1879.

Wijdicks EF. Brain death worldwide: accepted fact but no global consensus in diagnostic criteria. *Neurology*. 2002;58:20-25.

Wijdicks EF, Varelas PN, Gronseth GS, et al. Evidence-based guideline update: determining brain death in adults: report of the Quality Standards Subcommittee of the American Academy of Neurology. *Neurology*. 2010;74:1911-1918.

17

Prognosis in Neurocritical Care

David P. Lerner, MD and Saef Izzy, MD

Questions

Questions 1 and 2

An 87-year-old man with hypertension, coronary artery disease (prior coronary artery bypass grafting on aspirin), and chronic obstructive pulmonary disease presents to the emergency department (ED) after being found on the ground at home with slurred speech, right gaze deviation, and left-sided weakness. A head computed tomography (CT) was completed (shown below). The volume of hemorrhage was calculated to be approximately 75 mL without any intraventricular extension. His initial examination on arrival to the ED was as follows:

eyes opening to voice, oriented to self, severely dysarthric with, right gaze preference, left facial droop, no movement of the left arm or leg, and full strength of the right arm and leg.

1. What is his intracerebral hemorrhage (ICH) score?
   A. 1
   B. 2
   C. 3
   D. 4
   E. 5

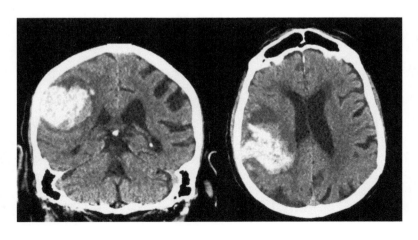

2. The patient survived his acute neurologic injury and was discharged from the intensive care four days after hemorrhage. He had a gastrostomy tube placed for enteral access and is ready for discharge from the hospital. Prior to discharge, a family discussion occurs. What is the chance of return to independent level of function at 90 day after the ICH?

 A. Approximately 0%

 B. Approximately 10%

 C. Approximately 40%

 D. Approximately 65%

 E. Approximately 80%

3. An 84-year-old man with coronary artery disease and arterial fibrillation had an ST-segment elevation myocardial infarction that was complicated by ventricular fibrillation cardiac arrest with 45 minutes of pulselessness. His initial management included evaluation in the cardiac catheterization lab with placement of a bare metal stent into the right coronary artery. He underwent 24 hours of cooling after cardiac arrest but, following this, he had limited neurologic recovery. On post arrest day 6, critical care unit staff called the neurointensivist to discuss the case. Which of the following statements is true?

 A. The most accurate prognostic test for poor neurologic outcome is electroencephalography (EEG).

 B. No corneal responses 6 days after cardiac arrest is consistent with no anticipated neurologic recovery.

 C. Neuron-specific enolase is not affected by cooling and can be used for prognosis at 6 days after cardiac arrest.

 D. Magnetic resonance imaging (MRI) can assist with prognosis, and the most commonly affected area of the brain is the cortical region.

 E. Unilateral presence of a somatosensory evoked potential is associated with poor neurologic recovery following cardiac arrest.

4. A 74-year-old man with coronary artery disease, severe aortic stenosis, hypertension, and chronic lymphocytic leukemia was brought to the ED from clinic for evaluation of progressive shortness of breath over 1 week. While in the ED, he had a cardiac arrest with an initial rhythm of ventricular fibrillation. Cardiopulmonary resuscitation was started, and he was treated with a single dose of epinephrine and 1 desynchronized defibrillation with return of spontaneous circulation. During the arrest, he was intubated for airway management. Approximately 45 minutes after arrest, his examination was pertinent for normal vital signs and an abbreviated neurology examination (Glasgow coma scale [GCS] 11t: E4, V1t, M6) with symmetric and reactive pupils, symmetric grimace, and antigravity movements in all extremities. You are consulted for recommendation on cooling the patient following cardiac arrest. Which of the following statements is correct regarding cooling in this patient?

 A. The patient is not an appropriate cooling candidate given he had a ventricular fibrillation arrest.

 B. The patient is not an appropriate cooling candidate given the likely inciting etiology is pulmonary.

 C. The patient is not an appropriate cooling candidate given his neurologic examination.

 D. The patient is not an appropriate cooling candidate given his life expectancy with his history of chronic lymphocytic leukemia.

 E. The patient is an appropriate cooling candidate and should be started on cooling with iced saline.

Questions 5 and 6

A 22-year-old woman was found unresponsive after a motorcycle accident. She was intubated in the field without use of any paralytic or sedating medication. Twelve hours after admission to the intensive care unit (ICU), an exam was completed. The patient was unarousable and unresponsive to painful stimuli. Vitals were stable. Family members arrived, and they wanted to know about the patient's clinical status.

5. The current consciousness state is considered as which of the following?

A. Stupor

B. Coma

C. Locked-in syndrome

D. Minimal conscious state

E. Persistent vegetative state

6. Seven days after aggressive ICU management, she has some awareness of environment but is not following commands; her sleep-wake cycle is now preserved. She also has normal brainstem autonomic functions. What is her consciousness state at this point?

A. Stupor

B. Coma

C. Locked-in syndrome

D. Minimal conscious state

E. Permanent vegetative state

7. A 69-year-old right-handed man with hypertension, hyperlipidemia, and bilateral carotid stenosis with right carotid endarterectomy 1 year prior to presentation presents with acute onset of aphasia and right hemibody weakness. He was not eligible for intravenous tissue plasminogen activator or intra-arterial thrombectomy given his last known well state was >12 hours from presentation to the ED. A head CT obtained at that time demonstrated early ischemic changes within the left middle cerebral artery territory, and a CT angiography (CTA) demonstrated a left middle cerebral artery occlusion in the M1 division. He was admitted to the neuro-ICU for blood pressure augmentation, frequent neurologic examinations, and monitoring for malignant cerebral edema. A repeat head CT was completed post stroke day 5 and is shown below.

The total ischemic stroke volume is 115 mL, and there are 2 locations of homogenous intraparenchymal hemorrhage within the posterior frontal lobe and basal ganglia. His examination shows the following: awake, limited mumbling of incoherent words, mimicking of movements, moderate right facial droop, movements of the right arm in the plain of the bed, full movement of the right leg, and normal strength of the left hemibody. There does not appear to be neglect of the right hemibody or space. Which of the following portends the worst prognosis for the patient?

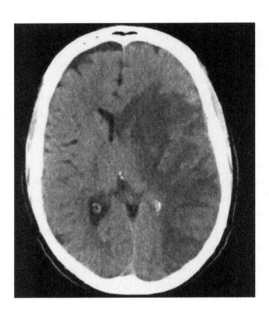

A. Age

B. Dominant-hemisphere lesion

C. Hemorrhagic conversion of ischemic stroke

D. Etiology of ischemic stroke

E. Ischemic stroke volume

8. A 49-year-old woman with no significant past medical history presents with 3 weeks of progressive headache. While out of the house with her husband, she had a witnessed loss of consciousness. She was taken to the ED, with the following initial vital signs: heart rate 72 bpm, blood pressure 95/50 mm Hg, temperature 97.5°F, oxygen saturation SpO$_2$ 98% on 2 L nasal cannula. Her neurologic examination findings were as follows: somnolent requiring repeated noxious stimulation to obtain a neurologic examination, antigravity and near full

strength movements, and limited antigravity movements on the left hemibody. A head CT was completed (shown below), which demonstrated diffuse subarachnoid hemorrhage with blood present in the basal cisterns, perimesencephalic, prepontine cisterns, and third and fourth ventricles. A CTA demonstrated a 6-mm basilar artery aneurysm. There was concern for early hydrocephalus attributed to her neurologic state, and a right frontal approach external ventricular drain was placed with an opening pressure estimated at 30 mm H$_2$O. After this, her examination improved, and she is now awake, interactive, and following commands with only left arm pronation and drift on examination. What is the patient's prognosis from her subarachnoid hemorrhage?

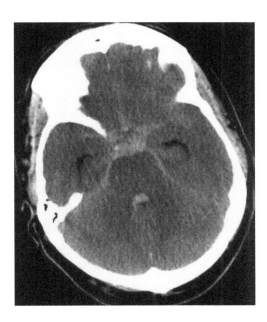

A. The patient's 30-day mortality is approximately 0%.
B. The patient's 30-day mortality is approximately 5%.
C. The patient's 30-day mortality is approximately 10%.
D. The patient's 30-day mortality is approximately 25%.
E. The patient's 30-day mortality is approximately 70%.

Questions 9 and 10

A 62-year-old man with history of hypertension was found unresponsive on the floor and had been down for an unclear amount of time. He was last known well 4 hours prior to being discovered down. Emergency medical services arrived to find him pulseless with an initial cardiac rhythm of ventricular fibrillation. Advanced cardiac life support was initiated, and return of spontaneous circulation was obtained in 15 minutes. On arrival to the hospital, the patient was intubated. "Off sedation," he was comatose with poorly reactive pupils, his eyes remained closed during examination, and no movements were noted to painful stimuli. The patient was admitted to the cardiac ICU, which contacted you for further recommendation.

9. What is your recommendation to the ICU team?
   A. Patient is likely seizing. Order EEG.
   B. Start hypothermia with goal temperature of 28°C to 32°C.
   C. Order MRI of the brain to assess prognosis.
   D. Start hypothermia for next 24 hours with target temperature of 32°C to 34°C.
   E. Recommend transition to hospice given poor neurologic examination.

10. Which of the following supports a poor prognostic outcome in this patient?
    A. Presence of pupillary response but absent corneal responses on day 3
    B. Single seizure and intermittent myoclonic jerks
    C. Somatosensory evoked potentials (SSEPs) with presence of bilateral N20 with median nerve stimulation
    D. MRI showing cortical ribbon distribution on diffusion restriction diffusion-weighted imaging (DWI) and apparent diffusion coefficient (ADC)
    E. EEG with generalized slowing at 2 to 4 Hz

11. A 49-year-old left-handed woman with no past medical history presented to the ED for acute onset of left hemibody weakness. Her initial National Institutes of Health Stroke Scale score was 25, consistent with a right middle cerebral artery stroke. A head CT was completed, which did not demonstrate any hemorrhage but did show a hyperdense right middle cerebral artery. She was treated with intravenous tissue plasminogen activator, and despite attempts at intra-arterial thrombectomy, the thrombus was unsuccessfully removed. Over the next 36 hours, there was slow progression of increased somnolence. A repeat CT scan was completed and is shown below. Prior to additional treatment decisions, a family meeting occurs to discuss the next steps in management. What information should be shared with the family?

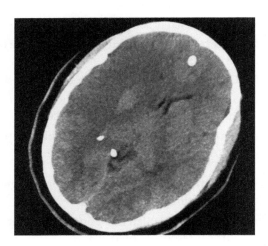

A. A hemicraniectomy will not be a life-saving intervention or change her clinical recovery given this is a dominant-hemisphere ischemic stroke.

B. A hemicraniectomy could be a life-saving intervention, but it will not change her clinical recovery given this is a dominant-hemisphere ischemic stroke.

C. A hemicraniectomy could be a life-saving intervention and will increase the likelihood of a good neurologic outcome given this is a dominant-hemisphere ischemic stroke.

D. A hemicraniectomy could be a life-saving intervention, but it will not change her clinical recovery given this is a non–dominant-hemisphere ischemic stroke.

E. A hemicraniectomy could be a life-saving intervention and will increase the likelihood of a good neurologic outcome given this is a non–dominant-hemisphere ischemic stroke.

12. A 28-year-old woman was a restrained passenger in a high-speed car versus telephone pole motor vehicle crash. Emergency medical services found the patient in the car and unresponsive. There was a prolonged extrication from the vehicle, and her initial neurologic examination revealed bilaterally unreactive pupils at 4 mm, agonal respirations, no gag or cough, and no movement in any extremity to noxious stimulation (GCS 3). She was intubated in the field without use of sedation or paralytic. Her initial vitals were heart rate 110 bpm and blood pressure 96/55 mm Hg. Her initial labs were remarkable for only a mild anemia with hemoglobin of 10.6 g/dL and a mildly elevated glucose of 165 mg/dL (9.2 mmol/L). A head CT was completed and demonstrated a right frontal and parafalcine subdural hemorrhage and a small left basal ganglia intraparenchymal hemorrhage. Which of the following is associated with the worst 6-month prognosis for this patient?

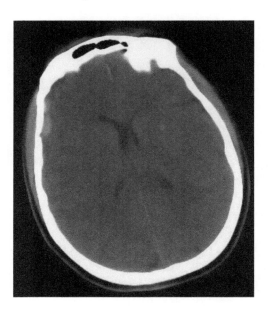

A. Age

B. Bilaterally nonreactive pupils

C. No motor movement to noxious stimulation

D. Hemoglobin value of 10.6 g/dL

E. Findings on head CT of subdural hemorrhages

Answers and Explanations

1. B; 2 B. The patient has a large, lobar hemorrhage. The intracerebral hemorrhage (ICH) score (Table 17-1) is a prognostic grading scale for 30-day mortality following primary ICH. The score uses **ALVIS: a**ge (< or > 80 years), **l**ocation (infratentorial or not), **v**olume of hemorrhage (< or > 30 mL), **i**ntraventricular hemorrhage (present or absent), Glasgow coma **s**cale score (15-13, 13-8, or <8). The 30-day mortality rates for patients with ICH scores of 1, 2, 3, and 4 were 13%, 26%, 72%, and 97%, respectively. In this patient's case, he receives points for age >80 years and volume of hemorrhage >30 mL, resulting in an ICH score of 2 and a 30-day mortality of 26%.

The prognostic score used to predict the functional outcome of a patient following a primary ICH is the FUNC score (Table 17-2). Same as the ICH score, the FUNC score uses **ALVIS: a**ge, **l**ocation of hemorrhage, **v**olume of hemorrhage, and Glasgow coma **s**cale. However, premorbid cognitive function is used in FUNC but not the ICH score. A higher score is associated with more likelihood of recovery to an independent state. The scores are grouped into 5 categories—<5, 5 to 7, 8, 9 to 10, and 11—which are associated with rates of functional independence at 90 days of 0%, 13%, 42%, 66%, and 82%, respectively.

Table 17-1. The Intracerebral Hemorrhage (ICH) Score

Component	Points	Total Points	30-Day Mortality (%)
Glasgow coma scale score			
3-4	2	5+	100
5-12	1		
13-15	0	4	97
ICH volume (mL)			
30	1	3	72
<30	0		
Interventricular hemorrhage			
Yes	1	2	26
No	0	1	13
Age (year)			
80	1	0	0
<80	0		
Infratentorial origin			
Yes	1		
No	0		

(Adapted from Hemphill JC 3rd, Bonovich DC, Besmertis L, Manley GT, Johnston SC. The ICH score: A simple, reliable grading scale for intracerebral hemorrhage. *Stroke*. 2001;32:891-897.)

Date of download: 01/30/17 from Neurology Collection: www.neurology.mhmedical.com. © McGraw-Hill Education. All rights reserved.

Reproduced with permission from Lee K. *The NeuroICU Book*. New York, NY: McGraw-Hill, 2012.

Table 17-2. FUNC Score

FUNC Score	Points
Glasgow coma score	
≥9	2
<9	0
Pre-ICH cognitive impairment	
No	1
Yes	0
ICH location	
Lobar	2
Deep	1
Infratentorial	0
Age (years)	
<70	2
71-79	1
>80	0
ICH volume (mL)	
<30	4
31-59	2
>60	0

Abbreviation: ICH, intracerebral hemorrhage.

3. **D.** The extent of brain injury is the key factor for prognostication after cardiac arrest. Clinical examination has been the staple of prognosis; prognostic findings such as absent pupillary reflexes, absent corneal reflexes and motor responses of extensor, and no movement to noxious stimulation have come into question in the era of cooling. Absence of corneal reflexes does not absolutely portend a poor prognosis. Although EEG can be used for the detection of seizures in the setting of cardiac arrest, the prognostication value has not been validated. Regarding myoclonic status, although generally strongly associated with poor outcome, there have been few reported cases of good outcome despite the myoclonic EEG findings. The absence of reactivity on EEG may be the most promising feature for predicting poor outcome. The largest study of somatosensory evoked potentials (SSEPs) found that bilaterally absent cortical sensory responses are associated with poor neurologic outcome. Pertinent biomarkers include neuron-specific enolase, which was studied alongside SSEP, and levels >33 µg/L predicted poor outcome, but this study was completed prior to cooling. Hypothermia can attenuate release of neuron-specific enolase, and there are reports of good outcome with levels >100 µg/L. Although there are limitations to imaging, many use MRI as a useful prognostication tool at 3 to 5 days after arrest. Common findings are diffuse cortical and basal ganglia restriction.

Evaluation after Cardiac Arrest

48-72 Hours	3-5 Days
Clinical examination	Clinical examination
Pupillary examination	Pupillary examination
Motor examination	Motor examination
EEG (if clinically indicated)	EEG (if clinically indicated)
Somatosensory evoked potential	
Evaluation for bilaterally absent N20	MRI (Diffuse restriction in basal ganglia and cortical ribbon)
Neuron-specific enolase (prior to cooling)	

Abbreviations: EEG, electroencephalography; MRI, magnetic resonance imaging.

4. **C.** Cooling patients after ventricular fibrillation and ventricular tachycardia arrests is a mainstay therapy to improve neurologic outcome and reduce mortality. Cooling trials have evaluated patients with ventricular fibrillation and ventricular tachycardia as the initial rhythm discovered during the arrest. There has yet to be an independent study evaluating the use of cooling in pulseless electrical activity and asystole, but pooled data indicate that cooling does not appear to have improved outcome in his cohort of patients. Exclusion criteria used in these trials include: coma from other etiology (noncardiac), with coma defined as GCS <8, intractable hemodynamic instability, suspected sepsis, major surgery within 14 days, active bleeding, major head trauma, and isolated respiratory arrest. Given this patient had a GCS >8, he is not an appropriate candidate for cooling. If he were, there are a number of different means of cooling, with early interventions consisting of ice packs to the groin and axilla and infusion of 30 mL/kg of 4°C saline.

5. **B; 6 D.** The initial patient evaluation is consistent with coma, which is defined as both unarousable and unresponsiveness. During this state, there is no noticeable sleep-wake, auditory, or visual communication functions, but reflexes and postural motor responses may still be present. A vegetative state is defined as unresponsiveness to self or environment. The difference between coma and vegetative state is a preservation of sleep-wake cycle and brainstem autonomic functions such as startle (brief orientation) response to visual or auditory stimuli. The term persistent vegetative state is used when this state lasts more than 1 month, and permanent vegetative state is used when this state lasts for >3 months in nontrauma cases and >1 year in traumatic brain injury cases. Minimal conscious state (MCS) is defined as severely impaired consciousness with minimal behavioral evidence of awareness to self and environment. Unlike vegetative state, MCS patients have partial preservation of conscious awareness. Stupor is a reduced level of consciousness, which requires constant and repeated external stimulation to arouse the patient to purposeful response. Locked-in syndrome is a state of quadriplegia and loss of lower cranial nerve function but with preservation of cognition, sensation, and eye movements.

7. **E.** The patient has sustained a large-vessel ischemic stroke most likely due to artery-to-artery emboli from his known atherosclerotic disease. There are

a number of clinical findings that are associated with poor prognosis. The most important prognostic indicator for this patient is the total volume of his ischemic stroke. On retrospective review of the Virtual International Stroke Trials Archive, there was a linear relationship between stroke volume size and modified Rankin score at 90 days, with larger ischemic strokes associated with worse functional outcome. Within this study, there was also association of poor outcome with age (also near linear, but significant increase in worse prognosis after age 80) and premorbid conditions including diabetes. There are mixed data regarding recovery following dominant versus nondominant hemisphere ischemic stroke. Several studies have shown there is improved stroke recovery following dominant-hemispheric ischemic stroke despite having significant language deficits. The major rehabilitation limitation with non–dominant-hemispheric strokes is the resulting neglect or inattention to the affected hemibody and hemiworld. With substantial inattention to the weak part of the body or world, there is limited rehabilitation potential. Although large, symptomatic hemorrhagic conversion is associated with worse outcome, the patient's small, asymptomatic hemorrhages are not associated with worse neurologic prognosis. Atherosclerotic disease does have a worse prognosis than microangiopathic disease (eg, lacunar stroke) but is similar to cardioembolic disease.

8. **C.** Mortality following aneurysmal subarachnoid hemorrhage is determined by the patient's clinical presentation. The Hunt and Hess grading scale was initially developed in the 1960s, and since then, it is the most widely used to prognosticate SAH mortality. With the progression of both critical care and neurocritical care, the mortality of aneurysmal subarachnoid hemorrhage has decreased. Recent studies have demonstrated a decrease in 30-day mortality of all aneurysmal subarachnoid grades. The table below reviews the grades, from asymptomatic to comatose. The patient's initial presentation is consistent with a Hunt and Hess grade of 4, but following external ventricular drain (EVD) placement, there is an improvement of 1 Hunt and Hess grade (now grade 3). The head CT demonstrates early signs of hydrocephalus with enlargement of the temporal horns of the lateral ventricles. When there is improvement in the Hunt and Hess

grade following EVD placement, these patients have outcomes similar to their post-EVD placement examination. In this case, the patient's new Hunt and Hess grade is associated with a 30-day mortality of 9%.

Hunt and Hess Grades

Hunt and Hess Grade	Description	Mortality (%)	Follow-Up Mortality (%)
1	Asymptomatic or minimal headache and slight nuchal rigidity	11	3
2	Moderate or severe headache, nuchal rigidity, no neurologic deficit other than cranial nerve palsy	26	3
3	Drowsiness, confusion, or mild focal deficit	37	9
4	Stupor, moderate to severe hemiparesis, possibly early decerebrate rigidity, and vegetative disturbance	71	24
5	Deep coma, decerebrate posturing, moribund appearance	100	71

9. **D; 10 D.** The Advanced Life Support Task Force recommendation from 2003 is to start hypothermia protocol (32°C-34°C) for 12 to 24 hours in unconscious adult patients with spontaneous circulation after out-of-hospital cardiac arrest when the initial rhythm was ventricular fibrillation. Hypothermia may also be beneficial for other rhythms or in-hospital cardiac arrest. There is high incidence of complications such as coagulopathy, arrhythmias, and infection, and these complications are more common if the core temperature falls considerably below 32°C.

Patients with hypoxic injury in the setting of cardiac arrest are at greater risk of seizures. At this point, the patient did not show clear signs of clinical seizure, so hypothermia needs to be started as soon as possible. EEG after weaning down hypothermia might be beneficial if the patient's exam remained poor. MRI of brain is not indicated on admission but will highly be considered during the hospital course to help with prognostication if the patient's exam remained poor. Although the patient's initial examination is poor, it is too early from the initial insult to make an accurate recommendation on transition of care to hospice.

Prognosis after cardiac arrest can be challenging; thus, relying on clinical examination and workup is warranted. The only answer that is clearly linked to poor neurologic outcome is D. The MRI findings describe profound, global hypoxia of the brain with resultant ischemic changes. The EEG changes discussed are indeterminate in assessing prognosis. A single seizure does not, by itself, portent a poor outcome. The myoclonic jerking associated with myoclonic status epilepticus is, however, associated with poor outcome. Continuous myoclonus is also associated with poor outcome despite intact brainstem functions. Generalized slowing on EEG does not portend a poor outcome. There is no clear association of biochemical marker S100 with poor outcome, especially in the setting of hypothermia.

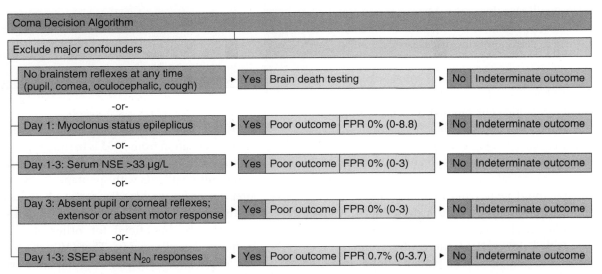

Reproduced with permission from Lee K. *The NeuroICU Book*. New York, NY: McGraw-Hill, 2012. Redrawn from Wijdicks EF, Hijdra A, Young GB, et al. Practice parameter: Prediction of outcome in comatose survivors after cardiopulmonary resuscitation (an evidence-based review): Report of the quality standards subcommittee of the American Academy of Neurology. *Neurology*. 2006;67:203-210.

11. C. The patient has malignant cerebral edema associated with a large ischemic stroke. There is limited right-to-left subfalcine herniation as shown on the CT of the head. The patient has experienced increased somnolence, likely due to ongoing increase in intracranial pressure. She is still quite early from her ischemic stroke but has a large territory of the right middle cerebral artery affected by the ischemic stroke. The use of a hemicraniectomy results in significantly lower mortality (30% vs 71%). In patients younger than age 60 years, there is also significantly reduced death or major disability, as defined by modified Rankin Scale >3 (74% vs 87%). The patient presented with profound aphasia and is left-handed, which marks the right hemisphere as the dominant hemisphere. Although there has been concern about interventions on the dominant hemisphere because they may leave patients alive but with profound aphasia and poor quality of life, long-term functional outcome of patients with large dominant and nondominant hemispheric infarction is not different.

12. **C.** The patient has sustained a severe traumatic brain injury due to her high-speed motor vehicle crash. The TBI-IMPACT prognostic score was developed using patient outcome data from multiple traumatic brain injury trials and is a prognostic model for mortality and unfavorable outcome at 6 months after injury. The model uses clinical, imaging, and laboratory data to calculate the probability of mortality and poor neurologic recovery. The clinical factors include age, motor score, and pupillary reactivity, with the most influential

being the lack of motor score. The addition of imaging and additional clinical findings increases the sensitivity, and these factors include hypoxia, hypotension, presence of traumatic subarachnoid hemorrhage, presence of epidural hematoma (protective), and severity of injury on CT scan. Finally, addition of laboratory data, hypoglycemia and anemia, can further refine the prognostic capability. The evaluation of this patient is shown in the table below, and with the available data, her predicted probability of 6-month mortality using clinical, imaging, and laboratory data is 32%, with an unfavorable outcome probability of 58%.

REFERENCES

Alexnder MP. Stroke rehabilitation outcome: a potential use of predictive variables to establish levels of care. *Stroke.* 1994;25:128-134.

Antigua H, Ortega-Gutierrez S, Schmidt JM, et al. Subarachnoid hemorrhage: who dies, and why? *Crit Care.* 2015;31:309-316.

Berkeley J, Geocadin, R. Coma and brain death. In: Torbey M, ed. *Neurocritical Care Book.* Cambridge, United Kingdom: Cambridge Press; 2009:227-235.

Bernard SA, Gray TW, Buist MD, et al. Treatment of comatose survivors of out-of-hospital cardiac arrest with induced hypothermia. *N Engl J Med.* 2002;346:557-563.

Booth CM, Boone RH, Tomlinson G, et al. Is this patient dead, vegetative, or severely neurologically impaired? Assessing outcome for comatose survivors of cardiac arrest. *JAMA.* 2004;291:870-879.

Dumas F, Grimaldi D, Zuber B, et al. Is hypothermia after cardiac arrest effective in both shockable and nonshockable patients? *Circulation.* 2011;123:877-886.

Graffagnino, C. Hypothermia: physiology and applications. In: Torbey M, ed. *Neurocritical Care Book.* Cambridge, United Kingdom: Cambridge Press; 2009:38-45.

Grau AJ, Weimar C, Buggle F, et al. Risk factors, outcome, and treatment in subtypes of ischemic stroke: the German Stroke Data Bank. *Stroke.* 2001;32:2559-2566.

Greer DM. Cardiac arrest and postanoxic encephalopathy. *Continuum.* 2015;21:1384-1396.

Gupta R, Connolly ES, Mayer S, et al. Hemicraniectomy for massive middle cerebral artery territory infarction: a systematic review. *Stroke.* 2004;35:539-543.

Hemphill JC, Bonovich DC, Besmertis L, et al. The ICH score: a simple, reliable grading scale for intracerebral hemorrhage. *Stroke.* 2001;32:891-897.

Hofmeijer J, Kappelle LJ, Algra A, et al. Surgical decompression for space-occupying cerebral infarction (the Hemicraniectomy after Middle Cerebral Artery infarction with Life-threatening Edema Trial [HAMLET]): a multicenter, open, randomized trial. *Lancet Neurol.* 2009;8:326-333.

Hunt WE, Hess RM. Surgical risks as related to time of intervention in the repair of intracranial aneurysms. *J Neurosurg.* 1968;28:14-20.

IMPACT-Prognostic Score for 6 Month Outcome After TBI

Clinical Characteristics	Imaging/ Additional Clinical Data	Laboratory Data
Age (0): <30 year old	Hypoxia (1): Suspected	Glucose (2): 9.2 mmol/L
Motor score (6): No movement	Hypotension (0): Not present	Hemoglobin (2): 10.6 mg/dL
Pupil reactivity (4): No pupil reacted	Computed tomography classification (2): Marshall grade II	
	Traumatic subarachnoid hemorrhage (0): Absent	
	Epidural hematoma (0): Absent	

Juttler E, Schwab S, Schmiedek P, et al. Decompressive Surgery for the Treatment of Malignant Infarction of Middle Cerebral Artery (DESTINY): a randomized, controlled trial. *Stroke.* 2007;38:2518-2525.

Kent DM, Hinchey J, Price LL, et al. In acute ischemic stroke, are asymptomatic intracranial hemorrhages clinically innocuous? *Stroke.* 2004;35:1141-1146.

Lehmann JF, DeLateur BJ, Fowler RS, et al. Stroke rehabilitation: outcome and prediction. *Arch Phys Med Rehabil.* 1997;56:375-382.

Leitherner C, Ploner CJ, Hasper D, et al. Dose hypothermia influence the predictive value of bilateral absent N20 after a cardiac arrest? *Neurology.* 2010;74:965-969.

Macciocchi SN, Diamond PT, Alves WM, et al. Ischemic stroke: relation of age, lesion location, and initial neurologic deficit to functional outcome. *Arch Phys Med Rehab.* 1998;79:1255-1257.

Marshall LF, Marshall SB, Klauber MR, et al. The diagnosis of head injury requires a classification based on computed axial tomography. *J Neurotrauma.* 1992;9(Suppl 1):S287-S292.

Nielsen N, Wetterslev J, Cronberg T, et al. Targeted temperature management at 33 C versus 36 C after cardiac arrest. *N Engl J Med.* 2013;369:2197-2206.

Nola JP, Morley PT, Vanden Hoek TL, et al. Therapeutic hypothermia after cardiac arrest: an advisory statement by the Advanced Life Support Task Force of the International Liaison Committee on Resuscitation. *Circulation.* 2003;108:118-121.

Ransom ER, Mocco J, Komotar RJ, et al. External ventricular drainage response in poor grade aneurysmal subarachnoid hemorrhage: effect on preoperative grading and prognosis. *Neurocrit Care.* 2007;6:174-180.

Rossetti AO, Oddo M, Logroscino G, et al. Prognostication after cardiac arrest and hypothermia. *Ann Neurol.* 2010;67:301-307.

Rost NS, Smith EE, Chang Y, et al. Prediction of functional outcome in patients with primary intracerebral hemorrhage: the FUNC score. *Stroke.* 2008;39:2304-2309.

Steyerberg EW, Mushkudiani N, Perel P, et al. Predicting outcome after traumatic brain injury: development and international validation of prognostic scores based on admission characteristics. *PLoS Med.* 2008;5:e165.

The Hypothermia After Cardia Arrest Study Group. Mild therapeutic hypothermia to improve the neurologic outcome after cardiac arrest. *N Engl J Med.* 2002;346:549-556.

Vahedi K, Vacaut E, Mateo J, et al. Sequential-design, multicenter, randomized, controlled trial of early decompressive craniectomy in malignant middle cerebral artery infarction (DECIMAL Trial). *Stroke.* 2007;38:2506-2517.

Vogt G, Laaage R, Shuaib A, et al. Initial lesion volume is an independent predictor of clinical stroke outcome at day 90: an analysis of the Virtual International Stroke Trials Archive (VISTA) database. *Stroke.* 2012;43:1266-1272.

Wijdicks EF, Hijdra A, Young GB, et al. Practice parameter: prediction of outcome in comatose survivors after cardiopulmonary resuscitation (an evidence-based review): report of the Quality Standards Subcommittee of the American Academy of Neurology. *Neurology.* 2006;67:203-210.

Wu O, Sorensen AG, Benner T, et al. Comatose patient with cardiac arrest: predicting clinical outcome with diffusion-weighted MR imaging. *Radiology.* 2009;252:173-181.

Yang MH, Lin HY, Fu J, et al. Decompressive hemicraniectomy in patients with malignant middle cerebral artery infarction: a systematic review and meta-analysis. *Surgeon.* 2015;13:230-240.

PART 2
Neurosurgical Management

18

Vascular Neurosurgery

Mark Dannenbaum, MD

Questions

1. Which of the following is branch of the meningo-hypophyseal trunk (MHT)?

   A. Vidian artery

   B. Caroticotympanic artery

   C. Inferior hypophyseal artery

   D. Superior hypophyseal artery

   E. Recurrent artery of Heubner

2. Which of the following segmental anatomic classifications correctly describes the second division of the middle cerebral artery (M2)?

   A. Sphenoidal segment

   B. Horizontal segment

   C. Insular segment

   D. Opercular segment

   E. Cortical segment

3. The blood supply to the cuneate and lingual gyri is provided by which artery?

   A. Anterior temporal artery

   B. Inferior temporal artery

   C. Medial posterior choroidal artery

   D. Parieto-occipital artery

   E. Calcarine artery

4. The below gadolinium-enhanced magnetic resonance imaging (MRI) scan and digital subtraction angiogram demonstrate which diagnosis?

   A. Right frontal lobe arteriovenous malformation

   B. Anterior ethmoidal dural arteriovenous fistula

   C. Carotid cavernous fistula

   D. Vein of Galen malformation

   E. Developmental venous anomaly

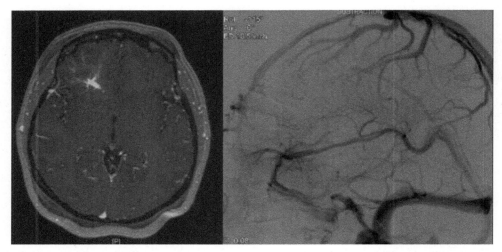

A. Axial T1 magnetic resonance image with contrast showing abnormal contrast enhancement in the deep right frontal lobe.
B. Digital subtraction angiogram in the venous phase showing abnormal venous drainage into the superior sagittal sinus.

5. The labyrinthine artery most frequently arises from which vessel?

   A. Posterior auricular artery

   B. Stapedial artery

   C. Caroticotympanic artery

   D. Anterior inferior cerebellar artery

   E. Basilar artery

6. The giant cavernous aneurysm shown below is most likely to present with which cranial neuropathy?

   A. Cranial nerve II

   B. Cranial nerve III

   C. Cranial nerve IV

   D. Cranial nerve V_3

   E. Cranial nerve VI

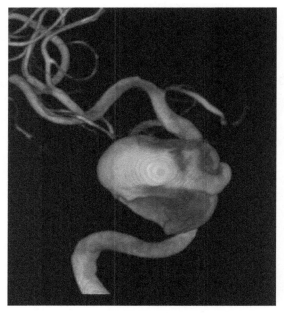

Anterior posterior computed tomography angiogram 3-dimensional reconstruction of internal carotid artery aneurysm at the cavernous sinus.

7. Which surgical approach will enable the most direct visualization of the left posterior inferior cerebellar artery aneurysm (PICA)?

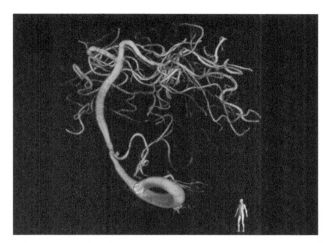

Oblique view of 3-dimensional reconstruction of a computed tomography angiogram of the left vertebral artery, basilar artery, and branches. There is small proximal posterior inferior cerebellar artery aneurysm.

A. Transsphenoidal/transclival
B. Left subtemporal
C. Left pterional (frontotemporal)
D. Left far lateral suboccipital
E. Midline suboccipital

8. A 39-year-old woman involved in a high-speed motor vehicle collision presents. After hemodynamic stabilization, a full neurologic examination is completed. The pertinent findings include left Horner's syndrome, vertigo, and ataxia, as well as sensory changes on the left side of the face and right side of the body. Which of the following is the most likely cause?

A. Left carotid artery dissection
B. Right carotid artery dissection
C. Left vertebral artery dissection
D. Right vertebral artery dissection
E. Right middle cerebral artery thrombosis

9. What is the best predictor of development of symptomatic clinical vasospasm after aneurysmal subarachnoid hemorrhage?

A. The amount of subarachnoid hemorrhage present on the admission head computed tomography (CT)
B. Long-standing history of cigarette smoking
C. Cocaine use
D. Age >50 years old
E. History of hypertension

10. The angiographic variant demonstrated below is best described as which of the following?

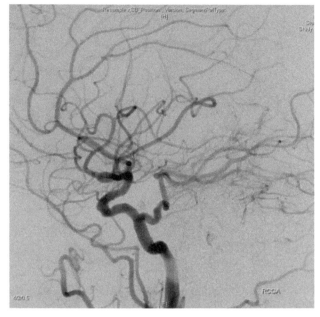

Digital subtraction angiogram: arterial phase in lateral projection of a right common carotid artery.

A. Fetal posterior cerebral artery
B. Primitive trigeminal artery
C. Persistent otic artery
D. Persistent hypoglossal artery
E. Proatlantal intersegmental artery

11. A patient presents to the office with a known history of recurrent epistaxis and mucocutaneous telangiectasias (see below). Which intracranial vascular pathology is associated with these findings?

    A. Dural arteriovenous fistula

    B. Brain arteriovenous malformation

    C. Carotid blowout secondary to dissection

    D. Direct carotid cavernous fistula

    E. Hemangioblastoma

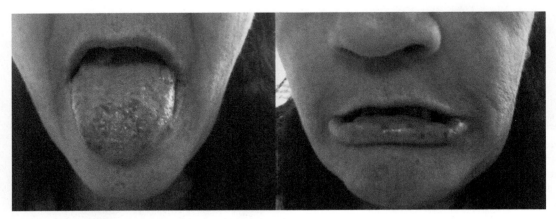

Multiple mucous membrane telangiectasias on labial and lingual surfaces.

12. What is the expected outcome for surgical resection of the arteriovenous malformation shown in the image (below) in experienced hands?

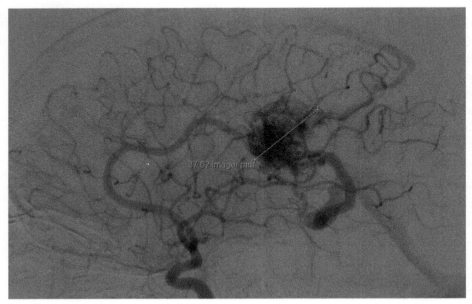

Digital subtraction angiography: Left internal carotid artery injection with lateral projection demonstrating an arteriovenous malformation with feeding vessel from middle cerebral artery and drainage into vein of Galen. This is located near the posterior superior temporal lobe.

	Minor Deficit (%)	Major Deficit (%)
A.	0	0
B.	5	0
C.	12	4
D.	20	7
E.	19	12

A. 9.0%

B. 14.6%

C. 26.0%

D. 38.2%

E. 66.1%

13. A 68-year-old man has a history of hypertension, hyperlipidemia, diabetes mellitus, and coronary artery disease with prior drug-eluting stent placed to the left descending coronary artery, all of which are now well-controlled diseases. He has 2 brief, transient episodes of right facial droop and "confusion" per his wife, which she describes further as inability to find the correct words within the last 90 days. Workup for a transient ischemic attack is revealing for the lesion shown below. What is the estimated stroke risk in 2 years with conservative management alone?

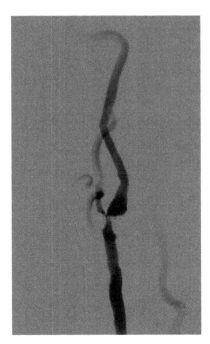

Digital subtraction angiogram: Early arterial phase of left common carotid artery injection. Image at the level of the left carotid artery bifurcation.

14. A 42-year-old woman presented to her primary care physician for paroxysmal shock-like pain in her right face that started while she was brushing her teeth. Over the course of several months, the pain became more persistent and required smaller amounts of stimulation to trigger it. She started carbamazepine with limited effect. She now wants to evaluate surgical options as she read that compression can sometimes cause her symptoms. Which artery is most often responsible for compression of the cranial nerve most likely causing her symptoms?

A. Superior cerebellar artery

B. Anterior inferior cerebellar artery

C. Posterior inferior cerebellar artery

D. Persistent trigeminal artery

E. Vidian artery

15. A 42-year-old man has new onset of migraine headache and is evaluated by his primary care physician. An MRI of the brain was completed as part of his workup and was abnormal, and he was sent to a neurosurgeon for further evaluation. A digital subtraction angiogram was completed and is shown below. What is the diagnosis?

A. Arteriovenous malformation (AVM)

B. Hemangioblastoma

C. Cavernous malformation

D. Capillary telangiectasia

E. Developmental venous anomaly

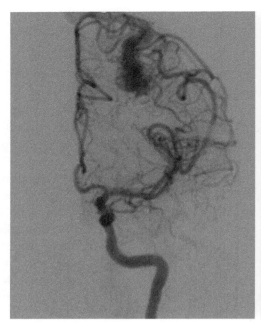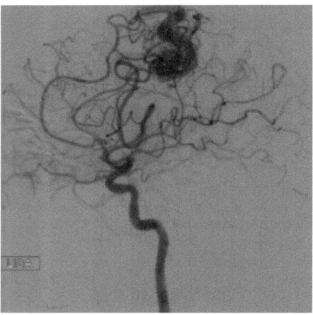

Digital subtraction angiogram: Left panel shows anterior-posterior projection of left internal carotid artery injection at mid-arterial phase. Right panel shows lateral projection of left internal carotid artery injection at mid-arterial phase.

Questions 16 and 17

A 48-year-old man was sent for evaluation of a palpable right neck mass near the angle of the mandible. He has no other symptoms at this time. A CT of the neck was completed, and this prompted an angiogram, shown below.

16. This lesion is most often supplied by which vessel?
   A. Internal carotid artery
   B. Ascending pharyngeal artery
   C. Vertebral artery
   D. Ascending cervical artery
   E. Superior thyroid artery

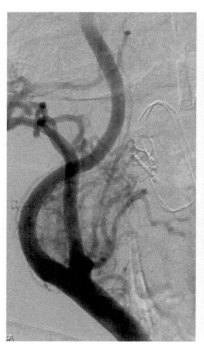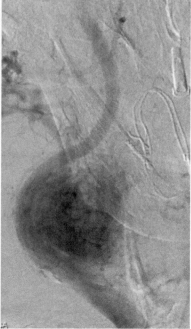

Digital subtraction angiogram of the lateral common carotid artery injection. Left panel shows early arterial phase image. Right panel shows late arterial phase image with intense blush of contrast.

17. Which of the following statements regarding the pathology demonstrated is true?

    A. They most often present as a palpable, painful neck masses.

    B. They are the most common anterior neck mass in children.

    C. They form under conditions of chronic hypoxia such as high altitudes, chronic obstructive pulmonary disease, or cyanotic heart disease.

    D. They are pathologically categorized as schwannomas.

    E. Ninety percent of patients will develop them as a result of genetic mutations, and they have a high likelihood for multiplicity.

18. The vascular lesion shown below directly drains into which of the following?

A. Basal vein of Rosenthal

B. Vein of Galen

C. Internal cerebral vein

D. Cavernous sinus

E. Straight sinus

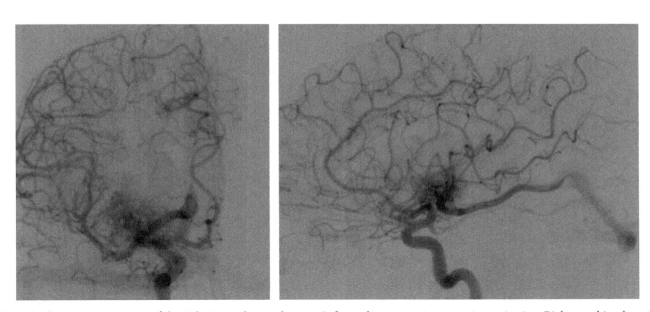

Digital subtraction angiogram of the right internal carotid artery. Left panel is an anterior-posterior projection. Right panel is a lateral projection.

19. A 16-year-old boy presented for evaluation of persistent difficulty with nasal breathing and recurrent episodes of severe epistaxis. He was found to have a juvenile nasopharyngeal angiofibroma that underwent liquid embolization. Following embolization, he underwent angiography, which is shown below. What is indicated by the white arrow?

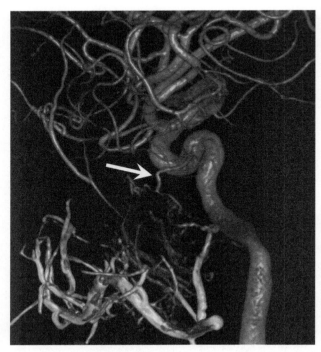

Digital subtraction angiogram 3-dimensional reconstruction of a left internal carotid artery injection after a liquid embolization of a juvenile nasopharyngeal angiofibroma (light grey).

A. Ophthalmic artery

B. Superior hypophyseal artery

C. Anterior choroidal artery

D. Meningohypophyseal trunk

E. Inferolateral trunk

20. A 37-year-old man is currently in the neurointensive care unit following a ruptured anterior communicating artery aneurysm that was successfully clipped. On day 4 of hospitalization, he developed a new left facial droop and arm weakness. He was transported to the angiography suite, and the initial image is shown below. What is the next best step in his care?

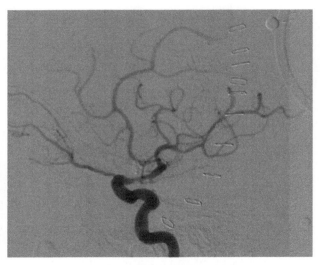

Digital subtraction angiogram. Right internal carotid artery injection with lateral projection in early arterial phase.

A. Return to operating room (OR) for clip repositioning

B. Transport to intensive care unit for electroencephalogram monitoring

C. Send cerebrospinal fluid for analysis and cultures

D. Balloon angioplasty

E. Return to OR for hematoma evacuation

21. What complication can be seen if metformin is continued following angiography?

A. Renal toxicity

B. Lactic acidosis

C. Induced hypercoagulable state

D. Arrhythmia onset

E. Accelerated contrast immune hyperactivity

22. A 71-year-old man develops severe dysphagia, respiratory distress, stridor, and labored respirations following a routine carotid endarterectomy. Physical exam showed swelling deep to the incision. What is the next best step?

   A. Intubate the patient in the recovery area (postanesthesia care unit [PACU])

   B. Place the patient on oxygen and return to the OR for elective intubation and possible neck exploration

   C. Open the surgical wound at the bedside emergently

   D. Send the patient to the neurointensive care unit on a non-rebreather assuming he is oxygenating properly

   E. Attempt beside drainage percutaneously with a 20-gauge needle

23. A 37-year-old woman developed an acute-onset dysarthria and right-sided weakness. On examination, there is lingual dysarthria, and on tongue protrusion, there is tongue deviation to the left, moderate right hemiparesis, and decreased sensation on the right hemibody. An MRI of the brain is completed and shown below. What is the most likely vessel affected as a result of her acute ischemic stroke?

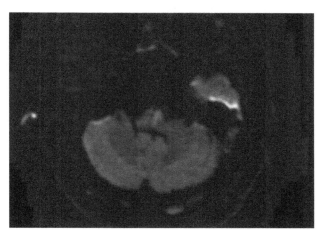

Magnetic resonance image (diffusion-weighted image): Axial cut at the level of the medulla with restricted diffusion in the left paramedian pontine distribution.

   A. Left vertebral artery

   B. Left posterior inferior cerebellar artery

   C. Anterior spinal artery

   D. Basilar artery trunk

   E. Left superior cerebellar artery

24. A 49-year-old woman with hypertension and ongoing tobacco use was found to have a right posterior communicating artery aneurysm that measured 9 mm with a wide-based neck. A right pterional craniotomy for clipping of a posterior communicating artery aneurysm is depicted below. What was the most likely clinical presentation?

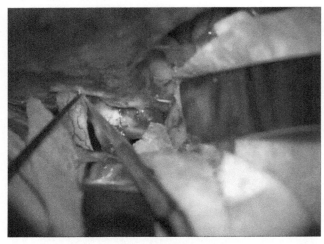

A right pterional craniotomy for clipping of a posterior communicating artery aneurysm, which as shown is about 9 mm with a wide-based neck.

A. Oculomotor nerve palsy, pupil sparing

B. Oculomotor nerve palsy, complete

C. Optic neuropathy

D. Cerebrospinal fluid (CSF) leak from erosion of a pneumatized anterior clinoid process

E. Epistaxis from erosion through the anterior clinoid process

25. A 6-year-old girl is taken to the emergency department via emergency medical services (EMS) after collapsing. On arrival of EMS, she was without a pulse, and cardiopulmonary resuscitation (CPR) was initiated. She required 20 minutes of CPR with eventual return of spontaneous circulation. What is the most likely cause of the imaging finding (shown below)?

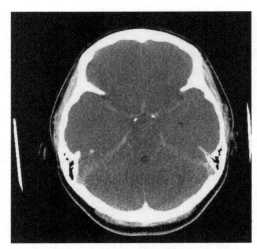

Noncontrast head computed tomography. Axial at the level of the midbrain.

A. Anoxia and underlying cerebral edema

B. Aneurysmal subarachnoid hemorrhage

C. Traumatic subarachnoid hemorrhage

D. Fungal meningitis

E. Tuberculous meningitis

26. Which of the following statements is correct regarding this spinal arteriovenous malformation (AVM) shown from a right T9 intercostal artery injection?

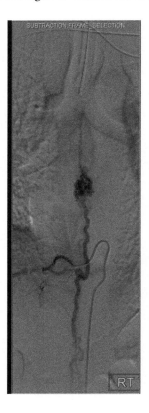

A. It is the most frequent spinal vascular malformation.

B. It has low pressure but high flow.

C. It rarely hemorrhages.

D. It is also referred to as a glomus type.

E. It is acquired.

27. A 58-year-old man with no past medical history presented to the emergency department (ED) from urgent care for evaluation of severe holocephalic headache. About 24 hours prior to presentation, he had abrupt onset of the headache that has not changed since that time. A head CT was completed in the ED and is shown below. Digital subtraction angiogram is also shown. What is the most likely etiology of the patient's hemorrhage?

A. A ruptured saccular right M1/M2 junction middle cerebral artery (MCA) aneurysm

B. A ruptured anterior communicating artery aneurysm filling from the right internal carotid artery (ICA)

C. A ruptured anterior communicating artery aneurysm filling from the left ICA

D. A dissecting aneurysm of the right M1 segment of MCA

E. A right anterior temporal artery aneurysm

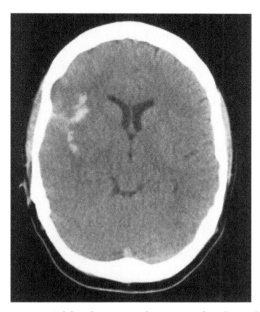

Noncontrast axial head computed tomography shows hyperdensity at the level of right Sylvian fissure.

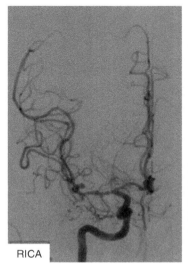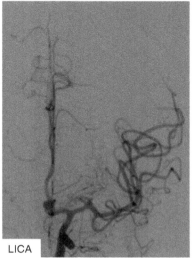

Digital subtraction angiogram. Left panel shows mid-arterial image of right internal carotid artery (RICA) injection in anterior-posterior projection. Right panel shows mid-arterial image of left internal carotid artery (LICA) injection in anterior-posterior projection.

28. Which of the following is true regarding MRI and subarachnoid hemorrhage evaluation within 1 week of onset?

    A. It is a less sensitive imaging modality for the acute detection of subarachnoid hemorrhage than CT (from 24-48 hours)

    B. Susceptibility-weighted image (SWI) sequences represent the sequence of choice for detecting blood in the subarachnoid space

    C. MRI is contraindicated due to the possibility of phase encoding artifact and potential precipitation of rupture

    D. Fluid-attenuated inversion recovery (FLAIR) sequence is the most useful sequence for detecting blood in the subarachnoid space.

29. A 36-year-old woman with 1 prior event of left facial numbness approximately 4 years ago that lasted for several months but improved presented to the ED for evaluation of left face and arm weakness and numbness. There was an abnormal head CT, and MRI was completed and is shown below. What is the most likely pathology based on her MRI?

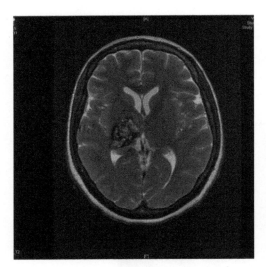

Axial T2 magnetic resonance imaging at the level of thalamus shows signs of reticulated mixed signal mass with a hemosiderin rim.

A. Hypertensive intraparenchymal hemorrhage

B. Arteriovenous malformation

C. Cavernous malformation

D. Capillary telangiectasia

E. Developmental venous anomaly

30. A 79-year-old man with hypertension, hyperlipidemia, coronary artery disease with prior right coronary artery myocardial infarction 9 months prior, peripheral vascular disease with known carotid occlusion of the right internal carotid artery, and prior C3-T1 cervical fusion presented to the ED for evaluation of transient expressive aphasia and right facial droop. Workup was revealing for the findings shown below. Which of the following would be an absolute contraindication for a carotid endarterectomy in this case?

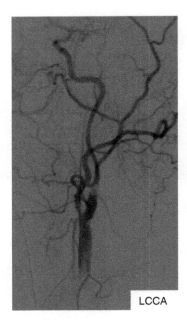

LCCA

Digital subtraction angiogram.

A. History of prior myocardial infarction

B. History of prior anterior cervical discectomy and fusion

C. Age >75 years

D. Presence of an unruptured ipsilateral intracranial aneurysm measuring 9 mm

E. Contralateral carotid stenosis of 60%

31. A 68-year-old man presented with new symptoms. A digital subtraction angiogram was completed and is shown below. Given the findings, which of the following was most likely his neurologic symptom?

A. High-volume epistaxis

B. Ischemia of the right hemisphere

C. Subarachnoid hemorrhage from retrograde cortical venous reflux

D. Intraparenchymal hemorrhage

E. Cranial nerve VI palsy

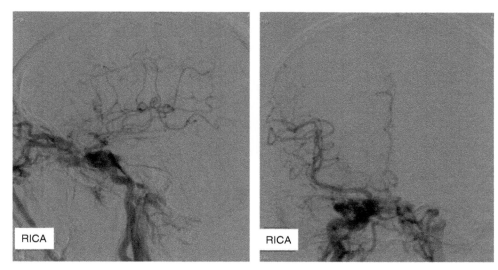

Digital subtraction angiogram. Left panel shows early arterial phase right internal carotid artery (RICA) injection in lateral projection. Right panel shows early arterial phase RICA injection in anterior-posterior projection.

32. A 57-year-old woman presented for new symptoms. A digital subtraction angiogram was completed and is shown below. Given the findings, which of the following was most likely her neurologic symptom?

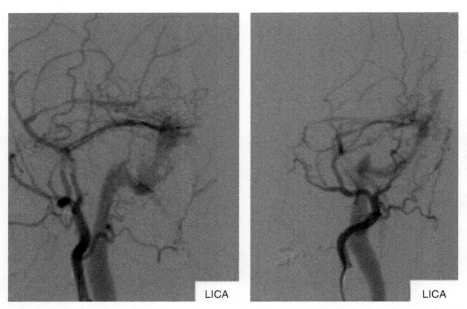

Digital subtraction angiogram. Left panel shows mid-arterial phase injection of the left internal carotid artery (LICA) in lateral projection. Right panel shows mid-arterial phase injection of the left internal carotid artery (LICA) in oblique projection.

    A. A lateral temporal intraparenchymal hemorrhage

    B. Pulsatile tinnitus

    C. Intractable vertigo and ataxia

    D. A seizure from venous congestion

    E. Spontaneous otorrhagia

33. A 38-year-old man who has ingested cocaine develops acute-onset dizziness, followed by headache, nausea, and vomiting. He goes to rest given he does not feel well. His friends go to check on him again 6 hours later and find him difficult to arouse. EMS is called, and he is brought to the ED for evaluation. He complains of substernal chest pain and appears terrified. A head CT is completed and shown below. What is the most likely etiology of the cerebellar infarction?

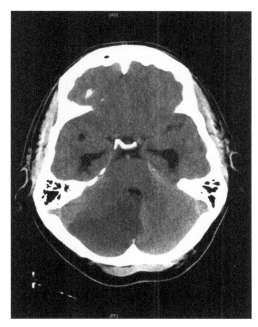

Noncontrast axial head computed tomography at the level of mid-pons.

    A. Right cervical vertebral artery dissection

    B. Rupture of a plaque from high-grade ostial stenosis of the right vertebral artery

    C. Fusiform aneurysm of the intradural right vertebral artery

    D. Focal vasospasm in the right posterior inferior cerebellar artery (PICA)

    E. Cardiogenic embolus

34. Six hours after a routine right frontotemporal craniotomy for clipping of an unruptured posterior communicating artery aneurysm, a patient develops acute left hemiplegia, left hemisensory loss, and a left homonymous hemianopsia. What is the most likely explanation?

    A. Acute embolic occlusion of the right M1 segment of the middle cerebral artery

    B. Acute occlusion of the right M1 segment of the middle cerebral artery secondary to vasospasm

    C. Hypoperfusion to right-sided lenticulostriate branches

    D. Surgical occlusion of the right anterior choroidal artery

    E. Venous infarction secondary to coagulation of the Sylvian vein

35. Which of the following glycoprotein IIb/IIIa inhibitors irreversibly inhibits its target?

    A. Abciximab

    B. Tirofiban

    C. Eptifibatide

    D. Clopidogrel

    E. Prasugrel

Answers and Explanations

1. **C.** The inferior hypophyseal artery arises as 1 of 3 branches of the meningohypophyseal trunk. The other 2 are the tentorial artery and dorsal meningeal. Choices A and B both arise from petrous internal carotid artery. Superior hypophyseal arises from the ophthalmic segment of the internal carotid artery. Recurrent artery of Heubner arises from anterior cerebral artery system.

2. **C.** The middle cerebral artery (MCA) is divided into 4 segments: sphenoidal, insular, opercular, and terminal/cortical (M1 to M4, respectively). The sphenoidal segment (M1) or horizontal segment has branches that supply the basal ganglia. The insular segment (M2) runs within the insula. The opercular segment (M3) extends laterally from the insula toward the cortex. The terminal segment (M4) begins at the external Sylvian fissure and extends distally to the cortex of the brain.

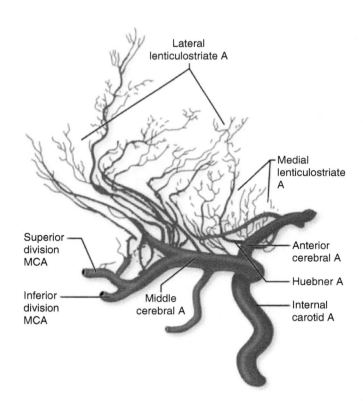

Reproduced with permission from Ropper AH, Samuel MA, Klein JP. *Adams and Victor's Principles of Neurology,* 10e. New York, NY: McGraw-Hill, 2014.

3. E. The cuneate and lingual gyri are portions of the occipital lobe, which are divided by the calcarine sulcus. These 2 gyri compose the primary visual cortex. The calcarine artery supplies this region of the brain. The anterior temporal artery typically branches from the M1 segment of the MCA and supplies the anterior third of the temporal gyri. The inferior temporal artery is typically a terminal branch off the posterior cerebral artery (PCA) via the lateral occipital artery. The medial posterior choroidal artery is a branch off the PCA second segment and supplies the midbrain, posterior thalamus, and pineal gland. The parieto-occipital branch is a terminal branch off the PCA that supplies the cuneus and precuneus.

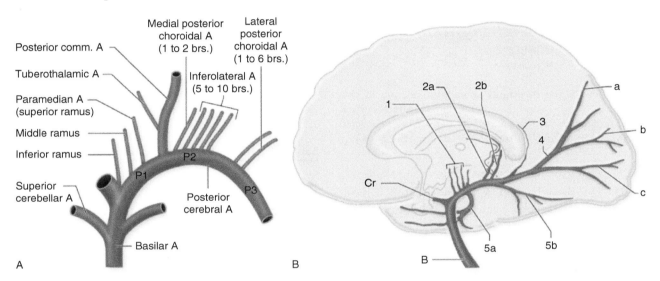

Reproduced with permission from Ropper AH, Samuel MA, Klein JP. *Adams and Victor's Principles of Neurology,* 10e. New York, NY: McGraw-Hill, 2014.

4. E. The digital subtraction angiogram (DSA) is shown in the venous phase. There are multiple veins collecting into a single central draining vein, which is consistent with developmental venous anomaly. This is the so-called "caput medusa appearance." There is no early venous drainage in the arterial phase, as would be seen in an arteriovenous malformation or fistula (not shown). However, based on the characteristic morphology on both the MRI and DSA, the diagnosis is certain, and the other entities are unlikely. A vein of Galen malformation will typically present in childhood or earlier with developmental delay, hydrocephalus, or potentially high-output cardiac failure. A carotid cavernous fistula is often secondary to trauma and commonly present with pulsatile exophthalmos.

5. D. The labyrinthine artery (or internal auditory artery) is most commonly a branch off the anterior inferior cerebellar artery (>85%) and less commonly a branch from the basilar artery (<15%), which courses with the vestibulocochlear nerve via the internal auditory meatus to supply the inner ear. The posterior auricular artery is a branch from the external carotid artery that supplies the auricle and the scalp posterior to the auricle. The stapedial artery is a branch from the posterior auricular artery that supplies the stapedius muscle. The caroticotympanic artery is a branch off the internal carotid artery that forms an anastomosis with the anterior tympanic branch and posterior tympanic branch arteries.

6. **E.** Within the cavernous sinus are cranial nerves III, IV, V_1, V_2, and VI as shown in the image below. The abducens nerve (cranial nerve VI) courses just inferior to the internal carotid artery and is the most susceptible to early compression and stretch, which can result in dysfunction.

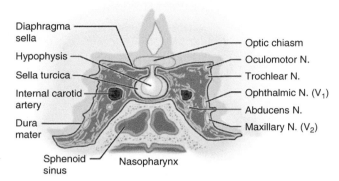

Coronal view of the cavernous sinus with relation of the internal carotid artery and the cranial nerves. (Adapted from Ropper A, Samuels M, Klein J. *Adams and Victor's Principles of Neurology*. 10th ed. New York, NY: McGraw-Hill; 2014.)

7. **D.** This is a left PICA aneurysm and is best approaches through a far lateral suboccipital corridor to achieve lateral exposure that will provide optimal visualization of the medulla, lower cranial nerves, vertebral artery, and proximal PICA. Subtemporal approach would best expose the temporal base, parasellar, retrochiasmatic, and anterolateral petroclival region. The transsphenoidal approach would best expose the sella and parasellar regions. The midline suboccipital approach would best expose the midline cerebellar structures. The pterional craniotomy provides access to the middle cranial fossa, anterior cranial fossa, and suprasellar/parasellar structures.

8. **C.** This patient has a left-sided Horner's syndrome, left facial sensation changes with crossed body sensation changes, and left cerebellar findings. These are classic findings in a lateral medullary (Wallenberg) syndrome. The common supply to the lateral medulla is the posterior inferior cerebellar artery, which commonly arises from the vertebral artery. Therefore, the most likely cause is a left vertebral artery dissection. A left carotid artery dissection

may cause a left-sided Horner's syndrome but will not explain the brainstem findings. A right MCA stroke will not produce these clinical manifestations.

9. **A.** The best predictor for symptomatic vasospasm following aneurysmal subarachnoid hemorrhage is the amount and distribution of subarachnoid hemorrhage on the initial head CT. The Fisher and, later, the modified Fisher scales (Table 18-1) were developed to assess the amount of hemorrhage and group patients into stratified risk groups. With increasing amount of hemorrhage, there is increased risk of vasospasm. Hypertension and smoking are risk factors for aneurysm development and rupture but do not increase the risk of symptomatic vasospasm. Cocaine can cause subarachnoid hemorrhage but does not increase the risk of symptomatic artery vasospasm. There are conflicting data regarding an association between age and symptomatic vasospasm. On a dichotomized scale, there is increased risk of vasospasm (with or without symptoms) in those who are younger than 50 years old.

Table 18-1. Modified Fisher Scale

Grade	Criteria on Computed Tomography	Incidence of Symptomatic Vasospasm
0	No SAH, no IVH	0%
1	Focal or diffuse, thin SAH; no IVH	24%
2	Thin focal or diffuse SAH, with IVH	33%
3	Thick focal or diffuse SAH; no IVH	33%
4	Thick focal or diffuse SAH, with IVH	40%

Abbreviations: IVH, intraventricular hemorrhage; SAH, subarachnoid hemorrhage.

10. **B.** The angiogram demonstrates a posterior projecting artery from the cavernous portion of the right internal carotid artery that anastomoses with the basilar artery. The location of the artery take-off and connection to the basilar artery is consistent with a primitive trigeminal artery. A persistent otic artery arises from the internal carotid artery within the carotid canal and joins the basilar artery inferiorly. Proatlantal artery can arise from the internal, external, or common (in descending frequency)

carotid artery and join with the ipsilateral vertebral artery. A persistent hypoglossal artery arises from the distal cervical internal carotid artery (ICA) and joins the inferior basilar artery. Fetal posterior cerebral artery arises from the terminal ICA and would project posteriorly to the PCA but not supply the basilar artery, as shown in the figure.

11. **B.** The history and examination findings are consistent with hereditary hemorrhagic telangiectasia (HHT), also known as Osler-Weber-Rendu syndrome. This is an autosomal dominate genetic disorder that leads to abnormal blood vessel formation. The most common vascular malformation within the brain is arteriovenous malformations.

12. **D.** The anticipated complications and complication rate of surgical resection of arteriovenous malformations (AVMs) depend on the Spetzler-Martin grade. The Spetzler-Martin grading system (Table 18-2) uses size, venous drainage, and location (in relation to eloquent cortex) to risk stratify surgical resection. The shown AMV Spetzler-Martin grade is 4: size is >3 cm but <6 cm (2 points); early venous drainage to the deep system is present (1 point); and it is located in or around receptive language areas (1 point for eloquent cortex).

Table 18-2. Spetzler-Martin Grading System

Category	No. of Points
AVM Size	
Small (<3 cm)	1
Medium (3-6 cm)	2
Large (>6 cm)	3
Localization	
Noneloquent	0
Eloquent	1
Venous drainage	
Superficial only	0
Deep	1

Abbreviation: AVM, arteriovenous malformation.

Adapted from Lee K. *The NeuroICU Book*. New York, NY: McGraw-Hill; 2012.

The Spetzler-Martin grade was originally validated in a study of 100 consecutive patients treated with microsurgical excision of AVMs. Morbidity rates were as follows:

Grade 1: 0%
Grade 2: 5% minor deficit, 0% major deficit
Grade 3: 12% minor deficit, 4% major deficit
Grade 4: 20% minor deficit, 7% major deficit
Grade 5: 19% minor deficit, 12% major deficit

13. **C.** The angiogram shown in this question demonstrates severe carotid stenosis at the level of the carotid bifurcation. The patient has multiple vascular risk factors, which are currently under control. Patients with symptomatic carotid stenosis should undergo revascularization to decrease the risk of ipsilateral ischemic stroke and death. In those who did not undergo carotid endarterectomy in the North American Symptomatic Carotid Endarterectomy Trial (NASCET), there was a 26% risk of ipsilateral stroke within 24 months.

14. **A.** The patient presents with paroxysmal, shock-like pain over her right face that is exacerbated by stimulation, which is consistent with trigeminal neuralgia. The most common cause of compressive trigeminal neuralgia is superior compression from the superior cerebellar artery (88% alone or in conjunction with additional compression) followed by the anterior inferior cerebellar artery (<25%). Given the lamination pattern of the fibers, medial compression will cause V_2 (maxillary division) syndrome; however, lateral compression may compress V_3 (mandibular branch). V_1 (ophthalmic branch) is rarely compressed.

Other compressive lesions can include basilar or vertebral arteries, aneurysm, persistent trigeminal neuralgia, or a petrous vein, but all of these are less common. Vidian artery, also known as artery of the pterygoid canal, acts as an internal-external carotid artery anastomosis.

15. **A.** The digital subtraction angiogram demonstrates a tangle of vessels with supply from a branch of the middle cerebral artery that has early venous drainage superficially. The connection between the arterial and venous structures without intervening capillaries is consistent with an AVM. The differential diagnosis includes hemangioblastoma, but there is lack of a central tumor blush that is typically seen. Cavernomas and capillary telangiectasias are angiography occult and will not be seen on an angiogram. A developmental venous anomaly shows multiple veins collecting into a single central

draining vein. This is the so-called "caput medusa appearance."

16. **B.** The imaging is most consistent with a carotid body tumor. This tumor is from the paraganglionic cells found within the carotid body. The common findings on angiogram are splitting of the internal and external carotid artery resulting in formation of the "lyre sign" (not shown) with intense early blush due to early venous shunting. The ascending pharyngeal artery is the main contributing artery.

17. **C.** This is a carotid body tumor. They develop under conditions of hypoxia. These rare lesions are usually a painless neck mass. They are uncommon in children. Histologically, they are paragangliomas. They rarely develop as a result of genetic mutations.

18. **A.** This AVM demonstrates deep venous drainage. The basal vein of Rosenthal can be clearly seen draining into the vein of Galen, which then drains to the straight sinus. Deep venous drainage is shown in the figure below.

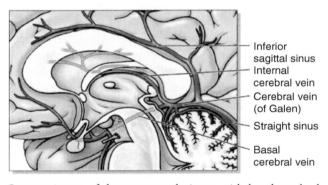

Cartoon image of deep venous drainage with basal cerebral vein (also known as vein of Rosenthal) draining into the vein of Galen and then straight sinus. (Adapted from Martin J: *Neuroanatomy Text and Atlas.* 4th ed. New York, NY: McGraw-Hill Education; 2012.)

19. **E.** The structure shown is the inferolateral trunk. It is laterally projecting and arises from the cavernous carotid. The superior hypophyseal system and the ophthalmic artery both arise more distally from the ophthalmic segment of the ICA. The anterior choroidal artery arises more distally from the communicating segment. The meningohypophyseal artery arises from the cavernous carotid; however, it projects posteriorly.

20. **D.** This patient has a neurologic deficit that is acute in onset and clearly matches the distribution of the spasm, which is shown here in the supraclinoid ICA. There is no other explanation such as postictal paralysis of completed infarction, and therefore, he should be treated aggressively.

21. **B.** Metformin is an oral medication for treatment of diabetes mellitus. There are limited data on complications in patients taking metformin who have received intravenous contrast, but in those who did have complications, there was substantial morbidity. In the setting of patients who have contrast-induced nephropathy and continue to take metformin, there is a risk of life-threatening lactic acidosis. Because contrast nephropathy is the precipitant cause to lactic acidosis, withholding metformin for 48 hours and knowing the renal function at that time can help guide re-administration of the medication. The 2015 guidelines from the American College of Radiology is as follows:

- Category I (estimated glomerular filtration rate [eGFR] >30 mL/min/1.73 m^2): Without evidence of acute kidney injury (AKI) and with eGFR >30, there is no need to discontinue metformin either prior to or following the intravenous administration of iodinated contrast media, nor is there an obligatory need to reassess the patient's renal function following the test.
- Category II (eGFR <30 mL/min/1.73 m^2): In those taking metformin who are known to have AKI or severe chronic kidney disease (stage IV or V), or who are undergoing arterial catheter studies that might result in emboli to the renal arteries, metformin should be temporarily discontinued at the time of or prior to the procedure, withheld for 48 hours subsequent to the procedure, and reinstituted only after renal function has been reevaluated.

22. **A.** Given the swelling following the operative case, there is the possibility of bleeding resulting in subcutaneous swelling and compression of the patient's airway. The sign of stridor is particularly concerning there is impending compromise of the airway from compression. Although drainage of potential blood may be required, the patient needs a secure airway prior to this. Following advanced cardiac life support guidelines, the airway comes first, and

in the setting of pending loss of airway, the patient should have his airway secured in the PACU.

23. **C.** The anterior spinal artery supplies the midline structures in the medulla, and these would include the hypoglossal nucleus and the corticospinal tracts. This patient could also have some deficits in vibration and proprioception as a result of damage to the medial lemniscus. This is medial medullary syndrome.

24. **B.** A large posterior communicating artery aneurysm most likely will present with a compression oculomotor neuropathy. Compressive neuropathies, if significant enough, can present with a complete nerve palsy and, on early presentation, would result in anisocoria. This is due to the anatomy of the oculomotor nerve. The parasympathetic fibers run along the periphery of the nerve and are early structures to become affected by compression. Pupil sparing is not usually seen in compressive lesions and is more characteristic of ischemic lesions.

Optic neuropathy is more characteristic in giant ophthalmic artery aneurysms. CSF leak and epistaxis are very unlikely.

25. **A.** Shown in the figure is a decrease in parenchymal attenuation, engorgement, and dilatation of the superficial venous structures due to elevated intracranial pressure. The fact that this is in a 6-year-old child and that there was a prolonged period of resuscitation makes anoxia the likely etiology. The key teaching point here is that the brain CT findings are very characteristic of pseudo-subarachnoid hemorrhage.

26. **D.** This is a glomus-type intramedullary AVM. This vascular lesion is congenital and is a high-pressure lesion. It is the most common intramedullary vascular malformation. However, type 1 dural AVMs that are extramedullary are much more common and are the most frequent spinal vascular malformation. There are 4 types of spinal AVMs:
   1. Single-coiled vessel (dural arteriovenous fistula)
   2. Intramedullary glomus (shown in figure)
   3. Juvenile
   4. Intradural perimedullary

27. **A.** Ruptured saccular right MCA aneurysm at junction of first and second segments (M1/2 MCA

aneurysm). The bleeding pattern for the subarachnoid hemorrhage is confined entirely within the right Sylvian fissure. There is no blood in the interhemispheric fissure, making rupture of an anterior communicating artery aneurysm much less likely. The other entities, including the dissecting morphology and right anterior temporal artery aneurysm, represent a much less common morphology and location, respectively.

28. **B.** When comparing MRI to CT scan, MRI is more sensitive in demonstrating subarachnoid hemorrhage than CT scan, but given the limited availability and delays associated with MRI imaging. CT is recommended for initial evaluation. When looking at different imaging sequences on MRI, the SWI sequence is more sensitive than FLAIR at demonstrating subarachnoid hemorrhage with particular improvement for interhemispheric and intraventricular hemorrhage.

29. **C.** This is a classic example of a reticulated mixed signal mass with a hemosiderin rim seen on T2 characteristic of a cavernous malformation. Although this is the correct location for a hypertensive hemorrhage, the complexity of the lesion is not consistent with this. Other common sites for hypertensive hemorrhage include the basal ganglia, pons, and cerebellum.

An arteriovenous malformation will have high-flow vessels present, which will result in flow voids on T2 imaging. A developmental venous anomaly has multiple veins collecting into a single central draining, so-called "caput medusa appearance." Capillary telangiectasias are most commonly found in the brainstem with high intensity on T2 imaging and typically numerous lesions, rather than a single lesion.

30. **E.** Although this patient is high risk for revascularization given his age, vascular disease, and contralateral carotid stenosis, none of these are absolute contraindications to revascularization. Carotid endarterectomy would require cross-clamping of the carotid to perform the atherectomy. There is high risk of embolization with cross-clamping given his atherosclerotic disease. If the contralateral carotid artery is occluded, as is the case in this patient, then occluding the ipsilateral carotid during surgery will possibly lead to ischemia.

The CREST trial excluded patients with ipsilateral intracranial aneurysms measuring >5 mm because there is increased risk of hemorrhage.

31. **E.** The angiogram demonstrates a large cavernous internal carotid artery aneurysm. This lesion would cause compression of other components of the cavernous sinus including cranial nerves III, IV, V_1, V_2, and VI. This lesion could erode into the sphenoid sinus, resulting in epistaxis and potential CSF leak. An aneurysm of this size could result in both arterial and subarachnoid hemorrhage.

   There is lower chance of intraparenchymal hemorrhage given that it is within a bony canal and low chance of decrease blood flow into the right hemisphere or ischemia.

32. **B.** The patient has a Borden type 1 dural arteriovenous fistula at the left transverse sigmoid junction with arterial supply from the middle meningeal and occipital arteries. This lesion does not have retrograde cortical vein reflux, which makes spontaneous hemorrhage unlikely. Patients with fistula in this location often present with pulsatile tinnitus because of the proximity to the auditory apparatus in the temporal bone.

33. **A.** The head CT demonstrates early ischemic changes in the right PICA territory. Given his chest pain, there is concern for possible aortic dissection, which could extend into the subclavian arteries. Stroke related to cocaine still has not been fully elucidated; however, dissection is known to result from cocaine use and can result in ischemic stroke. Of all the options listed for cerebellar stroke, a dissection of the vertebral artery is by far the most common etiology in a young or middle-age patient. Although vasospasm can occur from cocaine, the patient's clinical picture is more consistent with dissection.

34. **D.** The patient has a classical "triple H" deficit following anterior choroidal artery occlusion. Hemiplegia is the most consistent symptom because of ischemic infarction of the posterior limb of the internal capsule. Patients frequently experience hemisensory loss and a homonymous hemianopsia. A middle cerebral artery occlusion would result in additional findings of left gaze preference and neglect. Ischemia within the lenticulostriate branches would result in ischemia to the basal ganglia, which could result in hemiplegia and hypesthesia but would not result in a full hemianopsia. A venous infarction would result in a more cortical lesion near the Sylvian fissure, which would result in neglect symptoms.

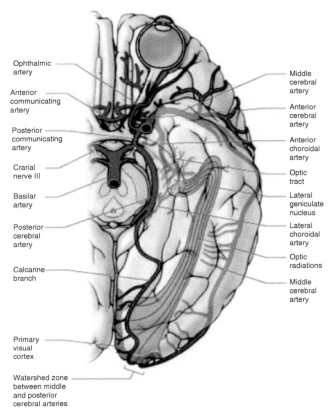

Reproduced with permission from Martin TJ, Corbett JJ. *Practical Neuroophthalmology.* New York, NY: McGraw-Hill, 2013.

35. **A.** Abciximab is a glycoprotein IIb/IIIa receptor antagonist that inhibits platelet aggregation irreversibly. It has rapid onset with a plasma half-life of approximately 10 minutes, but has effects on platelet function for ≥48 hours following administration given it is irreversible binding. Tirofiban and eptifibatide are reversible glycoprotein IIb/IIIa receptor antagonists.

   Prasugrel and clopidogrel are adenosine diphosphate receptor inhibitors.

REFERENCES

ACR Committee on Drugs and Contrast Media. *ACR Manual on Contrast Media.* 9th ed. Reston, VA: American College of Radiology;2013:1-128.

Alberquerque FC, Hu YC, Dashti SR, et al. Craniocervical arterial dissections as sequelae of chiropractic manipulation: patters of injury and management. *J Neurosurg.* 2011;115:1197-1205.

Antouniou GA, Kuhan G, Sfyroeras GS, et al. Contralateral occlusion of the internal carotid artery increases the risk of patients undergoing carotid endarterectomy. *J Vasc Surg.* 2013;57:1134-1145.

Bohnstedt BN, Kemp WJ 3rd, Li Y, et al. Surgical treatment of 127 anterior choroidal artery aneurysms: a cohort study of resultant ischemic complications. *Neurosurgery.* 2013;73:933-939.

Borden JA, Wu JK, Shucart WA. A proposed classification for spinal and cranial dural arteriovenous fistulous malformations and implications for treatment. *J Neurosurg.* 1995;82:166-179.

Brinjikji W, Iver VN, Wood CP, et al. Prevalence and characteristics of brain arteriovenous malformations in hereditary hemorrhagic telangiectasia: a systematic review and meta-analysis. *J Neurosurg.* 2016;21:1-9.

Dabbouseh NM, Ardelt A. Cocaine medicated apoptosis of vascular cells as a mechanism for carotid artery dissection leading to ischemic stroke. *Med Hypotheses.* 2011;77:201-203.

Davila VJ, Chang JM, Stone WM, et al. Current surgical management of carotid body tumors. *J Vasc Surg.* 2016;64:1703-1710.

De Campfleur NM, Langlois C, Ankenbrandt WJ, et al. Magnetic resonance imaging evaluation of cerebral cavernous malformations with susceptibility-weighted imaging. *Neurosurgery.* 2011;68:641-647.

Doppman JL, Di Chiro G, Oldfield EH. Origin of spinal arteriovenous malformation and normal cord vasculature from a common segmental artery: angiographic and therapeutic considerations. *Radiology.* 1985;154:687-689.

Frontera JA, Claassen J, Schmidt JM, et al. Prediction of symptomatic vasospasm after subarachnoid hemorrhage: the modified Fisher scale. *Neurosurgery.* 2006;59:21-27.

Fujita N, Shimada N, Takimoto H, et al. MR appearance of the persistent hypoglossal artery. *AJNR Am J Neuroradiol.* 1995;16:900-902.

Gaberel T, Borha A, di Palma C, et al. Clipping versus coiling in the management of posterior communicating artery aneurysms with third nerve palsy: a systematic review and meta-analysis. *World Neurosurg.* 2016;87:e4.

Geibprasert S, Pongpech S, Jiarakongmun P, et al. Radiologic assessment of brain arteriovenous malformations: what clinicians need to know. *Radiographics.* 2010;30:483-501.

Govani FS, Shouvlin CL. Hereditary hemorrhagic telangiectasia: a clinical and scientific review. *Eur J Human Gene.* 2009;17:860-871.

Hahn CD, Nicolle DA, Lownie SP, et al. Giant cavernous carotid aneurysms: clinical presentation in fifty-seven cases. *J Neuroophthalmol.* 2000;20:253-258.

Halbach VV, Hieshima GB, Higashida RT, et al. Carotid cavernous fistulae: indications for urgent treatment. *AJR Am J Roentegenol.* 1987;149:587-593.

Haller S, Etienne L, Kovari E, et al. Imaging of neurovascular compression syndromes: trigeminal neuralgia, hemifacial spasm, vestibular paroxysmia, and glossopharyngeal neuralgia. *AJNR Am J Neuroradiol.* 2016;37:1384-1392.

Harrigan MR, Deveikis JP, ed. *Handbook of Cerebrovascular Disease and Neurointerventional Technique.* 2nd ed. New York, NY: Humana Press; 2012.

Hashemzadeh M, Furukawa M, Goldsberry S, et al. Chemical structures and mode of action of intravenous glycoprotein IIb/IIIa receptor blockers: a review. *Exp Clin Cardiol.* 2008;13:192-197.

Hashemzadeh M, Goldsberry S, Furukawa M, et al. ADP receptor-blocker thienopyridines: chemical structures, mode of action and clinical use. *J Inv Cardiol.* 2009;21:406-412.

Ho VB, Smirniotopoulos JG, Murphy FM, et al. Radiologic-pathologic correlation: hemangioblastoma. *AJNR Am J Neuroradiol.* 1992;13:1342-1352.

Kale SP, Edgell RC, Alshekhlee A, et al. Age-associated vasospasm in aneurysmal subarachnoid hemorrhage. *J Stroke Cerebrovasc Dis.* 2013;22:22-27.

Khan UA, Thapar A, Shalhoub J, et al. Risk of intracerebral aneurysm rupture during carotid revascularization. *J Vasc Surg.* 2012;56:1739-1747.

Kim MJ, Kim MS. Persistent primitive trigeminal artery: analysis of anatomical characteristics and clinical significances. *Surg Radiol Anat.* 2015;37:69-74.

Konczalla J, Kashefiolasl S, Brawanski N, et al. Cerebral vasospasm and delayed cerebral infarctions in 225 patients with non-aneurysmal subarachnoid hemorrhage: the underestimated risk of Fisher 3 blood distribution. *J Neurointerv Surg.* 2016;pii:neurintsurg-2015-012153.

Krayenbuhl N, Guerrero C, Krisht AF. Technical strategies to approach aneurysm of the vertebral and posterior inferior cerebellar arteries. *Neurosurg Focus.* 2005;19:E4.

Krayenbuhl H, Yasargil MG, Huber P, et al. *Cerebral Angiography.* Stuttgart, Germany: Thieme; 1982.

Kurihara T. Abducens nerve palsy and ipsilateral incomplete Horner syndrome: a significant sign of locating the lesion in the posterior cavernous sinus. *Intern Med.* 2006;45:993-994.

Lee KY, Oh YW, Noh HJ, et al. Extraadrenal paraganglioma of the body: imaging features. *AJR Am J Roentgenol.* 2006;187:492-504.

Lee RR, Becher MW, Benson ML, et al. Brain capillary telangiectasia: MR imaging appearance and clinicohistological findings. *Radiology.* 1997;205:797-805.

Meurer WJ, Walsh B, Vilke GM, et al. Clinical guidelines for the emergency department evaluation of subarachnoid hemorrhage. *J Emerg Med.* 2016;50:696-701.

North American Symptomatic Carotid Endarterectomy Trial Collaborators. Beneficial effect of carotid endarterectomy in symptomatic patients with high-grade carotid stenosis. *N Engl J Med.* 1991;325:445-453.

O'Connor PS, Glaser JS. Intracavernous aneurysms and isolated sixth nerve palsy. In: Smith JL, ed. *Neuro-ophthalmology Focus.* New York, NY: Masson; 1981.

Osborn AG, ed. *Diagnostic Cerebral Angiography.* 2nd ed. Philadelphia, PA: Lippincott Williams & Wilkins; 1998.

Rhoton AL Jr. The cerebellar arteries. *Neurosurgery.* 2000;47(suppl 3):S7-S27.

Rouanet C, Reges D, Rocha E, et al. Main in the barrel syndrome with anterior spinal artery infarction due to vertebral artery dissection. *J Stroke Cerebrovasc Dis.* 2017;26:e41-e42.

Ruiz DSM, Yilmaz H, Gilloud P. Cerebral developmental venous anomalies: current concepts. *Ann Neurol.* 2009;66:271-283.

Sheffet AJ, Roubin G, Howard G, et al. Design of the Carotid Revascularization Endarterectomy vs. Stenting Trial (CREST). *Int J Stroke.* 2010;5:40-46.

Spetzler RF, Martin NA. A proposed grading system for arteriovenous malformations. *J Neurosurg.* 1986;65:476-483.

Tranvinh E, Heit JJ, Hacein-Bey L, et al. Contemporary imaging of cerebral arteriovenous malformations. *AJR Am J Roentgenol.* 2017;7:1-11.

Tubbs RS, Salter EG. Vidius Vidius: 1509-1569. *Neurosurgery.* 2006;59:201-203.

Umasankar U, Carroll TJ, Famubori A, et al. Vertebral artery dissection: not a rare cause of stroke in the young. *Age Ageing.* 2008;37:345-346.

Verma RK, Kotke R, Andereggen L, et al. Detecting subarachnoid hemorrhage: comparison of combined FLAIR/SWI versus CT. *Eur J Radiol.* 2013;82:1539-1545.

Waxman SG, ed. Cranial nerves and pathways. In: *Clinical Neuroanatomy.* 27th ed. New York, NY: McGraw-Hill Education; 2013.

Wong M, Shatzkes D. Brain capillary telangiectasia. *Appl Radiol.* 2013;2013:20-22.

Yuzawa H, Higano S, Mugikura S, et al. Pseudo-subarachnoid hemorrhage found in patients with postresuscitation encephalopathy: characteristics of CT findings and clinical importance. *AJNR Am J Neuroradiol.* 2008;29:1544-1549.

19

Brain Tumors and Hydrocephalus

Simon Hanft, MD

Questions

Questions 1-3

A 46-year-old man who has been suffering from worsening headaches over the past 1 to 2 weeks now presents with severe nausea and vomiting. His friend also notices that he has relatively significant gait imbalance. He is brought to the emergency department (ED) where a stat head computed tomography (CT) is performed and is shown below.

1. Based on this CT scan, what is the most likely diagnosis?

A. Obstructive mass at the level of the cerebral aqueduct

B. Intraventricular hemorrhage from the left-sided basal ganglia

C. Obstructive mass at the level of the foramen of Monro

D. Subarachnoid hemorrhage from a vascular lesion

E. Basilar meningitis

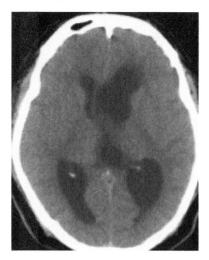 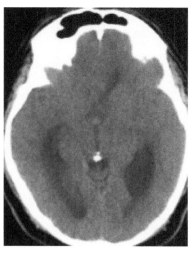

Computed tomography (CT) of the head, axial view, shows signs of severe asymmetric hydrocephalus with unilateral dilatation of the left-sided lateral ventricle.

2. After reviewing the CT scan, you recognize that there is a likely mass situated at the foramen of Monro. Clinically, the patient becomes noticeably more confused and then lethargic. His vital signs are stable, and he is protecting his airway. What is the next best step in management?

A. Stat magnetic resonance imaging (MRI) to better evaluate the mass for operative planning

B. Placement of bifrontal external ventricular drains for hydrocephalus treatment

C. Placement of a left frontal external ventricular drain for hydrocephalus treatment

D. Rapid administration of an osmotic diuretic such as mannitol

E. Hyperventilation

3. A ventriculostomy is performed at the bedside through a left frontal burr hole. There is spontaneous flow of high-pressure cerebrospinal fluid (CSF) through the catheter after it reaches the left frontal

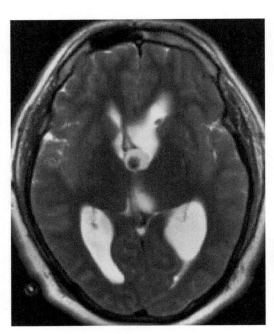

T2-weighted magnetic resonance imaging of the brain shows signs of central low T2 signal with higher peripheral T2 signal.

horn. The patient becomes much more awake and oriented. Since he is now stabilized, he is transported to the MRI suite for a contrasted study to better evaluate the mass lesion. A T2-weighted slice from this MRI is shown below. There is no evidence of contrast enhancement on the T1-weighted images. Based on the MRI, what is the most likely diagnosis?

A. Intra-axial tumor such as glioma

B. Colloid cyst

C. Subependymoma

D. Neurocysticercosis

E. Meningioma

Questions 4-6

A 24-year-old man complains of headaches to a friend and then suddenly collapses. He is intubated in the field by emergency medical services (EMS) and brought to an ED where a stat head CT is performed (shown below). On exam, the patient is afebrile and lethargic, with pupils equal, round, and reactive and with clear limited upward gaze; otherwise, there are no cranial nerves signs. There are no clear meningeal signs. The patient can move all extremities against gravity.

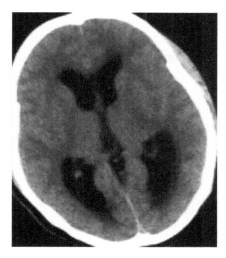
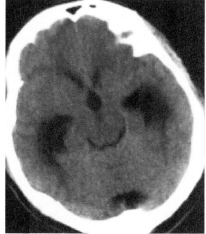

Computed tomography of the head reveals signs of very severe diffuse hydrocephalus.

4. If there is an underlying mass involved and not detected by CT of the head, where is it most likely to be located based on this pattern of hydrocephalus?

A. Frontal horn of the lateral ventricle

B. Temporal horn of the lateral ventricle

C. Third ventricle

D. Fourth ventricle

E. Prepontine cistern

5. A right frontal external ventricular drain is placed at the bedside to alleviate the elevated intracranial pressure from the hydrocephalus. The patient begins to follow commands as sedation is weaned. He is considered stable enough for an MRI. A standard contrasted MRI is performed, which locates a mass at the base of the fourth ventricle. This mass is best viewed on the sagittal cut (shown below). Which of the following would be the most appropriate next step in management?

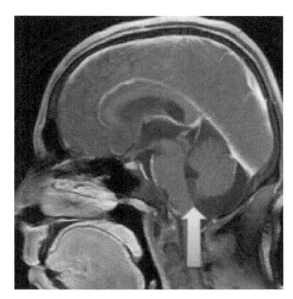

Magnetic resonance image of the brain: Fluid-attenuated inversion recovery (FLAIR) image, sagittal cut, shows mass at the base of the fourth ventricle.

A. Suboccipital craniotomy for resection of this mass

B. Endoscopic third ventriculostomy

C. Placement of a right ventriculoperitoneal shunt

D. Presumptive antihelminthic treatment with praziquantel

E. Progressive weaning of the external ventricular drain

6. The patient undergoes successful surgical extirpation of the cyst, and the immediate postoperative CT shows significant reduction in the degree of hydrocephalus (shown below). By the next morning, the patient has a moderate-sized fluid collection at the suboccipital surgical site. The external ventricular drain (EVD) had been kept at 10 cm H$_2$O above the external auditory meatus prior to surgery and immediately following. Given the appearance of the suboccipital surgical site collection, what should be done next?

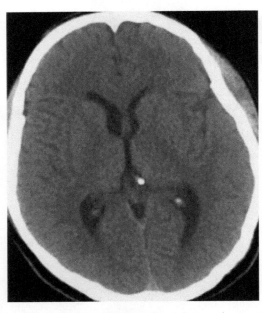

Computed tomography of the head, axial view, shows signs of improved hydrocephalus and external ventricular drain tip in place at the level of the third ventricle.

    A. Keep the EVD at 10 cm H$_2$O and continue to observe

    B. Lower the EVD to either 5 or 0 cm H$_2$O to increase CSF drainage

    C. Increase dexamethasone dosing to treat a likely aseptic meningitis

    D. Return to the operating room (OR) for wound repair

    E. Return to the OR for placement of a ventriculoperitoneal shunt

Questions 7-9

A 52-year-old woman with no significant past medical history presents with abrupt onset of seizure activity while at work. Her colleagues witness her collapse and then develop generalized convulsions. EMS is contacted, and the patient is brought to the local ED, where a head CT is performed (shown below). Patient is lethargic but oxygenating well without any additional symptoms. A few hours after admission, she is considered stable enough to undergo a contrasted MRI, which shows evidence of an infiltrative mass in the right frontal region with a small area of enhancement.

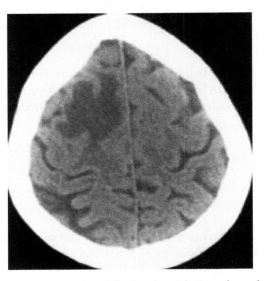

Computed tomography of the head, axial view, shows hypodensity in the right frontal lobe consistent with edema.

7. What is the most likely diagnosis?

    A. Cerebral abscess

    B. Metastasis

    C. Primary brain neoplasm

    D. Demyelinating disease

    E. Cerebral contusion

8. The patient undergoes an additional MRI that includes functional MRI and diffusion tensor imaging of the white matter tracts. The mass appears clearly in front of the motor cortex (shown below). Given the MRI findings, what is the next best step in management?

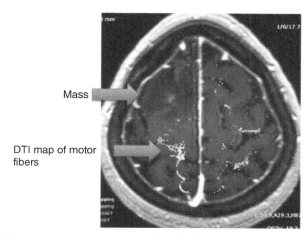

Magnetic resonance imaging (MRI) that includes functional MRI and diffusion tensor imaging (DTI) of the white matter tracts shows a right frontal mass that appears clearly in front of the motor cortex.

A. Video electroencephalography (EEG) for 24 to 48 hours

B. Open surgical resection of the mass

C. Stereotactic needle biopsy of the mass

D. Treatment with antiepileptic medications and a repeat MRI in 3 months

E. Radiation

9. The patient undergoes successful resection of the mass. Motor evoked potentials were preserved throughout surgery, and there is no evidence of residual tumor on the postoperative MRI. However, the patient wakes up with a dense hemiplegia involving the left face, arm, and leg. Sensation is preserved. She remains without any evidence of motor function on the left for the next 2 days while in the intensive care unit (ICU) prior to discharge. What is the most likely explanation for these postoperative symptoms?

A. Supplementary motor area (SMA) syndrome

B. Venous infarct

C. Arterial infarct

D. False localization during surgery and direct damage to the motor cortex and/or descending fibers

E. Todd paralysis

10. A 40-year-old woman presents with complaints of smelling burning rubber. This has been increasing in frequency and prompted an MRI of the brain, which revealed an enhancing mass in the left mesial temporal lobe (shown below). Clinical suspicion is high for a primary neoplasm. Given her young age and the presence of auras, the patient undergoes a resection of the mass. The surgery is uneventfully. Upon fully waking in the ICU, the patient is noted to have significant weakness involving the right side of the body, mainly the arm and leg. Immediate CT scan does not locate a hemorrhage or any mass-occupying lesion. What is the most likely diagnosis?

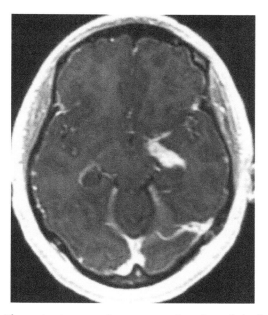

T1 with contrast magnetic resonance imaging of the brain, axial cut, shows enhancement of left mesial temporal lobe lesion.

A. Supplementary motor area (SMA) syndrome

B. Todd paralysis

C. Arterial infarct

D. Temporal lobe hematoma

E. Slow recovery from general anesthesia

Questions 11 and 12

A 70-year-old woman presents with declining mental status over the course of months. She has become more forgetful, is easily confused, and is not processing information as well as she had even a year prior. An MRI is ordered by her primary physician as part of a dementia workup, revealing a large dural-based mass (shown below). Due to the large size of the mass and the patient's symptoms, the patient undergoes surgical removal of the mass.

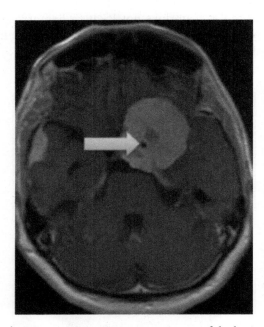

T1 with contrast magnetic resonance image of the brain, axial cut, shows sphenoid wing meningioma causing compression and edema of the adjacent left frontal and temporal lobes. The arrow indicates a black dot near the center of the mass.

11. What does the black dot indicated by the arrow in the MRI image likely represent?

A. Hemorrhage

B. Necrosis

C. Internal carotid artery flow void

D. Oculomotor nerve

E. Calcification

12. The patient undergoes a lengthy but ultimately successful removal of the tumor without any evidence of residual tumor by the end of the operation. The internal carotid artery (ICA) was successfully identified and spared. However, the patient wakes up hours after surgery with complete eyelid closure on the left. When the lid is raised, the pupil is fixed and dilated, and the eye is deviated laterally. What is the likely diagnosis?

A. Apraxia of lid opening

B. Arterial infarct

C. Venous infarct

D. Postoperative seizure activity

E. Cranial nerve injury

Questions 13-15

A 38-year-old man presents with progressive hearing loss in his left ear over the course of a few months. An MRI of the brain is ordered and shown below.

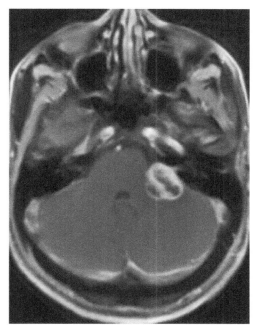

T1 with contrast magnetic resonance image of the brain, axial cut, shows a relatively large mass with heterogeneous enhancement in the cerebellopontine angle with extension into the internal acoustic canal.

13. Given the MRI appearance and associated symptoms, what is the most likely diagnosis?
   A. Acoustic neuroma
   B. Petroclival meningioma
   C. Clival chordoma
   D. Epidermoid
   E. Ependymoma

14. The patient undergoes successful suboccipital craniotomy for resection of tumor through a retrosigmoid approach. Later in the day on postoperative day 1, the patient starts to become obtunded. His postoperative MRI from early that morning reveals a cerebellar infarct (shown below). What is the most likely mechanism of his current clinical exam?

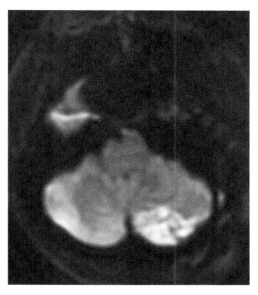

Magnetic resonance image of the brain, axial cut, diffusion-weighted image sequence shows left cerebellar acute stroke.

   A. Waxing and waning mental status associated with a large intracranial surgery
   B. Brainstem injury
   C. Hydrocephalus
   D. Pneumocephalus
   E. Aseptic meningitis

15. The head CT shows new ventricular dilatation of the lateral ventricles with rounding of the fourth ventricle, consistent with hydrocephalus. What is the most appropriate next step in management?
   A. Osmotic diuretic
   B. Repeat MRI
   C. Emergent return to the OR for cerebellar decompressive surgery
   D. Placement of an external ventricular drain (EVD)
   E. Placement of a lumbar drain

16. A 37-year-old man presents with worsening vision involving the right eye. He notes mainly peripheral visual loss, which is subsequently confirmed by his ophthalmologist on a visual fields exam. This prompts an MRI of the brain, which is shown below. The neurosurgeon performs a supraorbital craniotomy through an eyebrow approach to remove the mass. Postoperatively, the patient reports subjective improvement in his vision, but he develops a rapidly rising sodium level to 152 mEq/L. What is the most likely explanation for the hypernatremia?

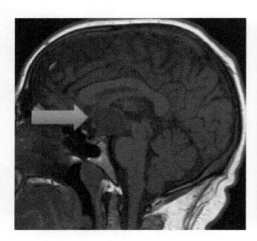 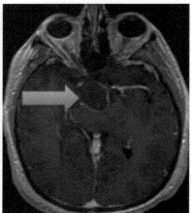

Magnetic resonance imaging of the brain. **A.** Sagittal fluid-attenuated inversion recovery sequence. **B.** Axial T1 with contrast sequence shows a large cystic mass in the suprasellar space.

    A. Diabetes insipidus

    B. Hypovolemia with resulting serum concentration of sodium

    C. Damage to the optic apparatus

    D. Use of hypertonic saline during the surgical procedure

    E. Release of tumor contents into the CSF space

Questions 17 and 18

A 58-year-old man develops severe sudden-onset headache and reports blurry vision. This brings him to his local ED where a CT scan reveals a hyperdense mass in the pituitary region suspicious for a hemorrhagic pituitary adenoma. He then undergoes an MRI with dedicated pituitary imaging that reveals a large, rim-enhancing mass in the pituitary region abutting and deforming the optic chiasm. There is hemorrhage present within the mass as seen on the T2 coronal image as well (shown below). The patient is admitted to the neuro-ICU where a full set of labs are drawn and the patient is stabilized from a cardiopulmonary standpoint.

during surgery by the neurosurgeon and collaborating ear, nose, and throat (ENT) surgeon. Around 12 hours after the operation while in the neuro-ICU, blood-tinged fluid begins to flow from the patient's nose. It is clearly exacerbated when the patient is tipped forward, indicating a persistent CSF leak. What is the next best step in management?

A. Bedside placement of a lumbar drain

B. Return to the OR for operative repair

C. Urgent CT scan

D. Lying the patient flat

E. Sending the fluid for a β_2-transferrin assay

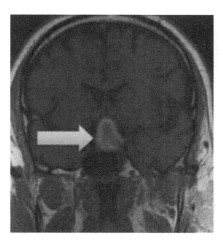 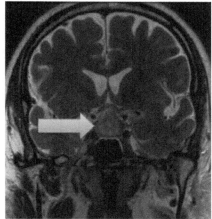

Magnetic resonance imaging of the brain, coronal cut. **A.** Fluid-attenuated inversion recovery sequence. **B.** T2 sequence that shows large, rim-enhancing mass in the pituitary region abutting and deforming the optic chiasm. Hemorrhage present within the mass is seen on the T2 coronal image as well.

17. What is the most appropriate next step?

A. Emergent transsphenoidal surgery for removal of the pituitary tumor

B. Administration of corticosteroid replacement

C. Repeat CT in 6 hours

D. CT angiography to assess for patency of the ICA and vasospasm

E. Visual fields testing

18. The patient undergoes successful endoscopic approach for tumor removal, and the postoperative MRI indicates complete resection with decompression of the optic nerves. Intraoperatively, a small hole was made through the arachnoid membrane, creating a low-flow CSF leak. This was repaired

Questions 19 and 20

A 34-year-old woman presents with 1 week of worsening headaches. On the day of admission, the headache has become so severe that she vomits and becomes obtunded. She was brought to the ED, where a CT of the head is performed (shown below). On examination, she is in extreme pain but is orienting well and communicating clearly. Therefore, she is considered safe to undergo an MRI to better evaluate this lesion. On MRI, the lesion in the midbrain has signal characteristics consistent with a cavernous malformation. She remains stable clinically.

20. The patient undergoes successful ETV surgery with significant resolution of hydrocephalus on the post-operative CT scan. However, in the days following surgery, she notes some issues with short-term memory. What is the most likely explanation for this finding?

A. Residual effect from the hydrocephalus

B. Midbrain injury

C. Thalamic injury

D. Forniceal injury

E. Septal injury

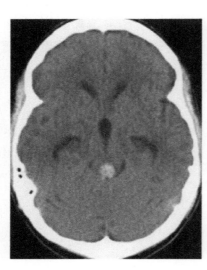 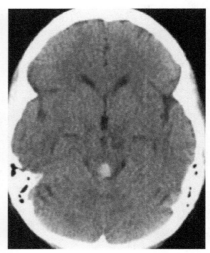

Computed tomography of the head, axial cut, reveals a hemorrhagic focus in the posterior midbrain and moderate hydrocephalus.

19. What is the next best step in management?

A. Emergent placement of an external ventricular drain at the bedside

B. Operative placement of a ventriculoperitoneal shunt

C. Operative resection of the cavernous malformation

D. Endoscopic third ventriculostomy (ETV)

E. Repeat CT in 6 hours

Questions 21 and 22

A 54-year-old man has been acting oddly over the past few weeks. He is occasionally disoriented to place and time. He is also having word-finding difficulty. On the morning of admission, he is extremely lethargic and barely rousing to noxious stimuli. His wife calls 911, and he is intubated in the field. CT of the head done emergently in the ED reveals signs of uncal herniation (shown below).

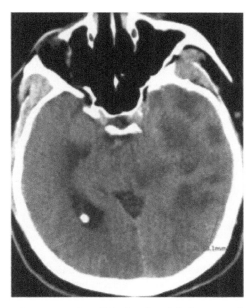

Computed tomography of the head, axial view, reveals a large left temporal mass with signs of uncal herniation.

21. What is the next best step in management?
  A. Emergent operative resection of the mass
  B. External ventricular drain
  C. Hemicraniectomy
  D. Placement of an intracranial pressure (ICP) monitor
  E. High-dose dexamethasone

22. After appropriate medical management, the patient becomes much more awake off sedation and follows commands. He is successfully extubated. An MRI is performed showing a likely high-grade glioma in the left temporal region (shown below). He undergoes temporal craniotomy for resection of tumor. Given the extent of posterior involvement in the left temporal lobe, what deficit might occur in the postoperative period?

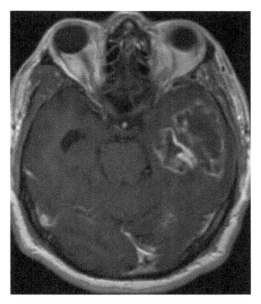

Magnetic resonance imaging of the brain, T1 with contrast sequence, shows heterogenous enhancement of left temporal mass.

  A. Cognitive functioning
  B. Aphasia
  C. Contralateral sensory loss
  D. Contralateral motor loss
  E. Bitemporal hemianopsia

Questions 23 and 24

A 51-year-old man presents with primarily head-aches over 1 to 2 weeks, but notes some imbalance as well. The headaches have become so severe that he brings himself to an ED where a CT head reveals a large thalamic mass (shown below). There is also resulting hydrocephalus. The patient remains clinically stable with only mild left arm and leg weakness on examination.

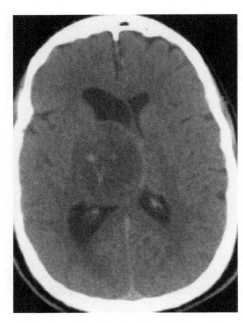

Computed tomography of the head, axial view, shows signs of right thalamic hypodensity and rim on hyperdensity, signs of lateral ventricular hydrocephalus, and midline shift near the mass.

23. What is the next best step in management?
    A. Emergent placement of an EVD at the bedside
    B. Emergency operation for resection of the mass
    C. Emergency operation for placement of a ventriculoperitoneal shunt
    D. MRI with contrast
    E. Elective biopsy

24. The patient undergoes an MRI revealing a very large necrotic mass situated in the right thalamus highly suspicious for a glioblastoma (shown below). The neurosurgeon elects to perform an endoscopic biopsy through the ventricle and then place a ventriculoperitoneal shunt. What must the surgeon take care to do as part of this planned operation?

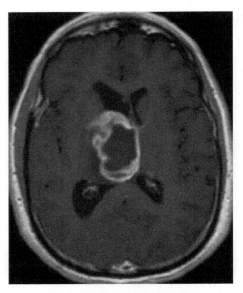

T1 with contrast magnetic resonance image of the brain, axial view, shows right thalamic hypointense lesion surrounded by hyperintense signal, as well as signs of hydrocephalus.

    A. Make sure the tip of the shunt is placed beyond the foramen of Monro into the third ventricle
    B. Make sure to fenestrate the septum pellucidum so that the lateral ventricles are connected
    C. Debulk enough of the tumor in the third ventricle so that the shunt is more likely to work
    D. Dilate the foramen of Monro to allow more CSF diversion
    E. Include a third ventriculostomy as another way of diverting CSF

Answers and Explanations

1. **C.** The CT scan shows severe asymmetric hydrocephalus with unilateral dilatation of the left-sided lateral ventricle. This is most consistent with obstruction at the level of the foramen of Monro. A mass situated at the cerebral aqueduct or fourth ventricle would cause symmetric dilatation of the lateral and third ventricles. In addition, there is a mass lesion located within the third ventricle as seen on the second CT slice. There is no evidence of hemorrhage in the ventricles, which can be a mechanism for asymmetric hydrocephalus, and there is also no subarachnoid hemorrhage. Basilar meningitis, although partially consistent with the presentation, would also cause diffuse hydrocephalus.

2. **C.** The patient is declining due to the hydrocephalus, and so this must be treated emergently at the bedside. Other measures to manage intracranial pressure (ICP) will be largely ineffectual in this case due to the prominence of the hydrocephalus. The CT reveals both severe hydrocephalus involving the left lateral ventricle only and a mass lesion at the foramen of Monro. In this case, the mass is selectively obstructing the foramen on the left, resulting in this asymmetric pattern, as the right lateral ventricle is not significantly dilated. Typically, lesions such as this at the foramen lead to obstruction at both foramina, which results in dilatation of both lateral ventricles. In these situations, bilateral external ventricular drains must be placed because a unilateral drain will not treat the hydrocephalus adequately. This is a case of compartmentalized hydrocephalus where a unilateral frontal drain from the left will be adequate to treat the problem.

3. **B.** There is some variability to the MRI appearance of a colloid cyst, but in conjunction with the presenting symptoms, colloid cyst stands out at the most likely diagnosis. These cysts are benign epithelial-lined congenital lesions and typically originate from the roof of anterior third ventricle. As is the case here, the patient can present with severe headaches and can rapidly deteriorate due to the sudden worsening of hydrocephalus. Colloid cysts can occasionally cause sudden death from such rapidly progressive hydrocephalus into brain herniation. The T2 image included here shows central low T2 signal with higher peripheral T2 signal, whereas the T1 image with contrast shows no rim enhancement (not shown).

    A subependymoma rarely presents with such severe and sudden hydrocephalus, although it is a mass that can be situated at the foramen of Monro, even though this is a less common location (more often found in the fourth ventricle and lateral ventricles). The other lesions would be atypical for this location.

4. **D.** The hydrocephalus pattern in this case involves both frontal horns, the temporal horns, and the third ventricle, which has a characteristic rounding appearance consistent with severe hydrocephalus. Since all of these compartments are equally affected, the "obstructive" lesion, which is not present on CT, is most likely to be situated at the level of the fourth ventricle. It could be located at the cerebral aqueduct or the inferior aspect of the ventricle; sometimes this location can be further narrowed down based on whether the fourth ventricle itself is dilated. In this case, the fourth ventricle is normal in caliber. If the lesion is at the outflow of the fourth ventricle, it can cause dilation of the fourth ventricle itself. This is much less likely for lesions located at the level of the cerebral aqueduct. The prepontine cistern is an atypical location for a brain mass and very rarely leads to the severe hydrocephalus that is depicted here.

5. **A.** The radiographic characteristics of this mass are consistent with the diagnosis of neurocysticercosis. The patient has a solitary cyst located in the inferior portion of the fourth ventricle, the most common

intraventricular location of these lesions. In addition, there is a small area of punctate enhancement (not shown) that is likely representative of an enhancing scolex. Since the diagnosis appears fairly clear, it is most appropriate to surgically remove this lesion. This will allow for diagnosis and subsequent appropriate antihelminthic treatment, and it will very likely treat the hydrocephalus. Both an endoscopic third ventriculostomy and shunt are reasonable options but do not directly address the mass, which is unlikely to respond to empiric antihelminthic drugs in its current vesicular form. Shunts have a high failure rate in this condition due to the inflammatory CSF from parasitic products. Without having treated the cause of the hydrocephalus, there is no point to weaning the external ventricular drain (EVD) as the patient will remain dependent on CSF diversion.

6. **B.** The fluid collection underneath the surgical incision represents a CSF collection referred to as a pseudomeningocele. Given the severe hydrocephalus, it is not surprising that in the immediate aftermath of surgery, there is some CSF accumulation. With the EVD still in place, the best maneuver is to lower the EVD so as to increase CSF diversion. This should decompress the pseudomeningocele and allow the wound to heal. The patient might have to keep the drain at this lower level for a few days before having it progressively weaned to see if the wound will tolerate it. Given the significant resolution of hydrocephalus, there is a high likelihood in this case that the collection will respond to increased drainage. If not, then the patient might need a ventriculoperitoneal shunt, but this option is reserved only if the patient clinically fails the EVD wean. Increasing steroid dosing could very well help with postoperative headaches, and there is an association with reduced seizure activity, but this will not help with the CSF accumulation. It is also premature to promptly revise the wound as it could very well heal with a few days of CSF diversion through the EVD.

7. **C.** The patient is in her early 50s without any prior medical history. Her initial presenting symptom was a seizure. The MRI shows an infiltrating mass with an area of enhancement. These all point to the patient having a primary brain tumor such as an astrocytoma or oligodendroglioma. Metastasis

is considered less likely given the lack of enhancement here, her relatively young age, and lack of cancer history. For similar reasons, an abscess would be considered extremely unlikely in healthy 52-year-old woman, and the MRI indicates otherwise as well. A cerebral contusion could appear edematous on CT, but this is an odd location for a contusion, and the enhancement argues against this diagnosis.

8. **B.** The MRI is strongly indicative of a primary neoplasm. Based on its location, it is in a surgically accessible region of the brain, directly anterior to the motor cortex without involvement of the descending motor fibers. With use of neuronavigation, scalp motor evoked potentials (MEPs), and intraoperative subcortical stimulation of the motor pathway, this is considered a safe operation and is strongly recommended for diagnostic and therapeutic purposes. The expectation of the surgeon in this case would be for gross total resection or near gross total if the motor fibers are encountered with stimulation during surgery. The evidence supporting safe aggressive removal of low-grade gliomas is mounting, and therefore, surgery is the correct next step. Video EEG is largely irrelevant as the source of the patient's new-onset seizure activity is clearly this mass, so the EEG is not needed for localization. A needle biopsy is typically reserved for cases where a complete resection cannot be safely achieved. An argument can be made for observation only, but a symptomatic brain mass in a healthy relatively young woman should be treated upfront. Demonstrated growth or increasing contrast enhancement on a 3-month MRI would delay necessary treatment and actually allow the tumor to transform to a higher grade entity. Radiation is likely to be needed postoperatively but is not first-line treatment for an undiagnosed mass that likely represents a low-grade glioma.

9. **A.** The postoperative MRI shows complete tumor removal, and the MEPs were unchanged during surgery. These facts argue strongly against direct injury to the motor region, as this type of injury would diminish the MEPs during surgery. Either a venous or arterial infarct can lead to this kind of postoperative weakness and should be high in the differential diagnosis, but the MRI can effectively rule these out by scrutiny of the diffusion-weighted images (DWI). These are also relatively uncommon

for the kind of surgery performed and would also lead to a reduction in the MEPs during surgery. A supplementary motor area (SMA) syndrome is actually expected in this case due to the location of the tumor in the SMA of the brain. Tumor resection in this region leads to a significant postoperative weakness involving the contralateral side. It is the leading diagnosis in this case given the location of the tumor, and in fact, the patient must be strongly counseled preoperatively about the severe weakness that will develop following surgery. Fortunately, the weakness nearly always resolves, and by her 2-week follow-up visit, this patient was fully ambulatory with antigravity strength in her left arm and restoration of facial symmetry. A Todd paralysis is possible but less likely in this case given the lack of any obvious intraoperative or postoperative seizure activity.

10. **C.** When a patient wakes up from a surgery in the mesial temporal region with a clear focal weakness, the index of suspicion for a stroke is very high. The immediate CT effectively rules out hemorrhage/hematoma, and a slow wakeup from anesthesia should not lead to such a clear focal deficit. The patient's postoperative MRI in this case reveals an anterior choroidal artery infarct involving the posterior limb of the internal capsule and thalamus,

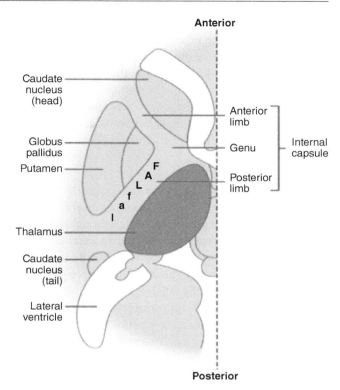

Reproduced with permission from Waxman S. *Clinical Neuroanatomy*. 28th ed. New York, NY: McGraw-Hill; 2017.

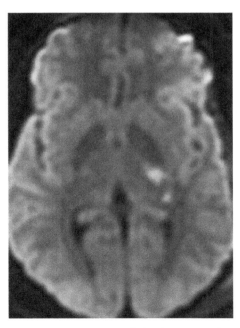

Magnetic resonance imaging of the brain, axial cut, DWI sequence shows choroidal artery infarct involving the posterior limb of the internal capsule and thalamus.

a known and feared complication of mesial temporal lobe surgery with an incidence of 1% to 2%. Although surgeries in the temporal lobe can be epileptogenic, the presence of an infarct on the postoperative MRI clearly rules out a Todd paralysis.

11. **C.** The black dot within the tumor represents the internal carotid artery as it courses through the center of the tumor. This is a significant finding in this case and makes complete surgical removal challenging and potentially too dangerous. It has serious clinical implications if injured, and may manifest as either an immediate stroke syndrome following surgery or as a delayed vasospasm from excessive manipulation during the case. The sequelae could therefore take hours to develop. These are important considerations in the postoperative assessment of a patient undergoing this operation for the treating intensivist.

12. **E.** This patient is suffering from a complete oculomotor nerve injury. She is unable to elevate the eyelid and has a fixed and dilated pupil with lateral deviation. In a tumor of this size, there was likely proximity, if not adhesion, to the third cranial

nerve as it travels underneath the tentorial edge. The likely mechanism here is direct injury to the oculomotor nerve during tumor removal. A stroke is unlikely to selectively cause this set of symptoms and can be ruled out by the postoperative MRI. The MRI will not, however, detect cranial nerve injury. Apraxia of lid opening should impact both eyelids and would ultimately be a diagnosis of exclusion in this case.

13. **A.** Acoustic neuromas, more properly referred to as vestibular schwannomas, commonly present with progressive hearing loss, although they can present with symptoms related to cerebellar and brainstem compression as well as hydrocephalus. This MRI shows characteristic heterogeneous enhancement likely related to a combination of cystic and hemorrhagic products within the tumor itself. The enhancement extends into the internal acoustic canal, which is strongly indicative of an acoustic neuroma with widening of the porus acusticus. This distinguishes the tumor from a meningioma. Clival chordomas involve the clivus and are not located in the cerebellopontine angle. The mass does not have imaging characteristics associated with the other tumors.

14. **C.** The cerebellar infarct is an important clue, as it is now causing swelling and compression of the fourth ventricle. This is leading to hydrocephalus, which in turn is causing the patient's declining clinical exam. The infarct could have been caused by retraction on the cerebellar hemisphere in order to access the tumor or by direct vascular injury to cerebellar arteries and/or veins. Answer choice A reflects a tendency that must be avoided in the neurointensive care unit. A young patient should not be steadily declining more than 24 hours after surgery, and a stat head CT must be obtained. The CT scan reveals the hydrocephalus. Brainstem injury, which can result from this operation, most commonly leads to an immediate clinical condition upon adequately waking from surgery, whether it is facial weakness or dysfunction with extraocular movements. Delayed decline in mental status is not related. Pneumocephalus can be a cause of agitation or altered mental status following surgery, but it is less likely to have such a profound effect as hydrocephalus. Aseptic meningitis, also referred to as a chemical meningitis, is more likely to lead

to headaches, nausea, and vomiting as opposed to gradually progressive lethargy. The head CT scan is critical to rule out these other entities.

15. **D.** Placement of an EVD through a right frontal approach will adequately treat the hydrocephalus in this situation. A lumbar drain is not indicated because the point of compression is at the level of the fourth ventricle, necessitating a proximal drain for CSF diversion. Repeat suboccipital craniectomy is an extreme response to this situation and is more likely to lead to additional morbidity. The cerebellar infarct is swelling, and this is a self-limited process. An EVD will likely be needed for a few days only to allow the cerebellar swelling to regress. Then it can be weaned or removed depending on the patient's clinical condition and repeat CT scan.

16. **A.** Craniopharyngiomas are very challenging surgical lesions despite their categorization as benign, slow-growing tumors. They are associated with significant perioperative morbidity and have a high recurrence rate. One of the classic complications with surgical removal of these tumors is seen in this case, diabetes insipidus. This can arise through manipulation of the tumor and indirect or direct damage to the hypothalamus or pituitary stalk and/or gland. The thirst mechanism can be compromised in these patients, so close attention must be paid to the sodium levels in the postoperative period to avoid severe hypernatremia. Administration of desmopressin is typically necessary to keep the sodium levels under control, and some patients require this medication long term. Optic nerve injury is not associated with a rising sodium level, nor is frontal lobe injury. Patients can develop a chemical meningitis from these surgeries, but hypernatremia is not a common byproduct of this process.

17. **B.** This patient is suffering from pituitary apoplexy, a rare presentation of a pituitary macroadenoma. Apoplexy results from either infarction of the tumor tissue or hemorrhage into the tumor itself. The exact mechanism remains a subject of debate. Once diagnosed, the first step is to stabilize the patient through administration of corticosteroid replacement. Failure to do so could lead to circulatory collapse as these patients are nearly always corticotropic deficient. Once the patient is

stabilized, he can then proceed to surgery through a transsphenoidal approach.

The dark center of the macroadenoma corresponds to a necrotic core with a rim of peripheral enhancement. This is a characteristic imaging finding in pituitary apoplexy. Repeat CT is relevant for typical intracranial bleeds that do not require urgent surgical decompression. CT angiography might have some application in these tumors but is absolutely not part of the standard initial assessment. Visual fields should be tested preferably prior to surgery, but in pituitary apoplexy, this can be deferred.

18. **A.** Postoperative CSF leaks are a well-known complication from transsphenoidal surgery. In this case, the surgeons felt that the intraoperative leak was small enough to be repaired primarily without a lumbar drain for CSF diversion. However, the leak persisted despite this closure, so the next step would be to place a lumbar drain in the ICU. It would be considered a bit premature to bring the patient back to the OR for an operative repair especially since a few days of lumbar drainage might seal the leak. If lumbar drainage fails, then the patient will have to be reexplored in the OR. A CT scan is not necessary in this case, and lying the patient flat is inadequate to treat active CSF rhinorrhea. In the setting of recent pituitary surgery where a CSF leak was encountered, there is no need to confirm that the fluid expressed from the nose is actual CSF with a β_2-transferrin assay, a time-consuming and costly study.

19. **D.** Clearly the patient needs to have her hydrocephalus treated; the question is how. Although an EVD is reasonable, the patient has demonstrated clinical stability, and so it does not need to be placed emergently at the bedside. A shunt is a reasonable option as well, but an ETV has the potential to cure the hydrocephalus without having to leave implanted hardware in the patient. Since the site of compression is at the cerebral aqueduct, an ETV is likely to work through bypassing the point of obstruction and opening a passage between the floor of the third ventricle and the prepontine cistern. The ETV success rate in treating hydrocephalus is somewhere between 70% and 80%, depending on the case series. The operation to remove this cavernous malformation is a huge undertaking and

is very likely to lead to morbidity given its location in the midbrain. It is more appropriate to treat the hydrocephalus first and then consider treatment approaches for the cavernoma down the road.

20. **D.** Although low risk, ETVs can be associated with various injuries related to the surgical approach and nearby anatomic structures. The patient has suffered an intrinsic midbrain injury due to the cavernoma hemorrhage, but this should not result in memory issues. The endoscope can cause direct injury to the fornix as it is passed en route to the floor of the third ventricle. Although not listed as a choice, injury to mammillary bodies, which define the posterior boundary of the area where the ventriculostomy is made through the third ventricle floor, can also lead to memory issues. Thalamic injury is a known complication, but memory is not usually impacted. Few septal injuries are associated with a memory deficit.

21. **E.** The CT scan shows severe edema and uncal herniation with proximity of the uncus to the midbrain. Although there appears to be an underlying mass, the edema is likely the main contributor to the degree of herniation. As such, high-dose dexamethasone is required (at least a 10 mg intravenous push and in some centers up to a 100 mg bolus). This should quickly treat the edema and reduce the degree of herniation over the course of a few hours. As the steroid effect increases, this will allow the treating neurosurgeon to obtain an MRI to better delineate the underlying mass lesion. This will make the surgery much safer and more effective. In addition, the steroids might help make the surgical corridor more manageable by diminishing the edema. Although emergency surgery is not completely wrong in this case, it could lead to significant morbidity and subtotal resection of the tumor, which will significantly impact prognosis. An EVD has no role due to the lack of hydrocephalus, and a hemicraniectomy is not recommended.

22. **B.** Since the tumor extends beyond 4.5 cm posterior to the anterior temporal tip, complete removal of the tumor and involved temporal lobe could result in aphasia, typically more of a receptive type. This patient would also very likely develop a superior quadrantopia due to disruption of the Meyer loop visual fibers, not bitemporal hemianopsia

pattern. Motor and sensation would be preserved, barring a significant vascular injury at surgery. Memory could also be impacted due to partial resection of the hippocampus, especially if it is the dominant hippocampus, which usually is on the left. However, overall cognitive executive functioning should be largely preserved.

23. **D.** Since the patient is stable, the best step is to obtain an MRI to better characterize this mass. This will allow the neurosurgeon to determine its true size, location, and relationship to critical anatomy, and whether or not this is a safely resectable lesion. Although the patient has significant hydrocephalus, it is causing headaches only, and he is not decompensating. Therefore, an EVD is not required, and clearly, an emergency surgery is not necessary. He may end up getting a biopsy only, but an MRI is needed to determine the proper operative approach.

24. **B.** The key in evaluating these cases of hydrocephalus is determining the site of obstruction. In this case, the thalamic mass is severely compressing the entire third ventricle. This is causing CSF buildup in both lateral ventricles, although the right appears more dilated. Placing a right frontal ventriculoperitoneal shunt runs the risk of inadequately diverting the CSF because the left frontal horn can continue to expand. By opening a hole in the septum pellucidum, which is a thin membrane dividing the 2 frontal horns, communication between the ventricles is established, and the shunt can lie in either of the 2 ventricles. Placing the shunt tip in the third ventricle is inadequate because it will become obstructed by the tumor. Debulking the tumor will introduce bleeding that could obstruct the shunt or even precipitate further complications. Some neurosurgeons would recommend attempted debulking of this mass. The option presented here is a biopsy and shunt approach, which should not include debulking unless the goal were resection of the mass. There is never an indication for dilating the foramen of Monro as this will lead to forniceal injury. Similar to placing the shunt in the third ventricle, an ETV is not an option here because the point of obstruction is at the level of the third ventricle and bilateral foramina of Monro, all of which is above the ETV site.

REFERENCES

Aldana PR, Kestle JR, Brockmeyer DL, et al. Results of endoscopic septal fenestration in the treatment of isolated ventricular hydrocephalus. *Pediatr Neurosurg.* 2003;38:286-294.

Banerjee C, Snelling B, Hanft S, et al. Bilateral cerebral infarction in the setting of pituitary apoplexy: a case presentation and literature review. *Pituitary.* 2015;18:352-358.

Bannur U, Rajshekhar V. Post-operative supplementary motor area syndrome: clinical features and outcomes. *Br J Neurosurg.* 2000;14:204-210.

Basso A, Carrizo A. Sphenoid ridge meningiomas. In: Schmidek HH, ed. *Operative Neurosurgical Techniques: Indications, Methods, and Results.* Philadelphia, PA: W.B. Saunders; 2000:316-324.

Benjamin V, McCormack B. Surgical management of tuberculum sellae and sphenoid ridge meningiomas. In: Schmidek HH, ed. *Operative Neurosurgical Techniques: Indications, Methods, and Results.* Philadelphia, PA: W.B. Saunders; 2000:305-315.

Betka J, Zvěřina E, Balogová Z, et al. Complications of microsurgery of vestibular schwannoma. *Biomed Res Int.* 2014;2014:315952.

Brotchi J, Bonnal JP. Lateral and middle sphenoid wing meningiomas. In: Al-Mefty O, ed. *Meningiomas.* New York, NY: Raven Press; 1991:413-425.

Chang EF, Clark A, Smith JS, et al. Functional mapping-guided resection of low-grade gliomas in eloquent areas of the brain: improvement of long-term survival. *J Neurosurg.* 2011;114:566-573.

Cohen AR. Endoscopic ventricular surgery. *Pediatr Neurosurg.* 1993;19:127-134.

Cuetter AC, Garcia-Bobadilla J, Guerra LG, et al. Neurocysticercosis: focus on intraventricular disease. *Clin Infect Dis.* 1997;24:157-164.

Duffau H, Lopes M, Arthuis F, et al. Contribution of intraoperative electrical stimulations in surgery of low grade gliomas: a comparative study between two series without (1985–96) and with (1996–2003) functional mapping in the same institution. *J Neurol Neurosurg Psychiatry.* 2005;76:845-851.

Elgamal E. CSF rhinorrhea after transsphenoidal surgery. *Int J Neurosurg.* 2007;1:5.

Esquenazi Y, Lo VP, Lee K. Critical care management of cerebral edema in brain tumors. *J Intensive Care Med.* 2017;32:15-24.

Ghirardello S, Hopper N, Albanese A, et al. Diabetes insipidus in craniopharyngioma: postoperative management of water and electrolyte disorders. *J Pediatr Endocrinol Metab.* 2006;19(suppl 1):413-421.

Gormley WB, Sekhar LN, Wright DC, et al. Acoustic neuromas: results of current surgical management. *Neurosurgery.* 1997;41:50-60.

Hadjipanayis CG, Schuette AJ, Nicholas B, et al. Full scope of options. *J Neurosurg.* 2010;67:197-205.

Hellwig D, Grotenhuis JA, Tirakotai W, et al. Endoscopic third ventriculostomy for obstructive hydrocephalus. *Neurosurg Rev.* 2005;28:1-38.

Hopf NJ, Grunert P, Fries G, et al. Endoscopic third ventriculostomy: outcome analysis of 100 consecutive procedures. *Neurosurgery.* 1999;44:795-804.

Jakimovski D, Bonci G, Attia M, et al. Incidence and significance of intraoperative cerebrospinal fluid leak in endoscopic pituitary surgery using intrathecal fluorescein. *World Neurosurg.* 2014;82:e513-e523.

Keles GE, Lundin DA, Lamborn KR, et al. Intraoperative subcortical stimulation mapping for hemispherical perirolandic gliomas located within or adjacent to the descending motor pathways: evaluation of morbidity and assessment of functional outcome in 294 patients. *J Neurosurg.* 2004;100:369-375.

Kucukyuruk B, Richardson RM, Wen WT, et al. Microsurgical anatomy of the temporal lobe and its implications on temporal lobe epilepsy surgery. *Epilepsy Res Treat.* 2012;2012:769825.

Langfitt JT, Rausch R. Word-finding deficits persist after left anteriotemporal lobectomy. *Arch Neurol.* 1996;53:72-76.

Marsh JC, Turian JV, Henkovic AM, et al. Temporal lobectomy for high grade gliomas: impact on outcomes and implications for postoperative radiation treatment field design. *Cancer Clin Oncol.* 2013;2:5-16.

Matushita H, Pinto FCG, Cardeal DD, et al. Hydrocephalus in neurocysticercosis. *Childs Nerv Syst.* 2011;27:1709-1721.

Mehta GU, Oldfield EH. Prevention of intraoperative cerebrospinal fluid leaks by lumbar cerebrospinal fluid drainage during surgery for pituitary macroadenomas. *J Neurosurg.* 2012;116:1299-1303.

Muthukumar N, Rossette D, Soundaram M, et al. Blindness following pituitary apoplexy: timing of surgery and neuro-ophthalmic outcome. *J Clin Neurosci.* 2008;15:873-879.

Nawar RN, Abdel Mannan D, Selman WR, et al. Pituitary tumor apoplexy: a review. *J Intensive Care Med.* 2008;23:75-90.

Pollock BE, Schreiner SA. A theory on the natural history of colloid cysts of the third ventricle. *Neurosurgery.* 2000;46:1077-1081.

Potgieser ARE, de Jong BM, Wagemakers M, et al. Insights from the supplementary motor area syndrome in balancing movement initiation and inhibition. *Front Hum Neurosci.* 2014;8:960.

Roth P, Wick W, Weller M. Steroids in neurooncology: actions, indications, side-effects. *Curr Opin Neurol.* 2010;23:597-602.

Ryken TC, McDermott M, Robinson PD. The role of steroids in the management of brain metastases: a systematic review and evidence-based clinical practice guideline. *J Neurooncol.* 2010;96:103-114.

Sanai N, Chang S, Berger MS. Low-grade gliomas in adults. A review. *J Neurosurg.* 2011;115:948-965.

Saski-Adams D, Hadar EJ. Temporal lobe epilepsy surgery: surgical complications. In: Luders HO, ed. *Textbook of Epilepsy Surgery.* Boca Raton, FL: CRC Press; 2008:1288-1299.

Schijman E, Peter JC, Rekate HL, et al. Management of hydrocephalus in posterior fossa tumors: how, what, when? *Childs Nerv Syst.* 2004;20:192-194.

Schroeder HW, Niendorf WR, Gaab MR. Complications of endoscopic third ventriculostomy. *J Neurosurg.* 2002;96:1032-1040.

Tu A, Tamburrini G, Steinbok P. Management of postoperative pseudomeningocele: an international survey study. *Childs Nerv Syst.* 2014;30:1791-1801.

Tubbs RS, Miller JH, Cohen-Gadol AA, et al. Intraoperative anatomic landmarks for resection of the amygdala during medial temporal lobe surgery. *Neurosurgery.* 2010;66:974-977.

Vaphiades M. The pituitary ring sign: an MRI sign of pituitary apoplexy. *Neuro-ophthalmology.* 2007;31:111-116.

Watts J, Box G, Galvin A, et al. Magnetic resonance imaging of meningiomas: a pictorial review. *Insights Imaging.* 2014;5:113-122.

20

Neurosurgical Emergencies

Ryan S. Kitagawa, MD

Questions

1. A 50-year-old man is brought into the emergency department (ED) after being stuck by a car moving at high speed. Upon arrival to the hospital, the patient is found to have no eye opening, verbal sounds, or motor movement to stimulation. Following intubation, resuscitation, and placement of an intracranial pressure monitor, the patient is admitted to the intensive care unit. His computed tomography (CT) and follow-up magnetic resonance imaging (MRI) scans are shown below. What is the source of the diffusion restriction seen in the corpus callosum and white matter on MRI?

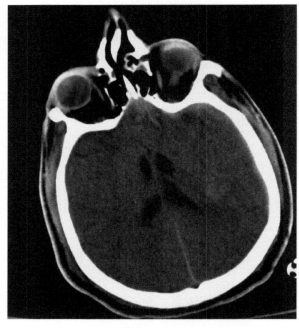

Axial head computed tomography at the level of the superior thalami.

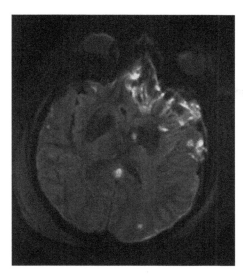

Axial magnetic resonance imaging of the brain diffusion weighted image (DWI) sequence at the level of the thalami and splenium of the corpus callosum.

A. Embolic infarctions from carotid dissection

B. Diffuse axonal injury

C. Hypoxic ischemic injury from the lack of timely intubation

D. Subclinical seizures

E. Intracranial hemorrhage from his trauma

2. A 50-year-old man suffered a traumatic brain injury with subsequent hemicraniectomy 3 months prior. He was transferred to an acute rehabilitation facility. On arrival, he was initially awake and able to participate in therapy, but the patient became progressively more somnolent. He was also noted to have intermittent tachycardia without fevers. A CT scan was obtained and is shown below. What is the source of the patient's altered mental status, and what is the appropriate treatment?

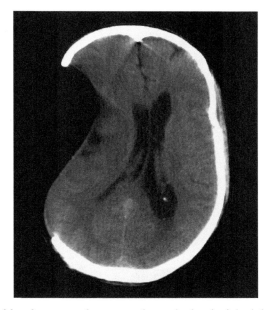

Axial head computed tomography at the level of the bilateral lateral ventricle atria.

A. Urinary tract infection; antibiotics

B. Hydrocephalus; ventriculoperitoneal shunt

C. Seizures; antiepileptic medications

D. Sympathetic storming; β-blocker medication

E. Syndrome of the trephined; cranioplasty

3. A 16-year-old girl is involved in a high-speed motor vehicle accident. She is intubated in the field and arrives with reactive pupils, no eye opening, and a withdraw response in all extremities. Her CT is displayed below. An intracranial pressure monitor is placed with an opening pressure of 40 mm Hg. Despite sedation, cerebrospinal fluid diversion, and hyperosmolar therapy, her intracranial pressure remains above 30 mm Hg. What intervention will decrease the likelihood of death in this patient with refractory elevated intracranial pressure?

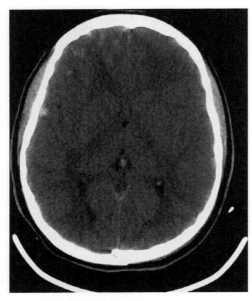

Axial head computed tomography at the level of the bilateral thalami.

A. Decompressive craniectomy
B. Pentobarbital coma
C. Hypothermia to 33°C
D. Neuromuscular paralytic
E. Intravenous steroids

4. A 19-year-old woman arrives to the hospital via emergency medical services (EMS) following a motorcycle crash. She is intubated in the field, and on her neurologic exam, her eyes are closed with reactive pupils, and she is flexor posturing bilaterally. She has numerous skull base fractures and cervical spine fractures. A CT of the brain was obtained and demonstrated frontotemporal contusions, and the CT angiogram demonstrated a grade IV internal carotid artery injury (based on

Biffl scale for blunt vascular injury). What is the proper treatment for the vascular lesion?

A. Observation with repeat imaging given the intracranial hemorrhage
B. Surgical intervention with carotid endarterectomy
C. Medical management with antiplatelet or anticoagulant agents when the hemorrhage is stable
D. No treatment or follow-up imaging is needed
E. Operative fixation of the cervical spine fracture.

5. A 39-year-old woman was found down and was taken to the hospital. Upon arrival to the ED, she is extensor posturing with a left-sided fixed and dilated pupil. Her CT scan is shown below. After surgical evacuation of her lesion, she is noted to improve to localization and eye opening. She has a marked decrease in her left-sided movements compared to her right. What is the source of this patient's weakness?

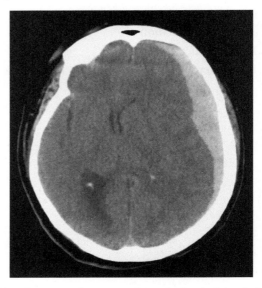

Axial head computed tomography at the level of the thalami.

A. Herniation stroke related to elevated intracranial pressure
B. Cervical spinal cord injury accompanying her trauma
C. Carotid dissection leading to ischemia
D. Compression of the contralateral cerebral peduncle
E. Posttraumatic seizure with Todd paralysis

6. A 25-year-old woman is brought into the hospital after a high-speed motor vehicle accident. She is intubated. On examination she is localizing bilaterally. Her CT is shown below. What is the source of the patient's hemorrhage?

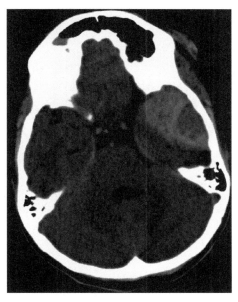

Axial head computed tomography at the level of the high pons.

A. Skull fracture with active arterial hemorrhage

B. Rupture of the Sylvian vein

C. Hemorrhage into a middle fossa arachnoid cyst

D. Temporal lobe contusion from impact into the temporal bone

E. Acute hemorrhage into a previous chronic subdural hematoma

7. A 42-year-old woman was hit by a car traveling at 40 miles per hour. Upon arrival to the ED, there was no eye opening and only flexor posturing of all extermities on exam. She was intubated and taken for CT imaging, where she was found to have multiple, small, extra-axial hemorrhages without mass effect. According to the Brain Trauma Foundation Guidelines, what is the next step in management?

A. Insertion of an intracranial pressure monitor

B. Hyperventilation

C. Hyperosmolar therapy with mannitol

D. Surgical decompression

E. Prophylactic hypothermia for neuroprotection

8. A 55-year-old man fell from a roof. On exam, he was withdrawing in all extremities, and so he was intubated. A CT scan was obtained, which showed multiple contusions and subarachnoid hemorrhage without mass effect. An intracranial pressure monitor was placed, and his pressure was elevated above 30 mm Hg despite intubation, cerebrospinal fluid diversion, and hyperosmolar therapy. Hypothermia with an intravascular cooling device was planned. Which of the following is true regarding hypothermia?

A. Hypothermia has been shown to have neuroprotective effects when administered shortly after injury.

B. Hypothermia has been shown to improve outcomes when administered prior to hyperosmolar therapy.

C. Patients who receive hypothermia have fewer complications in the immediate postinjury period.

D. Hypothermia is associated with reflexive tachycardia.

E. Hypothermia results in fewer third-tier interventions such as pentobarbital coma or decompressive craniectomy.

9. A 32-year-old man was assaulted with a baseball bat. He was initially opening his eyes to voice, not speaking, but localizing bilaterally. His CT showed a skull fracture with subarachnoid hemorrhage. He did not have any seizure-like activity at the time of admission. What is the appropriate duration of antiseizure medications?

A. He did not have a seizure; no antiseizure medication is needed

B. 1 year

C. 3 months

D. 1 month

E. 1 week

10. A 20-year-old man was shot in the head at close range. The patient had fixed and dilated pupils with no motor response. He was intubated, and a head CT scan was obtained. What CT features are associated with poor prognosis and likely fatal injury in a penetrating head injury patient?

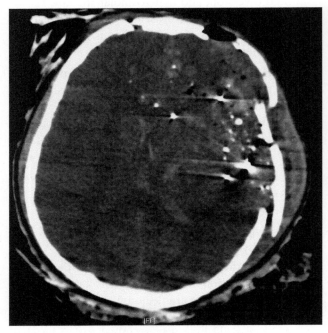

Axial noncontrast head computed tomography at the level of the splenium of the corpus callosum.

   A. Skull fracture
   B. Intracranial hemorrhage
   C. Epidural hematoma
   D. Hemispheric injury
   E. Ventricular involvement with hemorrhage

11. Following a gunshot wound to the head, a 50-year-old man had a bifrontotemporal craniectomy. He recovered to following commands bilaterally. Two weeks after his injury, he became acutely unresponsive with nonreactive pupils. He is taken for imaging, and his CT scan is shown below. What is the source of the patient's hemorrhage?

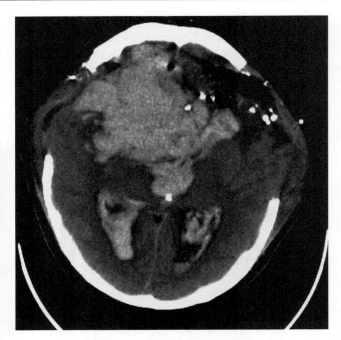

Noncontrast head computed tomography at the level of the bilateral lateral ventricle atria.

   A. Infection from the bullet fragments
   B. Hypertensive hemorrhage
   C. Rupture of an aneurysm
   D. Hemorrhagic transformation of an ischemic stroke
   E. Seizure

12. A 19-year-old woman is a victim of unwitnessed assault. She is intubated in the field and is transported to the hospital where she is found to have a fixed and dilated pupil with extensor limbs posturing. The patient had a CT scan of the head and cervical spine, which showed a large epidural hematoma with uncal herniation but no cervical spine fractures. She is taken emergently to the operating room where a craniotomy with evacuation of the hematoma was performed. The operation is uneventful with 250 mL of blood loss. In the recovery room, she remains chemically paralyzed, but upon transport to the intensive care unit, she becomes hemodynamically unstable. Her blood pressure is 75/40 mm Hg, and her heart rate is 160 bpm. What is a likely source of this patient's hemodynamic instability?

A. Hemorrhagic shock from undiagnosed hemorrhage source (such as intra-abdominal bleeding)

B. Undiagnosed cervical spine injury

C. Elevated intracranial pressure with herniation from malignant cerebral edema

D. Acute myocardial infarction (MI)

E. Lack of sedation with use of a neuromuscular paralytic

13. A 35-year-old man is involved in a motorcycle crash and was found to be extensor posturing at the scene. His blood pressure upon arrival to the ED was 85/45 mm Hg. Which of the following is contraindicated in this patient?

A. Intubation

B. Placement of intracranial pressure monitor

C. Intravenous steroid administration

D. Resuscitation to increase blood pressure

E. Imaging of the brain, cervical spine, and chest/abdomen/pelvis

14. An 87-year-old man with a history of atrial fibrillation presented with several weeks of progressive confusion with worsening left-sided weakness. He was scheduled for surgical evacuation of the lesion based on the below CT scan. Which of the following interventions has been shown to decrease the likelihood of subdural hematoma recurrence in a randomized, controlled trial?

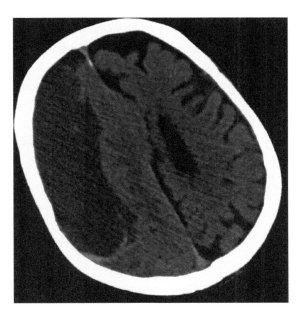

Axial head computed tomography.

A. Preoperative and postoperative steroid administration

B. Placement of a subdural drain at the time of surgery

C. Postoperative bedrest with head of bed flat

D. Multiple burr holes rather than a single burr hole

E. Placement of an intracranial pressure monitor

15. A 30-year-old man was involved in a high-speed motorcycle crash. He had no motor movement to stimulation and, therefore, was intubated in the field without medications. Upon arrival to the hospital, he has fixed and dilated pupils and no motor response. He is admitted to the intensive care unit, and his clinical exam that was performed by a qualified attending is consistent with brain death. He is normothermic with systolic blood pressure greater than 110 mm Hg, but he requires multiple vasopressors and significant ventilator support. Prior attempt at an apnea test resulted in hemodynamic instability. What is the next appropriate step to declare brain death?

A. None; his clinical exam is consistent with brain death

B. A second neurologic exam from another specialist

C. Attempt apnea test again

D. A nuclear medicine cerebral blood flow examination

E. Brain death cannot be declared in this patient

16. A 67-year-old man with a history of intravenous drug abuse, hypertension, and coronary artery disease presented with several weeks of severe neck pain. He is neurologically intact on exam. His MRI and CT are included below. What is the next course of action?

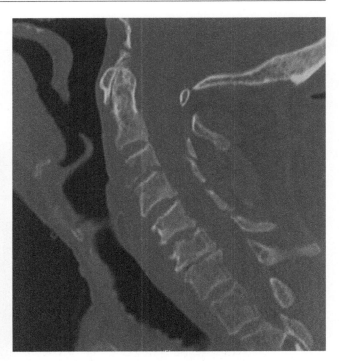

Saggital computed tomography of cervical spine (bone window).

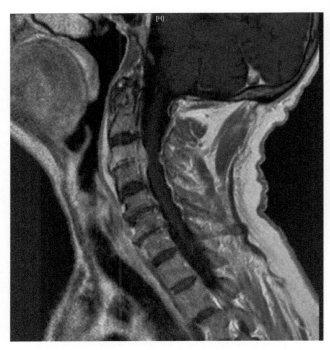

Saggital magnetic resonance imaging of cervical spine (T1 with contrast).

A. Schedule an elective cervical discectomy for degenerative disk disease when medically cleared

B. Interventional radiology-guided biopsy

C. Immediate anterior surgical decompression with stabilization

D. Intravenous antibiotics and observation

E. Physical therapy and epidural steroids

17. What are the most common cause and organism of osteomyelitis/discitis?

A. Surgical site infection; *Staphylococcus aureus*

B. Hematogenous; *S aureus*

C. Hematogenous; *Escherichia coli*

D. Direct spread of infection (eg, pyelonephritis or retropharyngeal); *S aureus*

E. Direct spread of infection; *E coli*

18. A 20-year-old man was involved in an altercation several weeks prior. He was found to have skull base fractures and cerebral contusions at that time. He was incarcerated but developed progressive altered mental status with high fever over the course of 2 weeks. He had a seizure and was intubated prior to arrival to the hospital. He had minimal withdraw in all extremities. An MRI scan was performed and is shown below. What is the best next appropriate action?

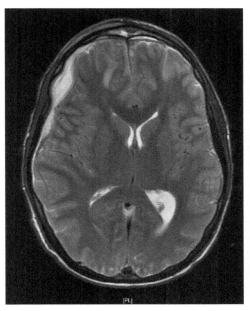 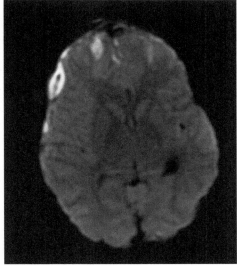

Axial magnetic resonance imaging of the brain. Left panel shows T2-weighted image at the level of a caduate head. Right panel shows diffusion-weighted image at the level of the caudate head.

 A. Continuous electroencephalography (EEG) and seizure control

 B. Lumbar puncture to rule out meningitis

 C. Immediate surgical evacuation

 D. Intracranial pressure monitoring

 E. Admission to the intensive care unit with serial imaging and neurological exams

19. A 65-year-old man with a past medical history of smoking and alcohol abuse presents with several weeks of progressive headaches followed by a several-day history of altered mental status and somnolence. Upon arrival to the hospital, the patient awakens to voice, has incomprehensible speech, and is localizing bilaterally. He had a CT followed by MRI, which are both shown below. From where did this lesion originate?

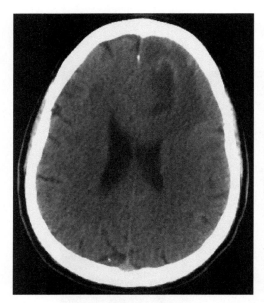

Axial head computed tomography shows left frontal hypodensity with small area of increased density.

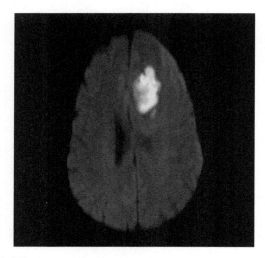

Axial diffusion-weighted magnetic resonance imaging of the brain with hyperintense lesion in the left frontal region.

A. Infected dental abscess
B. Primary lung mass
C. Cardiac embolus
D. Primary brain mass
E. Previous head injury

20. A 54-year-old man presents with a history of traumatic brain injury with craniectomy and ventriculoperitoneal shunt. He had a cranioplasty 6 weeks prior and now presents with progressive altered mental status. Upon arrival to the ED, he is arousable to voice with reactive pupils, incomprehensive sounds, localization on the left, and dense hemiparesis on the right. The motor exam is similar to before the cranioplasty. His CT is shown below. What is the appropriate next step?

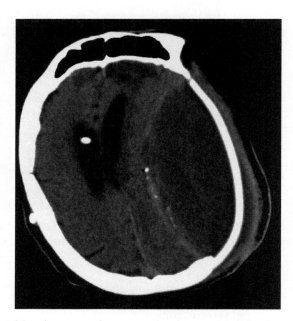

Axial head computed tomography shows mixed density epidural collection.

A. MRI to rule out infection
B. Shunt adjustment for overshunting
C. EEG to rule out seizures
D. Surgical exploration
E. Intravenous antibiotics

21. A 52-year-old man with a history of hypertension who just came back from a trip to South America, presented with progressive headaches and nausea with vomiting. He is somnolent but is able to follow commands in all extremities. Exam also shows papilledema on funduscopic exam. His CT is shown below. What is the source of this patient's hydrocephalus?

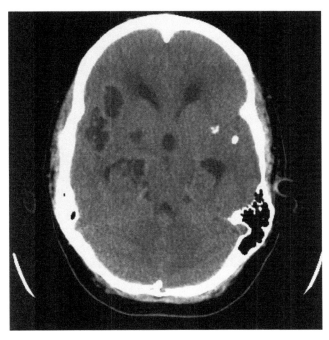

Axial head computed tomography.

A. Infection

B. Neoplasm

C. Aqueductal stenosis

D. Congenital

E. Meningitis

Questions 22 and 23

A 35-year-old man jumped into shallow water and immediately lost all motor function in his hands and legs after hitting his head on the riverbed. He was brought into the hospital and found to have no motor movement below C7 with no sensation and no rectal tone.

22. What is the correct steroid regimen?

A. Dexamethasone 10 mg intravenous once then 4 mg every 6 hours for 48 hours

B. Steroids are not indicated

C. A single bolus of methylprednisolone 30 mg/kg

D. 5.4 mg/kg/h of methylprednisolone for 48 hours

E. Both C and D

23. What is the patient's American Spinal Injury Association (ASIA) scale?

A. ASIA Impairment A

B. ASIA Impairment B

C. ASIA Impairment C

D. ASIA Impairment D

E. ASIA Impairment E

24. A 20-year-old man is involved in a high-speed motor vehicle accident. He arrives comatose and is extensor posturing bilaterally. His head CT shows evidence of diffuse axonal injury. EMS placed the patient in a cervical collar. What is the minimum necessary workup to clear and remove the cervical collar?

A. The cervical collar should remain until the patient is able to be clinically cleared

B. Flexion-extension x-rays with fluoroscopy

C. Cervical MRI without contrast

D. A thin-slice, high-resolution CT scan of the cervical spine

E. Plain x-rays of the cervical spine

25. A 26-year-old woman had a rollover motor vehicle accident with immediate loss of motor strength in her legs and hands. Upon arrival to the ED, she recalled the accident and gave a detailed history. She reported some sensation in all extremities and was able to move her arms with no strength below C7. Her blood pressure is 140/85 mm Hg, and heart rate is 60 bpm. Her CT scan is shown below. What is the appropriate next course of action?

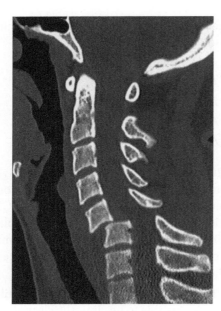

Sagittal cervical spine computed tomography (bone window).

A. A bolus of 30 mg/kg of methylprednisolone
B. Insertion of central venous access and vasopressors for spinal cord perfusion
C. Intubation for airway protection
D. MRI C spine followed by immediate fracture reduction and operative fixation
E. Admission to the intensive care unit for close observation of her respiratory and cardiac status

26. A 45-year-old man is involved in the motor vehicle accident with no loss of consciousness. He immediately noted severe thoracic back pain without weakness or numbness. He is neurologically intact on exam. His CT scan is shown below. What is the most appropriate treatment of this lesion?

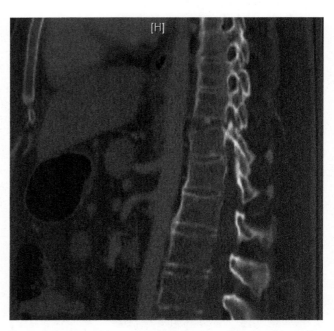

Sagittal thoracic spine computed tomography scan shows disruption of the ligaments and disk space in the thoracic spine.

A. No intervention is needed
B. Operative fixation
C. Bracing
D. Flexion-extension x-rays to determine the stability with possible surgical intervention
E. Intravenous steroids and neurologic observation

27. A 50-year-old man with a past medical history of hypertension developed acute lower back pain with sudden onset of inability to walk. He came to the ED and was noted to have saddle anesthesia with minimal movement in the feet. His rectal tone was diminished as well. His MRIs are shown below. What is the appropriate treatment for this patient?

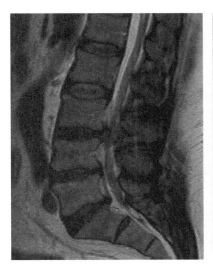 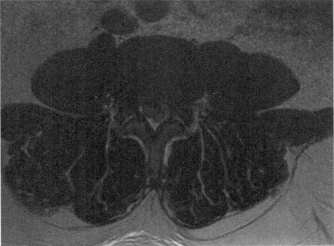

Magnetic resonance imaging of lumbar spine. T2 sequence with sagittal and axial images.

    A. Bedrest and steroids
    B. Physical therapy
    C. Microdiscectomy
    D. Posterior instrumentation and decompression
    E. Epidural steroid injection

28. Far lateral (extraforaminal) disk herniation at L3-4 will cause compression of which nerve root?
    A. L2
    B. L3
    C. L4
    D. L5
    E. None

29. A 19-year-old man with no past medical history has rapidly progressive headache, nuchal rigidity, photophobia, and fever. He lives in the college dormitory and reports that other students are also ill. On neurologic exam, he has high fevers and appears sick. He has presumed meningitis, and a lumbar puncture is planned. The patient is taken to interventional radiology following an aborted bedside attempt. The needle is passed, but no fluid is obtained. See the x-ray image below. Where is the needle tip located, and what is the correct adjustment?

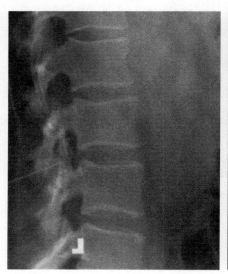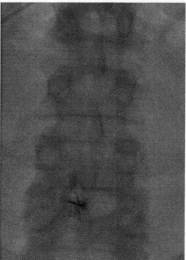

Lateral and anterior-posterior x-ray images of lumbar spine.

    A. Within the epidural spine; advance the needle

    B. Within the thecal sac; flush the needle

    C. On the lamina, lateral to the space; pull back and adjust medially

    D. On the lamina, inferior to the space; pull back and adjust superiorly

    E. On the spinous process; pick a new entry point

30. A fracture of the ring at C1 as a result of axial loading is known as a Jefferson fracture. By "Spence's rule," at what separation of the lateral masses relative to C2 is the transverse ligament likely ruptured?

    A. 3 mm

    B. 5 mm

    C. 7 mm

    D. 9 mm

    E. 11 mm

31. A 64-year-old man is involved in a motorcycle crash with multiple injuries including facial fractures, rib fractures, and multiple abdominal injuries. He is awake and alert, and his neurologic exam is unremarkable, with the exception of neck pain and cervical spine tenderness to palpation. His cervical CT is shown below. What is the cause of the patient's neck pain, and what is the proper management?

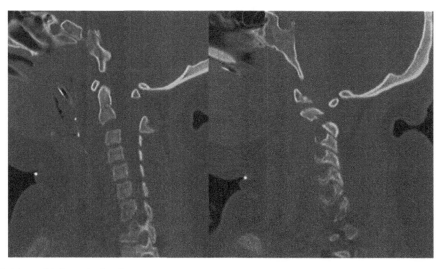

Left: cervical spine; right: sagittal cervical spine.

A. Hangman's fracture; operative stabilization

B. Type II odontoid fracture; operative stabilization

C. Type III odontoid fracture; cervical collar

D. No abnormality is present; maintain cervical collar until neck pain resolves

E. Degenerative changes without obvious fracture; obtain MRI of the cervical spine

32. A 60-year-old man undergoes an elective anterior cervical discectomy and fusion. Following an uneventful recovery in the postanesthesia care unit, he is transferred to the floor for his postoperative care. Several hours later, the patient is noted to be in respiratory distress with oxygen saturations of 85% on a non-rebreather mask. His cervical wound site appears to have ecchymosis with a mass that is palpable. What is the next appropriate step?

A. Continued observation with supplemental oxygen

B. Admission to the intensive care unit with non-invasive ventilation

C. Immediate intubation with mechanical ventilation

D. Bedside wound exploration, intubation, and formal operative revision

E. Angiogram for pseudoaneurysm

33. A 53-year-old woman presents with progressive bilateral lower extremity weakness with numbness and bowel and bladder incontinence. On her neurologic exam, she is awake and in no distress. She has full strength in her bilateral upper extremities without pathologic reflexes. She has modest, symmetric weakness in her bilateral lower extremities with upgoing Babinski reflexes with hyperreflexia. Her MRIs of the cervical and thoracic (with intravenous contrast) spine are shown below. What is the source of the patient's symptoms, and what is the appropriate treatment?

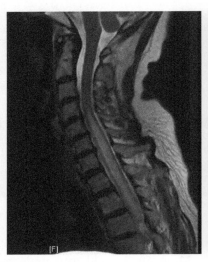 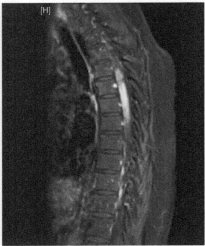

Magnetic resonance imaging of the spine. Left panel shows short tau inversion recovery (STIR) image of cervical spine. Right panel shows postcontrast T1 image of thoracic spine.

A. Transverse myelitis; steroids
B. Spinal cord infarction; vascular workup
C. Hydromyelia; cerebrospinal fluid diversion
D. Intradural extramedullary neoplasm; resection
E. Intramedullary neoplasm; biopsy with consideration of resection

Answers and Explanations

1. **B.** In patients with high-energy injuries, diffuse axonal injury is a common source of poor neurologic exam. These lesions may be present in multiple locations and are best visualized on MRI. The diffusion-weighted sequence will classically show restricted diffusion lesions in the gray-white junction, corpus callosum, and brainstem. These classic locations make embolic infarcts, seizures, and hemorrhage less likely.

2. **E.** Delayed neurologic deterioration in a patient with traumatic brain injury has a challenging differential diagnosis, and any of the listed choices is possible. Loss of cerebral volume combined with the weight of the skin against the brain can frequently cause "sinking skull flap syndrome" or "syndrome of the trephined." The signs and symptoms are highly variable and can include headaches, focal neurologic deficits, hemodynamic alterations, and clinical herniation. Radiographic signs include midline shift away from the craniectomy site. The symptoms may be transiently treated with bedrest with the head of the bed flat or down, but the definitive treatment is cranioplasty.

3. **A.** Multiple clinical trials for the treatment of malignant intracranial hypertension have failed to show benefit. Pentobarbital coma and neuromuscular paralytic have not shown outcome benefit. Hypothermia and intravenous steroids have been shown to worsen the outcome in traumatic brain injury patients with elevated intracranial pressure. In the RescueICP trial, decompression craniectomy was associated with decreased mortality.

4. **C.** Blunt cerebrovascular injury has been increasingly recognized as a source of cerebral infarction. The Biffl (or Denver) Classification System separates these lesions into 5 grades, with grade IV being complete occlusion of the artery (Table 20-1). This lesion represents an extremely high risk for

Table 20-1. Biffl Classification System and Prognosis

Grade	Vessel Injury	Prognosis
I	Mild intimal injury or irregular intima	Heals regardless of therapy
II	Dissection with raised intimal flap, intraluminal thrombosis	70% of dissections or hematomas with luminal stenosis progress despite heparin therapy
III	Pseudoaneurysm	8% of pseudoaneurysms heal with heparin and 90% resolve with stenting
IV	Vessel occlusion/thrombosis	Occluded arteries do not recanalize early
V	Vessel transection	Lethal and refractory to therapy

embolization, and therefore, treatment with antiplatelet or anticoagulant agent is appropriate when safe from a systemic injury standpoint.

5. **D.** Although all of the options are possible complications of severe traumatic brain injury, this patient arrived with herniation syndrome. This condition

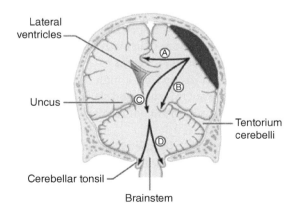

Schematic of different herniation types. **A.** Subfalcine. **B.** Uncal. **C.** Transtentorial. **D.** Tonsillar. (Adapted from Berkowitz AL. *Clinical Neurology and Neuroanatomy: A Localization-Based Approach.* New York, NY: McGraw-Hill; 2016.)

includes ipsilateral cranial nerve III dysfunction with pupillary involvement and coma. Postoperatively, the patient had a false lateralizing sign with ipsilateral motor weakness known as the Kernohan notch.

6. **A.** This imaging represents active arterial hemorrhage as represented by the "swirl sign" on the CT. This is an area of hypodensity within an acute hemorrhage. Given the location of the hemorrhage within the temporal fossa and the shape, an epidural hemorrhage is suspected. The most common cause of a temporal epidural hemorrhage is a fracture of the squamous temporal bone with laceration of the middle meningeal artery.

7. **A.** The acute management of severe traumatic brain injury has become increasingly standardized with the introduction of the Brain Trauma Foundation Guidelines. Prophylactic hyperventilation and hyperosmolar therapy are not recommended in the absence of herniation symptoms. Neuroprotection via prophylactic craniectomy or hypothermia has also failed to demonstrate benefit in this population. Insertion of an intracranial pressure monitor in a comatose patient continues to be the gold standard for treatment of severe traumatic brain injury without surgical mass lesion.

8. **E.** A multitude of clinical trials have examined hypothermia in severe traumatic brain injury. Repeated studies, including NABISH II, have failed to demonstrate improved outcomes when prophylactic hypothermia is used for neuroprotection for the general population. In the Eurotherm3235 trial, hypothermia was specifically used for elevated intracranial pressure. This study failed to show benefit of hypothermia in terms of outcomes, and the hypothermia group had a high rate of complications. However, this study did show fewer third-tier interventions in the hypothermia group.

9. **E.** Posttraumatic seizure prophylaxis may be used in traumatic brain injury. In the study by Timken et al, in patients with moderate or severe traumatic brain injury, seizure prophylaxis decreased the incidence of seizures for 1 week but failed to demonstrate long-term benefit. 7 days seizure prophylaxis is recommended per 2016 Neurotrauma foundation guideline. The exact agent and the use of these

medications in mild traumatic brain injury remain controversial.

10. **E.** Outcome prediction in penetrating head injury is essential to the management of these patients. In some studies, the prehospital mortality may be as high as 90%, and the in-hospital mortality of the survivors may be up to 50%. In comatose patients, ventricular involvement is associated with a poor prognosis. Other predictors include:
    - Bihemispheric injury
    - Effacement of the basal cisterns
    - Diffuse fragmentation
    - Posterior fossa involvement

    Choices A to D are not associated with poor outcome and are not the correct answers.

11. **C.** Posttraumatic pseudoaneurysm formation is a potential complication of penetrating head injuries and is the most likely cause of hemorrhage in this patient. Screening for these lesions is needed following injury.

12. **A.** This patient is suffering from acute, posttraumatic shock, which may have a variety of contributing factors. Elevated intracranial pressure and lack of appropriate sedation would typically induce hypertension and are unlikely. A young, healthy individual would also be unlikely to be suffering an acute MI in the setting of trauma. The accompanying tachycardia would imply a lack of intravascular volume, which would be consistent with an undiagnosed hemorrhagic lesion such as an intra-abdominal injury. Following volume resuscitation, an appropriate workup with an ultrasound or CT followed by possible operative intervention or endovascular embolization is needed.

13. **C.** All of the interventions with the exception of steroids are recommended in severe traumatic brain injury. In the CRASH trial of steroids in traumatic brain injury, a worse outcome was demonstrated in patients treated with steroids, and therefore, their use is contraindicated in this patient.

14. **B.** A multitude of interventions have been attempted to decrease the recurrence of chronic subdural hemorrhage after surgical evacuation. Steroid administration, bedrest, and multiple burr

holes have been studied in retrospective reviews. However, the only intervention that has been shown to be of benefit in a randomized, controlled trial is the insertion of a subdural drain at the time of surgery.

15. **D.** To declare an adult patient brain dead, several requirements are needed. The patient should be normothermic and without any sedating agents. A neurologic exam that is consistent with brain death followed by confirmatory testing as needed if unable to complete a full neurologic examination and apnea test. Both an apnea test and a nuclear medicine cerebral blood flow examination are possible. In this particular patient, his hemodynamic instability would prevent an apnea test.

16. **C.** The patient has radiographic evidence of osteomyelitis with discitis. The bony erosion and enhancing epidural mass would not favor a degenerative process, and therefore, an elective surgical intervention or medical management would not be appropriate. The presence of cervical stenosis and spinal cord compression would argue against medical management without surgery for the infection.

17. **B.** Although all of these choices are possible, hematogenous spread of *S aureus* is the most common.

18. **C.** The patient has clinical and radiographic evidence of a subdural empyema. This lesion may result from hematogenous spread or could be the result of direct violation of the skull and dura (as would be the case in this patient). His history of trauma would explain the subacute contusions, but the radiographic features, rapid progression of symptoms, and poor neurologic exam would favor infection over subacute subdural hemorrhage. A subdural empyema is a surgical emergency and requires immediate exploration.

19. **A.** The lesion shows restricted diffusion on MRI, which would favor a proteinaceous fluid or subacute blood products. The most likely diagnosis is intracranial abscess. The CT would not be typical of trauma or cardiac embolus, and the relatively fast progression of symptoms would favor the diagnosis of infection over a primary brain mass. Surgical exploration is the most appropriate next step of management.

20. **D.** The patient has a mixed density epidural collection. In the subacute postoperative period, the most likely cause of this lesion is infection. Overshunting extra-axial hemorrhage is possible, but the dilated ventricles on imaging make this possibility less likely. An MRI and laboratory testing would aid in the diagnosis of infection, but mass effect and midline shift make surgical exploration the appropriate intervention. Intravenous antibiotics would not correct the mass effect and are unlikely to be effective when a purulent mass is present.

21. **A.** The patient had multiple intracranial lesions of differing densities. This represents neurocysticercosis at various stages with obstructive hydrocephalus. The appropriate treatment is cerebrospinal fluid diversion followed by medical treatment of his infection.

22. **B.** The use of steroids in spinal cord injury is a controversial topic. In the National Acute Spinal Cord Injury Studies, some benefit was found in a post hoc analysis, but no randomized, placebo-controlled trial has shown a true outcome improvement. The current guidelines for acute spinal cord injury from the American Association of Neurological Surgeons recommend against the use of steroids, and this treatment has largely been abandoned in clinical practice.

23. A. The patient has complete loss of motor and sensory function below C7. The lack of motor and sensory function including lack of sacral segments (as demonstrated by lack of rectal tone) is consistent with ASIA Impairment A.

ASIA Impairment Scale (AIS)

A = Complete. No sensory or motor function is preserved in the sacral segments S4-5.

B = Sensory Incomplete. Sensory but not motor function is preserved below the neurological level and includes the sacral segments S4-5 (light touch or pin prick at S4-5 or deep anal pressure) AND no motor function is preserved more than three levels below the motor level on other side of the body.

C = Motor Incomplete. Motor function is preserved at the most caudal sacral segments for voluntary and contraction (VAC) OR the patient meets the criteria for sensory incomplete status (sensory function preserved at the most caudal sacral segments (S4-S5) by LT, PP or DAP), and has some sparing of motor function more than three levels below the ipsilateral motor level on either side of the body.
(This includes key or non-key muscle functions to determine motor incomplete status.) For AIS C – less than half of key muscle functions below the single NLI have a muscle grade ≥ 3.

D = Motor Incomplete. Motor incomplete status as defined above, with at least half (half or more) of key muscle functions below the single NLI having a muscle grade ≥ 3.

E = Normal. If sensation and motor function as tested with the ISNCSCI are graded as normal in all segments, and the patient had prior deficits, then the AIS grade is E. Someone without an initial SCI does not receive an AIS grade.

Using ND: To document the sensory motor and NLI levels the ASIA impairment Scale grade, and/or the zone of partial preservation (ZPP) when they are unable to be determined based on the examination results.

American Spinal Injury Association (ASIA) Impairment Scale. (Adapted from Salardini A, Biller J. *The Hospital Neurology Book.* New York, NY: McGraw-Hill; 2016.)

24. D. Clearance of the cervical collar of a comatose patient is a controversial issue. The definitive imaging study for cervical spine clearance would be an MRI, but several studies, including the meta-analysis by Panczykowski et al, demonstrate that in a majority of cases, a high-resolution, thin-slice CT that demonstrates no acute fractures or dislocations is sufficient for clearance of the cervical spine and removal of the collar.

25. D. The patient has sustained an incomplete spinal cord injury with ongoing compression of the spinal cord. The current guidelines for spinal cord injury do not recommend steroids for the treatment of this lesion. Because the patient is maintaining her mean arterial pressure >85 mm Hg and is protecting her airway, intubation and vasopressors are not needed. Given the ongoing compression, immediate intervention is appropriate. Closed or open reduction followed by operative fixation is the standard of care.

26. B. The patient has sustained a disruption of the ligaments and disk space in the thoracic spine. This is a biomechanically unstable lesion and should be treated with surgical intervention. The use of steroids is not recommended in this neurologically intact patient, and flexion-extension films are contraindicated. There are multiple classification systems for thoracic and lumbar injuries. The most commonly used are the AO classification system and the Thoracolumbar Injury Classification and Severity (TLICS) system, but by both systems, this lesion should be treated with surgery.

27. C. The patient has acute cauda equina syndrome with imaging that is consistent with a herniated disk at L3-4. This is a surgical emergency and requires immediate decompression. There are no radiographic signs of instability, and therefore, stabilization is not indicated. For symptomatic nerve root compression without overt neurologic deficit, medical management with epidural steroids and physical therapy are reasonable options.

28. B. A far lateral disk herniation will cause compression of the L3 nerve root, whereas a disk herniation within the spine canal will cause compression of the L4 nerve root.

29. A. The lateral x-ray demonstrates that the needle is too shallow, but the anteroposterior view demonstrates that the trajectory is appropriate. Advancing the needle past the epidural space should yield cerebrospinal fluid.

30. C. "Spence's rule" states that a sum of greater than 7 mm of excursion of C1 beyond C2 for both sides combined likely represents a rupture of the transverse ligament.

31. A. The patient has suffered a hangman's fracture. This is an extension-distraction injury at the C2 level involving the pars interarticularis without involvement of the odontoid process. This lesion may require operative intervention depending on the separation of the fracture fragments and relative degree of forward subluxation of C2 on C3. In this particular patient, the relative degree of separation requires operative stabilization.

32. D. The patient has a postoperative neck hematoma, which is a surgical and airway emergency. Intubation is appropriate, but the lesion itself may compress the airway. An immediate evacuation of the hematoma is needed, followed by a formal exploration.

33. E. The cervical spine MRI demonstrates hydromyelia. Tubular cavitation of the spinal cord, and progressive neurologic symptoms make the case unusual for transverse myelitis, spinal cord infarction, or extramedullary lesion. The presence of an enhancing mass on the thoracic MRI implies that the hydromyelia results from a neoplasm. The lesion is likely a primary neoplasm, and the pathology of the mass would determine the degree of surgical intervention with gross total resection being the treatment of choice for ependymoma.

REFERENCES

American College of Surgeons Committee on Trauma. Shock. In: *Advanced Trauma Life Support ATLS Student Course Manual.* Chicago, IL: American College of Surgeons Committee on Trauma; 2012:73.

Andrews PJ, Sinclair HL, Rodriguez A, et al. Hypothermia for intracranial hypertension after traumatic brain injury. *N Engl J Med.* 2015;373:2403-2412.

Ardolino A, Sleat G, Willett K. Outcome measurements in major trauma: results of a consensus meeting. *Injury.* 2012;43(10):1662-1666.

Biffl WL, Moore EE, Offner PJ, et al. Blunt carotid arterial injuries: implications of a new grading scale. *J Trauma.* 1999;47:845-853.

Bracken MB, Shepard MJ, Holford TR, et al. Administration of methylprednisolone for 24 or 48 hours or tirilazad mesylate for 48 hours in the treatment of acute spinal cord injury. Results of the Third National Acute Spinal Cord Injury Randomized Controlled Trial. National Acute Spinal Cord Injury Study. *JAMA.* 1997;277:1597-1604.

Brain Trauma Foundation. *Guidelines for the Management of Severe Traumatic Brain Injury.* 4th ed. Portland, OR: Oregon Health & Science University; 2016.

Brouwer MC, van de Beek D. Management of bacterial central nervous system infections. *Handb Clin Neurol.* 2017;140:349-364.

Clifton GL, Valadka A, Zygun D, et al. Very early hypothermia induction in patients with severe brain injury (the National Acute Brain Injury Study: Hypothermia II): a randomised trial. *Lancet Neurol.* 2011;10:131-139.

Cothren CC, Biffl WL, Moore EE, et al. Treatment for blunt cerebrovascular injuries: equivalence of anticoagulation and antiplatelet agents. *Arch Surg.* 2009;144:685-690.

Cuetter AC, Garcia-Bobadilla J, Guerra LG, et al. Neurocysticosis: focus on intraventricular disease. *Clin Infect Dis.* 1997;24:157-164.

Dabdoub CB, Adorno JO, Urbano J, Silveira EN, Orlandi BM. Review of the management of infected subdural hematoma. *World Neurosurg.* 2016;87:663.e1-8.

Darouiche RO. Spinal epidural abscess. *N Engl J Med.* 2006;355:2012.

Deyo RA, Mirza SK. Clinical practice herniated lumbar intervertebral disk. *N Engl J Med.* 2016;374(18):1763-1772.

Edwards P, Arango M, Balica L, et al. Final results of MRC CRASH, a randomised placebo-controlled trial of intravenous corticosteroid in adults with head injury: outcomes at 6 months. *Lancet.* 2005;365:1957-1959.

Gornet ME, Kelly MP. Fractures of the axis: a review of pediatric, adult, and geriatric injuries. *Curr Rev Musculoskelet Med.* 2016;9(4):505-512.

Hurlbert RJ, Hadley MN, Walters BC, et al. Pharmacological therapy for acute spinal cord injury. *Neurosurgery.* 2015;76(suppl 1):S71-S83.

Hutchinson PJ, Kolias AG, Timofeev IS, et al. Trial of decompressive craniectomy for traumatic intracranial hypertension. *N Engl J Med.* 2016;375:1119-1130.

Matushita H, Pinto FCG, Cardeal DD, et al. Hydrocephalus in neurocystersarcosis. *Childs Nerv Syst.* 2011;27:1709-1721.

Panczykowski DM, Tomycz ND, Okonkwo DO. Comparative effectiveness of using computed tomography alone to exclude cervical spine injuries in obtunded or intubated patients: meta-analysis of 14,327 patients with blunt trauma. *J Neurosurg.* 2011;115:541-549.

Radcliffe KE, Sonagli MA, Rodrigues LM, et al. Does C$_1$ fracture displacement correlate with transverse ligament integrity? *Orthop Surg.* 2013;5:94-99.

Rosenfeld JV, Bell RS, Armonda R. Current concepts in penetrating and blast injury to the central nervous system. *World J Surg.* 2015;39:1352-1362.

Ryken TC, Hurlbert RJ, Hadley MN, et al. The acute cardiopulmonary management of patients with cervical spinal cord injuries. *Neurosurgery.* 2013;72(suppl 2):84-92.

Santarius T, Kirkpatrick PJ, Ganesan D, et al. Use of drains versus no drains after burr-hole evacuation of chronic subdural haematoma: a randomised controlled trial. *Lancet.* 2009;374:1067-1073.

Sendi P, Bregenzer T, Zimmerli W. Spinal epidural abscess in clinical practice. *QJM.* 2008;101:1-12.

Timken NR, Dikmen SS, Wilensky AJ, et al. A randomized, double-blind study of phenytoin for the prevention of post-traumatic seizures. *N Engl J Med.* 1990;323:497-502.

Vaccaro AR, Lehman RA Jr, Hurlbert RJ, et al. A new classification of thoracolumbar injuries: the importance of injury morphology, the integrity of the posterior ligamentous complex, and neurologic status. *Spine (Phila Pa 1976)*. 2005;30:2325-2333.

Vaccaro AR, Oner C, Kepler CK, et al. AOSpine thoracolumbar spine injury classification system: fracture description, neurological status, and key modifiers. *Spine (Phila Pa 1976)*. 2003;38:2028-2037.

Wijdicks EF, Varelas PN, Gronseth GS, et al. Evidence-based guideline update: determining brain death in adults: report of the Quality Standards Subcommittee of the American Academy of Neurology. *Neurology*. 2010;74:1911-1918.

Wu J, Armstrong TS, Gilbert MR. Biology and management of ependymomas. *Neuro Oncol*. 2016;18(7):902-913.

PART 3
Medical Critical Care

21

Pulmonary Diseases

Abduljabbar Dheyab, MD, Jason Kovacevic, MD, Hassan Anbari, MD, and Scott Kopec, MD

Questions

1. A 35-year-old patient with history of heroin abuse was found unresponsive and developed aspiration pneumonia after an overdose. His pneumonia was complicated by acute respiratory failure, and he required intensive care unit (ICU) admission with intubation, after which he developed severe acute respiratory distress syndrome (ARDS) (chest radiograph shown below). His initial vent settings were volume assist-control ventilation with a tidal volume of 840 (12 mL/kg of ideal body weight), a respiratory rate of 12 breaths/min, a positive end-expiratory pressure (PEEP) of 10 cm H_2O, and a fraction of inspired oxygen (FiO_2) of 0.5. His plateau pressure is 38 cm H_2O, pH is 7.40, partial pressure of carbon dioxide (PCO_2) is 46 mm Hg, and arterial partial pressure of oxygen (PaO_2) is 68 mm Hg. Given his current clinical picture, he is placed on the National Institutes of Health ARDS Network protocol, which reduces his tidal volume to 6 mL/kg of ideal body weight with an accompanying increase in respiratory rate. He maintains an acceptable partial pressure of arterial carbon dioxide ($PaCO_2$) and pH while the ARDS protocol is instituted. What will be the effect on lung compliance and oxygenation in the next 48 to 72 hours?

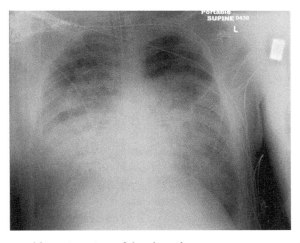

A portable supine view of the chest demonstrates asymmetrical confluent bilateral patchy airspace opacities suggestive of acute respiratory distress syndrome.

    A. Both lung compliance and oxygenation will improve.

    B. Both lung compliance and oxygenation will worsen.

    C. Lung compliance will improve, but oxygenation will not be affected.

    D. Neither will be affected.

2. A previously healthy 50-year-old man is admitted to the ICU for progressively worsening respiratory failure secondary to acute postviral bacterial pneumonia. He eventually required mechanical ventilation with deep sedation and neuromuscular blockade. He is currently being maintained on volume-control ventilation with tidal volume of 6 mL/kg of ideal body weight, FiO_2 of 100%, and PEEP of 14 cm H_2O over the first 24 hours to maintain oxygen saturations of 91%. His peak pressures are 42 cm H_2O, and his plateau pressures are between 34 and 38 cm H_2O. Which of the following treatment options should be initiated?

A. Inhaled prostaglandin

B. Oscillatory ventilation (high-frequency oscillatory ventilation)

C. Prone positioning

D. Pressure-control ventilation

E. Increase PEEP to 20 cm H_2O

3. A 24-year-old woman with history of asthma presented to the emergency department (ED) with signs of respiratory distress. She has had asthma since childhood and is generally asymptomatic; however, she has had several instances of sudden-onset severe attacks requiring intubation on 3 prior occasions. No clear trigger for her attacks has been elicited. After each attack, she is extubated the following day, and pulmonary function testing has been normal after each discharge.

Her home maintenance therapy includes fluticasone (2 puffs twice a day) with albuterol rescue inhaler. She can exercise without difficulty and has never had nocturnal respiratory symptoms. Due to her worsening respiratory status, she is unable to give any further history, but her coworkers state that she had complained of dyspnea and throat tightness throughout the day. Audible wheezing was also noted.

On clinical exam, she is tachypneic with a respiratory rate of 36 breaths/min and tachycardic to around 120 bpm. Lung exam reveals inspiratory and expiratory wheezing. She is placed on 50% Venturi mask and is given 6 nebulizers with albuterol and ipratropium. Her chest x-ray is normal. Despite nebulized treatment, she begins to tire and is intubated in the ED and admitted to the ICU. She is placed on volume-control ventilation with tidal volume of 450 mL with PEEP of 5 cm H_2O.

Following intubation, her wheezing improves, and her peak and plateau pressures are 20 and 18 cm H_2O, respectively. She is eventually extubated the next day and discharged soon after. Which of the following interventions would likely most benefit this patient in the future?

A. Referral for possible bronchial thermoplasty

B. Prescription for EpiPen to be used at the beginning of next attack

C. Referral to ear, nose, and throat (ENT) specialist and speech pathologist

D. Switching her fluticasone to combined steroid/long-acting β-agonist inhaler

4. A 55-year-old woman is evaluated in the ED for status asthmaticus. She has had several attacks in the past requiring ED visits. A methacholine challenge test performed 1 month prior to admission demonstrated severe bronchial hyperreactivity with a PC_{20} (provocative concentration of methacholine causing a 20% drop in forced expiratory volume in 1 second) of 0.88 mg/mL.

In the ED, she receives stacked nebulizers with albuterol and ipratropium via a spacer device 20 minutes apart. She also receives 125 mg of intravenous (IV) Solu-Medrol. On exam, she remains markedly tachypneic, with use of accessory muscles noted, and has sinus tachycardia to 120 bpm. Her blood pressure is stable at 122/76 mm Hg. She has diffuse expiratory wheezing noted.

An arterial blood gas performed while on 50% oxygen via face mask shows a pH of 7.39, PCO_2 of 15 mm Hg, PO_2 of 205 mm Hg, and a bicarbonate of 16 mEq/L. Her serum lactate was 88 mg/dL (9.8 mmol/L). Serum chemistries and complete blood count are within normal limits. Arterial blood gas done during previous ED visit showed pH of 7.35, PCO_2 of 19 mm Hg, PO_2 of 170 mm Hg, bicarbonate of 17 mEq/L, and serum lactate of 153 mg/dL. Currently, what additional therapy would you recommend?

A. Stop albuterol and give subcutaneous epinephrine

B. Give a trial of noninvasive positive-pressure ventilation

C. Give a trial of IV magnesium sulfate

D. Stop albuterol and switch to a long-acting β-agonist

5. A 65-year-old man is being mechanically ventilated for ARDS. His FiO_2 is currently 0.7, pH is 7.30, PCO_2 is 50 mm Hg, and PO_2 is 62 mm Hg. He is on low tidal volume ventilation with 6 mL/kg of ideal body weight, PEEP is 14 cm H_2O, and his plateau pressure is 32 cm H_2O. The ICU team decides to place the patient in the prone position. Most recent trial data suggest that to improve mortality, the patient will need which of the following?

   A. Reduction in FiO_2

   B. To remain in the prone position for at least 16 hours daily

   C. Continuous rotation between prone positioning and supine

   D. An increase in tidal volume

6. An 86-year-old woman undergoes ultrasound-guided central venous catheter placement after being admitted to the ICU for septic shock secondary to cholangitis. Placement of the central venous catheter was difficult. After the procedure, the ultrasound was used to check for pneumothorax. What ultrasonography finding is reassuring that no pneumothorax was caused by difficult placement of the central line?

   A. Seashore sign on M-mode ultrasound

   B. Lung point seen on B-mode ultrasound

   C. Absence of lung sliding on B-mode ultrasound

   D. "Barcode" sign on M-mode ultrasound

7. A 38-year-old woman is evaluated for a 5-day history of worsening dyspnea and hemoptysis. She has no known pulmonary disease and has a remote smoking history. Further history is obtained, and the patient has also endorsed dark, concentrated urine. Her diffusing capacity of the lungs for carbon monoxide (DL_{CO}) is 110% of predicted. High-resolution computed tomography (CT) of the chest is obtained and shows diffuse ground-glass opacities with interlobular septal thickening. Laboratory evaluation obtained on admission shows mild decrease in hemoglobin (Hgb) to 10.1 g/dL, white blood cell (WBC) count of 9.0×10^9/L, platelet count of 350×10^9/L, blood urea nitrogen (BUN) of 50 mg/dL, and creatinine (Cr) of 3.2 mg/dL. Urinalysis shows a pH of 5.2, 3+ protein with dysmorphic red blood cells, and red blood cell casts. Both cytoplasmic and perinuclear antineutrophil cytoplasmic antibodies are negative. Antiglomerular basement membrane antibody was positive. What should the initial treatment regimen include for this patient?

   A. Cyclophosphamide plus rituximab

   B. Rituximab plus prednisone

   C. Plasmapheresis

   D. Plasmapheresis in addition to cyclophosphamide and prednisone.

8. A 46-year-old man with a history of IV drug use was recently admitted for bacterial endocarditis. Blood cultures done on admission revealed infection with methicillin-resistant *Staphylococcus aureus*. The patient had a peripherally inserted central catheter placed for long-term antibiotic therapy. A 4- to 6-week course with vancomycin was initially intended; however, the patient recounted having a severe allergy to vancomycin, so his antibiotic was changed to daptomycin. Therapy with daptomycin 6 mg/kg/d was initiated, and 3 days into therapy with his new antibiotic, the patient developed dyspnea, fever, rigors, and dry cough. His other medications included acetaminophen as needed for pain, lisinopril for hypertension, and atorvastatin for hyperlipidemia.

   His symptoms continued to progress, and he again presented to the hospital for evaluation. Physical exam was performed showing temperature of 38.3°C, respiratory rate of 26 breaths/min, and oxygen saturations of 90% on room air. Lung auscultation demonstrated diffuse crackles. No jugular venous distention (JVD) or lower extremity edema was noted. The patient denied any orthopnea or paroxysmal nocturnal dyspnea. The peripherally inserted central catheter line was intact, and insertion site was without evidence of infection. The chest x-ray showed upper lung zone predominant opacities that were bilateral. Laboratory studies showed WBC of 12.0×10^9/L, and automated cell differential was normal. Echocardiogram showed ejection fraction of 65% with no significant valvular abnormalities. Bronchoscopy with bronchoalveolar lavage was performed with negative cultures but elevated eosinophil count to 65%. Which of the following medications is likely responsible for the patient's current lung findings?

   A. Lisinopril

   B. Atorvastatin

   C. Daptomycin

   D. Acetaminophen

9. A 28-year-old woman with a history of severe asthma presents to the pulmonary clinic for her first injection of omalizumab. She receives the injection and within minutes becomes acutely distressed. A rapid response is called, and on evaluation by the rapid response team, the patient describes diffuse itching and shortness of breath. Her blood pressure has decreased from 126/80 mm Hg on admission to 94/66 mm Hg, her heart rate is 124 bpm and regular, she has diffuse urticaria noted over her arms and chest, wheezing is noted on auscultation, and swelling of her lips is noted. What is the most appropriate next step that should be taken by the rapid response team?

A. IV magnesium infusion

B. Nebulizer with albuterol and ipratropium

C. Intramuscular (IM) epinephrine

D. IV methylprednisolone

10. A 67-year-old former smoker with advanced chronic obstructive pulmonary disease (COPD) who is currently on maximal medical therapy and continuous oxygen presents for evaluation following the fourth exacerbation of his COPD in the past year. Pulmonary function tests demonstrate a forced expiratory volume in 1 second (FEV_1) of 27% of predicted. CT scan of the chest shows predominantly upper lobe emphysema. Arterial blood gas at rest shows PaO_2 of 54 mm Hg and PCO_2 of 50 mm Hg. His past medical history is otherwise only significant for well-controlled hypertension. What surgical option is most appropriate for the management of his COPD?

A. Lung volume reduction surgery

B. Lung transplantation

C. Heart-lung combined transplantation

D. Clinical observation without surgery

11. A 30-year-old man who developed severe ARDS secondary to acute alcohol-induced pancreatitis is currently decompensating with mechanical ventilation. Arterial blood gas shows pH of 7.25, PCO_2 of 53 mm Hg, and PO_2 of 48 mm Hg. He is currently on low tidal volume protocol for ARDS but continues to require 100% FiO_2 and PEEP of 16 mm Hg. His plateau pressure is 35 cm H_2O. Given his worsening clinical status, initiation of venovenous extracorporeal membrane oxygenation is planned. What

can be expected regarding the patient's ventilator settings?

A. Supplemental oxygen and PEEP can be stopped.

B. Tidal volume can be increased.

C. Supplemental oxygen and PEEP can be reduced but will still be required.

D. The ventilator should continue at the current settings.

12. A 50-year-old woman is admitted to the ICU with septic shock related to severe *Clostridium difficile* infection after receiving antibiotics for upper respiratory infection 1 week prior to admission. Inferior vena cava assessment via ultrasound was performed on admission showing complete collapse during the respiratory cycle. The patient received adequate volume resuscitation with 30 mL/kg of crystalloid solution, but she remains hypotensive, with cuff pressure of 65/40 mm Hg. What vasoconstrictor and mean arterial pressure (MAP) goal would be most appropriate for this patient?

A. IV epinephrine; MAP >90 mm Hg

B. Vasopressin; MAP 65-70 mm Hg

C. Dopamine; MAP 80-85 mm Hg

D. Norepinephrine; MAP 65-70 mm Hg

13. A 70-year-old woman with a history of myasthenia gravis currently being treated with pyridostigmine is admitted to the ICU with sepsis secondary to pneumonia. Her preliminary sputum culture results show *Pseudomonas* species. The patient has already received vancomycin. Which additional antibiotics should be started while waiting for the final speciation and sensitivities of her sputum culture?

A. Imipenem plus tobramycin

B. Piperacillin-tazobactam plus amikacin

C. Cefepime plus levofloxacin

D. Ceftazidime plus meropenem

14. A 40-year-old alcoholic with cirrhosis complicated by ascites develops severe alcohol withdrawal and is transferred to the ICU. He is intubated for airway protection because he requires high doses of benzodiazepines and barbiturates to control his withdrawal. He also has history of asthma, and bronchodilator therapy has been continued

during ICU admission. During his ICU admission, the patient suddenly becomes unstable with hypotension, tachycardia, and decrease in urine output. In addition, physical exam is notable for a distended firm abdomen and decrease in bowel sounds. Significant changes are noted in airway pressures: plateau pressures are 28 to >40 cm H_2O, and peak pressures are 30 to >46 cm H_2O. Bladder pressure has been measured and is noted to be 26 cm H_2O. Diagnostic paracentesis is negative for spontaneous bacterial peritonitis. Bedside ultrasound of the chest wall is done and shows seashore sign on M-mode ultrasound. Chest x-ray remains unchanged from admission. Which of the following is the likely diagnosis?

A. Bronchospasm

B. Pneumothorax

C. Abdominal compartment syndrome

D. Obstruction of ventilator tubing

15. A 47-year-old woman with history of methadone dependency was admitted to the ICU with respiratory failure secondary to multilobar pneumonia. She was started on broad-spectrum antibiotic treatment with vancomycin, ceftazidime, and azithromycin. During the night in the ICU, she was agitated, so her sedatives were increased and she was given doses of fentanyl and propofol to improve her synchrony with the ventilator; she also received IV doses of haloperidol. By the second day in the ICU, she had received a total of 8 L of normal saline IV fluids, and her chest x-ray was showing signs of fluid overload, so she underwent diuresis with furosemide. She developed arrhythmia (shown in the figure below). Her labs were as follows: potassium 3.2 mmol/L, calcium 8.5 mg/dL, and magnesium of 2 mg/dL. Which of the following combinations is likely responsible for her arrhythmia?

A. Haloperidol, methadone, and azithromycin

B. Vancomycin, propofol, and fentanyl

C. Ceftazidime, furosemide, and propofol

D. Hypokalemia, fentanyl, and vancomycin

16. A 37-year-old man is rescued from a fire at a plastics factory. When initially found, he was awake and mildly confused, with first-degree burns to his face, neck, right upper extremity, and chest. The patient's mustache is partially burned off. He received 100% FiO_2 at the scene. Upon arrival to the hospital, he is lethargic, with heart rate of 132 bpm, blood pressure of 140/80 mm Hg, respiratory rate of 32 breaths/min, and oxygen saturation (SpO_2) of 97% on 100% non-rebreather mask. Due to the altered mental status, tachypnea, and concern for upper airway edema, the patient is successfully intubated with an 8-0 endotracheal tube. On assist-control (AC) ventilation of 16 breaths/min, 100% FiO_2, and PEEP of 5 cm H_2O, the patient's arterial blood gas demonstrates a $PaCO_2$ of 27 mm Hg and a PaO_2 of 213 mm Hg. Other labs of note include carboxyhemoglobin of 8.1%, mixed venous saturation of 89%, lactate of 14 mmol/L, creatinine of 0.9 mg/dL, and potassium of 4.5 mEq/dL. What is the most appropriate management of this patient?

A. Administer hyperbaric oxygen

B. Administer sodium thiosulfate and hydroxocobalamin

C. Administer methylene blue

D. Start emergent hemodialysis

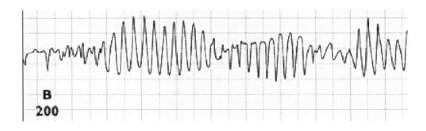

17. A 68-year-old railroad worker is exposed to large amounts of chlorine gas while transferring the gas from one tanker car to another. Upon arrival to the hospital, the patient is lethargic, dyspneic, and tachycardic. He is intubated and placed on mechanical ventilation and undergoes appropriate decontamination. He is on AC with a rate of 16 breaths/min, tidal volume of 6 mL/kg of ideal body weight, 100% FiO$_2$, and PEEP of 5 cm H$_2$O, resulting in a PaO$_2$ of 81 mm Hg. Portable chest x-ray revealed appropriately placed ETT and diffuse infiltrates consistent with ARDS. You conclude that the patient most likely has acute lung injury from inhalation of chlorine gas. Which of the following interventions would be considered contraindicated in this patient?

A. Inhaled sodium bicarbonate

B. Inhaled budesonide

C. Systemic glucocorticoids

D. All of the above

18. A 67-year-old woman is transferred to the ICU for hypotension on postoperative day 3 after undergoing a left pneumonectomy for stage IIA squamous cell carcinoma of the lung. The patient's initial surgery was uncomplicated aside from developing atrial fibrillation requiring intermittent doses of an IV β-blocker for rate control before spontaneously converting to normal sinus rhythm by postoperative day 2. On postoperative day 1, the patient had her left-sided chest tube removed and was ambulating with assistance on 3 L of oxygen. On the day of transfer to the ICU, the patient started to develop progressively worsening tachycardia and hypotension. Initially, the hypotension transiently improved with a 1-L bolus of normal saline, but at transfer, the patient's systolic blood pressure was in the low 80s. Upon arrival to the ICU, the patient had the following findings: afebrile, blood pressure

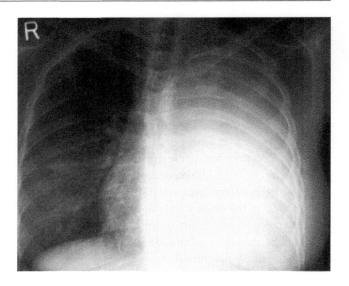

of 78/60 mm Hg, sinus tachycardia with a heart rate of 130 bpm, respiratory rate of 20 breaths/min, and SpO$_2$ on 4 L nasal cannula of 93%. Exam was notable for absent breath sounds on the left, but clear breath sounds on the right, with some evidence of jugular venous distention and no lower extremity edema. Labs of note included a stable WBC of 12.1 × 10^9/L, Hgb of 10.1 g/dL, BUN of 35 mg/dL, creatinine of 0.9 mg/dL, and troponin of 0.01 ng/mL. Electrocardiogram confirmed sinus tachycardia without any ischemic changes. Portable chest radiograph is shown below. What is the most likely etiology of the patient's hypotension?

A. Sepsis associated with a postpneumonectomy empyema

B. Spontaneous hemorrhage into the postpneumonectomy space

C. Acute pulmonary embolism

D. Chylous fluid filling the postpneumonectomy space

19. A 70-year-old man is admitted with septic shock and ARDS stemming from gallstone pancreatitis. He underwent successful stone removal via emergent endoscopic retrograde cholangiopancreatography (ERCP), and over the past 12 hours, he has been weaned off norepinephrine, and his ventilator support has been weaned from 70% FiO_2 and PEEP of 15 cm H_2O to 50% FiO_2 and PEEP of 10 cm H_2O. You are notified by the patient's nurse that the high airway pressure alarm is going off on the patient's ventilator. You find the patient to be agitated but not following commands. He is mildly tachycardic with a heart rate of 110 bpm, his blood pressure is 140/86 mm Hg, and his SpO_2 reads 91%; all of these values have not significantly changed over the past 2 hours. Auscultating breath sounds over the ventilator alarm is difficult, but you do hear breath sounds bilaterally. The respiratory therapist confirms the peak airway pressure to be 75 cm H_2O, with a plateau airway pressure of 27 cm H_2O. Airway pressures recorded 3 hours earlier revealed a peak airway pressure of 29 cm H_2O and a plateau airway pressure of 24 cm H_2O. What is the most likely cause of the patient's elevated airway pressure?

A. Patient biting down on the endotracheal tube

B. An air leak in the ventilator tubing

C. Development of a tension pneumothorax

D. The endotracheal tube migrating into the right mainstem bronchus

Answers and Explanations

1. **B.** Based on the ARDS Network trial published in 2007, a mortality benefit was found by using a low tidal volume strategy of 6 mL/kg of ideal body weight. However, despite having a mortality benefit, both respiratory system compliance and PaO_2/FiO_2 ratios are worse in low tidal volume protocols. Although reduced tidal volumes and lower plateau pressures are considered to be lung protective in the setting of ARDS, they adversely affect lung physiology. With low tidal volumes, lung recruitment and minute ventilation are both negatively affected, resulting in permissive hypercapnia, increased atelectasis, poor lung compliance, and an increase in ventilation/perfusion (V/Q) mismatch. These effects are often viewed as an acceptable trade-off if ventilator-induced lung injury can be avoided. Despite these negative effects on lung physiology in the first 24 to 48 hours, after 72 hours, the differences between low tidal volume and high tidal volume strategies are minimal, and patients on low tidal volume protocols demonstrate improved survival.

2. **C.** This patient should be placed in the prone position. Patients with a diagnosis of moderate to severe ARDS benefit from prone positioning as a result of a redistribution of the blood flow from the dorsal to the ventral regions of the lung. Gravity influences its redistribution equally, and dorsal recruitment prevails over ventral recruitment because of the chest anatomy and causes a more homogeneous lung inflation with change to lung perfusion. The initiation of prone positioning should be based on the severity of ARDS. Prone positioning in addition to lung protective strategies, such as low tidal volumes, should be applied for at least 16 hours daily. Prone positioning improves mortality in patients with severe ARDS by decreasing the degree of ventilator-associated lung injury and by improving oxygenation.

    Inhaled prostaglandin has not been associated with improvement in mortality, despite it being used sometimes to improve V/Q mismatch. Choice B has not been shown to improve mortality; in one study, high-frequency oscillatory ventilation applied early in moderate to severe ARDS, compared to low tidal volume ventilation and high PEEP, had no mortality benefit and may have worsened outcome. As for switching the mode of ventilation, pressure-control ventilation seems to be a more physiologic way of ventilating patient, but it does not have an impact on the mortality of patients with ARDS. While the final option appears very intriguing and it can be argued that increasing the PEEP is the first step in treatment of ARDS along with low tidal volume. However, this patient has high plateau of 34 cm H_2O, and based on the ARDS Network protocol, the plateau should be kept below 30 cm H_2O, and increasing the PEEP to 20 cm H_2O would not serve to reduce that but, instead, could worsen barotrauma potential. Finding appropriate PEEP in an ARDS patient can be tricky, and although not routinely applied in practice, esophageal balloon catheters that measure pleural pressure have been used to estimate transpulmonary pressure (which is the airway pressure minus pleural pressure) in order to determine the optimal level of PEEP in patients with ARDS. Guiding the ventilator setting with the use of esophageal pressures to estimate the transpulmonary pressure was shown to significantly improve oxygenation and compliance in a study of ARDS patients (PaO_2/FiO_2 ratio at 72 hours was 88 mm Hg higher in the esophageal pressure–guided group than in the control group).

3. **C.** This patient should be referred to otolaryngology and speech pathology for evaluation for vocal cord dysfunction (VCD). Her constellation of symptoms including sudden-onset dyspnea, wheezing, and throat tightness in the setting of normal pulmonary function tests and mechanics after intubation are highly suggestive of vocal cord dysfunction. Patient should be referred to ENT in this setting for direct laryngoscopy for accurate diagnosis and then referral to speech pathology for continued therapy.

VCD prevalence is unknown as it can mimic other conditions, making an accurate diagnosis more difficult. It is suggested that the condition is more common in women and healthcare workers. When this condition coexists with asthma, suspicion should be raised when the symptoms and need for rescue inhalers are out of proportion on pulmonary function tests. The most common symptoms are dyspnea, wheezing, and stridor. Stridor is an important clinical finding and is most suggestive of the condition when it is present.

The patient does not have severe or poorly controlled asthma, so changing her medications would not be beneficial at this time. Bronchial thermoplasty similarly would not help with a diagnosis of VCD. The use of injected epinephrine would also not be helpful because this patient does not demonstrate any evidence of anaphylaxis, in which vocal cord edema can happen, leading to stridor; below is an imaging example of vocal cord edema on computed tomography (CT) scan of the neck.

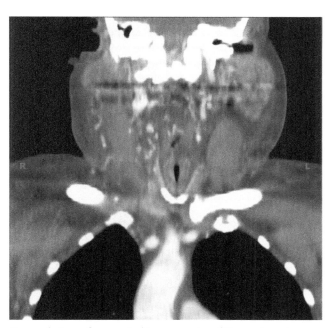

Coronal view of computed tomography of the neck and upper thorax with contrast shows swelling of the vocal cords and subglottic region consistent with angioedema.

4. **C.** Lactic acidosis can be seen in the setting of severe asthma exacerbation due to hypoxemia and underperfusion of tissues. In the patient described in this case, blood pressure is stable and arterial oxygen was above normal limits on 50% mask,

so this is unlikely the cause of her lactic acidosis. Lactic acidosis in the setting of hypoperfusion is most likely due to type A lactic acidosis. Given that she had an elevated lactate during a previous ED visit, her elevated lactate is likely secondary to type B lactic acidosis. Type B lactic acidosis has been reported with β-agonists in asthmatics and when used as a tocolytic in premature labor. Treatment involves removing the offending agent such as a short-acting β-agonist. Subcutaneous epinephrine has been associated with type B lactic acidosis and would not be a suitable substitute in this case. There is no role for noninvasive ventilation as the patient does not show evidence of tiring, her PCO_2 is low, and there is no evidence of hypoventilation. So, in this case, a trial of IV magnesium would be appropriate in addition to stopping her β-agonist.

5. **B.** Placing patients with severe ARDS in the prone position while mechanically ventilated has numerous benefits. Cardiac weight is relieved on the posterior lung regions. Diaphragmatic movement is improved with breath delivery. Finally, chest wall compliance is reduced, which helps to redistribute PEEP and tidal volume. The combination of these effects helps to improve gas exchange and decreases ventilator-associated lung injury.

A recent large trial that recruited patients with very severe lung injury ($PaO_2/FiO_2 < 150$) evaluated the effects of prone positioning for longer duration. Patients were assigned to either the supine or prone group, and patients randomized to the prone group spent 16 hours daily in the prone position. This duration is longer than had been used in previous studies, which may account for the improvement in mortality that was observed in this trial.

Choices A and D are incorrect as these settings are generally set similar to those in the supine position and would likely not need to be altered significantly after prone positioning.

6. **A.** Ultrasound is becoming a more commonly used tool in the identification of pneumothorax after procedures. Recent controlled trials have shown that ultrasound is superior to supine portable chest x-ray for the detection of pneumothorax. On chest wall evaluation, lung sliding seen on B-mode ultrasound and seashore sign (wave on the beach) on M-mode are signs that are seen with the normal opposition of parietal and visceral pleura. Thus, answer A is correct.

Lung point indicates a point where sliding of the pleura is no longer seen, which is pathognomonic of pneumothorax. As described earlier, total absence of lung sliding is also indicative of pneumothorax. Barcode sign refers to absence of sliding noted on M-mode ultrasound, which indicates a static state of the visceral and parietal pleura and also indicates a pneumothorax.

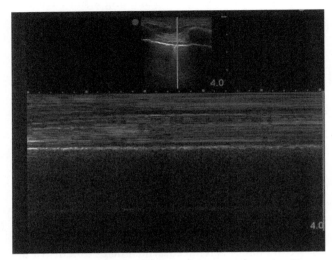

M-mode linear probe lung ultrasound shows seashore sign. Reproduced with permission from Grippi MA, Elias JA, Fishman JA, Kotloff RM, Pack AI, Senior RM, Siegel MD. *Fishman's Pulmonary Diseases and Disorders* 5e. New York, NY: McGraw-Hill, 2015.

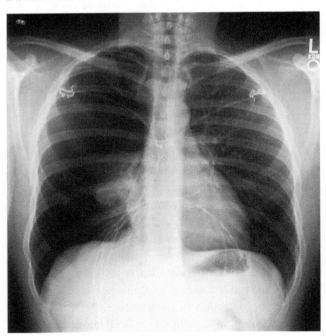

Posteroanterior view of the chest demonstrates large right pneumothorax with total collapse of the lung. There is no leftward mediastinal or tracheal shift.

7. **D.** The patient in this scenario has been diagnosed with antiglomerular basement membrane disease with concomitant diffuse pulmonary hemorrhage. Given the severity of her lung disease, she requires rapid therapy with immune-modulating medications and plasmapheresis to salvage her remaining renal function and to decrease her hemoptysis, which could quickly lead to acute respiratory failure. The combination of plasmapheresis plus cyclophosphamide and steroids works to remove circulating antibodies while decreasing production of new antibodies; thus, answer choice D is correct. Rituximab, which is an anti-CD20 monoclonal antibody, is used as second-line treatment for antiglomerular basement membrane disease and should not be used with plasmapheresis as it will be removed during this process.

8. **C.** The patient likely has acute eosinophilic pneumonia (AEP) secondary to daptomycin administration. AEP is most commonly associated with medications, other inhaled toxins, and radiation therapy. AEP should be suspected if a patient presents with febrile illness of less than 5 days in duration from inciting factor, diffuse bilateral pulmonary opacities, evidence of hypoxemia, bronchoalveolar lavage demonstrating >25% eosinophils, or eosinophilic pneumonitis. The

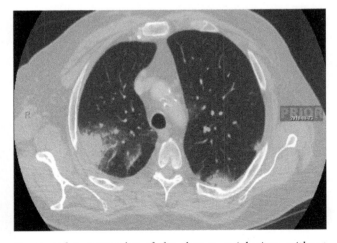

Computed tomography of the thorax, axial view, without contrast demonstrates bilateral airspace consolidations and surrounding ground-glass opacities with thickening of bronchovascular bundle. Findings are suggestive of eosinophilic pneumonia in the appropriate clinical setting.

diagnosis also requires exposure to a source known to cause AEP, exclusion of infectious causes of eosinophilic pulmonary opacities, improvement with cessation of offending agent, and recurrence with rechallenge.

Of the choices listed, daptomycin is most closely linked with AEP. Therefore, the correct answer is C. Daptomycin currently carries a warning label regarding the risk of developing AEP with administration of this medication.

9. **C.** The patient is currently having an anaphylactic reaction to omalizumab administration. She has wheezing on exam with an acute decrease in blood pressure and notable skin changes. Thus, the most appropriate course of action is IM administration of epinephrine. For adults, the dose of epinephrine is 0.3 to 0.5 mg (dilution is 1 mg/mL of 1:1000), which is usually injected into the thigh muscle. Slow infusion of epinephrine is also acceptable in 1:10,000 dilution if IV is readily available.

Other pharmacologic interventions that should also be administered include histamine-blocking agents of both H_1 and H_2 receptors and IV steroids. Although these agents do help with the symptoms of allergic reaction, they will not help in acute anaphylaxis.

10. **A.** The patient described in this scenario is a good candidate for lung volume reduction surgery. He currently meets the parameters described by the National Emphysema Treatment Trial, which state that patients should ideally be <75 years of age, have upper lobe predominant disease, and have an FEV_1 between 20% and 45% of predicted, PaO_2 >45 mm Hg on room air, and $PaCO_2$ <60 mm Hg. Patients who receive long volume reduction surgery demonstrate improvements in exercise tolerance, quality of life, and possibly survival. He is not a candidate for lung transplantation as he does not have evidence of cor pulmonale or pulmonary hypertension, and his FEV_1 is not <20% of predicted. Combined heart and lung transplant is also not a viable option as he exceeds the recommended age of 55. He also does not meet the criteria of left ventricular dysfunction with irreversible right-sided dysfunction. The chest radiographs below show features of hyperinflation and emphysematous changes of COPD.

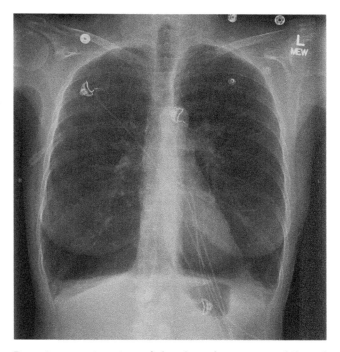

Posterior anterior view of the chest demonstrates bilateral increased lung lucency and hyperinflation with good penetration consistent with emphysematous changes related to COPD. Bibasilar lung scarring is seen. Cardiac silhouette and pulmonary arteries appear unremarkable.

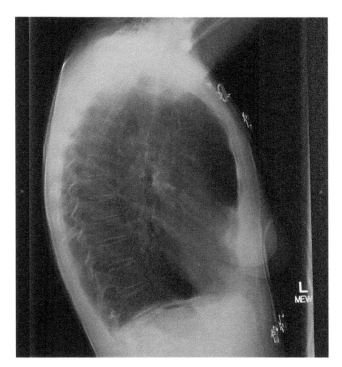

Lateral view of the chest demonstrates increased anteroposterior diameter and flattening of the diaphragm consistent with emphysema.

11. **C.** The patient currently has severe ARDS and is decompensating with mechanical ventilation alone, and thus, venovenous extracorporeal membrane oxygenation (ECMO) is being considered. This patient will require a double lumen catheter to be placed into the great veins, after which blood will be pumped through an oxygenator and back into the venous system. By this system, the patient's carbon dioxide will achieve adequate clearance, but because a significant portion of the cardiac output does not flow through the oxygenator, the patient will still require supplemental oxygen and PEEP.

In this patient, ECMO will allow the mechanical ventilation settings to be reduced to safer levels despite not being able to completely oxygenate the patient. Therefore, increase in tidal volumes is not necessary as ECMO will clear the patient's carbon dioxide. In addition, as noted earlier, since the patient's blood will only be partially oxygenated, supplemental oxygen and PEEP will still be required, eliminating choice A, but they can be decreased to safer levels, eliminating choice D.

12. **D.** The patient should be treated with norepinephrine as the first-line vasoconstrictor after adequate volume resuscitation. The target MAP should be between 65 and 70 mm Hg. Studies comparing dopamine and norepinephrine have shown a higher mortality with the use of dopamine in all forms of shock. Dopamine was also shown to have a higher rate or arrhythmia. Epinephrine and vasopressin are also incorrect because they are not used as first-line vasoconstrictors.

MAP targets of 65 to 70 mm Hg have been compared to higher MAP goals, and there was no mortality benefit found. Patients who had MAPs of 80 to 85 mm Hg had a higher incidence of atrial fibrillation and other arrhythmias while requiring longer duration of vasopressors.

13. **D.** This patient has history of myasthenia gravis and infection with *Pseudomonas* requiring prompt initiation of 2 antipseudomonal antibiotics until sensitivities are known. In this case, the most appropriate combination is meropenem and ceftazidime, as this combination is less likely to worsen her myasthenia gravis. Many medications are known to increase muscular weakness including many antibiotics. Aminoglycosides are one such category, with the known adverse effect of blockade of the neuromuscular junction. Other antibiotics that should be avoided in patients with myasthenia gravis include fluoroquinolones, macrolides, and tetracyclines.

14. **C.** This patient likely has abdominal compartment syndrome secondary to large-volume ascites. Abdominal compartment syndrome is defined as intra-abdominal pressures >20 cm H_2O associated with new organ dysfunction. The patient described in this scenario has evidence of increased abdominal pressure with firm tense abdomen, decrease in bowel sounds, increased airway pressures, and significantly elevated bladder pressure. The effect on the pulmonary system results in an increase in both peak and plateau pressures, as seen in this case. The increase in abdominal pressure leads to a decrease in chest wall compliance and decreased movement of the diaphragm.

Pneumothorax could also lead to changes in pressures; however, unchanged chest x-ray and bedside ultrasound point to a different cause. The other choices would lead to elevation in peak pressures and not an increase in plateau pressures.

15. **A.** Of the choices listed, choice A is the most likely to explain the arrhythmia the patient developed. The patient had developed torsade de pointes arrhythmia, which is a wide complex ventricular arrhythmia that has been associated with increased QT duration and the occurrence of Q on T, where a new contraction in the ventricles ensues before full repolarization has occurred, triggering this arrhythmia to propagate.

Of the choices listed, macrolide antibiotics have been associated with QT prolongations, and other antibiotics such as fluoroquinolone and sulfamethoxazole-trimethoprim have also been implicated. Choice A also includes haloperidol, which is a drug known for its QT prolonging effect. Methadone, a long-acting narcotic, has also been implicated in QT prolongation. Choice B does not include a medication that has been strongly associated with QT prolongation, as vancomycin, propofol, and fentanyl are not strongly associated with QT prolongation. The same applies to choices C and D, although hypokalemia can worsen QT prolongation along with hypomagnesemia and hypercalcemia, but choice A includes more medications that can induce QT prolongation, making it the likely choice for this patient's arrhythmia.

16. **B.** The patient is suffering from cyanide poisoning. Cyanide poisoning is not uncommon in survivors of fires, especially if large amounts of plastics or rubber are burned in the fire. The major clues are the history and the elevated lactate and mixed venous saturation associated with appropriate oxygenation as measured by the PaO_2 on the arterial blood gas. Cyanide rapidly binds to mitochondrial cytochrome oxidase, blocking oxidative phosphorylation and the production of adenosine triphosphate (ATP). Cells then switch to anaerobic metabolism, resulting in the production of lactic acid. Despite adequate levels of oxygen, cells are unable to use oxygen in the production of ATP. Signs and symptoms of cyanide poisoning include altered mental status, tachypnea, tachycardia, flushing, seizures, hypotension, and lactic acidosis. Patients typically have adequate PaO_2 levels, and thus, cyanosis is not seen with cyanide poisoning. Antidotes are available for cyanide poisoning and include sodium nitrite, amyl nitrate, sodium thiosulfate, and hydroxocobalamin. Sodium nitrite and amyl nitrate work by causing the oxidation of iron in hemoglobin, producing methemoglobinemia. Cyanide then binds to methemoglobin instead of mitochondrial cytochrome oxidase. Sodium thiosulfate works as an antidote to cyanide poisoning by donating sulfur groups to the enzyme rhodanese, which in turn transforms cyanide into thiocyanide. Thiocyanide is less toxic than cyanide and is excreted in the urine, so patients with abnormal renal function may require hemodialysis after receiving sodium thiosulfate to assist in its removal. Hydroxocobalamin binds intracellular cyanide with a much higher affinity than cyanide binds with mitochondrial cytochrome oxidase. This results in the formation of cyanocobalamin, which is nontoxic and excreted in the urine. It is probably best to treat patients with cyanide poisoning with more than 1 antidote. Studies suggest that using sodium thiosulfate and hydroxocobalamin concurrently is the most effective and safest therapy for cyanide poisoning.

17. **C.** The use of systemic glucocorticoids in the management of inhalation injuries is of no value and is considered contraindicated because they have not been shown to lessen the degree of airway edema and lung inflammation and may increase the risk of developing superimposed pneumonia. Treatment of inhalation injuries is mostly supportive. Supplemental oxygen should be administered. Inhaled β-agonists may be helpful in reversing some bronchoconstriction and may aid in pulmonary toilet by increasing mucociliary clearance and inducing a more productive cough. Patients with chlorine gas exposure may benefit from treatment with inhaled budesonide. Nebulized solutions of 3.75% or 4.2% sodium bicarbonate have also been proposed in the treatment of chlorine gas exposure. Further studies are warranted to evaluate their effectiveness. Although the benefits of inhaled budesonide and sodium bicarbonate may not be firmly established, there are very few, if any, contraindications.

18. **D.** This is an uncommon complication of a pneumonectomy, occurring in about 1% of cases, and is due to direct injury of the thoracic duct at the time of surgery. The key to making the diagnosis is identifying the rapid filling of the postpneumonectomy space as seen on chest x-ray, coupled with the hypotension and tachycardia due to intravascular volume loss. Immediately following pneumonectomy, air fills the space. Within 24 hours, the ipsilateral hemidiaphragm becomes slightly elevated, the mediastinum shifts slightly toward the postpneumonectomy space, and fluid starts accumulating in the postpneumonectomy space. Generally, fluid accumulates at a rate of approximately 2 rib spaces per day. After 2 weeks, 80% to 90% of the space is filled with fluid. Complete opacification of the hemithorax after pneumonectomy takes an average of approximately 4 months, with a range from 3 weeks to 7 months. Rapid filling of the postpneumonectomy space suggests either hemorrhage or the leaking of chyle into the space. Since the patient's Hgb had been stable, hemorrhage into the space is very unlikely. A postpneumonectomy space empyema certainly can present with sepsis, but it will not be associated with complete filling of the postpneumonectomy space by postoperative day 3. A pulmonary embolism is not an uncommon complication of any major surgery such as a pneumonectomy and may explain the initial atrial fibrillation, sinus tachycardia, and hypotension, but would not explain the chest radiograph findings.

19. **A.** The patient is biting down on the endotracheal tube, resulting in the sudden rise in the peak airway pressures with little change in the plateau

airway pressures. Peak airway pressures are, in part, dependent on the resistance of the airways, the chest wall, and the lungs, with plateau airway pressures, in part, dependent of the resistance of the chest wall and lungs. The obvious difference between the peak and plateau airway pressures is the pressure needed to overcome the resistance of the airways, including the endotracheal tube. This difference is typically 5 to 8 mm H_2O. Although an air leak in the ventilator tubing will most likely result in a decrease in peak and plateau airway pressures, the other 3 choices will all result in a significant increase in the peak airway pressure. However, choices C and D will also result in a similar rise in the plateau airway pressures.

REFERENCES

Acute Respiratory Distress Syndrome Network, Brower RG, Matthay MA, et al. Ventilation with lower tidal volumes as compared with traditional tidal volumes for acute lung injury and the acute respiratory distress syndrome. *N Engl J Med*. 2000;342:1301-1308.

Allen J. Acute eosinophilia pneumonia. *Semin Respir Crit Care Med*. 2006;27(2):142-147.

An G, West MA. Abdominal compartment syndrome: a concise clinical review. *Crit Care Med*. 2008;36(4):1304-1310.

Asfar P, Mexiani F, Hamel JF, et al; SEPSISPAM Investigators. High versus low blood-pressure target in patients with septic shock. *N Engl J Med*. 2014;370(17):1583-1593.

Aziz F, Penupolu X, Xu X, He J. Lung transplant in end-staged chronic obstructive pulmonary disease (COPD) patients: a concise review. *J Thorac Dis*. 2010;2(2):111-116.

Bahrainwala AH, Simon MR. Wheezing and vocal cord dysfunction mimicking asthma. *Curr Opin Pulm Med*. 2001;7(1):8-13.

Balkissoon R, Kenin K. Asthma: vocal cord dysfunction (VCD) and other dysfunctional breathing disorders. *Semin Respir Crit Care Med*. 2012;33(6):595-605.

Barillari A, Fioretti M. Lung ultrasound: a new tool for the emergency physician. *Intern Emerg Med*. 2010;5(4):335-340.

Baud FJ, Barriot P, Toffis V, et al. Elevated blood cyanide concentrations in victims of smoke inhalation. *N Engl J Med*. 1991;325:1761-1766.

Benoit SR, Mendelsohn AB, Nourjah P, et al. Risk factors for prolonged QTc among US adults: Third National Health and Nutrition Examination Survey. *Eur J Cardiovasc Prev Rehabil*. 2005;12(4):363-368.

Borron SW, Baud FJ, Barriot P, et al. Prospective study of hydroxocobalamin for acute cyanide poisoning in smoke inhalation. *Ann Emerg Med*. 2007;49:794-801.

Combes A, Bacchetta M, Brodie D, Muller T, Pellegrino V. Extracorporeal membrane oxygenation for respiratory failure in adults. *Curr Opin Crit Care*. 2012;18(1):99-104.

Cui Z, Zhao J, Jia XY, et al. Anti-glomerular basement membrane disease: outcomes of different therapeutic regimens in a large single-center Chinese cohort study. *Medicine (Baltimore)*. 2011;90(5):303-311.

De Backer D, Biston P, Devriendt J, et al. Comparison of dopamine and norepinephrine in the treatment of sock. *N Engl J Med*. 2010;362(9):779-789.

Dhand UK. Clinical approach to the weak patient in the intensive care unit. *Respir Care*. 2006;51(9):1024-1040.

Dodda VR, Spiro P. Can albuterol be blamed for lactic acidosis? *Respir Care*. 2012;57(12):2115-2118.

Drew BJ, Ackerman MJ, Funk M, et al. Prevention of torsade de pointes in hospital settings: a scientific statement from the American Heart Association and the American College of Cardiology Foundation. *J Am Coll Cardiol*. 2010;55(9):934-947.

Dreyfuss D, Savmon G. Ventilator induced lung injury: lessons from experimental studies. *Am J Resp Crit Care Med*. 1998;157:294-323.

Ferguson ND, Cook DJ, Guyatt GH, et al. High-frequency oscillation in early acute respiratory distress syndrome. *N Engl J Med*. 2013;368(9):795.

Gattinoni L, Carlesso E, Langer T. Clinical review: extracorporeal membrane oxygenation. *Crit Care*. 2011;15(6):243-253.

Grasso S, Stripoli T, De Michele M, et al. ARDSnet ventilator protocol and alveolar hyperinflation: role of positive end-expiratory pressure. *Am J Resp Crit Care Med*. 2007;176:761-767.

Guerin C, Reignier J, Richard JC, et al. Prone positioning in severe acute respiratory distress syndrome. *N Engl J Med*. 2013;368(23):2159-2168.

Hedenstierna G, Larsson A. Influence of abdominal pressure on respiratory and abdominal organ function. *Curr Opin Crit Care*. 2012;18(1):80-85.

Idrees M, Fitzgerald JM. Vocal cord dysfunction in bronchial asthma. A review article. *J Asthma*. 2014;20:1-9.

Jani-Acsadi A, Lisak RP. Myasthenic crisis: guidelines for prevention and treatment. *J Neurol Sci*. 207;261(1-2):127-133.

Johnson JP, Moore J Jr, Austin HA 3rd, Balow JE, Antonovych TT, Wilson CB. Therapy of anti-glomerular basement membrane antibody disease: analysis of prognostic significance of clinical, pathologic and treatment factors. *Medicine (Baltimore)*. 1985;64(4):219-227.

Kopec SE, Irwin RS, Umali-Torres CB, et al. The postpneumonectomy state. *Chest*. 1998;114:1158-1184.

Lafci G, Budak AB, Yener AU, Cicek OF. Use of extracorporeal membrane oxygenation in adults. *Heart Lung Circ*. 2014;23(1):10-23.

Levine BA, Petroff PA, Slade CL, et al. Prospective trials of dexamethasone and aerosolized gentamicin in the treatment of inhalational injury in the burned patient. *J Trauma*. 1978;18:188-193.

Lewis L, Ferguson I, House SL, et al. Albuterol administration is commonly associated with increases in serum lactate in patients with asthma treated for acute exacerbation of asthma. *Chest*. 2014;145(1):53-59.

Lieberman P, Nicklas RA, Oppenheimer J, et al. The diagnosis and management of anaphylaxis practice parameter: 2010 update. *J Allergy Clin Immunol*. 2010;126(3):477-480.

Mallow-Corbett S, Herlihy A, Sessler CN. Drug-induced acute respiratory failure. In: Papadopoulos J, Cooper B,

Kane-Gill S, Mallow-Corbett S, Barletta J, eds. *Drug-Induced Complications in the Critically Ill Patient: A Guide for Recognition and Treatment.* Mount Prospect, IL: Lippincott; 2012:87-105.

Mayo PH, Doelken P. Pleural ultrasonography. *Clin Chest Med.* 2006;27(2):215-227.

Miller BA, Gray A, Leblanc TW, Sexton DJ, Martin AR, Slama TG. Acute eosinophilic pneumonia secondary to daptomycin: a report of three cases. *Clin Infect Dis.* 2010;50(11):e63-e68.

Moon RE, Camporesi EM. Respiratory monitoring. In: Miller RD, ed. *Anesthesia.* 4th ed. New York, NY: Churchill Livingstone; 1994:1253-1292.

National Emphysema Treatment Trial Research Group. Patients at high risk of death after lung-volume-reduction surgery. *N Engl J Med.* 2001;345(15):1075-1083.

National Institutes of Health. ARDS Network Ventilation and lower tidal volumes as compared with traditional tidal volumes for acute lung injury and the acute respiratory distress syndrome. *N Engl J Med.* 2000;342:1301-1308.

Orens JB, Estenne M, Arcasoy S, et al. International guidelines for the selection of lung transplant candidates: 2006 update: a consensus report from the Pulmonary Scientific Council of the International Society for Heart and Lung Transplantation. *J Heart Lung Transplant.* 2006;25(7):745-755.

Pedcenko V, Bondar O, Fogo AB, et al. Molecular architecture of the Goodpasture autoantigen in anti-GBM nephritis. *N Engl J Med.* 2010;363(4):343-354.

Roden DM. Drug-induced prolongation of the QT interval. *N Engl J Med.* 2004;350:1013-1022.

Russell JA, Walley KR, Singer J, et al. Vasopressin vs norepinephrine infusion in patients with septic shock. *N Engl J Med.* 2008;358(9):877-887.

Schmidt M, Tachon G, Devilliers C, et al. Blood oxygenation and decarboxylation determinants during veno-venous ECMO for respiratory failure in adults. *Int Care Med.* 2013;39:838-846.

Simons KJ, Simons FE. Epinephrine and its use in anaphylaxis: current issues. *Curr Opin Allergy Clin Immunol.* 2010;10(4):354-361.

Sud S, Friedrich JO, Adhikari NK, et al. Effect of prone positioning during mechanical ventilation on mortality among patients with acute respiratory distress syndrome: a systemic review and meta-analysis. *CMAJ.* 2014;186(10):E381-E390.

Talmor D, Sarge T, Malhotra A, et al. Mechanical ventilation guided by esophageal pressure in acute lung injury. *N Engl J Med.* 2008;359(20):2095.

US Army Institute of Surgical Research. Joint theater trauma system clinical practice guideline, Inhalational injury and toxic industrial chemical exposure. 2008. http://www.usaisr.amedd.army.mil/cpgs/Inhalation_Injury_and_Toxic_Industrial_Chemicals_7_Jun_%2012.pdf. Accessed June 24, 2017.

Volpicelli G. Sonographic diagnosis of pneumothorax. *Intensive Care Med.* 2011;37(2):224-232.

Wilkerson RG, Stone MB. Sensitivity of bedside ultrasound and supine anteroposterior chest radiographs for the identification of pneumothorax after blunt trauma. *Acad Emerg Med.* 2010;17(1):11-17.

Wang J, Zhang L, Walther SM. Administration of aerosolized terbutaline and budesonide reduces chlorine gas-induced acute lung injury. *J Trauma* 2004;56:850-862.

22

Gastroenterology and Liver Diseases

Manhal Izzy, MD, Christopher Velez, MD, Yasir Azzawi, MD, and Lawrence J. Brandt, MD, MACG, AGA-F, FASGE

Questions

1. A 71-year-old man presented to the emergency department (ED) for productive cough, dyspnea, and subjective fevers. He has mild intermittent asthma for which he takes albuterol as needed. Vital signs showed a fever of 101°F, respiratory rate of 38 breaths/min, heart rate of 112 bpm, and blood pressure of 86/45 mm Hg. Chest x-ray showed right lower lobe infiltrates. A diagnosis of septic shock secondary to severe pneumonia was made, and the patient was subsequently intubated and admitted to the intensive care unit (ICU). His hemodynamic status had initially improved, but on the third day of admission, while still in the ICU, the patient started passing melena and his hemoglobin (Hgb) dropped to 8 mg/dL from 11 mg/dL at the time of admission. His blood urea nitrogen (BUN) was 36 mg/dL, with a serum creatinine of 0.7 mg/dL. Esophagogastroduodenoscopy (EGD) was done and showed multiple superficial gastric ulcers (shown below). What is the likely underlying etiology for the ulcers?

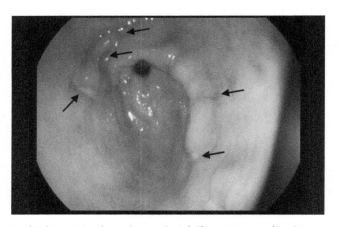

Multiple gastric ulcers (*arrows*) at different stages of healing.

A. Nonsteroidal anti-inflammatory drugs (NSAIDs)

B. *Helicobacter pylori* gastritis

C. Stress ulcer

D. Malignancy

E. Cytomegalovirus

2. A 67-year-old man presented to the ED after 1 episode of syncope and 24 hours of passing "dark" stool. He takes over-the-counter ibuprofen for knee pain. On admission, his vital signs were remarkable for a blood pressure of 89/51 mm Hg and heart rate of 110 bpm, and he was found to have maroon-colored stool. Hgb level was 7.6 g/dL compared with 13.6 g/dL on a visit to his primary care doctor 6 weeks previously. BUN was 31 mg/dL, with a creatinine of 0.95 mg/dL. Platelet count was $310 \times 10^3/\mu L$, and international normalized ratio (INR) was 0.9. Blood pressure normalized after a 1-L bolus of normal saline. An 80-mg bolus of intravenous (IV) pantoprazole was given, followed by infusion of 8 mg/h, and a dose of IV erythromycin 250 mg was also started. EGD was performed and showed a 1.5-cm duodenal ulcer with an oozing visible vessel (shown below) that was successfully treated with epinephrine injection and heater probe. What is the most appropriate next step in management?

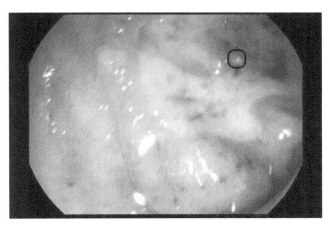

Duodenal ulcer with an oozing visible vessel (*circle*).

    A. Maintain pantoprazole for 48 hours

    B. Start solid diet

    C. Switch to daily oral pantoprazole

    D. Discharge home

    E. Start clear liquid diet

3. A 43-year-old previously healthy man presented to the ED with epigastric pain and dark-colored stool for 2 days. He was not on any medication. His vital signs on admission were heart rate of 79 bpm, blood pressure of 122/73 mm Hg, respiratory rate of 17 breaths/min, and normal temperature. On exam, he was found to have melenic stool. His Hgb was 8.9 g/dL, and his BUN was 26 mg/dL, with creatinine of 1 mg/dL. IV proton pump inhibitor (PPI) was started, and EGD was performed, showing 1-cm duodenal bulb ulcer with a flat pigmented spot (shown below). Gastric biopsy to rule out *H pylori* was obtained. What is the best course of management of this patient?

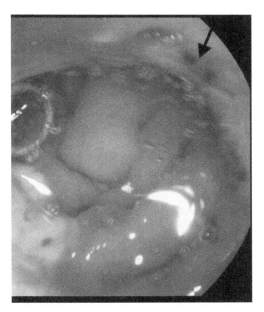

Duodenal ulcer with a flat pigmented spot (*arrow*).

    A. Continue IV PPI

    B. Switch to daily oral PPI

    C. Discharge home

    D. Admit to ICU

    E. Add a histamine 2 (H_2)-receptor antagonist

4. A 54-year-old man presented to the ED after 4 episodes of hematemesis at home, the last of which was 6 hours prior to presentation. His medical history is remarkable for obesity and hypertension. Home medications are aspirin, valsartan, and multivitamin. He has no history of liver disease or prior upper gastrointestinal (UGI) bleeding. His vital signs on arrival were blood pressure of 116/73 mm Hg, heart rate of 89 bpm, respiratory rate of 16 breaths/min, and normal temperature. Physical examination revealed mild epigastric tenderness and tarry stool. Laboratory testing showed Hgb of 7.2 g/dL, platelet of $300 \times 10^3/\mu L$, INR of 1.0, BUN of 40 mg/dL, and creatinine of 1.1 mg/dL. During his last admission for asthma exacerbation 3 months ago, his laboratory testing showed an Hgb of 13 g/dL, creatinine of 0.9 mg/dL, and BUN of 12 mg/dL. IV pantoprazole was started. What is the best next step in management?

A. Perform upper endoscopy

B. Perform transfusion of packed red blood cells

C. Insert nasogastric tube for a gastric lavage

D. Send urine electrolytes

E. Discharge home and follow up as outpatient since the patient is stable

5. An 81-year-old man presented to the hospital with 2 days of worsening abdominal pain that was mostly right-sided. No rectal bleeding or other gastrointestinal (GI) symptoms were reported. His medical history is remarkable for coronary artery disease, diabetes mellitus, hypertension, and hyperlipidemia. His medications included nifedipine, aspirin, sitagliptin, and atorvastatin. Vital signs were normal except for tachycardia of 106 bpm. Physical examination was notable for right quadrant abdominal tenderness without rebound. Blood testing revealed the following: Hgb 18 mg/dL, BUN 18 mg/dL, lactate dehydrogenase 25 U/L, sodium 137 mEq/l, and white blood cell (WBC) count $17 \times 10^3/\mu L$. Abdominal computed tomography (CT) showed thickening of the right colon suspicious for ischemic colitis. No radiologic abnormalities were seen in other areas of the colon. Which of the following is the best next step in the patient's management?

A. Abdominal ultrasound with duplex study

B. Colonoscopy

C. CT angiography (CTA)

D. Observation

E. Surgery consultation

6. A 79-year-old woman was sent from a nursing home for 3 days of diarrhea, which was described as 8 loose nonbloody bowel movements a day. She was recently in the hospital for treatment of pneumonia and was discharged 3 weeks previously. Vital signs on arrival were temperature of 101°F, blood pressure of 90/50 mm Hg, heart rate of 98 bpm, and respiratory rate of 22 breaths/min. Physical examination revealed abdominal tenderness with present bowel sounds and without distension. There was no change in mental status from baseline. Laboratory testing was remarkable for positive *Clostridium difficile* stool testing, albumin 2.5 g/dL, WBC $17 \times 10^3/\mu L$, lactate 2.9 mmol/L, and creatinine 1.9 mg/dL. These tests were normal upon discharge 3 weeks ago. The patient's blood pressure normalized after a bolus of normal saline. What is the best next step in management?

A. Oral metronidazole

B. Oral vancomycin

C. Vancomycin enemas

D. Oral vancomycin with IV metronidazole

E. Fecal microbiota transplantation

7. A 52-year-old man is brought to the hospital with epigastric pain that began 12 hours previously. He described it as sharp, radiating to the back, and associated with nausea and nonbloody vomiting. His medical history is notable for type 2 diabetes mellitus for which he is on sitagliptin. The patient denies drinking alcohol or having similar illness in the past. Vital signs were normal. Abdominal examination showed epigastric tenderness without rebound tenderness. Bowel sounds were present.

Hgb	13.2 mg/dL
BUN	30 mg/dL
Lipase	1289 U/L
Alkaline phosphatase	85 IU/L
Aspartate aminotransferase (AST)	16 U/L
Alanine aminotransferase (ALT)	20 U/L
Bilirubin	0.9 mg/dL
Triglyceride	99 mg/dL

Chest x-ray and right upper quadrant ultrasound were unremarkable. His laboratory testing is shown below. What is the best next step in management?

A. Albumin infusion

B. Magnetic resonance cholangiopancreatography (MRCP)

C. Upper endoscopy

D. Lactated Ringer's infusion

E. CT of the abdomen

8. A 48-year-old man presents to the ED with hematemesis. He vomited bright red blood 12 hours previously and initially had delayed coming to the hospital until his wife insisted. He has had no prior episodes of bleeding. He complains of mild epigastric discomfort. He currently does not feel nauseated, and he has not vomited for 12 hours. He has a past medical history significant for chronic hepatitis C infection for which he has declined treatment. He does not take NSAIDs.

His initial triage vital signs are remarkable for a heart rate of 110 bpm, a blood pressure of 80/50 mm Hg, and a respiratory rate of 20 breaths/min. On physical examination, pallor is noted as well as dried blood around his mouth. He has abdominal distention with dullness to percussion over the flanks and with central tympany. There is shifting dullness but no abdominal tenderness. There is bilateral pitting lower extremity edema. Digital rectal exam shows brown stool.

Initial laboratory studies are pending. However, annual laboratory testing performed 6 months ago showed the following:

Hemoglobin 10 g/dL

WBC 4000/μL

Platelets 135,000/μL

Sodium 130 mEq/L

BUN 34 mg/dL

Creatinine 1.1 mg/dL

ALT 36 IU/L

AST 34 IU/L

Total bilirubin 2.1 mg/dL

Alkaline phosphatase 130 IU/L

INR 1.4

Fluid resuscitation was just initiated. What is the next appropriate step in management?

A. Initiate massive transfusion protocol

B. Emergent upper endoscopy

C. Administer prothrombin complex concentrate (PCC)

D. Administer parenteral somatostatin analogue (such as octreotide)

E. Administer fresh frozen plasma to address coagulopathy

9. A 52-year-old West African woman is admitted to the hospital for her next cycle of chemotherapy. She has a past medical history significant for Burkitt lymphoma and chronic hepatitis B complicated by cirrhosis. Her medical history is also notable for large esophageal varices, for which she has been prescribed nadolol for primary prophylaxis of esophageal variceal bleeding. During her admission, she has developed pancytopenia and has received multiple transfusions of blood products to address profound anemia and thrombocytopenia.

You are called overnight because the patient complains of epigastric discomfort and weakness. Suddenly, she begins to have large-volume hematemesis (estimated to be approximately 500 mL) and becomes hemodynamically unstable, with a heart rate of 90 bpm and a nadir blood pressure of 60/40 mm Hg. She is becoming increasingly diaphoretic, has conjunctival pallor, and is having fluctuating mental status. She continues to vomit bright red blood.

In addition to ensuring appropriate IV access, starting volume resuscitation, and intubating the patient, which of the following interventions is the most appropriate at this time?

A. Order replacement blood products

B. Emergently place a transjugular intrahepatic portosystemic shunt (TIPS)

C. Insert a Minnesota tube for balloon tamponade effect

D. Begin octreotide infusion

E. Begin vasopressors and titrate to a target mean arterial pressure (MAP) of at least 65 mm Hg

10. You are asked to evaluate a 25-year-old man in the ED who was sent in by his primary care doctor for excruciating abdominal pain. He presented for a walk-in appointment having been brought in by his wife for abdominal pain that began the night previously, but worsened this morning. The pain was so severe that the patient had difficulty focusing during the medical interview. He attributes his symptoms to something he ate the night prior when celebrating a work colleague's birthday. He has had no bowel movement since the prior day and has no nausea or vomiting. There is a history of type 1 diabetes mellitus and a history of appendectomy as a child. He drinks alcohol occasionally, does not smoke, and denies illicit substance use. When his wife is excused for the physical exam, he admits to occasional cocaine usage when out with friends. His physical exam is notable for a heart rate of 95 bpm, a blood pressure of 160/100 mm Hg, and a temperature of 100.2°F. He grimaces during palpation of the abdomen, which appears to be somewhat distended. He requests to be discharged with antibiotics just in case he has food poisoning and some oxycodone so he can return to work for an important client meeting. Which of the following should be recommended to the ED staff?

A. Do not administer antibiotics.

B. Order CTA of the abdomen and pelvis and discuss case with the surgical service.

C. Discharge the patient with narcotic analgesia and instructions to return if he does not improve within 48 hours.

D. Perform an abdominal plain film to evaluate for bowel obstruction.

E. Perform an electrocardiogram (ECG) to rule out acute coronary syndrome.

11. An 82-year-old woman is admitted to a monitored setting for a new diagnosis of atrial fibrillation, and you are reviewing her history prior to discharge home tomorrow. In terms of her hospital course, she was started on parenteral heparin, and long-term anticoagulation with warfarin was planned due to intracardiac thrombus. Her atrial fibrillation has been adequately rate controlled with metoprolol. She has additional medical history consisting of chronic kidney disease and an abdominal abscess, for which she has had abdominal surgery, although she does not recall which type. She no longer

undergoes cancer screening given her age, but believes that her most recent colonoscopy 7 years ago was normal. She has no allergies, and she took only amlodipine at home prior to her admission. Overnight, you are called for profuse hematochezia. She has never suffered from such bleeding before. When you see her, she is diaphoretic, tachycardic (120 bpm), and hypotensive at 90/50 mm Hg. There is a large vertical scar over the patient's abdomen; palpation elicits no complaint of pain. There is no stool being evacuated, and in her diaper, you only see fresh bright red blood. Hemoglobin level is 10 g/dL, down from a baseline value of 13 g/dL. The remainder of the laboratory results are normal. What is the most likely diagnosis for this patient?

A. Diverticular bleeding complicated by hemorrhagic shock

B. Ischemic colitis

C. Bleeding from angioectasia

D. Hemorrhage from previously asymptomatic colon cancer

E. Hemorrhoidal bleeding

12. A 45-year-old obese woman is transferred to the ICU after developing healthcare-associated pneumonia complicated by respiratory distress during a prolonged hospitalization for repair of an incarcerated inguinal hernia. Currently, the patient is being treated with piperacillin-tazobactam as well as prophylactic pantoprazole and subcutaneous heparin, in addition to propofol for sedation. The patient has a history of type 2 diabetes mellitus, hypertension, and nonalcoholic fatty liver disease. Her home medications include metformin and lisinopril.

Her respiratory status improves with treatment, but when sedation is lightened to prepare for extubation, she begins grimacing. Palpation of the right upper abdominal quadrant causes her the most distress. Laboratory studies show the following:

WBC 9000/μL

ALT 38 IU/L

AST 60 IU/L

Total bilirubin 1.6 mg/dL

Direct bilirubin 0.7 mg/dL

Alkaline phosphatase 140 IU/L

Amylase 130 U/L

Lipase 120 IU

INR 1.1

Ultrasound of the abdomen shows a thickened gallbladder wall as well as a borderline elevated common bile duct diameter at 7 mm. There do not appear to be any calculi. However, the radiologist reading the study cautions that it was limited by the patient's body habitus. What is the next appropriate diagnostic step?

A. MRCP to assess for choledocholithiasis

B. Endoscopic retrograde cholangiopancreatography

C. CT to evaluate for other intra-abdominal processes

D. Switch piperacillin-tazobactam to another antibiotic

E. Cholecystostomy tube or cholecystectomy if patient's condition worsens

13. An 80-year-old man is admitted to the ICU with urinary tract infection complicated by septic shock and altered mental status. He has a prior history of benign prostate hypertrophy. The patient has a chronic indwelling catheter and has been admitted several times for suspected infection. Prior bacterial culture sensitivities suggested resistance to most routinely used parenteral antibiotics including piperacillin-tazobactam. He remains tachycardic and hypotensive despite aggressive crystalloid administration. Based on previous sensitivities, meropenem is selected, with some initial clinical improvement. His initial leukocytosis improves, as do his mental status and hemodynamics.

After 24 hours of receiving meropenem, the patient begins to decompensate again. He complains of feeling weak, light headed, and clammy, and has continued suprapubic pain. In addition to worsening leukocytosis, he has the following pattern of liver tests:

ALT 100 IU/L

AST 130 IU/L

Total bilirubin 4.1 mg/dL

Direct bilirubin 2.6 mg/dL

Alkaline phosphatase 220 IU/L

Urine culture shows >100,000 colony-forming units of *Enterobacter cloacae*. Antibiotic sensitivities are pending. Abdominal ultrasound (AUS) is unremarkable. INR is normal. What is the most likely diagnosis for the patient's abnormal liver tests?

A. Ischemic hepatopathy

B. Ascending cholangitis

C. Acute cholecystitis

D. Cholestasis of sepsis

E. Acetaminophen overdose

14. A 40-year-old man is admitted to the neurosurgical ICU due to traumatic brain injury sustained after falling in the setting of a tonic-clonic seizure while out with friends. The patient had been recently diagnosed with a seizure disorder and had been started on phenytoin 6 weeks previously. He reports only occasional alcohol drinking. Head imaging shows epidural hemorrhage, and he subsequently undergoes craniotomy. His postoperative course is unremarkable, but he remains intubated. He is continued on phenytoin. His laboratory studies are as follows:

ALT 420 IU/L

AST 200 IU/L

Total bilirubin 1.4 mg/dL

Direct bilirubin 1.0 mg/dL

Alkaline phosphatase 190 IU/L

INR 1.0

WBC 12,100/μL

The patient remains intubated, with normal vital signs except for mild fever of 100.6°F. Abdominal ultrasound is unremarkable. Review of liver tests and viral hepatitis profile from 2 months ago reveals normal results. What is the next appropriate step in management?

A. Administer systemic glucocorticoids

B. Withdraw phenytoin and switch to levetiracetam

C. Perform liver biopsy

D. Continue to monitor liver tests

E. Start pentoxifylline

15. A 49-year-old man was admitted to the hospital with altered mental status after his wife found him to be lethargic. The wife stated that the patient had not seen his doctor for almost 2 months. The patient's medical history is remarkable for cirrhosis secondary to nonalcoholic steatohepatitis. His vital signs in the ED showed a temperature of 99.1°F, blood pressure of 110/75 mm Hg, heart rate of 65 bpm, and respiratory rate of 14 breaths/min. On physical exam, the patient was confused and jaundiced and had asterixis. Abdominal exam showed mild ascites but no tenderness. CT scan of the head did not show any signs of acute ischemia or injury. Drug screen was negative. Labs were as follows:

Hgb	14 g/L
WBC	$8 \times 10^3/\mu L$
Platelet	$121 \times 10^3/\mu L$
Hematocrit (Hct)	39%
Bands	8 %

Sodium (Na)	130 mEq/L
Potassium (K)	3.6 mEq/L
Chloride (Cl⁻)	100 mEq/L
Creatinine (Cr)	1.8 mg/dL
BUN	32 mg/dL
Bicarbonate	20 mEq/L
Glucose	180 mg/dL

ALT	39 IU/L
AST	40 IU/L
Total bilirubin	4.2 mg/dL
Alkaline phosphatase	158 IU/L
Albumin	3.0 g/dL
Ammonia	200 μg/dL

What medication should be started as the next step in the management?

A. Lactulose

B. Vancomycin

C. Rifaximin

D. Probiotics

E. Cefazolin

16. A 29-year-old woman presented to the ED with nausea and vomiting of 1 day in duration. She stated that she took around 30 tablets of pain medicine for her backache but could not remember the name of the drug. Her initial vital signs showed a temperature of 99.2°F, blood pressure of 108/68 mm Hg, pulse rate of 92 bpm, and respiratory rate of 24 breaths/min. The physical exam was remarkable for right upper quadrant (RUQ) tenderness and mild icterus. She had asterixis but was oriented to time and place. Serologic studies showed a sodium of 136 mEq/L, creatinine of 3.5 mg/dL, chloride of 100 mmol/L, BUN of 30 mg/dL, potassium of 4.0 mEq/L, and bicarbonate of 12 mmol/L. Liver tests showed an ALT of 5250 IU/L, AST of 5600 IU/L, total bilirubin of 2.2 mg/dL, and alkaline phosphatase of 158 IU/L. Her serum alcohol level was elevated, and her serum acetaminophen level was 31 mg/dL. INR was 3.0, and an arterial pH was 7.25. After admitting the patient to the ICU, what is the next step in the management?

A. Start N-acetylcysteine

B. Start bicarbonate drip

C. Provide supportive care

D. Proceed with hemodialysis

E. Start penicillin G

17. A 64-year-old man was admitted to the ICU for stage 4 hepatic encephalopathy and hypoxemia requiring intubation and mechanical ventilation. His medical history was remarkable for cirrhosis secondary to chronic hepatitis C. His initial vital signs showed a temperature of 99.5°F, blood pressure of 95/55 mm Hg, respiratory rate of 18 breaths/min, and heart rate of 85 bpm. His urine and blood bacteriology cultures did not show any growth. Lactulose was started. His serum creatinine level increased from his baseline of 1.5 mg/dL to 3.1 mg/dL the next day. Other laboratory findings are listed below. Ultrasound examination of the kidneys did not show any signs of obstruction, and his fractional excretion of sodium (FE_{Na}) was 0.1%. Albumin infusion was given for 48 hours without improvement in creatinine. What is the best next treatment option?

Na	128 mEq/L
K	3.6 mEq/L
Cl⁻	100 mEq/L
Cr	3.1 mg/dL
BUN	50 mg/dL
Bicarbonate	22 mEq/L
Ammonia	200 µg/dL
Glucose	180 mg/dL

A. Norepinephrine bitartrate (Levophed)

B. Octreotide

C. Kidney transplantation

D. Hemodialysis

E. Furosemide

18. A 64-year-old woman was admitted to the ICU with RUQ pain, jaundice, and fever. She had asthma and diabetes mellitus type 2 for which she was taking metformin. Vital signs showed a temperature of 101°F, blood pressure of 85/58 mm Hg, heart rate of 108 bpm, and respiratory rate of 20 breaths/min. Physical exam was notable for RUQ tenderness and altered mental status. Initial blood work showed an AST of 91 IU/L, ALT of 129 IU/L, alkaline phosphatase of 331 IU/L, total bilirubin of 5.8 mg/dL, WBC count of $24 \times 10^3/\mu$L with 30% bands, Hgb of 13 g/L, and platelet of $152 \times 10^3/\mu$L. Gram stains of blood showed gram-negative bacteria. Ultrasound examination of the RUQ demonstrated stones in the gallbladder and intrahepatic and extrahepatic biliary ductal dilatation with a common bile duct diameter of 1.3 cm. The patient is currently being treated with saline infusion and piperacillin-tazobactam. What is the next step in the management of this patient?

A. Schedule endoscopic retrograde cholangiopancreatography (ERCP) next week.

B. Perform ERCP within the next 24 hours.

C. Perform percutaneous transhepatic cholangiography within the next 24 hours.

D. Add vancomycin.

E. Add amoxicillin.

19. A 60-year-old man presented to the ED with lower abdominal pain. His medical history is remarkable for cirrhosis caused by chronic hepatitis C virus infection. His vital signs were a temperature of 99.6°F, blood pressure of 90/55 mm Hg, heart rate of 108 bpm, and respiratory rate of 19 breaths/min. On physical exam, the patient was found to have a moderate amount of ascites and to be diffusely tender on palpitation. Paracentesis was performed with removal of 3 L of nonbloody ascitic fluid. His initial lab data are shown in the table below. What is the best treatment option?

Ascitic	Result
Fluid Analysis	
WBC	500 cells/µL
Neutrophil	80%
Albumin	1.2 g/dL
Protein	1.0 g/dL

Hgb	14 g/L
WBC	$20 \times 10^3/\mu$L
Platelet	$121 \times 10^3/\mu$L
Hct	39%
Bands	28%

Na	130 mEq/L
K	3.6 mEq/L
Cl⁻	100 mEq/L
Cr	1.3 mg/dL
BUN	28 mg/dL
Bicarbonate	20 mEq/L
Glucose	180 mg/dL

A. Vancomycin

B. Cefotaxime and albumin

C. Cefotaxime only

D. Fluconazole

E. Trimethoprim-sulfamethoxazole

20. A 69-year-old man presented to the hospital with abdominal pain of 3 days in duration. The pain was sharp, severe, epigastric, associated with nausea and vomiting, and radiating to the back. Over the past few months, he had increased his "usual" alcoholic intake after he lost his wife in a motor vehicle accident. The lipase level on admission was 1310 U/L, BUN was 25 mg/dL, and his WBC was $8 \times 10^3/\mu L$. On day 3, due to an unsatisfactory clinical response to IV hydration, contrast-based CT was done revealing acute pancreatitis and pancreatic necrosis without a defined wall (shown below). The rate of IV hydration and pain medication was increased, resulting in symptomatic improvement; oral intake was resumed. On day 8, his epigastric pain significantly worsened, and his vital signs showed a temperature of 100.9°F, blood pressure of 88/65 mm Hg, heart rate of 110 bpm, and respiratory rate of 18 breaths/min. His blood tests are listed below. Repeat contrast-enhanced CT scan showed expansion of the pancreatic necrosis compared to the initial CT. He was subsequently transferred to the ICU, and aggressive fluid replacement was initiated. What is the next best treatment option?

Na	130 mEq/L
K	3.6 mEq/L
Cl⁻	100 mEq/L
Cr	2.0 mg/dL
BUN	32 mg/dL
Bicarbonate	20 mEq/L
Glucose	180 mg/dL

ALT	35 IU/L
AST	55 IU/L
Total bilirubin	2.2 mg/dL
Alkaline phosphatase	158 IU/L
Albumin	2.8 g/dL

A. Endoscopic debridement of the necrotic tissue

B. CT-guided fine-needle aspiration (FNA) of the pancreatic necrosis

C. Surgical debridement of the necrotic tissue

D. Start vancomycin

E. Start piperacillin-tazobactam

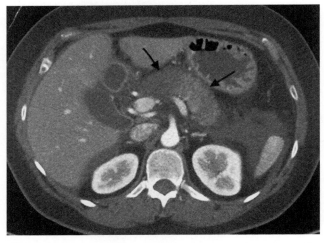

Abdominal computed tomography demonstrating pancreatic necrosis (*left arrow*) and pancreatic inflammation (*right arrow*).

Hgb	14 g/L
WBC	$19 \times 10^3/\mu L$
Platelet	$321 \times 10^3/\mu L$
Hct	48%
Bands	25%

21. A 58-year-old woman presented to the hospital with chest pain and dizziness. Her medical history was notable for hypertension, hyperlipidemia, and diabetes mellitus. She was taking metformin, lisinopril, and pravastatin. She described the pain as sharp, retrosternal, and radiating to the left shoulder. Her initial electrocardiogram showed ST elevation in leads II and III. Vital signs showed a heart rate of 110 bpm, blood pressure of 85/45 mm Hg, respiratory rate of 14 breaths/min, and temperature of 98.0°F. Laboratory testing in the ED revealed a normal complete blood count, comprehensive metabolic panel, and coagulation parameters; her serum troponin level was 4 μg/L. The patient had percutaneous coronary intervention and stent placement, and she subsequently stabilized in the cardiac ICU.

The patient's blood tests 1 day later showed the results outlined below. Testing for viral and autoimmune hepatitis was unremarkable. Doppler ultrasound examination of the liver showed a normal liver morphology, patent hepatic vasculature, and normal blood flow. What is the likely diagnosis?

Hgb	14 g/L
WBC	$6 \times 10^3/\mu L$
Platelet	$350 \times 10^3/\mu L$
Hct	42%
Bands	4%

Na	135 mEq/L
K	3.6 mEq/L
Cl⁻	100 mEq/L
Cr	2.8 mg/dL
BUN	32 mg/dL
Bicarbonate	16 mEq/L
Glucose	110 mg/dL

ALT	2550 IU/L
AST	3330 IU/L
Total bilirubin	2.2 mg/dL
Alkaline phosphatase	158 IU/L
Albumin	3.4 g/dL
Lactic acid dehydrogenase	650 U/L
INR	2.2

A. Ischemic hepatitis

B. Drug-induced liver injury

C. Portal vein thrombosis

D. Acute hepatitis B

E. Acute exacerbation of autoimmune hepatitis

Answers and Explanations

1. C. The likely etiology for this patient's ulcers is critical illness–related stress. Stress ulcers, also called stress-related mucosal injury, are seen in critically ill patients and are thought to result from mucosal ischemia and diminished mucosal protection. The most common location of such ulcers is the stomach, but they can also occur in other sites of the gastrointestinal (GI) tract (eg, duodenum and rectum). Bleeding stress ulcers are estimated to occur in 1.5% of critically ill patients. The risk factors are mechanical ventilation, coagulopathy, prior upper GI (UGI) bleeding, sepsis, prolonged ICU admission, and high-dose steroids. A large multicenter study has shown that oral omeprazole and intravenous (IV) cimetidine are equally effective in preventing bleeding in these patients. In this patient, however, since ulcers already were present, proton pump inhibitor (PPI)-based therapy is preferred over histamine receptor blocker.

The patient is not on NSAIDs (choice A) and is not known to have an immunosuppressive illness that would predispose to cytomegalovirus (choice E). In view of the high prevalence of *H pylori* in the community, this patient could have *H pylori* gastritis (choice B), but the temporal presentation of his ulcer bleeding during his ICU stay is most consistent with ongoing critical illness being the trigger. The acute presentation argues against malignancy as a cause for this patient's presentation (choice D).

2. E. This patient has an NSAID-induced ulcer that bled and resulted in overt GI bleeding with symptomatic anemia. Endoscopic therapy of peptic ulcer is warranted when high-risk features (eg, visible vessel, active bleeding, or adherent clot) are noted on the endoscopic exam. Once endoscopic therapy has been performed, IV PPI should be continued for 72 hours followed by a twice-daily oral PPI regimen to be continued upon discharge, and therefore, limiting PPI-based therapy to 48 hours (choice A) is insufficient for treatment of a recently bleeding

peptic ulcer. After endoscopy, these patients should be maintained on a clear liquid diet (choice E), and if there is no evidence of recurrent GI bleeding, diet can be advanced. In view of the high risk of recurrent bleeding in patients with peptic ulcer and a visible vessel, solid diet should be avoided (choice B) after the procedure in case performing repeat EGD is urgently needed because of rebleeding. Clear liquid diet allows sedation or anesthesia to be administered within 2 hours after the last ingestion in case urgent EGD is needed. It is premature to switch to oral therapy before the 72-hour interval has lapsed (choice C). Patients with hemodynamically significant UGI bleeding treated with endoscopic therapy should be monitored in the inpatient setting for at least 3 days, and therefore, the patient cannot be sent home at this time (choice D). It is noteworthy that erythromycin was given in this case as a prokinetic agent to help empty the stomach of any blood prior to endoscopy.

3. B. This patient suffered duodenal ulcer bleeding that spontaneously ceased, and his ulcer currently exhibits a flat pigmented spot, which denotes low risk of rebleeding; thus, no endoscopic therapy is warranted. Since no endoscopic therapy was pursued, there is no need for IV PPI (choice A), and therefore, daily oral PPI would suffice (choice B). The patient should stay in the hospital for 1 to 2 days and be maintained on clear liquid diet for 1 day. Continued IV PPI (choice A) would have been indicated if the patient were found to have high-risk ulcer features (eg, active bleeding, visible vessel, or adherent clot), which require endoscopic therapy. Although patients with clean-based ulcers can be discharged home, patients with a flat pigmented spot should stay in the hospital for 1 to 2 days to be monitored for further bleeding. Admission to the ICU (choice D) is not required in this hemodynamically stable patient with a low-risk ulcer for which no endoscopic therapy was appropriate. There is no utility of adding cimetidine for patients with bleeding peptic ulcer when a more effective therapy (ie, PPI) has already been started. Of note, this patient's ulcer is likely secondary to *Helicobacter* infection.

4. **A.** The patient clearly has UGI bleeding. After ensuring hemodynamic stability and starting IV PPI, endoscopic evaluation is warranted (choice A). The source of bleeding in this case is likely peptic ulcer disease secondary to aspirin use. Blood transfusion in UGI bleeding (choice B) should be avoided when the Hgb is >7 mg/dL in the absence of coronary artery disease (CAD) or ongoing massive GI bleeding. This patient does not have ongoing massive GI bleeding given hemodynamic stability and the fact that the last vomiting episode was 6 hours prior to presentation. A large randomized controlled study showed that a restrictive transfusion strategy (Hgb <7 g/dL) results in significantly better outcomes than liberal transfusion strategy (Hgb <9 mg/dL) in terms of survival, rebleeding, and adverse events. Gastric lavage (choice C) is not indicated in the management of patients with UGI bleeding because studies have shown that 18% of UGI bleedings can be missed when gastric lavage is relied upon. The elevated BUN-to-creatinine ratio (accelerated azotemia) is secondary to UGI bleeding and does not represent a renal insult; therefore, obtaining urine studies is not required in this case (choice D). Discharging a patient who has had a recent overt UGI bleeding prior to endoscopic evaluation is inappropriate (choice E).

5. **C.** Ischemic colitis is commonly observed in the elderly, especially in those with atherosclerotic cardiovascular disease. In most cases, ischemic colitis is attributed to nonocclusive local hypoperfusion since no causative anatomic abnormalities are found. Ischemic colitis usually presents with rectal bleeding and abdominal pain; however, isolated right-sided ischemic colitis (IRIC) can present with abdominal pain in the absence of rectal bleeding and is an indicator of poor prognosis. The superior mesenteric artery supplies both the right colon and the small bowel, and therefore, patients with isolated right-sided colon ischemia also may be at high risk of impending acute mesenteric ischemia (small bowel ischemia). Thus, whenever IRIC is suspected, it is crucial to first rule out superior mesenteric artery occlusion with CT angiography

(CTA) or magnetic resonance angiography (MRA). If CTA or MRA shows superior mesenteric artery (SMA) occlusion, surgery (choice E) and interventional radiology consultations are warranted. In cases of suspected IRIC in which SMA occlusion is excluded or in cases where there is no isolated right-sided involvement, colonoscopy with biopsy (choice B) should be pursued to confirm the diagnosis. Antibiotic therapy should be considered if there are 3 or more of the following: male sex, hypotension (systolic blood pressure <90 mm Hg), tachycardia (heart rate >100 bpm), abdominal pain without rectal bleeding, BUN >20 mg/dL, Hgb <12 g/dL, lactate dehydrogenase >350 U/L, serum sodium <136 mEq/L (mmol/L), or white blood cell (WBC) >15 × 10^3/μL. Duplex study (choice A) is an inappropriate test because it cannot assess the superior mesenteric artery in its entirety. Observation (choice D) is inappropriate in this patient who has a potentially life-threatening condition.

6. **D.** *Clostridium difficile* infection (CDI) is an increasingly common cause of GI-related hospital admissions. Patients with recent hospital admission or recent antibiotic use and elderly individuals who are residents of long-term care facilities are at higher risk for this infection. This patient was recently treated with antibiotics for pneumonia and is now being admitted to the ICU for severe and complicated CDI. The criteria for severe disease are serum albumin <3 g/dL with WBC ≥15 × 10^3/μL and/or abdominal tenderness; usually, severe CDI is treated with oral vancomycin alone (choice B). The criteria for severe and complicated CDI are any of the following: admission to ICU, hypotension with or without use of vasopressors, fever ≥101.3°F, ileus or significant abdominal distention, mental status changes, WBC ≥35 × 10^3/μL or <2000 × 10^3/μL, serum lactate levels >2.2 mmol/L, or end organ failure. Patients with severe and complicated CDI should be treated with oral vancomycin 125 mg every 6 hours and IV metronidazole 500 mg every 8 hours (choice D). Additionally, vancomycin enemas (choice C) and surgical consultation should be considered in these patients. Oral metronidazole can be considered in mild cases of CDI (choice A) without any of the aforementioned criteria. Oral or rectal vancomycin alone is insufficient for treating this patient. Fecal microbiota transplantation (choice E) is a highly successful therapy that

is reserved for cases of recurrent CDI or severe cases that are unresponsive to medical therapy; it is, therefore, inappropriate in this clinical scenario.

7. **D.** Acute pancreatitis is a frequently encountered GI disease, and it was reported in 2009 to be the most common GI discharge diagnosis in the United States. The most common causes of acute pancreatitis are alcohol abuse and gallstones. Less common causes are hypertriglyceridemia and medications. Sitagliptin (Januvia) has been recently reported to be associated with acute pancreatitis. In every case of pancreatitis, it is crucial to obtain a detailed history about alcohol use and current medications, sonographic imaging of the biliary tree (to exclude gallstones), and a triglyceride level. The diagnosis of acute pancreatitis requires 2 of the following criteria: lipase and/or amylase level more than 3 times the upper limit of normal; abdominal pain consistent with the disease; and radiologic evidence of pancreatic inflammation. Aggressive hydration with isotonic crystalloid solution should be started in all patients (except those with cardiovascular or renal comorbidities) in the first 24 hours of presentation. The preferred solution is lactated Ringer's solution except in patients with hypercalcemia. Lactated Ringer's solution was found to be more effective than normal saline in resolving the systemic inflammatory response syndrome within 24 hours in these patients. Albumin (choice A) is, therefore, not the appropriate hydration solution in this clinical scenario. The fluid rate should be reassessed and potentially changed every 6 hours depending on the BUN level. The goal is to decrease BUN to baseline. Upper endoscopy (choice C) has no utility in the management of acute pancreatitis. Although frequently performed, abdominal imaging by CT or magnetic resonance imaging (choices B and E) should be reserved for patients with insufficient evidence of acute pancreatitis (suggestive pain or only elevated pancreatic enzymes) or in patients who fail to improve after 48 hours of admission.

8. **D.** In this case, the patient is presenting with hemodynamic instability in the setting of UGI bleeding. It is very likely that the patient has cirrhosis; he has a risk factor for chronic liver disease (hepatitis C) and has physical exam signs and laboratory studies that are typically found in cirrhosis. As such, it is critical to identify variceal bleeding as a likely source of UGI hemorrhage. Somatostatin analogues such as octreotide administered intravenously are the next appropriate step in management for suspected variceal bleeding. Octreotide promotes splanchnic vasoconstriction, which reduces portal blood flow and, as a result, can ease variceal bleeding. It also reduces secretion of gastric acid. This allows time for more definitive treatment (such as endoscopic therapy or transjugular intrahepatic portosystemic shunt) to be planned.

Massive transfusion protocol (choice A) can be indicated for hemorrhage of any type associated with hemodynamic instability. However, overtransfusion can increase portal pressure even higher than baseline, thus increasing the risk of rebleeding. Before pursuing upper endoscopy, the patient first should be resuscitated and given agents such as somatostatin analogues since variceal bleeding is suspected. Although the patient could be mildly coagulopathic as a result of cirrhosis, correction of coagulopathy (choices C and E) is generally not warranted if INR is less than 1.5. It is noteworthy that a recent meta-analysis has shown PCC to be superior to fresh frozen plasma in the setting of warfarin-related coagulopathy reversal, in terms of rapid effect, smaller administered volume, and all-cause mortality; there was no increase in thromboembolic events in the PCC group.

9. **C.** The patient's rapid decompensation associated with hematemesis should raise concern for variceal bleeding that is life-threatening. Therefore, insertion of a Minnesota tube for balloon tamponade of the varices is the next appropriate step in management. A Minnesota tube consists of a gastric balloon and an esophageal balloon, either or both of which can be inflated to compress a bleeding varix. Incorrect placement of the gastric balloon into the esophagus or inflation of just the esophageal balloon can result in esophageal perforation. The Minnesota tube relies on tension of the tethered gastric balloon to tamponade bleeding varices at the gastroesophageal junction. In patients with such severe variceal bleeding, concomitant endotracheal tube intubation is generally recommended, not only for airway protection, but also to protect against migration of the esophageal balloon. It is a temporizing measure to be used only during immediately life-threatening bleeding and usually is not kept inflated for longer than 24 hours, by which

time a more definitive intervention such as endo-scopic therapy or TIPS placement is performed.

Blood products and octreotide infusion (choices A and D) are certainly components of this patient's management. However, the patient is at imminent risk of circulatory collapse and requires immediate cessation of bleeding. Overtransfu-sion may also exacerbate her variceal bleeding by increasing portal hypertension. TIPS (choice B) is incorrect because endoscopic management, not TIPS placement, would be the most appropriate next therapeutic intervention. If endoscopic ther-apy fails, then TIPS can be considered. Vasopressor support (choice E) is inappropriate at this time as it is most important to halt the bleeding and expand the circulatory volume prior to using vasopressors. Vasopressors might be eventually required in this patient if the colloid-based volume resuscitation and blood transfusion fail to normalize the patient's blood pressure.

10. **B.** It is critical in this case to recognize that the patient has acute onset of abdominal pain with only mild tenderness and that the pain is out of propor-tion to the findings on exam. This presentation is typical of acute mesenteric ischemia. This patient likely has cocaine-induced nonocclusive acute mesenteric ischemia due to vasospasm. Labora-tory abnormalities can include elevated hematocrit (due to volume depletion), leukocytosis, metabolic acidosis, and elevated serum lactate, as well as ele-vated serum amylase, aspartate aminotransferase, and lactate dehydrogenase, although all of these abnormalities develop late, usually after intestinal gangrene has occurred. Advanced abdominal imag-ing with angiography (choice B) is warranted to diagnose acute mesenteric ischemia, evaluate for occlusion of the superior mesenteric artery, and exclude other nonischemic disorders. Although the patient is likely suffering from nonocclusive acute mesenteric ischemia, medical management is gen-erally similar to that of occlusive acute mesenteric ischemia, including IV crystalloids, oxygen supple-mentation, maintaining NPO (nothing by mouth) status, and a vasodilating agent such as papaverine. Occlusive mesenteric ischemia might require addi-tional interventions depending on its etiology, such as the administration of anticoagulant in the case of acute thrombus. Once acute mesenteric ischemia is recognized, worsening abdominal pain, fever, and

bloody diarrhea should prompt consideration for surgical intervention.

Patients will frequently relate abdominal pain to food (choice A) but pointing away from infec-tious etiologies are the severity of pain and the lack of other symptoms such as nausea, vomiting, and diarrhea. Although the patient may request nar-cotic analgesia (choice C), given the possibility of mesenteric infarction, this would not be appropri-ate. Arguing against bowel obstruction (choice D) are the lack of vomiting and pronounced abdominal distention even though the childhood appendec-tomy would put him at risk for bowel obstruction due to adhesions. Finally, although an ECG (choice E) would not be incorrect as myocardial infarction in diabetic patients can present atypically as abdom-inal pain (especially inferior wall infarctions), the diagnosis of mesenteric ischemia would still be missed.

11. **A.** The patient's clinical picture of painless but significant rectal bleeding is most compatible with diverticular bleeding. Diverticula form due to weaknesses in the colon wall where arterioles penetrate the wall to supply the organ. Her age is what predisposes her most to diverticulosis, which is present in over half of patients above the age of 80. Anticoagulation in this case exacerbates the bleeding severity.

Ischemic colitis (choice B), especially in elderly patients, should be considered. However, the lack of abdominal pain and severity of bleeding would be atypical. Although an angioectasia (choice C) can be a source of both upper and lower GI bleeding, the patient's profuse pattern of bleeding is unusual as angioectasia bleeding tends to be slower and less likely to be brisk. While the patient has (appropri-ately) stopped colorectal cancer screening at the age of 75, colon cancer presenting with painless brisk hematochezia would be uncommon (choice D). Finally, the severity of bleeding is out of proportion for hemorrhoidal bleeding (choice E).

In terms of management, because this patient is hemodynamically unstable, while she is being resuscitated, anticoagulation should be reversed and EGD should be considered to rule out brisk UGI bleeding. Should this be negative and the patient continue to be hemodynamically unstable, diagnostic and possible therapeutic modalities such as CTA should be employed? If the patient is more hemodynamically stable after EGD, rapid bowel preparation should be administered (consisting of 4-6 L of polyethylene glycol–containing bowel purging agents) over 3 to 4 hours until the rectal effluent is clear. Colonoscopy is the modality of choice for diagnosis and treatment with continued bleeding.

12. **E.** The patient's clinical picture and finding of a thickened gallbladder wall suggest acute cholecystitis. Abdominal ultrasound (AUS) is a sensitive and specific diagnostic modality for calculus gallbladder disease (84% and 95%, respectively). AUS for cholecystitis is somewhat less sensitive and specific (81% and 83%, respectively), with some studies suggesting wider variability in sensitivity ranging as low as 50% to as high as 100% compared to AUS for gallstones. The finding of cholecystitis and an absence of gallstones should, in this critically ill patient, heighten suspicion for acalculous cholecystitis. There is no pattern of liver test abnormality that is specific for acalculous cholecystitis. It is thought that acalculous cholecystitis composes more than 15% of acute cholecystitis cases, with pathogenesis thought to be due to bile stasis and ischemia resulting in infection and inflammation that can progress to frank gangrene. Whereas cholecystectomy is definitive treatment for calculus cholecystitis, cholecystostomy tube placement can be considered for acalculous cholecystitis, especially if the patient is too sick for surgery. Although this patient is at risk for gallstone disease (obese body habitus, age, female sex), the absence of gallstones on ultrasonography and only borderline elevation of the common bile duct diameter in the setting of normal alkaline phosphatase should point away from further workup for choledocholithiasis, making choices A and B incorrect. There is no need to pursue CT scan (choice C) because cholecystitis is the most likely etiology for the patient's abdominal pain located typically in the right upper quadrant. Although piperacillin-tazobactam (choice D) can be associated with liver injury, this cannot explain gallbladder wall edema.

13. **D.** The patient is in septic shock, possibly from a carbapenem-resistant *Enterobacter* (CRE) as he has decompensated on meropenem after initial improvement. It has been estimated that bilirubin, alkaline phosphatase, and transaminase elevations occur in 12% of patients diagnosed with sepsis and that more than 20% of jaundice in the community setting is due to sepsis. Gram-negative organisms have been implicated in the vast majority of these cases. Hepatic bilirubin metabolism can be disturbed with sepsis (especially if hemolysis is occurring due to immunologically mediated red blood cell injury) as a result of impaired bilirubin uptake, canalicular and basolateral transport of bile acids, and bilirubin clearance.

Ischemic hepatopathy (choice A) can be associated with septic shock but would typically result in much more severe transaminase elevations (at least 1000 IU/L). Although ascending cholangitis (choice B) can be associated with hyperbilirubinemia, leukocytosis, and septic shock, in the absence of elevated alkaline phosphatase, right upper quadrant (RUQ) abdominal pain, or radiologic features, this is less likely. Acute cholecystitis is similarly unlikely (choice C) in this abdominal pain-free patient, and it does not typically present with such derangements in liver tests. Finally, a missed acetaminophen overdose (choice E) causing this degree of decompensation would not be likely without more severe (even if downtrending) elevations in serum transaminases and without elevation in INR to suggest liver failure.

14. **B.** The patient has abnormal liver tests of a hepatocellular pattern (ie, predominant ALT elevation) that likely reflect drug-induced liver injury (DILI) given his normal liver tests prior to starting phenytoin. After any new medication is initiated, the clinician should be concerned about DILI. Patient-specific variables (eg, age, sex, comorbidities, especially diabetes, underlying alcohol or tobacco abuse) and polypharmacy can increase the risk of DILI. Antiepileptic agents such as phenytoin can induce an anticonvulsant hypersensitivity syndrome consistent with hepatocellular (predominantly elevated transaminases) or cholestatic (predominantly elevated alkaline phosphatase and bilirubin) liver injury with fever and rash. The phenytoin-induced liver injury typically occurs 2 to 8 weeks after initiation of the drug and starts to resolve several days after discontinuation of it. When phenytoin-related DILI is suspected, phenytoin should be discontinued and another antiepileptic agent should be used.

Administering systemic glucocorticoids (choice A) would only be appropriate if there was strong suspicion for severe alcoholic hepatitis, which is unlikely given the provided history, trend of liver tests (alcohol injury causes predominant AST elevation, rather than ALT), and normal prothrombin time/INR. Steroids would be indicated in severe alcoholic hepatitis because they improve short-term mortality (evidence is more limited for improvement in long-term mortality). Liver biopsy (choice C) can be considered, especially if withdrawal of phenytoin does not improve liver tests, but is not appropriate at this time. Continuing to monitor liver tests (choice D) is not appropriate given ongoing significant liver injury. Pentoxifylline administration (choice E) is incorrect because even if he were suffering from severe alcoholic hepatitis, recent evidence suggests that pentoxifylline is not associated with improved outcomes.

A useful database is maintained by the National Institutes of Health that catalogues medications and data regarding their risk of provoking liver injury (https://livertox.nih.gov/).

15. **A.** Hepatic encephalopathy (HE) is a reversible neuropsychiatric illness in patients with hepatic decompensation and is divided into covert and overt subclasses. The covert subtype can only be detected using neuropsychiatric special testing, whereas the overt type is detected clinically and ranges from lethargy to coma. It is very important in the management of HE to recognize any precipitating factors such as infections, GI bleeding, overdiuresis, electrolyte imbalance, or constipation. Patients with suspected HE should be promptly started on enteral lactulose. Lactulose (choice A) works by preventing the absorption of the free ammonia (NH_3) into the blood by converting it to the ammonium (NH_4) form. Rifaximin (choice C), a nonabsorbable antibiotic, has been demonstrated to benefit patients with recurrent HE as studies showed that rifaximin reduces the risk of developing new episodes when added to lactulose. Since there is no report of recurrent HE in this patient, rifaximin would not be warranted at this time. Probiotics (choice D) work by altering the gut microbiota and have not been shown yet to improve HE. Although infection can precipitate HE, it is premature to initiate antibiotics prior to having any evidence of infection; thus, vancomycin and cefazolin are inappropriate answers (choices B and E). It is notable that high ammonia does not add any diagnostic or prognostic value in the management of HE as high levels of ammonia neither confirm nor exclude the diagnosis; a normal serum ammonia level, however, should raise the suspicion that an alternative diagnosis might be the cause of altered mental status.

16. **A.** This patient has acute liver failure due to an acetaminophen overdose and should be admitted to an ICU because of the high morbidity and mortality in this patient population. Acute liver failure is defined by deterioration in the ability of the liver to produce coagulation factors and is characterized by an increase in the INR in addition to mental status changes in a patient with acute liver damage and no features suggesting cirrhosis or chronic liver disease in the past 26 weeks. Because the patient's mental status can further decline and may develop a more severe form of hepatic encephalopathy, ICU admission should be considered, and a transplant center should be notified. King's College criteria are used to identify patients with acute liver failure who have poor prognosis:

- pH <7.3
- OR in 24 hours:
- INR >6 (platelet >100/µL) AND
- Cr >300 mmol/L AND
- Grade 3 or 4 encephalopathy

Acetaminophen, when administered in appropriate amounts, is metabolized in the liver mainly by conjugation with sulfate or glucuronide to form nontoxic compounds that are excreted by the kidneys. A small fraction of the acetaminophen is metabolized by hepatic cytochrome 450 into a highly toxic metabolite, *N*-acetyl-*p*-benzoquinoneimine (NAPQI). To enable urinary excretion of this highly toxic compound, the hepatocyte conjugates it with glutathione. In cases of acetaminophen overdose, a large fraction of the acetaminophen is metabolized into excessive amounts of NAPQI, which causes acute liver injury due to depletion of glutathione stores and attenuation of the conjugation process. *N*-acetylcysteine works by restoring glutathione in the liver cells and boosting sulfate conjugation, which result in decreasing the toxic effect of acetaminophen overdose. Patients with acetaminophen toxicity should be started on *N*-acetylcysteine (choice A), given either orally or by IV route.

Supportive care (choice C) alone is inappropriate in patients with acute liver failure secondary to acetaminophen toxicity, and treatment with *N*-acetylcysteine is warranted. Bicarbonate drip and hemodialysis (choices B and D) can be appropriate measures for patients with severe acidosis but not as first-line treatment for acute liver failure. Penicillin G (choice E) has been recommended for patients with acute liver failure secondary to mushroom poisoning but not for acetaminophen toxicity.

17. **A.** This patient presented with hepatorenal syndrome (HRS), which is defined as worsening kidney function in the presence of cirrhosis with clinically significant portal hypertension leading to splanchnic vasodilation and consequent renal vasoconstriction and hypoperfusion. HRS can also develop in the setting of fulminant hepatic failure or acute alcoholic hepatitis. Major criteria for the diagnosis of HRS include cirrhosis with ascites, serum creatinine >1.5 mg/dL, no improvement despite diuretic withdrawal and albumin infusion (1 g/kg) for 48 hours, absence of shock or recent use of hepatotoxic drugs, and no features of parenchymal kidney disease as indicated by proteinuria >500 mg/d, microhematuria, and/or abnormal renal ultrasonography. A recent study suggested that urine albumin >100 mg/dL and FE_{Na} >0.5% favor acute tubular necrosis (ATN) over HRS. Conversely, low urine albumin and FE_{Na} <0.1% favor HRS. Patients with suspected diagnosis of HRS who show unsatisfactory response to albumin challenge should be transferred to a monitored setting and started on norepinephrine or vasopressin. Vasopressors have been shown to improve outcomes in these patients by reversing the splanchnic vasodilation, which eventually leads to increasing blood flow to the kidneys. If a monitored bed is not available, patients can be maintained on midodrine, octreotide (choice B), and albumin infusions in the interim.

Neither hemodialysis nor renal transplantation (choices C and D) is appropriate for this patient because they will not reverse the contributing pathophysiology, which is the clinically significant portal hypertension. Hemodialysis could be considered if there is no response to vasopressors and as a bridge until transplantation. Diuretics (choice E) could be appropriate in the setting of ATN, but they are detrimental in the case of HRS.

18. **B.** This is a patient with acute cholangitis, which is a bacterial infection of the biliary tree in the setting of bile stasis secondary to biliary obstruction. As a result, patients typically present in 50% to 75% of instances with fever, jaundice, and RUQ pain, an occurrence known as the Charcot triad; when hypotension and confusion are added to these symptoms, it is called the Reynolds pentad.

The most common risk factors for cholangitis are obstruction of the biliary tract through choledocholithiasis followed by benign biliary stenosis, especially in patients with primary sclerosing cholangitis. The role of the ERCP (answer B) is vital in the management of acute cholangitis, especially in the first 24 hours of the admission. Stone extraction and/or stent insertion is the treatment of choice for establishing biliary drainage in acute cholangitis. Urgent endoscopic intervention in these patients reduces the mortality rate and shortens hospital stay. Percutaneous transhepatic cholangiography (choice C) is second-line therapy and should be considered if ERCP failed or is not available at the facility. Vancomycin and amoxicillin (choices D and E) are appropriate antibiotics for gram-positive bacteria, but in our patient, who has the typical gram-negative bacteremia of ascending cholangitis, they would be inappropriate.

19. **B.** Spontaneous bacterial peritonitis (SBP) is infection of the ascitic fluid in patients with cirrhosis in the absence of identifiable intra-abdominal infection, inflammation, perforation, or recent instrumentation. SBP is diagnosed by an elevation in the ascitic fluid absolute polymorphonuclear leukocyte (PMN) count to ≥250 cells/μL. Most patients with SBP present with abdominal pain and fever, whereas a minority have hypotension and septic shock; note that 6% of SBP patients have neither abdominal pain nor tenderness on presentation. The American Association for the Study of Liver Diseases (AASLD) recommends antibiotic treatment with cefotaxime, which covers the most common 3 bacteria contributing to SBP: *Escherichia coli*, *Klebsiella pneumoniae*, and *Streptococcal pneumoniae*. AASLD also recommends that albumin infusion should be given if the creatinine is >1 mg/dL, the BUN is >30 mg/dL, or the total bilirubin is >4 mg/dL as studies showed an increased survival rate in patients who had received albumin on days 1

and 3 of the treatment; therefore, cefotaxime alone (choice C) is an inappropriate answer in this case.

Vancomycin (choice A) does not cover gram-negative bacteria. Although fluconazole (choice D) is an antifungal medication, fungi are very rare cause of the SBP. Starting trimethoprim-sulfamethoxazole (choice E) is recommended for SBP prophylaxis but not for acute infection.

20. **B.** This patient has severe acute pancreatitis complicated by pancreatic necrosis causing severe systemic inflammatory response and organ failure. Less than 10% of patients with acute pancreatitis develop pancreatic necrosis, and approximately one-third develop infections in the necrotic fluid collection. Infected pancreatic necrosis should be suspected in any patient with pancreatic necrosis on imaging who fails to improve or deteriorates after 7 to 10 days of hospitalization. Both infected necrosis and sterile necrosis can present with leukocytosis, fever, and organ failure, and the only approach to separate these entities is CT-guided FNA. The FNA in this patient should be followed by administration of broad-spectrum antibiotics until infection is confirmed or excluded based on the aspirate analysis. Some experts suggested that FNA should only be performed in patients who do not respond to empiric antibiotics. The American College of Gastroenterology recommends either 1 of these 2 approaches (FNA followed by antibiotics vs empiric use of antibiotics) in patients with suspected infected pancreatic necrosis. The most common organisms in infected pancreatic necrosis are gram-negative bacteria (eg, *Klebsiella* and *E coli*). Carbapenems (not vancomycin or piperacillin-tazobactam; choices D and E) are the antibiotic class of choice in the treatment of infected pancreatic necrosis because of better penetration of pancreatic tissue resulting in better outcomes. Debridement (surgical or endoscopic; choices A and C) is usually delayed until 4 weeks after presentation, as long as the patient is responding to antibiotics and remains clinically stable; this delay would allow the development of a wall around the necrosis (walled-off pancreatic necrosis).

21. **A.** This patient had ischemic hepatitis (also known as shock liver or hypoxic hepatitis), which is characterized by significant and rapid elevation in the liver enzymes more than 10 times the upper normal limit in critically ill patients who suffer hemodynamic instability. It is also characterized by significant rise in lactate dehydrogenase. The remarkable increase in the liver enzymes 24 to 48 hours after the ischemic insult is characteristic of this clinical entity and serves to differentiate it from other hepatitides, especially in the setting of unremarkable serologic (viral and autoimmune) testing for liver disease; therefore, choices D and E are incorrect. Portal vein thrombosis (PVT; choice C) also can present with elevation in the liver enzymes and is usually diagnosed by Doppler ultrasound of the liver and confirmed by contrast CT scan or magnetic resonance imaging. Our patient had a normal duplex examination with normal blood flow in the portal and hepatic vasculature, making the diagnosis of PVT unlikely. The remarkable rapid rise in liver tests in the setting of hypotension favors ischemic hepatitis (choice A) over drug-induced liver injury (choice B). The management of ischemic hepatitis is mainly supportive, and the liver enzymes are expected to normalize within 7 to 10 days.

REFERENCES

Agrawal A, Sharma BC, Sharma P, et al. Secondary prophylaxis of hepatic encephalopathy in cirrhosis: an open-label, randomized controlled trial of lactulose, probiotics, and no therapy. *Am J Gastroenterol.* 2012;107:1043-1050.

Akriviadis EA, Runyon BA. The value of an algorithm in differentiating spontaneous from secondary bacterial peritonitis. *Gastroenterology.* 1990;98:127-133.

Als-Nielsen B, Gluud LL, Gluud C. Non-absorbable disaccharides for hepatic encephalopathy: systematic review of randomised trials. *BMJ.* 2004;328:1046.

American College of Gastroenterology guideline: management of acute pancreatitis. *Am J Gastroenterol.* 2013;108(9):1400-1416.

Ansaloni L, Pisano M, Coccolini F, et al. 2016 World Society of Emergency Surgery guidelines on acute calculous cholecystitis. *World J Emerg Surg.* 2016;11:25.

ASGE Standards of Practice Committee. The role of endoscopy in the evaluation of suspected choledocholithiasis. *Gastrointest Endosc.* 2010;71:1-9.

Banks P, Bollen T, Dervenis C, et al. Classification of acute pancreatitis–2012: revision of the Atlanta classification and definitions by international consensus. *Gut.* 2013;62:102-111.

Belcher JM, Sanyal AJ, Peixoto AJ, et al. Kidney biomarkers and differential diagnosis of patients with cirrhosis and acute kidney injury. *Hepatology.* 2014;60:622-632.

Birrer R, Takuda Y, Takara T. Hypoxic hepatopathy: pathophysiology and prognosis. *Intern Med.* 2007;46(14):1063-1070.

Brandt LJ, Feuerstadt P, Longstreth GF, Boley SJ. ACG clinical guideline: epidemiology, risk factors, patterns of presentation, diagnosis, and management of colon ischemia (CI). *Am J Gastroenterol.* 2015;110:18-44.

Chai-Adisaksopha C, Hillis C, Siegal DM, et al. Prothrombin complex concentrates versus fresh frozen plasma for warfarin reversal: a systematic review and meta-analysis. *Thromb Haemost.* 2016;116:879-890.

Chand N, Sanyal AJ. Sepsis-induced cholestasis. *Hepatology* 2007;45(1):230-241.

Conrad SA, Gabrielli A, Margolis B, et al. Randomized, double-blind comparison of immediate-release omeprazole oral suspension versus intravenous cimetidine for the prevention of upper gastrointestinal bleeding in critically ill patients. *Crit Care Med.* 2005;33:760-765.

Cohen JA, Kaplan MM. Left-sided heart failure presenting as hepatitis. *Gastroenterology.* 1978;74(3):583-587.

Cook DJ, Fuller HD, Guyatt GH, et al. Risk factors for gastrointestinal bleeding in critically ill patients. Canadian Critical Care Trials Group. *N Engl J Med.* 1994;330:377-381.

de Franchis R. Evolving consensus in portal hypertension report of the Baveno IV Consensus Workshop on methodology of diagnosis and therapy in portal hypertension. *J Hepatol.* 2005;43:167-176.

de Franchis E. Expanding consensus in portal hypertension report of the Baveno VI Consensus Workshop: stratifying risk and individualizing care for portal hypertension. *J Hepatol.* 2015;63:743-752.

Eckerwall G, Olin H, Andersson B, et al. Fluid resuscitation and nutritional support during severe acute pancreatitis in the past: what have we learned and how can we do better? *Clin Nutr.* 2006;25:497-504.

Feldman M, Friedman LS, Brandt LJ. *Sleisenger and Fordtran's Gastrointestinal and Liver Disease.* 10th ed. New York, NY: Saunders; 2015.

Felisart J, Rimola A, Arroyo V, et al. Randomized comparative study of efficacy and nephrotoxicity of ampicillin plus tobramycin versus cefotaxime in cirrhotics with severe infections. *Hepatology.* 1985;5:457-462.

Ferenci P, Lockwood A, Mullen K, et al. Hepatic encephalopathy—definition, nomenclature, diagnosis, and quantification: final report of the working party at the 11th World Congresses of Gastroenterology, Vienna, 1998. *Hepatology.* 2002;35:716-721.

Fontana RJ. Pathogenesis of idiosyncratic drug-induced liver injury and clinical perspectives. *Gastroenterology* 2014;146(4):914-928.

Forrest JA, Clements JA, Prescott LF. Clinical pharmacokinetics of paracetamol. *Clin Pharmacokinet.* 1982;7(2):93-107.

Garcia-Tsao G, Sanyal AJ, Grace ND, Carrey WD. Prevention and management of gastroesophageal varices and variceal hemorrhage in cirrhosis. Practice Guidelines Committee of the American Association for the Study of Liver Diseases. *Am J Gastroenterol.* 2007;102(9):2086-2102.

Gluud LL, Christensen K, Christensen E, Krag A. Systemic review of randomized trials of vasoconstrictor drugs for hepatorenal syndrome. *Hepatology.* 2010;51:576-584.

Hoefs JC, Canawati HN, Sapico FL, et al. Spontaneous bacterial peritonitis. *Hepatology.* 1982;2:399-407.

Jensen DM, Machicado GA, Jutabha R, Kovacs TO. Urgent colonoscopy for the diagnosis and treatment of severe diverticular hemorrhage. *N Engl J Med.* 2000;342(2):78-82.

Keays R, Harrison PM, Wendon JA, et al. Intravenous acetylcysteine in paracetamol induced fulminant hepatic failure: a prospective controlled trial. *BMJ.* 1991;303:1026-1029.

Kozuch PL, Brandt LJ. Review articles: diagnosis and management of mesenteric ischaemia with an emphasis on pharmacotherapy. *Aliment Pharmacol Ther.* 2005;21:201-215.

Lai EC, Mok FP, Tan ES, et al. Endoscopic biliary drainage for severe acute cholangitis. *N Engl J Med.* 326;24:1582-1586.

Laine L. Upper gastrointestinal bleeding due to a peptic ulcer. *N Engl J Med.* 2016;374(24):2367-2376.

Laine L, Jensen DM. Management of patients with ulcer bleeding. *Am J Gastroenterol.* 2012;107(3):345-360.

Lee WM, Stravitz RT, Larson AM. Introduction to the revised American Association for the Study of Liver Diseases Position Paper on acute liver failure 2011. *Hepatology.* 2012;55(3):965-967.

Lipsett PA, Pitt HA. Acute cholangitis. *Front Biosci.* 2003;8:1229-1239.

Liumbruno GM, Bennardello F, Lattanzio A, et al. Recommendations for the transfusion of patients in the peri-operative period: the intraoperative period. *Blood Transfus.* 2011;9:189-217.

Matrana MR, Margolin DA. Epidemiology and pathophysiology of diverticular disease. *Clin Colon Rectal Surg.* 2009;22(3):141-146.

National Library of Medicine. Piperacillin-tazobactam. https://livertox.nlm.nih.gov//PiperacillinandTazobactam.htm. Accessed June 24, 2017.

Nesseler N, Launey Y, Aninat C, Morel F, Malledant Y, Seguin P. Clinical review: the liver in sepsis. *Crit Care.* 2012;16(5):235.

O'Grady JG, Alexander GJ, Hayllar KM, et al. Early indicators of prognosis in fulminant hepatic failure. *Gastroenterology.* 1989;97:439-445.

Ostapowicz G, Fontana RJ, Schiødt FV, et al. Results of a prospective study of acute liver failure at 17 tertiary care centers in the United States. *Ann Intern Med.* 2002;137:947-954.

Patidar KR, Bajaj JS. Antibiotics for the treatment of hepatic encephalopathy. *Metab Brain Dis.* 2013;28:307-312.

Practice Parameters Committee of the American College of Gastroenterology. ACG clinical guideline: the diagnosis and management of idiosyncratic drug-induced liver injury. *Am J Gastroenterol.* 2014;109(7):950-966.

Ryu JK, Ryu KH, Kim KH. Clinical features of acute acalculous cholecystitis. *J Clin Gastroenterol* 2003;36(2):166-169.

Saik RP, Greenburg AG, Farris J, et al. Spectrum of cholangitis. *Am Surg.* 1975;130(2):143-150.

Salerno F, Gerbes A, Gines P, Wong F, Arroyo V. Diagnosis, prevention and treatment of the hepatorenal syndrome in cirrhosis: a consensus workshop of the international ascites club. *Gut.* 2007;56:1310-1318.

Singh N, Gayowski T, Yu VL, et al. Trimethoprim-sulfamethoxazole for the prevention of spontaneous bacterial peritonitis in cirrhosis: a randomized trial. *Ann Intern Med.* 1995;122:595-598.

Sort P, Navasa M, Arroyo V, et al. Effect of intravenous albumin on renal impairment and mortality in patients with cirrhosis and spontaneous bacterial peritonitis. *N Engl J Med.* 1999;341:403-409.

Strate LL, Gralnek IM. ACG clinical guideline: management of patients with acute lower gastrointestinal bleeding. *Am J Gastroenterol.* 2016;111(4):459-474.

Surawicz CM, Brandt LJ, Binion DG, et al. Guidelines for diagnosis, treatment, and prevention of *Clostridium difficile* infections. *Am J Gastroenterol.* 2013;108(4):478-498.

Tapper EB, Sengupta N, Bonder A. The incidence and outcomes of ischemic hepatitis: a systematic review with meta-analysis. *Am J Med.* 2015;128(12):1314-1321.

Tenner S, Baillie J, DeWitt J, Vege SS; American College of Gastroenterology. American College of Gastroenterology guideline: management of acute pancreatitis. *Am J Gastroenterol.* 2013;108(9):1400-1416.

Thursz MR, Richardson P, Allison M, et al. Prednisolone or pentoxifylline for alcoholic hepatitis. *N Engl J Med.* 2015;372(17):1619-1628.

Tilsed JV, Casamassima A, Kurihara H, et al. European Society for Trauma and Emergency Surgery guidelines: acute mesenteric ischaemia. *Eur J Trauma Emerg Surg.* 2016;42:253-270.

Tzakis AG, Gordon RD, Shaw BW, Iwatsuki S, Starzl TE. Clinical presentation of hepatic artery thrombosis after liver transplantation in the cyclosporine era. *Transplantation.* 1985;40:667-671

van Santvoort HC, Bakker OJ, Bollen TL, et al. A conservative and minimally invasive approach to necrotizing pancreatitis improves outcome. *Gastroenterology.* 2011;141(4):1254-1263.

Villanueva C, Colomo A, Bosch A, et al. Transfusion strategies for acute upper gastrointestinal bleeding. *N Engl J Med.* 2013;368(1):11-21.

Vilstrup H, Amodio P, Bajaj J, et al. Hepatic encephalopathy in chronic liver disease: 2014 Practice Guideline by the American Association for the Study of Liver Diseases and the European Association for the Study of the Liver. *J Hepatol.* 2014;61(3):642-659.

Witzke O, Baumann M, Patschan D, et al. Which patients benefit from hemodialysis therapy in hepatorenal syndrome? *J Gastroenterol Hepatol.* 2004;19:1369-1373.

Wu BU, Hwang JQ, Gardner TH, et al. Lactated Ringer's solution reduces systemic inflammation compared with saline in patients with acute pancreatitis. *Clin Gastroenterol Hepatol.* 2011;9(8):710-717.

23

Renal, Infectious, Electrolytes, and Other General Critical Care Questions

Jason L. Sanders, MD, PhD, Nicole Ruopp, MD, Alyssa Y. Castillo, MD, Julia Ann Roberts, MD, Max W. Adelman, MD, Caitlin Lee Cohen, MD, and Saef Izzy, MD

Questions

1. A patient presents after a several-day history of abdominal pain and diarrhea, accompanied by minimal food and fluid intake due to feeling "unwell." Initial laboratory evaluation reveals the following. What is the acid-base abnormality in this patient?

pH	7.30
PCO$_2$	30 mm Hg
HCO$_3^-$	16 mmol/L
Anion gap	17 mmol/L

   A. Anion gap metabolic acidosis

   B. Anion gap metabolic acidosis and respiratory acidosis

   C. Normal anion gap metabolic acidosis and respiratory acidosis

   D. Anion gap metabolic acidosis and metabolic alkalosis

   E. Anion gap metabolic acidosis and normal anion gap metabolic acidosis

2. A patient is admitted to the intensive care unit (ICU) after being found down next to several empty pill bottles. She is unarousable to voice and noxious stimuli, with significant metabolic disarray noted on laboratory evaluation. After conversing with her parents, you suspect that the patient has ingested large amounts of aspirin. You would expect her labs to reflect which of the following?

   A. Anion gap metabolic acidosis

   B. Normal anion gap metabolic acidosis

   C. Anion gap metabolic acidosis and respiratory alkalosis

   D. Anion gap metabolic acidosis and respiratory acidosis

   E. Normal anion gap metabolic acidosis and metabolic alkalosis

3. A patient is admitted to the hospital with profound nausea and emesis and is found to have a small bowel obstruction. Prior to a definitive diagnosis, the patient is started on piperacillin-tazobactam, metronidazole, and vancomycin. Several days into his hospital course, laboratory evaluation reveals the below values. Serum pH returns to normal with infusion of sodium chloride (NaCl). Which of the

following is likely to be the cause of this patient's metabolic alkalosis?

pH	7.52
PCO_2	44 mm Hg
HCO_3^-	30 mmol/L

A. Excessive use of calcium carbonate ($CaCO_3$) for nausea

B. Mineralocorticoid excess

C. Use of piperacillin-tazobactam

D. Frequent nasogastric (NG) tube suctioning

E. Hypomagnesemia

4. A patient is brought to the emergency department (ED) with nausea, vomiting, and altered mental status after a presumed toxic ingestion. Initial labs reveal the below values. Which substance did this patient most likely ingest?

pH	7.25
PCO_2	33 mm Hg
Sodium (Na)	140 mmol/L
Potassium (K)	3.9 mmol/L
Chloride (Cl^-)	101 mmol/L
HCO_3^-	18 mmol/L
Blood urea nitrogen (BUN)	67 mg/dL
Creatinine (Cr)	2.4 mg/dL
Glucose	100 mg/dL
Anion gap	20 mmol/L
Plasma osmolality	298 mOsm/kg H_2O
Serum ethanol (EtOH)	<10 mg/dL

A. Ethylene glycol

B. Acetaminophen

C. Salicylates

D. Methanol

5. A patient presents to the hospital feeling "short of breath." She carries a diagnosis of chronic obstructive pulmonary disease (COPD) and is found to be wheezing with a respiratory rate of 26 breaths/min upon physical exam. You worry that she is having an acute exacerbation of her baseline COPD. Labs

obtained upon presentation (room air) are shown below. What can you determine about this patient's clinical status?

pH	7.28
$PaCO_2$	65 mm Hg
PaO_2	80 mm Hg
Na	142 mmol/L
K	3.8 mmol/L
Cl^-	101 mmol/L
HCO_3^-	34 mmol/L
BUN	15 mg/dL
Cr	0.9 mg/dL
Glucose	98 mg/dL

A. Her hypercarbia likely indicates an acute COPD exacerbation.

B. Her obstructive lung disease is likely at baseline; look for other causes of dyspnea.

C. This patient is tachypneic in response to a metabolic acidosis, which should be identified and addressed.

D. This patient has a metabolic alkalosis and is retaining carbon dioxide (CO_2) as a compensatory response.

6. A 42-year-old man is transferred from an outside hospital with a white blood cell (WBC) count of 81,000 cells/μL with circulating blasts, mild anemia, and thrombocytopenia. His labs are also notable for a sodium of 150 mmol/L. He complains of a tongue hematoma, fatigue for 3 months, and extreme thirst. His blood smear was purportedly positive in the outside records for bilobed blasts, azurophilic granules, and Auer rods, but the original report and the slides were not sent with the patient. He arrives at 2:00 a.m. when no hematologist or pathologist is available to review his blood smear. What is the most appropriate treatment overnight?

A. Start cytarabine

B. Start all-*trans*-retinoic acid

C. No treatment until your hospital's hematologist reviews the slide or flow cytometry returns

D. Start desmopressin

E. Start leukapheresis

7. A 62-year-old woman with rheumatoid arthritis on chronic prednisone is admitted to the ICU with 4 days of bloody diarrhea. On hospital day 2, a computed tomography (CT) scan of the abdomen shows diffuse colitis. She is started on ciprofloxacin and metronidazole, and on hospital day 3, she has a seizure and is treated with intravenous (IV) lorazepam. She has 2 subsequent seizures and is intubated for airway protection, sedated with propofol, and transferred to the ICU. Her labs are notable for a Cr 3.7 mg/dL (from baseline 0.86 mg/dL), potassium of 5.4 mmol/L, international normalized ratio (INR) 1.1, hemoglobin (Hgb) 8.3 g/dL, WBC 21,000 cells/µL, and platelets 41,000/µL. Lactate dehydrogenase (LDH) is elevated, and haptoglobin is pending. Electroencephalography (EEG) shows epileptiform activity any time propofol is weaned. She requires norepinephrine and vasopressin to maintain mean arterial pressure (MAP) >65 mm Hg. On hospital day 4, her stool studies come back positive for Shiga toxin, and cultures grow *Escherichia coli* O157:H7. Urine output has dropped to 300 mL/d over the past 2 days. In addition to suppressing seizure, what is the most important next management?

A. Start eculizumab

B. Initiate plasmapheresis

C. Broaden from ciprofloxacin/metronidazole to meropenem/metronidazole

D. Transfuse platelets

E. Initiate continuous venovenous hemofiltration

8. A 72-year-old man is admitted to the ICU from the endoscopy suite after esophagogastroduodenoscopy for duodenal ulcer complicated by a gastrointestinal bleed requiring transfusion of 2 units of packed red blood cells (PRBCs). The ulcer is deep, but hemostasis is achieved with clipping during endoscopy. On hospital day 4, he has a large-volume melena followed by gross hematemesis. His blood pressure drops from 98/56 mm Hg to 75/44 mm Hg during this episode, and he is given 6 L of normal saline as well as 8 units of O⁻ blood in the 45 minutes it takes to prepare the interventional radiology (IR) suite. He is taken to the IR, but despite best efforts, hemostasis is not achieved and he dies. Which of the following would be most likely to have helped achieve hemostasis?

A. Transfusing plasma, platelets, and PRBCs in a 1:1:1 ratio

B. Transfusing plasma, platelets, and PRBCs in a 1:1:2 ratio

C. Less aggressive crystalloid use

D. Use of bicarbonate to correct acidosis

9. A 66-year-old man is found unconscious in a snow bank. His vitals are as follows: temperature 92.5°F, blood pressure 102/56 mm Hg, pulse 46 bpm, and respiratory rate 10 breaths/min. His blood alcohol level is elevated. Labs are notable for Cr 1.5 mg/dL, K 5.9 mmol/L, INR 1.6, partial thromboplastin time (PTT) 58.4 seconds, WBC 14,000 cells/µL, Hgb 10.1 g/dL, and platelets 24,000/µL. Liver function tests are pending. His chest x-ray shows right middle and right lower lobe patchy opacities concerning for aspiration pneumonia. He has red blood in the Foley catheter and blood at the corners of his mouth. A wound on his right calf is continually trickling, and his feet appear dusky. What is the best treatment to improve his bleeding?

A. Give antithrombin III

B. Broad-spectrum antibiotics

C. Use of heating pads and warm saline gastric lavage

D. Transfusion of fresh frozen plasma

E. Transfusion of platelets

10. A 77-year-old woman presents with 3 months of fatigue, headache, blurred vision, and intermittent nosebleeds. Her vitals are as follows: temperature 97.8°F, blood pressure 147/86 mm Hg, pulse 78 bpm, and respiratory rate 18 breaths/min. Her initial labs are notable for hemoglobin 10.6 g/dL, WBC 8300 cells/μL, platelets 124,000/μL, INR 1.1, and PTT 52.7 seconds. Basic metabolic panel is notable only for Cr 1.1 mg/dL and Na 132 mEq/L (unknown baseline). Urinalysis is notable for 1+ proteinuria. She has 5-beat nystagmus and a palpable spleen on exam. Appropriate laboratories are sent, but while waiting for their return, the patient develops a blind spot in her left eye. Fundoscopic exam at this time reveals a small retinal hemorrhage and sausaging of the arteries. Which of the following therapies should you start immediately?

   A. Plasmapheresis

   B. Laser ablation of the hemorrhage

   C. Rituximab

   D. Antihypertensives

   E. IV fluids

11. A 67-year-old woman is admitted to the ICU with a right lower lobe pneumonia. She is hypotensive with a blood pressure of 94/66 mm Hg and tachycardic to 150 bpm. An electrocardiogram (ECG) is obtained, and she is found to have new-onset atrial fibrillation. Antibiotics and IV fluids are given. Thyroid studies are obtained with the results shown below. Given these findings, what is the recommended treatment?

	Results	Reference Range
Thyroid-stimulating hormone (TSH)	3 mIU/mL	2-11 mIU/mL
Total thyroxine (T$_4$)	4 μg/dL	5-12 μg/dL
Free T$_4$	0.5 ng/dL	0.8-2.84 ng/dL
Triiodothyronine (T$_3$)	75 ng/dL	90-200 ng/dL
Reverse Triiodothyronine (rT$_3$)	93 ng/dL	13-50 ng/dL

   A. Continue antibiotics and supportive care only

   B. Start IV levothyroxine

   C. Start IV levothyroxine and hydrocortisone

   D. Start propranolol, methimazole, and hydrocortisone

12. A 55-year-old man presents to the ED obtunded with a new left lower lobe pneumonia in the setting of several months of progressive fatigue. He has hypertension, hyperlipidemia, and hypothyroidism. His family reports increasing apathy and lethargy over the past several months, which has culminated in more recent weight gain and confusion prior to onset of his respiratory symptoms. Vitals are notable for a temperature of 35°C, blood pressure of 94/56 mm Hg, heart rate of 42 bpm, respiratory rate of 8 breaths/min, and oxygen saturation (SpO$_2$) of 97% on 3 L nasal cannula. On exam, he is altered and lethargic, but arousable to sternal rub. His pulmonary exam is notable for crackles in his left base. You also note a well-healed thyroidectomy scar on his neck. Laboratory exam is notable for the following: WBC 15,000 cell/μL with 90% polymorphonuclear leukocytes, Na 128 mEq/L, and glucose 65 mg/dL. TSH is 27.54 mIU/mL, and free T$_4$ is 0.356 ng/dL. ECG reveals sinus bradycardia. Antibiotics and IV fluids are initiated. What is the next best step in management?

   A. Administer atropine

   B. Administer IV levothyroxine and hydrocortisone

   C. Administer IV levothyroxine

   D. Place a warming blanket

13. A 62-year-old woman with type 2 diabetes mellitus is admitted to the ICU with septic shock attributed to a urinary tract infection. IV fluids and antibiotics are initiated, and her vital signs stabilize. A blood glucose is checked and returns at 350 mg/dL. The team initiates an insulin drip targeting a blood glucose level of <110 mg/dL. Which of the following is true regarding intensive insulin therapy (IIT) in the ICU?

   A. Mortality is decreased.

   B. ICU length of stay is reduced.

   C. Ventilator-free days are increased.

   D. Hypoglycemia is a more frequent occurrence.

14. A 66-year-old woman is admitted to the ICU with altered mental status and severe hyperglycemia following outpatient initiation of prednisone for a mild COPD exacerbation 3 days prior. Past medical history is significant for diabetes mellitus type 2 controlled with multiple oral antihyperglycemics and hypertension, for which she takes metoprolol. Laboratory evaluation is notable for the following:

Sodium (mEq/L)	149
Potassium (mEq/L)	4.3
Chloride (mEq/L)	115
Bicarbonate (mEq/L)	22
Glucose (mg/dL)	916
Serum osmolality (mOsm/kg)	329
Lactate (mg/dL)	0.4

Chest x-ray is normal. Patient is given 1 L of normal saline and 10-unit IV bolus of regular insulin, and an insulin infusion is started. Which of the following is true regarding management of this patient's hyperosmolar hyperglycemic state compared to diabetic ketoacidosis (DKA)?

A. Insulin requirements are usually greater than in DKA.

B. Fluid requirements are less than in DKA.

C. Serum and urine ketones are frequently positive.

D. Transition to subcutaneous insulin should occur upon closure of anion gap.

15. A 56-year-old man is admitted to the ICU with alcohol-induced severe pancreatitis. He requires massive fluid resuscitation for refractory hypotension and briefly required vasopressor support. During fluid resuscitation, he develops worsening hypoxia and work of breathing requiring intubation, but he ultimately stabilizes hemodynamically. Over the next 48 hours, he develops worsening hypotension with blood pressure of 85/52 mm Hg and heart rate of 125 bpm. He remains ventilated; however, his peak pressures have uptrended from 20 to 41 cm H_2O with stable tidal volumes, and his urine output has decreased from 30 to 8 mL/h. On exam, he is moving air well throughout his chest, but exam is notable for a tense, distended abdomen and anasarca. Laboratory exam reveals BUN has increased from 31 to 55 mg/dL and Cr has increased from 1.4 to 3.2 mg/dL. A bladder pressure is obtained and is noted to be 23 mm Hg. Which of the following is most likely to lead to an improvement in his renal failure?

A. 1 L bolus of normal saline (NS)

B. Diagnostic paracentesis

C. Therapeutic paracentesis

D. Initiation of vasopressors

Questions 16 and 17

A 68-year-old woman with hypothyroidism, alcohol abuse disorder, and alcoholic cirrhosis presents to the ED following a fall at home. She reports feeling poorly for 2 days prior to the fall with symptoms of nausea, vomiting, and poor oral intake. Her home medications include levothyroxine, lactulose, nadolol, furosemide, and spironolactone. On exam, she is afebrile, heart rate is 68 bpm, blood pressures is 112/62 mm Hg, and SpO_2 is 94% on room air. She has spider angiomas and a mildly distended abdomen without fluid wave. Mucous membranes are dry. She is alert and oriented and is following commands; there is no asterixis. Admission labs are notable for a serum Na of 107 mEq/L, K of 4.2 mEq/L, and Cr of 2.3 mg/dL (baseline 0.7 mg/dL). A chest x-ray and noncontrast CT scan of the head show no abnormalities.

16. What additional laboratory studies are required to identify the source of this patient's hyponatremia?

  I. Serum osmolality

  II. Urine osmolality and urine Na

  III. TSH and serum glucose

  IV. Triglycerides

  V. Aldosterone level

A. Only I

B. I and II

C. I, II, and III

D. I, II, III, and IV

E. I, II, III, IV, and V

17. Further testing demonstrates a serum osmolality of 245 mOsm/kg, urine osmolality of 348 mOsm/kg, and urine Na of 15 mEq/L. TSH is stable from prior value at 2.45 U/mL. Based on these studies, what is the most likely etiology of her hyponatremia?

   A. Low effective arterial blood volume 2/2 decompensated cirrhosis

   B. Syndrome of inappropriate antidiuretic hormone (SIADH)

   C. Hypovolemia

   D. Beer potomania

   E. Low-solute diet ("tea and toast diet")

Questions 18 and 19

A 21-year-old woman is brought to the ED by her family for nausea, vomiting, abdominal pain, and confusion. Her mother reports that she has been urinating frequently and complaining of burning with urination; the patient is unable to provide any further history. Her vital signs are temperature of 98.8°F, pulse of 110 bpm, blood pressure of 90/60 mm Hg, respiratory rate of 30 breaths/min, and SpO_2 of 98% on room air. Her exam is notable for dry mucous membranes, deep and rapid breathing, and a fruity smell on her breath. Presenting labs show the following: serum Na 141, K 3.1, Cl⁻ 102, CO_2 15, and glucose 631. Arterial blood gas (ABG) shows pH 7.17, PCO_2 24 mm Hg, and PO_2 of 59 mm Hg.

18. What is the best initial treatment for this patient?

   I. Aggressive fluid resuscitation with 3 L NS

   II. Potassium supplementation of 40 mEq/L NS

   III. Regular insulin bolus of 10 U IV followed by regular insulin gtt at 0.1 U/kg/h

   IV. Sodium bicarbonate IV infusion

   A. I and II

   B. I, II, and IV

   C. I, II, and III

   D. All of the above

19. The patient is transferred to the ICU for DKA management and frequent lab monitoring. She is treated with aggressive fluid resuscitation, potassium repletion, and started on an insulin gtt. Twenty-four hours later, her anion gap has closed to 8 mEq/L, and her serum glucose level is 270 mg/dL. What is the next best step in management?

   A. Continue insulin gtt until glucose is <150 mg/dL

   B. Discontinue insulin gtt and give 0.5 U/kg long-acting insulin subcutaneously (SC)

   C. Continue insulin gtt and give 0.5 U/kg long-acting insulin SC

   D. Discontinue insulin gtt and begin scheduled mealtime short-acting insulin SC

20. A 72-year-old woman with a history of coronary artery disease, paroxysmal atrial fibrillation on warfarin, and mild COPD was found down at home. She was brought by ambulance to the ED. She was intubated for airway protection. Non-contrast enhanced head CT showed a moderately large frontal intraparenchymal hemorrhage. She was admitted to the neuro-ICU for neuromonitoring and blood pressure control. After 1 week, she showed some neurologic recovery but failed a spontaneous breathing trial and was unable to be extubated. Four days later, she developed a fever to 100.8°F that responded to acetaminophen, and then 2 episodes of mild, brief hypotension that were responsive to fluid boluses. Blood, urine, and sputum cultures were drawn. Chest x-ray was indeterminate for pneumonia versus atelectasis. She was started on vancomycin and piperacillin-tazobactam for a presumed hospital-acquired infection. She remained euvolemic and hemodynamically stable on similar ventilator settings. Cultures showed no growth to date. Three days later, she developed acute kidney injury. Microscopic examination of the urine showed some WBC casts, no red cell casts, and no crystals. What is the most appropriate next step in management of her acute kidney injury?

   A. Additional volume resuscitation

   B. Initiate hemodialysis

   C. Discontinue antibiotics

   D. Obtain abdominal CT angiogram

   E. Continue to monitor

21. A 32-year-old man with paraplegia is admitted to the hospital for suicide attempt by consuming 50 pills of sertraline. He suffered a motor vehicle collision 3 years ago. His course was complicated by paraplegia, which was further complicated by multiple ventilator-associated pneumonias and need for tracheostomy, which has since been reversed. Tissue and blood cultures have previously been positive for multidrug-resistant gram-positive and gram-negative organisms. Paraplegia worsened his underlying depression, and he has required psychiatric hospitalizations due to suicide attempts. On admission, he is noted to have worsening decubitus and heel ulcers with purulent drainage. Based on prior culture data, he is started on linezolid, ceftazidime, and metronidazole.

On day 4 of admission, he develops tachycardia with a heart rate of 115 bpm and a fever to 100.8°F. Physical exam is notable for agitation, dry mucous membranes, flushed skin, and mild tremor in his upper extremities. What is the next best step in management?

A. Administer lorazepam
B. Change ceftazidime to meropenem
C. Discontinue linezolid
D. Administer fluid bolus
E. Administer acetaminophen

22. A 68-year-old man with a history of congestive heart failure, coronary artery disease, hypertension, bipolar disorder, and schizophrenia who lives in a group home is brought to the ED by his roommate. The roommate found him talking incoherently for the entire afternoon. The roommate notes that the patient has had intermittent headaches for several days. Upon arrival to the ED, vitals are as follows: temperature 100.8°F, heart rate 92 bpm, blood pressure 110/65 mm Hg, and SpO$_2$ 99% on room air. His initial lab work shows the following:

Na (mEq/L) 134
K (mEq/L) 3.5
Cl$^-$ (mEq/L) 88
HCO$_3^-$ (mEq/L) 22
BUN (mg/dL) 12
Cr (mg/dL) 0.9
WBC (cells/μL) 12.5

A noncontrast head CT shows no acute process. A lumbar puncture is performed, which is notable for opening pressure of 24 mm H$_2$O, glucose of 48 mg/dL, and protein of 75 mg/dL (normal <45 mg/dL). He is started on vancomycin, ceftriaxone, and acyclovir empirically. His neurologic status rapidly declines. He is intubated for inability to protect his airway. An orogastric tube and urinary catheter are placed. He is admitted to the neuro-ICU. He remains hemodynamically stable and euvolemic. Infectious studies are pending. On day 3 of admission, his creatinine is 3.3 mg/dL, and his urine output decreases. Bladder scan shows no residual. What is the next best step in management?

A. Aggressive fluid resuscitation
B. Discontinue acyclovir
C. Replace the urinary catheter
D. Discontinue vancomycin
E. Obtain renal ultrasound

23. A 76-year-old woman with a history of mild Alzheimer dementia, gastroesophageal reflux disease, and osteoporosis is found at home by her children muttering incoherently. They take her to the ED. On arrival, vitals are as follows: temperature 101.7°F, heart rate 115 bpm, blood pressure 85/40 mm Hg, and SpO$_2$ 98% on room air. Initial labs show the following:

Na (mEq/L) 132
K (mEq/L) 3.2
Cl$^-$ (mEq/L) 85
HCO$_3^-$ (mEq/L) 16
BUN (mg/dL) 45
Cr (mg/dL) 2.3
Lactate (mg/dL) 3.9
WBC (cells/μL) 14.5
Hgb (g/dL) 10.1
ABG: pH 7.25, PCO$_2$ 30 mm Hg, PO$_2$ 110 mm Hg

Blood cultures and urine cultures are drawn. She is diagnosed with sepsis due to a urinary tract infection. She is resuscitated with IV crystalloid. Over the next 2 days, her condition improves, she is weaned off pressors, she requires no further fluid resuscitation, and her acute kidney injury nearly resolves. She no longer requires intensive care. She is awaiting transfer to the floor. Blood and urine cultures show the following:

Anaerobic bottle: *Enterobacter cloacae* **complex**

Antibiotic	Mean Inhibitory Concentration (mg/L)	Interpretation
Amikacin	<2	Susceptible
Amoxicillin/ clavulanate	>32	Resistant
Ampicillin	>32	Resistant
Aztreonam	<1	Susceptible
Cefazolin	>64	Resistant
Cefepime	<1	Susceptible
Ceftriaxone	<1	Susceptible
Ciprofloxacin	<0.25	Susceptible
Ertapenem	<0.5	Susceptible
Gentamicin	<1	Susceptible
Imipenem	<0.25	Susceptible
Levofloxacin	<0.12	Susceptible
Meropenem	<0.25	Susceptible
Piperacillin/ tazobactam	<4	Susceptible
Tetracycline	<1	Susceptible
Trimethoprim/ sulfamethoxazole	<20	Susceptible

What is the most appropriate antibiotic for ongoing treatment?

A. Trimethoprim-sulfamethoxazole

B. Doxycycline

C. Ceftriaxone

D. Ciprofloxacin

E. Cefepime

24. A 52-year-old man presents to the ED with 2 days of mildly progressive facial pain and nasal drainage. Beginning the morning of presentation, he noted redness, swelling, and pain of the right inferior orbit. He has coronary artery disease, hypertension, and diabetes mellitus. He had rapidly progressive renal disease and, after being on hemodialysis, received a renal transplant 3 years ago. He has done well since then without complication and has not required dialysis after transplant. He is compliant with all his medications.

In the ED, vitals are as follows: temperature 100.7°F, heart rate 93 bpm, blood pressure 135/84 mm Hg, and SpO$_2$ 99% on room air. Exam reveals purulent nasal drainage, right inferior orbit swelling with overlying erythema, and sinus tenderness. He has full extraocular motions without pain. He is diagnosed with sinusitis complicated by preseptal cellulitis. Cultures of the nares and eye are obtained. IV vancomycin, ceftazidime, and metronidazole are started, and the patient is admitted. Over the next 12 hours, his symptoms worsen, and his pain becomes intense. He has intermittent low-volume epistaxis. What is the next best step in management?

A. Switch ceftazidime to cefepime

B. Begin sinus irrigation

C. Obtain CT of the face

D. Obtain urgent surgical consultation

E. Continue to monitor awaiting culture data

25. A 75-year-old man with hypertension, hyperlipidemia, chronic kidney disease, diabetes, severe COPD, prior myocardial infarction, and prior transient ischemic attacks suddenly collapses while shopping in the grocery store. Emergency services arrive, and on scene, his finger stick blood glucose is 125 mg/dL. He is not moving his left arm or left leg and is slurring his words. In the ED, his initial vitals are as follows: heart rate 78 bpm, blood pressure 147/84 mm Hg, respiratory rate 12 breaths/min, and SpO$_2$ 94% on room air. He weighs 80 kg. He is diagnosed with an acute ischemic stroke. Stat noncontrast head CT shows no acute process, and tissue plasminogen activator (tPA) is given.

   Thirty minutes later, he suddenly complains of a headache. He becomes unresponsive but maintains pulses. His SpO$_2$ worsens to 85% but improves with jaw thrusting and application of supplemental oxygen. He is intubated for airway protection. Initial settings for assist-control, volume-control ventilation are tidal volume 800 mL, rate 16, positive end-expiratory pressure (PEEP) 10 cm H$_2$O, and fraction of inspired oxygen (FiO$_2$) 60% to maintain SpO$_2$ >94%. Another stat noncontrast head CT shows an intraparenchymal hemorrhage. He is taken to the neuro-ICU for further care. An hour after arrival, his blood pressure declines to 105/77 mm Hg, and then to 95/74 mm Hg. He is given a bolus of crystalloid. He then suffers a cardiac arrest; the monitor shows pulseless electrical activity (PEA). What may have prevented his cardiac arrest?

   A. Placement of an intraventricular drain

   B. Earlier volume resuscitation

   C. Empiric antibiotics

   D. Disconnecting the ventilator temporarily

   E. Administration of aspirin

26. A 60-year-old woman with a 120-pack-year smoking history, severe COPD, anxiety, hypertension, and prior gastric bypass surgery is admitted to the ICU with sepsis due to a urinary tract infection. She is initially hypotensive and requires volume resuscitation. Normally, she requires 2 L of oxygen by nasal cannula (NC) at all times to maintain SpO$_2$ >92%. She develops increased work of breathing. Her SpO$_2$ is 92% on 6 L NC. She is anxious and asks for more oxygen. She is given 1 mg of lorazepam, and her oxygen is increased to 10 L NC. Oxygen saturation increases to 98%. Chest x-ray shows hyperinflated lungs. She remains at this level of inspired oxygen. Three hours later, her respiratory rate declines, and her oxygen saturation declines to 92%. She appears more somnolent. Bilevel positive airway pressure (BiPAP) noninvasive ventilation is initiated. Her oxygen saturation improves to 96%, but she remains somnolent. Out of concern for inability to protect her airway, she is intubated. Under what circumstance could intubation have been prevented?

   A. If she was not given lorazepam for anxiety

   B. If she was not volume resuscitated

   C. If she was placed on BiPAP earlier

   D. If her oxygen was not increased from 6 to 10 L

Answers and Explanations

1. E. This patient presents with a serum pH of 7.30, indicative of acidemia. Lab values of bicarbonate (HCO_3^-; 16 mmol/L) and partial pressure of carbon dioxide (PCO_2; 30 mm Hg) reveal a metabolic acidosis with adequate respiratory compensation. The elevated anion gap at 17 mmol/L further describes the presence of an anion gap metabolic acidosis, potentially due to lactic acidosis or ketosis in the setting of poor oral intake. Examination of the "gap-gap" ratio, however, reveals the following:

$$\text{Anion gap (AG) excess}/HCO_3^- \text{ deficit}$$
$$= (AG - 12)/(24 - HCO_3^-)$$
$$= (17 - 12)/(24 - 16) = 5/8$$

Thus, the gap-gap ratio is <1, signaling a greater decrease in HCO_3^- than increase in anion gap. This signals the co-existence of a normal anion gap (hyperchloremic) metabolic acidosis in this patient, likely due to the patient's preceding history of diarrhea.

2. C. Aspirin, or acetylsalicylic acid, is a salicylate. Ingestion of high amounts of salicylates (>150 mg/kg) triggers both a primary metabolic acidosis and a primary respiratory alkalosis, resulting in a mixed acid-base disorder with normal pH. Salicylic acid uncouples oxidative phosphorylation within mitochondria, spurring lactic acid production via anaerobic metabolism to create an anion gap metabolic acidosis. Salicylic acid also acts directly on the respiratory neurons within the brainstem, driving an increase in minute ventilation that produces a respiratory alkalosis. Over time, the metabolic acidosis will worsen due to accumulating lactic acid, driving a decrease in serum pH.

3. D. Although all of the answers can result in metabolic alkalosis, only 1 of these causes is fluid responsive—frequent NG tube suctioning. This patient has developed a metabolic alkalosis over the course of his hospitalization. Return of the serum pH to normal following administration of normal saline demonstrates the presences of a chloride-responsive metabolic alkalosis. Conditions underlying chloride-responsive metabolic alkaloses include:

- Vomiting
- Frequent NG tube suctioning (due to loss of hydrogen chloride in gastric fluid)
- Extracellular volume loss and loop/thiazide diuretic use (due to overall chloride depletion)

Mineralocorticoid excess is classified as a chloride-resistant metabolic alkalosis and would not be expected to improve with NaCl infusion. Excessive use of $CaCO_3$ (antacids) can result in metabolic alkalosis as carbonate acts as a base. Some antibiotics can cause metabolic alkalosis, and although exceedingly rare, piperacillin-tazobactam can cause a non–fluid-responsive metabolic alkalosis. Lastly, hypomagnesemia results in potassium and acid wasting in the kidney and a non–fluid-responsive metabolic alkalosis.

4. A. This patient presents with an anion gap metabolic acidosis after presumed toxic ingestion. The formula for calculated plasma osmolality is:

$$\text{Plasma osmolality} = (2 \times [Na^+]) + [glucose]/18 + BUN/2.8$$

Thus, this patient's calculated plasma osmolality is 309 mOsm/kg H_2O. Measured plasma osmolality is 290 mOsm/kg H_2O. Therefore, this patient's osmolar gap is 19 mOsm/kg H_2O (normal <10 mOsm/kg H_2O). The presence of an osmolar gap raises suspicion for either ethylene glycol or methanol ingestion. Of these 2 possibilities, the presence of renal dysfunction makes ethylene glycol the more likely ingested substance. The main ingredient in antifreeze, ethylene glycol metabolism results in the formation of oxalic acid, which then combines with calcium to form calcium oxalate crystals. These insoluble crystals precipitate within the tubular lumen, causing damage to the renal tubules. Examination of the urine for crystalluria may reveal thin, needle-shaped calcium oxalate monohydrate crystals.

5. **B.** Examination of this patient's arterial blood gas (ABG) shows a primary respiratory acidosis. A serum HCO_3^- of 34 mmol/L suggests a degree of metabolic compensation compatible with chronic respiratory acidosis, rather than acute.

The expected metabolic compensation for an acute respiratory acidosis is:

$$\Delta\, HCO_3^- = 0.1 \times \Delta\, PaCO_2 = 0.1 \times 25 = 2.5$$

The expected HCO_3^- in adequate compensation for acute respiratory acidosis would be 24 + 2.5 = 26.5.

The expected metabolic compensation for a chronic respiratory acidosis is:

$$\Delta\, HCO_3^- = 0.4 \times \Delta\, PaCO_2 = 0.4 \times 25 = 10$$

The expected HCO_3^- in adequate compensation for a chronic respiratory acidosis would be 24 + 10 = 34.

Thus, this patient has appropriately compensated for a chronic respiratory acidosis. She likely has baseline hypercarbia in the setting of COPD that has not acutely worsened. Other causes for her dyspnea should be sought.

6. **B.** This patient likely has acute promyelocytic leukemia (APML), which has not been confirmed but is highly suggested by the presence of Auer rods at an outside hospital. APML should be treated as early as possible with all-*trans*-retinoic-acid (ATRA). ATRA is a fairly benign form of chemotherapy, although a systemic inflammatory response syndrome (SIRS)–like response called differentiation syndrome can occur. Starting ATRA as soon as possible is preferred over waiting for flow cytometry or a second read because APML is a highly treatable condition, and many of those who die from it die from early hemorrhagic complications before starting treatment.

Cytarabine is used for acute myeloid leukemia (AML) and has many side effects and should not be started until APML is ruled out. Indications for leukapheresis include the following:

- WBC count of >100,000/μL in the acute setting
- WBC count of >300,000/μL in the chronic setting
- Hyperviscosity such as myocardial infarction, confusion, diffuse alveolar hemorrhage, or pulmonary edema

Leukostasis does seem to be more common in APML than AML, so these patients should be monitored closely with frequent WBC and symptom checks. With a sodium of 150 mmol/L, this patient is likely exhibiting central involvement of APML and a central diabetes insipidus, a rare but known complication of APML. Desmopressin is a reasonable treatment for this central diabetes insipidus, but a sodium of 150 mmol/L is unlikely to cause long-term harm to the patient, whereas a hemorrhagic complication of APML might.

7. **E.** This patient's hyperkalemia, renal failure, and oliguria are indicative that she will imminently need renal replacement therapy, and her blood pressures likely will not support typical hemodialysis.

Eculizumab is a c5-complement inhibitor that has been researched in atypical hemolytic-uremic syndrome (HUS), but only minimally studied for Shiga-like toxic *E coli* (STEC) HUS. It is still used sometimes in early STEC-HUS with neurologic involvement, but the evidence is not sufficient in patients with multiple organ failure.

Antibiotics in HUS are still a highly contentious topic, with many practitioners believing that use of antibiotics for enterohemorrhagic *E coli* worsens the risk of HUS by increasing Shiga toxin production, based on in vitro studies and several studies of children with STEC-HUS. However, a larger German study of an *E coli* O104 outbreak indicated that antibiotics (multiple agents used, most commonly meropenem/metronidazole) were associated with a lower incidence of seizure or death; however, this is a flawed study on a different strain. However, in a patient who has HUS and is already been on antibiotics, adding more antibiotics is unlikely to substantively improve or worsen outcomes.

Plasmapheresis is indicated in thrombotic thrombocytopenic purpura (TTP) or undifferentiated TTP/HUS. For known STEC-HUS, plasmapheresis is not indicated. Prednisone should not be stopped suddenly in this patient because stopping it is unlikely to worsen her HUS and it could cause relative adrenal insufficiency. Platelet transfusion is not indicated in HUS unless someone has a critical bleed because it is a consumptive process that would likely consume any transfused platelets, exposing the patient to risk without any clear benefit.

8. A. The current recommendation for replacing blood products in the setting of hemorrhagic shock is to use a 1:1:1 ratio of plasma, platelets, and PRBCs for any patient who requires massive transfusion. A phase III, multisite, randomized clinical trial of 680 severely injured patients who arrived at level I trauma centers in North America showed that using a 1:1:1 strategy, versus 1:1:2 strategy, was associated with an improvement of hemostasis and mortality rates, but not in all other causes of mortality at 24 hours and 30 days. This study mostly looked at the trauma population, which is likely to be a population more at risk for hypercoagulability and bleeding diathesis than the population with gastrointestinal bleeding, but the results can be extrapolated for all patients with massive hemorrhage who require blood product transfusions.

9. C. This patient's low platelets and high INR might be explained by his alcohol use but could also indicate disseminated intravascular coagulation (DIC) in this instance. Active bleeding is indicative of a bleeding diathesis, likely DIC in the setting of hypothermia, although sepsis from pneumonia could also be attributed. He does not have any life-threatening bleeding at this point, however, and transfusion of blood products is unlikely to help. Active rewarming is the answer to correcting his bleeding diathesis. Antibiotics should likely be started, but will not immediately improve his bleeding, especially if he remains cold. Antithrombin III, initially thought to be helpful as a result of its anti-inflammatory and antithrombotic properties, is generally not used in DIC because it increases the risk of bleeding without reduction in risk of mortality.

10. E. This patient is presenting with hyperviscosity syndrome (spontaneous mucous membrane bleeding, headache, retinopathy, fatigue), likely from Waldenström macroglobulinemia. Hyperviscosity can also be seen in polycythemia, multiple myeloma, leukemia, sickle cell disease, and sepsis, but the patient does not have any lab findings to suggest these options.

A serum protein electrophoresis, serum viscosity, and immunoglobulin (Ig) M level should all be sent, and plasmapheresis should be considered given the concern for retinal hemorrhage. However, IV fluid is a fast and effective temporizing measure to prevent further retinal damage while plasmapheresis is being prepared. It is not necessary to pherese someone down to a normal viscosity; the goal of either IV fluids or pheresis is to achieve plasma viscosity of <2.5 while waiting for the initiation of chemotherapy.

11. A. The patient has nonthyroidal illness syndrome (NTIS), previously known as euthyroid sick syndrome, which is a common finding in ICU patients. No treatment is indicated. This syndrome is characterized by normal or low levels of free thyroxine (T_4), low triiodothyronine (T_3), and high reverse triiodothyronine (rT_3). Thyroid-stimulating hormone (TSH) may be normal or low. It was previously felt that these patients represented a euthyroid state, but this has not been substantiated by data. Given the frequency of NTIS in critical illness, it is recommended that thyroid function studies only be checked in patients in whom there is a high index of suspicion for thyroidal illness. Levothyroxine and levothyroxine with hydrocortisone would be indicated in primary hypothyroidism or myxedema coma, respectively; however, TSH would be high in these entities. Propranolol, methimazole, and hydrocortisone would be indicated in thyroid storm; however, one would expect low TSH and high free T_4 in this setting.

Disease	TSH	T_4	Free T_4	rT_3
Primary hypothyroidism	↑	↓	↓	↓
Secondary hypothyroidism	↔ or ↓	↓	↓	↓
Primary hyperthyroidism	↓	↑	↑	↑
Secondary hyperthyroidism	↑	↑	↑	↑
Sick euthyroid	Variable	↔ or ↓	Variable	↔ or ↑

12. **B.** This patient has presented with profound hypothyroidism and requires prompt initiation of IV levothyroxine and hydrocortisone. Severe or inadequately treated hypothyroidism can progress to myxedema coma or may be precipitated following exposure to an infectious stressor, myocardial infarction, exposure to extreme cold, or administration of sedative medications.

Some of the common signs and symptoms of myxedema coma include:

- Sinus bradycardia
- Hypothermia
- Hypoventilation
- Hyponatremia
- Hypoglycemia
- Lethargy and fatigue, which can progress to altered mental status and even frank coma

Treatment must be initiated rapidly and includes IV forms of T_4 or T_3. Additionally, patients are at significant risk for concomitant adrenal insufficiency, and thus, stress dose steroids must also be initiated at onset of treatment.

Atropine could be considered for symptomatic bradycardia; however, this patient's bradycardia is secondary to hypothyroidism and will respond to IV levothyroxine. A warming blanket would address this patient's hypothermia but would not correct the underlying etiology.

13. **D.** Intensive insulin therapy (IIT) as an ICU glucose management strategy has been evaluated by several randomized controlled trials and 2 meta-analyses. NICE-SUGAR was a large, multicenter randomized controlled trial containing both medical and surgical ICU patients who were randomized to conventional glucose control (target blood glucose <180 mg/dL) versus IIT (target blood glucose 81-108 mg/dL). In this study, although the IIT group was noted to have lower blood glucoses (115 vs 144 mg/dL), they were also noted to have significantly higher 90-day mortality (odds ratio, 1.14; 95% confidence interval [CI], 1.02-1.28) and higher risk of hypoglycemia. This was further validated by a subsequent meta-analysis, comprising 26 randomized controlled trials including NICE-SUGAR. The meta-analysis found a similar mortality among IIT patients compared to conventional glucose control (relative risk of death 0.93; 95% CI, 0.83-1.04), and the pooled relative risk for hypoglycemia with IIT was 6.0 (95% CI, 4.5-8.0). There was a slight benefit in surgical ICU patients with IIT. No difference was found in ICU length of stay or ventilator-free days.

14. **A.** Hyperosmolar hyperglycemic state (HHS), also known as hyperosmolar nonketotic coma (HONKC), is characterized by the following triad of symptoms:

- Hyperosmolality
- Severe hyperglycemia
- Dehydration

Patients frequently present with blood glucose >600 mg/dL and serum osmolality of >320 mOsm/kg. Unlike in DKA, ketoacidosis is typically absent, but encephalopathy is more prominent secondary to the notable hyperosmolality. DKA and HHS frequently exist on a spectrum, with some patients having aspects of both. Treatment centers around IV fluid resuscitation, insulin, and correcting electrolyte imbalances. Typically, fluid requirements are greater in HHS due to the severity of hyperosmolality and secondary osmotic diuresis. Insulin requirements also tend to be higher in HHS than in DKA as these patients have higher levels of insulin resistance. Insulin infusions are continued until osmolality is normalized and the patient's mental status is corrected.

15. **C.** This patient has abdominal compartment syndrome (ACS), which has compromised his renal function, leading to acute kidney injury. ACS is diagnosed by demonstration of intra-abdominal pressures (IAP) ≥20 mm Hg with new organ dysfunction or organ failure.

ACS results from decreased perfusion and oxygen delivery of intra-abdominal organs and can manifest as hypovolemic shock, acute kidney injury, increased intrathoracic pressures with associated respiratory failure, increased intracranial pressure, and hepatic failure.

The ascertainment of intra-abdominal pressures is obtained indirectly by measurement of a urinary bladder pressure. Normal IAP is approximately 5 to 7 mm Hg, although morbidly obese individuals often have higher baseline pressures, ranging from 9 to 14 mm Hg. Intra-abdominal hypertension is defined as IAP ≥12 mm Hg.

Medical management centers around abdominal decompression, most commonly via decompression of solid organ or hollow viscera or space-occupying lesions (eg, ascites, blood, tumors), or correcting conditions that limit abdominal wall expansion.

Medical management of ACS in this patient would include therapeutic paracentesis as a first-line therapy. Refractory cases or severe cases usually require surgical decompression. The massive fluid resuscitation required in this patient in the setting of active capillary leak likely contributed to the development of ACS; thus, further volume resuscitation would likely only further worsen his ACS.

Vasopressor initiation may improve this patient's MAPs and thus may transiently improve renal function; however, this would not be the definitive management of his ACS. Diagnostic paracentesis has no role in the management of ACS.

16. **D.** To rule out pseudohyponatremia, triglyceride levels and a serum glucose are required. A corrected serum Na can be calculated by adding 2.4 to the measured Na for every increase of 100 in the glucose value. Given her history of hypothyroidism, a TSH should be checked to ensure no underlying endocrinopathy. Serum osmolality, urine osmolality, and urine Na are required to determine if antidiuretic hormone is activated and if the kidneys are in a sodium-avid state. An aldosterone level is not required in the evaluation of hyponatremia.

17. **C.** The serum osmolality is less than the urine osmolality, indicating that antidiuretic hormone (ADH) is activated. Her urine Na is less than 20 to 30 mEq/L, indicating that the kidney is in a salt-avid state. Given her dry mucous membranes and acute kidney injury, she is most likely hypovolemic due to her nausea/vomiting, poor oral intake, and concurrent diuretic use. Her chemistries could suggest low effective arterial blood volume (EABV) due to decompensated cirrhosis, but there are no signs of volume overload on her exam. Given that her kidneys are in a sodium-avid state, SIADH can be ruled out; SIADH typically is associated with urine Na >20 to 30 mEq/L.

Beer potomania and low-solute diet are both associated with deactivation of ADH and a urine osmolality of <100 mOsm/kg.

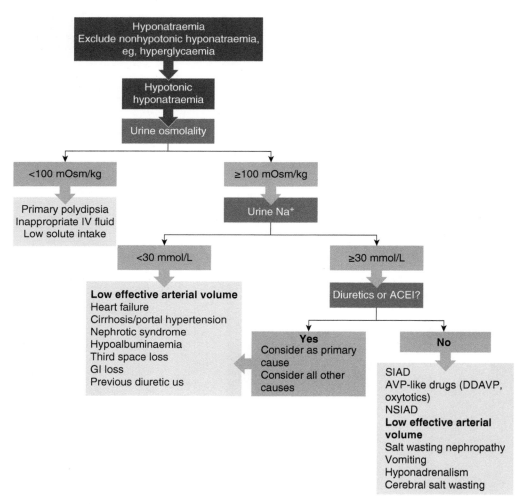

Reproduced with permission from Ball SG. How I approach hyponatraemia. *Clin Med.* 2013 Jun: 13(3):291-295.

18. **A.** This patient has presented in diabetic ketoacidosis (DKA), with grossly elevated serum glucose associated with signs and symptoms of severe dehydration. The foundation of initial treatment in DKA is aggressive fluid resuscitation, as most patients have a 5- to 8-L total body water deficit at the time of presentation. Similarly, patients often have a total body deficit of 300 to 600 mEq of potassium at the time of presentation, requiring aggressive potassium supplementation of 20 to 40 mEq/L with IV fluid resuscitation.

An insulin gtt should not be initiated until the potassium is >3.3 mEq/L, as this puts the patient at risk of severe and potentially life-threatening hypokalemia. There is no evidence to support the use of bicarbonate infusion in patients with a pH of >6.9.

19. **C.** The anion gap has closed, and it is thus safe to begin the transition to subcutaneous (SC) insulin. The correct answer is to continue the insulin infusion and begin weight-based SC long-acting insulin. It is critical to overlap the insulin infusion and SC insulin by approximately 2 to 4 hours in order to prevent the anion gap from reopening. This patient likely has a new diagnosis of type 1 diabetes mellitus and thus will require basal insulin; scheduled mealtime short-acting insulin alone will not be sufficient.

20. **C.** The antibiotics should be discontinued. In an ICU patient with fever and hypotension, it is often warranted to empirically begin anti-infectives while awaiting the results of an infectious workup. Nonetheless, not all fevers or brief episodes of hypotension are due to infection. Piperacillin-tazobactam, in combination with vancomycin, has been associated with acute kidney injury. The mechanism is not fully understood. Preliminary evidence suggests injury may occur through acute tubular necrosis due to direct toxic effect of these antibiotics when given in combination. Moreover, in this case, after more than 48 hours of no culture growth, stable hemodynamics and ventilator settings, and no additional fevers, it is less likely that she had a true infection requiring anti-infectives.

Although hypotension increases risk of renal ischemic injury, brief, mild episodes that are volume responsive and do not require pressors imply that hypotension injury is less likely. Moreover, she has remained euvolemic and hemodynamically stable.

Hemodialysis is not necessary because the patient does not meet criteria for medically refractory renal failure, hyperkalemia, acidosis, uremia, or volume overload.

The patient has an increased risk of thromboembolism due to age, critical illness, immobility, and history of atrial fibrillation now off anticoagulation due to her intracerebral hemorrhage. Although possibly due to thromboembolic causes, isolated renal infarct is nonetheless rare. CT angiogram will be less helpful.

21. **C.** This question requires recognizing that the patient is in the early stages of serotonin syndrome. He is at high risk for serotonin syndrome given his overdose of the selective serotonin reuptake inhibitor (SSRI) sertraline. Co-administration of linezolid and SSRIs has been associated with serotonin syndrome. Although there is sparse description of the pattern of interaction between these agents, some studies suggest a median onset of symptoms of approximately 4 to 10 days. As with any case of serotonin syndrome, the first step is discontinuing any medications that can worsen the syndrome. After this, administration of benzodiazepines is indicated. Remaining care is supportive.

22. **B.** This patient presented with symptoms and signs concerning for meningitis. He is treated empirically for common bacterial causes of meningitis, as well as for possible herpes meningitis with acyclovir. His initial serum laboratories suggest normal renal function. On day 3 of admission, he develops acute kidney injury. Providers should have a systematic approach to acute kidney injury to aid diagnosis and management. Typically, the differential is divided into:

- Prerenal causes
- Intrinsic renal causes
- Postrenal causes

In this patient, postrenal causes are unlikely given his placement of a Foley catheter on admission, which we assume was functioning well. Thus, replacing the Foley catheter would not improve his renal function.

Common prerenal causes of acute kidney injury are decreased circulating volume, which can occur from sepsis, dehydration, or the cardiorenal syndrome, and medications causing afferent vessel constriction (eg, angiotensin-converting enzyme inhibitors, nonsteroidal anti-inflammatory drugs). This patient is euvolemic on exam, and there is no suggestion of sepsis, nor is there any mention of medications affecting his afferent vessels. Along with his history of heart failure, for which fluid balance must be weighed carefully, these findings suggest that aggressive fluid resuscitation would not be the first step to improve his renal function. Vancomycin infrequently causes acute kidney injury, although its clearance is markedly affected by renal function. This patient likely has intrinsic kidney injury due to crystalline nephropathy, a known toxic effect of acyclovir. It usually presents within several days of beginning acyclovir. Risk is higher with IV administration, presumably from faster rate of crystal accumulation within the kidney. Although hydration is a mainstay of treatment for crystalline nephropathy, the first step is stopping the offending agent.

23. **D.** This elderly woman is recovering from urosepsis due to *Enterobacter cloacae*. *Enterobacter* is part of a larger group of gram-negative bacteria, the Enterobacteriaceae. These organisms, which also include *Serratia*, *Proteus*, *Klebsiella*, *Acinetobacter*, *Citrobacter*, *Escherichia*, and *Pseudomonas*, among others, increasingly harbor drug-resistance mechanisms that inactivate even broad-spectrum antibiotics. Choice of antibiotic, particularly when narrowing from empiric treatment, must take into account host factors, infection location, organisms, minimum inhibitory concentration (MIC), administration route, and resistance patterns, including possible inducible resistance. One common form of inducible resistance is the presence of the *AmpC* gene, an inducible factor that can lead to cephalosporin resistance. Resistance to third-generation cephalosporins, such as ceftriaxone, can occur quickly with hyper-*AmpC*–producing mutants. Although ceftriaxone may initially treat the infection, the organism may become resistant quickly. Fourth-generation cephalosporins, such as cefepime, are generally effective against these organisms, but there are notable cases with inducible resistance. Nonetheless, the patient likely does not require an antibiotic with as wide a spectrum as cefepime when other options are available, and narrowing is a safe option without increased mortality under the auspices of an antibiotic stewardship program. Ciprofloxacin, doxycycline, and trimethoprim-sulfamethoxazole are all available orally and intravenously. The fluoroquinolones, such as ciprofloxacin, have the same bioavailability orally as intravenously and, in general, are the only effective oral option for treatment of bacteremia. Subsequently, narrowing to ciprofloxacin is the correct decision.

24. **C.** This patient presents with symptoms and signs concerning for a sinus infection and coexisting preseptal cellulitis. Although sinus infections are common, and preseptal cellulitis often stems from a sinus infection, bacterial sinusitis does not often rapidly progress over 2 to 3 days to cause such intense pain and epistaxis. Bacterial sinusitis is typically caused by *Staphylococcus aureus*, *Streptococcus*, coagulase-negative *Staphylococcus*, *Moraxella*, or anaerobes. When due to gram-negative organisms, particularly in a diabetic, there is concern for pseudomonal infection. Vancomycin, ceftazidime, and metronidazole should adequately cover these common community-acquired organisms. Nonetheless, this patient is at high risk for other invasive organisms, particularly due to his diabetes, solid organ transplant necessitating immune suppression, and exposure working construction. Given these risk factors, rapidly progressive sinus infection leading to intense pain, tissue ischemia, and bleeding is concerning for mucormycosis. Definitive diagnosis is made by histopathology and culture, but culture is slow and often yields no growth, necessitating a high index of suspicion and urgent invasive testing. This should occur before ordering additional diagnostics, such as imaging, given that mucormycosis can severely worsen in only hours. The fastest way to obtain invasive testing, as well as expedite debridement of the angioinvasive fungus, is urgent surgical evaluation. In concert with surgical evaluation, the first-line antifungal treatment for mucormycosis is liposomal amphotericin B.

25. **D.** This man with severe COPD suffered an ischemic stroke that converted to a hemorrhagic stroke after administration of tPA. He required mechanical ventilation for airway protection. He then suffered a PEA arrest. Patients with COPD require careful attention to their ventilatory parameters. They usually have slightly higher lung volumes, but they nonetheless are best served by tidal volume

ventilation that minimizes barotrauma, atelectatic trauma, and overdistension, to lower their risk of developing acute respiratory distress syndrome (ARDS). In general, low tidal volume ventilation targeting 6 to 8 mL/kg has become standard of care after demonstrating mortality benefit in several large clinical trials.

COPD patients also require longer expiratory phases, and thus lower respiratory rates, due to their native obstructive lung disease. This gentleman did not develop ARDS. He was placed on a tidal volume of 800 mL, or 10 mL/kg, and a respiratory rate higher than his native respiratory rate. Combined, these 2 settings led to overdistension and air trapping, also known as auto-PEEP. Patients with COPD are at higher risk for air trapping. Air trapping increases intrathoracic pressure and decreases venous return to the heart. Blood pressure will eventually decline and can lead to cardiac arrest. If a patient with air trapping is in impending danger from increased intrathoracic pressure, a reliable and quick maneuver to relieve trapped air is disconnecting the ventilator from the endotracheal tube. This allows trapped air to exit quickly, decreases intrathoracic pressure, and increases venous return. The ventilator should then be reattached with more optimal settings to minimize air trapping.

26. **D.** This question relates to ventilation/perfusion (V/Q) matching in a COPD patient. The partial pressure of oxygen at the alveolar capillary governs capillary vasodilation. Regional oxygen variation in the lung causes blood to shunt away from poorly oxygenated zones to more highly oxygenated zones. This optimizes V/Q matching. The alveoli in COPD patients are abnormal and cannot optimally participate in gas exchange. Increasing the partial pressure of oxygen in inspired air in a COPD patient vasodilates alveolar capillaries in lung units that cannot adequately ventilate and therefore leads to global reduction in ventilation. Ultimately, the PCO_2 will rise, despite potentially increasing PO_2. This is the reason why overoxygenating a patient with COPD can lead to increased PCO_2 and hypercarbia, or "oxygen narcosis," often manifested as somnolence. This patient does not require oxygen saturation above her native resting saturation. Although there is disagreement on specific lower limits, patients with COPD, especially when severe, usually do not require oxygen saturations above 88% to 92%. Her

chest x-ray does not suggest cardiogenic pulmonary edema from overresuscitation or ARDS. Her somnolence, which led to intubation, was most likely caused by increasing her inspired oxygen to target an SpO_2 far above her baseline, leading to worse V/Q matching and increased PCO_2.

REFERENCES

Adrogué HJ, Madias NE. Hyponatremia. *N Engl J Med.* 2000;342(21):1581-1589.

Ali AM, Mirrakhimov AE, Abboud CN, Cashen AF. Leukostasis in adult acute hyperleukocytic leukemia: a clinician's digest. *Hematol Oncol.* 2016;34(2):69-78.

Chiha M, Samarasighe S, Kabaker AS. Thyroid storm: an updated review. *J Intensive Care Med.* 2015;30(3):131-140.

Cho KC. Electrolyte and acid-base disorders. In: Papadakis MA, McPhee SJ, Rabow MW, eds. *Current Medical Diagnosis & Treatment 2017.* New York, NY: McGraw-Hill; 2017.

Danion F, Aguilar C, Catherinot E, et al. Mucormycosis: new developments into a persistently devastating infection. *Semin Respir Crit Care Med.* 2015;36(5):692-705.

De Waele JJ, De Laet I, Kirkpatrick AW, Hoste E. Intraabdominal hypertension and abdominal compartment syndrome. *Am J Kidney Dis.* 2011;57(1):159-169.

DuBose TD Jr. Acidosis and alkalosis. In: Kasper D, Fauci A, Hauser S, Longo D, Jameson J, Loscalzo J, eds. *Harrison's Principles of Internal Medicine.* 19th ed. New York, NY: McGraw-Hill; 2014.

Farmakiotis D, Kontoyiannis DP. Mucormycosis. *Infect Dis Clin North Am.* 2016;30(1):143-163.

Fliers E, Bianco AC, Langouche L, et al. Thyroid function in critical illness. *Lancet Diabetes Endocrinol.* 2015;3(10):816-825.

Giuliano CA, Patel CR, Kale-Pradhan PB. Is the combination of piperacillin-tazobactam and vancomycin associated with development of acute kidney injury? A meta-analysis. *Pharmacotherapy.* 2016;36(12):1217-1228.

Griesdale DEG, de Souza RJ, van Dam RM, et al. Intensive insulin therapy and mortality among critically ill patients: a meta-analysis including NICE-SUGAR study data. *CMAJ.* 2009;180(8):821-827.

Guo Y, Gao W, Yang H, et al. De-escalation of empiric antibiotics in patients with severe sepsis or septic shock: a meta-analysis. *Heart Lung.* 2016;45(5):454-459.

Hammond DA, Smith MN, Li C, et al. Systematic review and meta-analysis of acute kidney injury associated with concomitant vancomycin and piperacillin/tazobactam. *Clin Infect Dis.* 2016;10:ciw811.

Holcomb JB, Tilley BC, Baraniuk S et al; PROPPR Study Group. Transfusion of plasma, platelets, and red blood cells in a 1:1:1 vs a 1:1:2 ratio and mortality in patients with severe trauma: the PROPPR randomized clinical trial. *JAMA.* 2015;313(5):471-482.

Jiranantakan T, Anderson IB. Ethylene glycol and other glycols. In: Olson KR, eds. *Poisoning & Drug Overdose.* 6th ed. New York, NY: McGraw-Hill; 2012.

Karpman D, Loos S, Tati R, Arvidsson I. Haemolytic uraemic syndrome. *J Intern Med.* 2017;281(2):123-148.

Kaufman DC, Kitching AJ, Kellum JA. Acid-base balance. In: Hall JB, Schmidt GA, Kress JP, eds. *Principles of Critical Care.* 4th ed. New York, NY: McGraw-Hill; 2014.

Kibble JD, Halsey CR, eds. Renal physiology and acid-base balance. In: *Medical Physiology: The Big Picture.* New York, NY: McGraw-Hill; 2014.

Kitabchi AE, Umpierrez GE, Murphy MB, Kreisberg RA. Hyperglycemic crises in adult patients with diabetes: a consensus statement from the American Diabetes Association. *Diabetes Care.* 2006;29(12):2739-2748.

Klubo-Gwiezdzinska J, Wartofsky L. Thyroid emergencies. *Med Clin North Am.* 2012;96(2):385-403.

Kwaku MP, Burman KD. Myxedema coma. *J Intensive Care Med.* 2007;22(4):224-231.

Laghi F, Tobin MJ. Chapter 4. Indications for mechanical ventilation. In: Tobin MJ, eds. *Principles and Practice of Mechanical Ventilation.* 3rd ed. New York, NY: McGraw-Hill; 2013.

Latcha S. Electrolyte disorders in critically ill patients. In: Oropello JM, Pastores SM, Kvetan V, eds. *Critical Care.* New York, NY: McGraw-Hill; 2017.

Leatherman JW. Chapter 30. Mechanical ventilation for severe asthma. In: Tobin MJ, eds. *Principles and Practice of Mechanical Ventilation.* 3rd ed. New York, NY: McGraw-Hill; 2013.

Legendre CM, Licht C, Muus P, et al. Terminal complement inhibitor eculizumab in atypical hemolytic-uremic syndrome. *N Engl J Med.* 2013;368(23):2169-2181.

Narita M, Tsuji BT, Yu VL. Linezolid-associated peripheral and optic neuropathy, lactic acidosis, and serotonin syndrome. *Pharmacotherapy.* 2007;27(8):1189-1197.

Navalkele B, Pogue JM, Karino S, et al. Risk of acute kidney injury in patients on concomitant vancomycin and piperacillin-tazobactam compared to those on vancomycin and cefepime. *Clin Infect Dis.* 2017;64(2):116-123.

Mahajan SL, Myers TJ, Baldini MG. Disseminated intravascular coagulation during rewarming following hypothermia. *JAMA.* 1981;245(24):2517-2518.

Marcucci G, Bloomfield CD. Acute myeloid leukemia. In: Kasper D, Fauci A, Hauser S, Longo D, Jameson J, Loscalzo J, eds. *Harrison's Principles of Internal Medicine.* 19th ed. New York, NY: McGraw-Hill; 2014.

Morales-Molina JA, Mateu-de Antonio J, Marín-Casino M, Grau S. Linezolid-associated serotonin syndrome: what we can learn from cases reported so far. *J Antimicrob Chemother.* 2005;56(6):1176-1178.

NICE-SUGAR Study Investigators. Intensive versus conventional glucose control in critically ill patients. *N Engl J Med.* 2009;360(13):1283-1297.

Pasquel FJ, Umpierrez GE. Hyperosmolar hyperglycemic state: a historic review of the clinical presentation, diagnosis, and treatment. *Diabetes Care.* 2014;37:3124-3131.

Perazella MA. Drug-induced renal failure: update on new medications and unique mechanisms of nephrotoxicity. *Am J Med Sci.* 2003;325(6):349-362.

Powers AC. Diabetes mellitus: management and therapies. In: Kasper D, Fauci A, Hauser S, Longo D, Jameson J, Loscalzo J, eds. *Harrison's Principles of Internal Medicine.* 19th ed. New York, NY: McGraw-Hill; 2014.

Rindone JP, Mellen C, Ryba J. Does piperacillin-tazobactam increase the risk of nephrotoxicity when used with vancomycin: a meta-analysis of observational trials. *Curr Drug Saf.* Epub ahead of print on October 24, 2016.

Siedner MJ, Galar A, Guzmán-Suarez BB, et al. Cefepime vs other antibacterial agents for the treatment of *Enterobacter* species bacteremia. *Clin Infect Dis.* 2014;58(11):1554-1563.

Sugrue M. Abdominal compartment syndrome. *Curr Opin Crit Care.* 2005;11:333-338.

Taylor JJ, Wilson JW, Estes LL. Linezolid and serotonergic drug interactions: a retrospective survey. *Clin Infect Dis.* 2006;43(2):180-187.

Vincent JL, Bassetti M, François B, et al. Advances in antibiotic therapy in the critically ill. *Crit Care.* 2016;20(1):133.

Wada H, Matsumoto T, Yamashita Y. Diagnosis and treatment of disseminated intravascular coagulation (DIC) according to four DIC guidelines. *J Intensive Care.* 2014;2(1):15.

Yeung S, Manzullo EF. Oncologic emergencies. In: Kantarjian HM, Wolff RA, eds. *The MD Anderson Manual of Medical Oncology.* 3rd ed. New York, NY: McGraw-Hill.

PART 4
Surgical Critical Care

24

Intrathoracic Diseases

Barry Kelly, MD and Somnath Bose, MD

Questions

1. A 28-year-old pregnant woman is brought emergently to the emergency department (ED) trauma bay by emergency medical services (EMS) following a head-on motor vehicle accident in which she was the sole occupant of the vehicle. The driver of the other vehicle died at the scene. Upon arrival to the trauma bay, you observe a woman in the advanced stages of pregnancy. She is immobilized in a cervical spine collar on a spinal board. She is crying, and has bilateral cubital fossa intravenous access placed by EMS. Her initial vital signs are a heart rate of 130 bpm, sinus rhythm, noninvasive blood pressure of 70/40 mm Hg, and oxygen saturation (SpO_2) of 88% on a 100% oxygen nonrebreather mask. She becomes acutely diaphoretic, and you displace the uterus to the patient's left side by placing a wedge beneath the spinal board. Her blood pressure improves to 90/65 mm Hg. She complains of severe sternal pain and has marked bruising on her right anterior chest. Auscultation reveals absence of breath sounds and dullness to percussion on the right with normal breath sounds and percussion on the left. What is the next most appropriate step in her management?

   A. Obtain an urgent computed tomography (CT) scan of thorax, abdomen, and pelvis

   B. Obtain an urgent obstetrics consult

   C. Intubate the patient to secure the airway

   D. Perform an emergency tube thoracotomy on the right side

2. An 83-year-old woman sustains multiple rib fractures to the right rib cage following a mechanical fall on ice. Which of the following interventions is most likely to prevent respiratory complications from her rib fractures?

   A. Splinting the rib cage with external compressive supports

   B. Nonsteriodal anti-inflammatory medications for pain, bedrest, and physiotherapy

   C. Surgical plating of the affected ribs

   D. Thoracic epidural plus IV patient controlled analgesia (PCA) and physiotherapy

3. A young boy is brought emergently to the ED after he was "shot" with a nail gun by his younger brother while playing in their father's workshop. The patient is sobbing, stating that the nail in his chest "really hurts." The patient is sitting upright on a resuscitation stretcher. You note the following vital signs: heart rate of 130 bpm with variable-sized QRS complexes, blood pressure of 120/80 mm Hg, and SpO_2 of 100% on a non-rebreather mask. Auscultation of bilateral lung fields reveals equal breath sounds with scattered wheezes. The head of a nail is evident protruding from the left lower sternal edge. The patient is deemed stable to be transported to radiology for a CT scan of the thorax. As the patient is being transferred to radiology, a healthcare worker lowers the upright angle of the stretcher. The patient becomes acutely distressed and dyspneic. What is the most likely pathology causing this acute deterioration?

A. Tension pneumothorax

B. Acute aspiration from esophageal rupture

C. Pericardial tamponade

D. Decompensated hemorrhagic shock from hemothorax

4. As the intensivist on call in a small community hospital, you are paged by the orthopedic resident to urgently assess a 34-year-old non–English-speaking man who was brought in by the EMS, having been found semiconscious under a collapsed brick wall. Upon arrival to the ED, the patient is in a cervical spine collar and is pale and barely conscious. You note noisy breathing beneath a 100% rebreather mask. His initial vital signs are a temperature of 89.6°F, heart rate of 110 bpm, sinus tachycardia, and blood pressure of 100/88 mm Hg; his SpO_2 is not obtainable. Marked ecchymosis is evident across his chest. His right lower limb is grossly deformed, and a bony fragment protrudes through the legging of his work trousers. The orthopedic resident confirms a compound fracture of the right femur and absence of all arterial pulses below the right knee.

The attending orthopedist has been informed and wishes to take the patient to the operating room (OR) for open reduction and internal fixation as a matter of urgency. As you perform a primary survey, the ED nurse informs you that the patient's vitals have changed with a heart rate of 140 bpm and blood pressure of 70/40 mm Hg. You notice marked subcutaneous emphysema on the right chest, and breath sounds are diminished on the right compared to the left. The orthopedic resident suggests you bring him directly to the OR for intubation and stabilization to allow early anatomic correction of the right leg. What is the next *most* appropriate intervention?

A. Give a 1-L bolus of crystalloid

B. Obtain a definitive airway with midline stabilization in the ED

C. Perform an emergent needle thoracentesis on the right side followed by chest tube insertion

D. Proceed to the OR for intubation and stabilization

5. A 35-year-old man developed progressively worsening shortness of breath on the floor and was transferred to the intensive care unit. He was awaiting a planned video-assisted thoracoscopy (VATS) and pleurodesis for the management of a persistent bronchopleural fistula. He is now 2 weeks post extensive chest trauma secondary to a motor vehicle accident. His injuries included bilateral pneumothoraces requiring bilateral chest tube insertion. His left-sided chest tube has been removed, and chest imaging shows complete resolution of the pneumothorax on that side. His right-sided pneumothorax persists despite having been managed with two 28-Fr chest tubes with negative pressure suction and multiple clamp trials. Two chest tubes remain in situ on the right side. Upon examination, you find the patient to be tachypneic with a respiratory rate of 30 breaths/min, using accessory muscles of respiration. His SpO_2 is 90% on a non-rebreather mask. The thoracic surgeon on call points out that

the leak has progressively worsened over the past 6 hours and decides to do an urgent VATS pleurodesis. You decide to assist the anesthesiologist to secure the airway in the intensive care unit in view of impending respiratory failure and anticipated emergent surgery. You plan to insert a single lumen tube with a bronchial blocker for lung isolation to facilitate effective ventilation. After an uneventful induction, direct laryngoscopy reveals a Cormack-Lehane grade 1 view. After insertion of a size 8.5-mm cuffed endotracheal tube, you promptly realize that you are unable to ventilate the patient. A capnography trace is not detectable. The patient is well perfused with absence of cyanosis. What is the most likely reason for the absent capnography trace?

A. Cardiac arrest due to a tension pneumothorax

B. Right-sided endobronchial intubation

C. Anaphylaxis with pulseless electrical activity (PEA) arrest

D. Esophageal intubation

6. A young professional race car driver is brought to the ED after a crash at a nearby race circuit. The vehicle he was driving slid off the track while failing to negotiate a turn and collided head on with a safety barrier. The driver was wearing a helmet and did not lose consciousness. All air bag protection devices were deployed. The steering wheel of the vehicle became dislodged from its mount. In the trauma bay of the ED, with the exception of moderate chest pain, the primary survey is essentially normal. As an adjunct to the primary survey, a chest x-ray is suspicious for a widened mediastinum. An aortic disruption/dissection is high on the differential, so a CT aortogram is requested. If the CT confirms the suspicion of an aortic injury, where is the most likely site of the injury?

A. The sinotubular junction

B. The abdominal aorta

C. The junction of the ascending aorta and the innominate (brachiocephalic) artery

D. The junction of the left subclavian artery and the descending aorta

7. A 14-year-old boy is emergently brought by air ambulance from an outside hospital after having sustained a severe penetrating trauma to his upper chest and neck. He was riding an all-terrain vehicle at 30 mph when he drove into a chain-link barrier to a property entrance. He was catapulted from the bike. Despite sustaining severe penetrating injury to his neck and bruising to his upper chest, he was able to contact 911 with his cell phone. On arrival to ED, the boy is stridorous and in distress, but is hemodynamically stable. He has an open wound to his anterior neck and has marked subcutaneous emphysema. The severity of his stridor is increasing. Which of the following is the safest approach to secure his airway?

A. Await the results of a CT scan to define the anatomy of the injury.

B. Perform a rapid sequence induction in the ED trauma bay.

C. Perform an emergent cricothyroidotomy in the ED trauma bay.

D. Expedite transfer to the OR for an inhalational induction and fiberoptic-guided endotracheal intubation with the trauma surgeons, cardiac surgeons, and perfusionist in the OR.

8. A previously healthy 62-year-old man was out on a strenuous hike when he tripped on a descent. His upper abdomen made contact with a large boulder. He did not lose consciousness or experience any other trauma. However, he experienced moderate chest and epigastric pain for the remainder of the descent, which alerted him to call the EMS on return to his vehicle. He was brought to a local ED. His primary survey was essentially normal, but his chest x-ray revealed some air in his mediastinum and a left-sided pleural effusion but no evidence of a pneumothorax. Given this history, what is the most likely cause for his pneumomediastinum, and how can the diagnosis be confirmed?

A. Flailed chest with bronchopleural fistula diagnosed with CT of the chest

B. Tension pneumothorax diagnosed with CT of the chest

C. Esophageal rupture diagnosed with a contrast swallow study

D. Small bowel perforation on CT of the abdomen

Answers and Explanations

1. **D.** The woman in this scenario is verbalizing, so her airway is patent. An endotracheal tube is not an obligation at this point. A potential distractor is the fact that she is pregnant. Caval compression has been addressed, and she remains hypotensive in the setting of obvious chest trauma. Her jugular veins are most likely very difficult to assess in the context of the cervical spine collar. The clinical findings on her chest exam are consistent with a significant hemothorax. As per advanced trauma life support (ATLS) guidelines, she is in shock and the diagnosis of a life-threatening hemothorax should be confirmed by the emergent placement of a chest tube. This diagnosis, if time permits, can be confirmed by performing an urgent chest x-ray as an adjunct to the primary survey. Urgent surgical exploration by thoracotomy is indicated if >1.500 mL of blood has accumulated and/or an ongoing production of >200 mL of blood per hour to control the source of bleeding. She is too unstable for safe transfer for more advanced diagnostic imaging.

2. **D.** Pain on motion following rib injury typically results in splinting of the thorax, which impairs ventilation and effective coughing. Atelectasis and pneumonia are a particular concern in the elderly population and mandate a thoughtful approach to pain management. Trauma guidelines encourage the use of neuraxial analgesia in the form of a thoracic epidural or paravertebral blockade, especially in the elderly population in the absence of contraindications. Taping, rib belts, and external splints are contraindicated. Limited evidence supports the routine use of surgical fixation.

3. **C.** The site of injury and positional orthopnea are consistent with a diagnosis of pericardial effusion and potential tamponade physiology. The right ventricle is positioned most anteriorly in the mediastinum and, as such, is most vulnerable to penetrating trauma. In contrast to the left ventricle, which lies more posterior, the right ventricle supplies the low-pressure pulmonic circulation. Penetrating trauma to the right ventricle results in a lower rate of bleeding compared to the left ventricle, which is often fatal. Tamponade can result from continued bleeding into the pericardial sac. The pericardial sac normally contains about 10 to 30 mL of serous fluid. In the acute setting, as little as 50 to 100 mL of blood may result in tamponade and cardiogenic shock. The presence of orthopnea relieved by sitting up is a clinical clue to the underlying diagnosis of tamponade physiology. The penetrating object should only be removed following sternotomy and surgical exploration. This clinical scenario is extremely challenging to the anesthesiologist as induction of general anesthesia and introduction of positive-pressure ventilation may result in decrease of right-sided cardiac chamber pressures and cardiac arrest due to tamponade. A senior anesthesiologist, ideally with subspecialty training in cardiac anesthesia and perioperative echocardiography, should supervise induction of general anesthesia. The patient should be draped with all invasive access and monitoring devices placed prior to induction. Maintenance of spontaneous ventilation should be a priority to prevent chamber collapse. Alternative sites of cannulation for cardiopulmonary bypass should be considered and draped a priori.

4. **C.** The scenario described is one of polytrauma in a young man who is hemodynamically unstable with multiple concurrent etiologies. ATLS primary survey guidelines obligate the clinician to follow a sequential diagnostic pathway to rule out and treat life-threatening conditions. The scenario here describes a trauma patient with a possible unstable airway mobilized in a cervical spine collar with clinical signs that are highly suspicious for a tension pneumothorax. Complicating the management is

the "distracting" injury of a compound fracture that the orthopedists urgently wish to operate upon. In stabilizing this patient, the natural response is to follow the Airway, Breathing, Circulation, Disability, Exposure algorithm. However, recognition and treatment of a potential tension pneumothorax is the highest priority because the patient is hemodynamically unstable. Securing the airway and institution of positive-pressure ventilation in this patient prior to relieving the circulatory compromise due to the tension pneumothorax could result in a cardiac arrest. The priority here is to needle decompress the pneumothorax and insert a chest tube after improvement in hemodynamics.

5. **B.** This scenario describes an unusual complication associated with nonroutine anesthesia equipment. A large endotracheal tube (ETT; size 8.5 mm) with a bronchial blocking device is often used for ease of insertion and lung isolation instead of a double lumen tube, especially in small patients with limited mouth opening. The pathology here is a bronchopleural fistula resulting in direct connection between the patient's upper airway and the pleural space. The pleural space, in turn, is in direct connection with an external underwater seal device. Because the patient has 2 large-bore chest drains in situ, the likelihood is that the ETT is in the right main bronchus and the majority of the tidal volumes are passing directly to the underwater seal. High suspicion and quick recognition will allow the clinician to observe marked air bubbling in the underwater chambers with each tidal volume. The patient is well perfused, so a cardiac arrest is unlikely. Because the insertion of a bronchial blocker involves direct guidance with a bronchoscope, this situation can be rapidly diagnosed and treated by confirming that the ETT is endobronchial, withdrawing the ETT to above the carina, and correctly inserting a bronchial blocker into the right main bronchus to allow isolated ventilation of the left lung. Recognition of this complication is crucial to the safety of this patient as treatment is relatively simple, but failure to recognize it may lead the clinician down an alternative treatment pathway that may be detrimental to the patient's safety.

6. **D.** This scenario describes the classic deceleration injury in which varied intrathoracic forces can result in aortic disruption at the site called the isthmus. The isthmus corresponds to the site of attachment of the ligamentum arteriosus, which is the remnant of the patent ductus arteriosus. Traumatic rupture of the aorta is a common cause of death at the scene. Survivors tend to have incomplete laceration when continuity is maintained by an intact adventitial layer, which results in a contained hematoma. Classic radiologic findings on chest x-ray include a widened mediastinum, obliteration of the aortic knob adjacent to the left pulmonary artery, and apical capping with a left-sided pleural effusion. A helical CT scan of the aorta is the diagnostic investigation of choice because sensitivity and specificity approach 100%. Traditionally, the repair of an aortic hematoma involved sternotomy and cardiopulmonary bypass with placement of an interpositional graft. However, in certain circumstances, endovascular stenting is the preferred approach.

7. **D.** This situation is arguably the most challenging situation any anesthesiologist or an intensivist will face throughout his or her career. This young boy has clinical evidence of a tracheocutaneous fistula, and his airway patency is becoming increasingly compromised. An overenthusiastic anesthesiologist/intensivist may opt to secure the airway early without a clear understanding of potential complications. Undoubtedly, securing the airway is of paramount importance given the clinical history and should prioritize obtaining any further diagnostic imaging. Committing to a definitive airway with rapid sequence induction is perilous, as loss of spontaneous breathing and muscle tone may result in acute airway occlusion and inability to ventilate. Although direct laryngoscopy may allow intubation of the vocal cords with an endotracheal tube, unfortunately, direct passage of the tube cannot be guaranteed in the presence of tracheobronchial disruption. The safest method to adequately secure the airway in this grave situation is an inhalation induction in the OR with an asleep fiberoptic intubation to confirm correct distal placement of the endotracheal tube. The importance of a surgical backup plan to include an urgent surgical tracheostomy and access to cardiopulmonary bypass should not be understated, in case more distant bronchial injury is present.

8. C. This scenario describes a man who sustained blunt trauma to his abdomen when performing strenuous activity. His radiologic findings are supportive of a visceral perforation as the lung fields display no evidence of hematoma. Trauma to the upper abdomen with persistent sternal pain and pneumomediastinum warrants an upper gastrointestinal study. The diagnosis is confirmed when contrast is seen in the mediastinum. Depending on timing of presentation, repair performed within a few hours of injury leads to a much better prognosis. Otherwise, treatment consists of wide drainage of the pleural space and mediastinum with direct repair of the injury via thoracotomy.

REFERENCES

Banki F, Estrera AL, Harrison RG, et al. Pneumomediastinum: etiology and a guide to diagnosis and treatment. *Am J Surg*. 2013;206(6):1001-1006.

Bulger EM, Edwards T, Klotz P, Jurkovich GJ. Epidural analgesia improves outcome after multiple rib fractures. *Surgery*. 2004;136(2):426-430.

Campos J, Ueda K. Update on anesthetic complications of robotic thoracic surgery. *Minerva Anestesiol*. 2014;80(1):83-88.

Chapdelaine J, Beaunoyer M, Daigneault P, et al. Spontaneous pneumomediastinum: an extensive workup is not required. *J Am Coll Surg*. 2014;219(4):713-717.

Demetriades D, Velmahos GC, Scalea TM, et al. Operative repair or endovascular stent graft in blunt traumatic thoracic aortic injuries: results of an American Association for the Surgery of Trauma Multicenter Study. *J Trauma*. 2008;64(3):561-570.

Dulchavsky SA, Schwarz KL, Kirkpatrick AW, et al. Prospective evaluation of thoracic ultrasound in the detection of pneumothorax. *J Trauma*. 2001;50(2):201-205.

Dunham CM, Barraco RD, Clark DE, et al. Guidelines for emergency tracheal intubation immediately after traumatic injury. *J Trauma*. 2003;55(1):162-179.

Dyer DS, Moore EE, Ilke DN, et al. Thoracic aortic injury: how predictive is mechanism and is chest computed tomography a reliable screening tool? A prospective study of 1,561 patients. *J Trauma*. 2000;48(4):673-682.

Ekeh AP, Peterson W, Woods RJ, et al. Is chest x-ray an adequate screening tool for the diagnosis of blunt thoracic aortic injury? *J Trauma*. 2008;65(5):1088-1092.

Grocott HP, Gulati H, Srinathan S, Mackensen GB. Anesthesia and the patient with pericardial disease. *Can J Anesth*. 2011;58:952-966.

Horlocker TT, Wedel DJ, Rowlingson, JC, et al. Anticoagulation 3rd edition. https://www.asra.com/advisory-guidelines/article/1/anticoagulation-3rd-edition. Accessed June 25, 2017.

Karalis DG, Victor MF, Davis GA, et al. The role of echocardiography in blunt chest trauma: a transthoracic and transesophageal echocardiographic study. *J Trauma*. 1994;36(1):53-58.

Karmy-Jones R, Jurkovich GJ, Nathens AB, et al. Timing of urgent thoracotomy for hemorrhage after trauma: a multicenter study. *Arch Surg*. 2001;136(5):513-518.

Moon MR, Luchette FA, Gibson SW, et al. Prospective, randomized comparison of epidural versus parenteral opioid analgesia in thoracic trauma. *Ann Surg*. 1999;229(5):684-691.

Naghibi K, Hashemi SL, Sajedi P. Anesthetic management of tracheobronchial rupture following blunt chest trauma. *Acta Anaesthesiol Scand*. 2003;47(7):901-903.

Ramzy AI, Rodriguez A, Turney SZ. Management of major tracheobronchial ruptures in patients with multiple system trauma. *J Trauma*. 1988;28(9):1353-1357.

Simon BJ, Cushman J, Barraco R, et al. Pain management guidelines for blunt thoracic trauma: an EAST Practice Management Guidelines Workgroup. *J Trauma*. 2005;59(5):1256-1267.

Stafford RE, Linn J, Washington L. Incidence and management of occult hemothoraces. *Am J Surg*. 2006;192:722-726.

25

Ventilation and Pulmonary Mechanics

Juan Perrone, MD, and Abraham Sonny, MD

Questions

1. A 50-year-old man underwent a craniotomy for subdural hematoma evacuation. Muscle relaxants were used throughout the case but were not pharmacologically reversed. He was brought to the intensive care unit (ICU) intubated. He had spontaneous breathing efforts shortly after ICU admission and is now being assessed for extubation. Which is the best indicator of return of neuromuscular function prior to extubation?

   A. Ability to follow commands with a strong handgrip

   B. Spontaneous breathing trial showing adequate gas exchange with normal tidal volumes and a respiratory rate of 20 breaths/min

   C. A quantitative train-of-4 ratio of 0.9

   D. Inspiratory force of –20 cm H_2O

2. After placement of a subclavian central venous catheter in a mechanically ventilated patient, you obtain the following ultrasonographic image along the anterior and lateral chest walls. What is the arrow emphasizing?

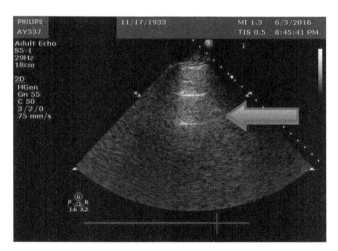

Ultrasound (axial image) of the thoracic cavity.

   A. Normal lung parenchyma

   B. Pneumothorax

   C. Pleural effusion

   D. Lung infiltrates

3. A 62-year-old morbidly obese woman is 2 days after an extensive head and neck oncologic procedure with free-flap reconstruction and tracheostomy. While in the surgical ICU, she becomes agitated, and her tracheostomy is dislodged. She becomes acutely hypoxic. What is the most appropriate management of this patient?

   A. 100% oxygen via tracheostomy mask over stoma

   B. Immediate tracheostomy tube replacement

   C. Return to operating room for tracheostomy revision

   D. Oral tracheal intubation

4. A 71-year-old man with a history of coronary artery disease, chronic obstructive pulmonary disease (COPD), and severe peripheral vascular disease remains intubated in the ICU after an aortobifemoral bypass procedure. What does the ventilator flow waveform (shown below) demonstrate?

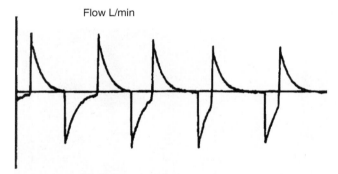

Flow L/min

Schematic representation of ventilator waveform over time.

   A. Patient-ventilator dyssynchrony

   B. Normal pressure support ventilation

   C. Normal assist control ventilation

   D. Occult positive end-expiratory pressure (PEEP)

5. Which of the following patients is the best candidate for noninvasive positive-pressure ventilation?

   A. A 60-year-old man with severe COPD exacerbation and mild lethargy, blood pressure (BP) of 140/92 mm Hg, heart rate (HR) of 110 bpm, respiratory rate (RR) of 30 breaths/min, pulse oximetry of 96% on non-rebreather mask, arterial blood gas (ABG) pH of 7.20, partial pressures of carbon dioxide ($Paco_2$) of 70 mm Hg, and partial pressure of oxygen (Pao_2) of 120 mm Hg

   B. A 50-year-old man with ST-segment elevation myocardial infarction, pulmonary edema, BP of 90/64 mm Hg, HR of 110 bpm, RR of 25 breaths/min, pulse oximetry of 90% on non-rebreather mask, ABG pH of 7.28, $Paco_2$ of 45 mm Hg, and Pao_2 of 58 mm Hg

   C. A 30-year-old woman with asthma exacerbation, BP of 102/56 mm Hg, HR of 108 bpm, RR of 26 breaths/min, pulse oximetry of 95% on 4-L nasal cannula, ABG pH of 7.44, $Paco_2$ of 36 mm Hg, and Pao_2 of 120 mm Hg

   D. A 70-year-old man with bronchiectasis, worsening shortness of breath, significant ongoing hemoptysis, BP of 110/68 mm Hg, HR of 105 bpm, RR of 32 breaths/min, pulse oximetry of 92% on non-rebreather mask, ABG pH of 7.42, $Paco_2$ of 30 mm Hg, and Pao_2 of 65 mm Hg

6. A 55-year-old man is intubated for severe acute respiratory distress syndrome (ARDS). Current settings are as follows: tidal volume 450 mL, RR 28 breaths/min, and PEEP 15 cm H_2O. Plateau pressure is 30 cm H_2O. What is the respiratory system compliance?

   A. 60 mL/cm H_2O

   B. 45 mL/cm H_2O

   C. 30 mL/cm H_2O

   D. 15 mL/cm H_2O

7. Which of the following will not improve oxygenation and survival in patients with severe ARDS?

   A. Neuromuscular blockade

   B. Low tidal volume ventilation

   C. Steroids

   D. Prone positioning

8. A 25-year-old man with severe traumatic brain injury remains intubated in the ICU 4 days after decompressive craniectomy. Which of the following statements is true regarding tracheostomy in this patient?

   A. Early tracheostomy will likely decrease the incidence of ventilator-associated pneumonia and mortality.

   B. Early tracheostomy will require a second procedure to close the stoma.

   C. Percutaneous tracheostomy kits are associated with increased procedural cost.

   D. Timing of tracheostomy remains a subjective decision based on the anticipated disease course or difficult ventilator weaning.

9. A 55-year-old morbidly obese man develops ARDS after a motor vehicle collision. He is being ventilated with a tidal volume of 5 mL/kg, RR of 18 breaths/min, and PEEP of 15 cm H_2O. Peak airway pressure is 45 cm H_2O, and plateau pressure is 30 cm H_2O. What is the transpulmonary pressure?

   A. 15 cm H_2O, the difference between peak and plateau pressures

   B. 15 cm H_2O, the difference between PEEP and plateau pressure

   C. 30 cm H_2O, the difference between peak pressure and PEEP

   D. Cannot be estimated with the information given

10. A 45-year-old man with no prior history of cardiopulmonary problems undergoes an uneventful elective craniotomy for tumor resection. During the procedure, he is given 3 L of crystalloid and 2 units of packed red blood cells. Emergence from anesthesia is notable for agitation, and he is observed biting at the endotracheal tube. He is extubated, and during transport to the ICU, he develops coughing of copious pink frothy sputum and profound oxygen desaturation requiring reintubation. What is the most likely diagnosis?

    A. Acute neurogenic pulmonary edema

    B. Transfusion-associated circulatory overload

    C. Negative-pressure pulmonary edema

    D. Transfusion-related acute lung injury

11. A 47-year-old man, with a height of 180 cm, weight of 76.2 kg, and hypertension, was brought to the emergency department after a loss of consciousness without return to normal. He was intubated by emergency medical services en route to the hospital for hypoxia. A head computed tomography scan was completed in the emergency department and demonstrated diffuse thick subarachnoid hemorrhage. His vitals while in the emergency department were as follows: HR 112 bpm, BP 178/102 mm Hg, and oxygen saturation 89% on 100% fraction of inspired oxygen (FiO_2). His ventilator settings are as follows: volume assist control, set rate 16, volume 600 mL, and PEEP 5 mm Hg. A portable chest x-ray was completed in the emergency department and is shown below. What is the next best step in management for this patient?

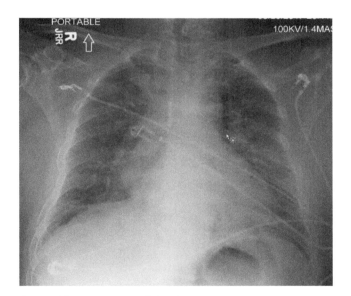

A portable supine view of the chest.

   A. Start intravenous furosemide at 80 mg every 6 hours for goal fluid balance of −2 L

   B. Start intravenous cisatracurium for improved ventilator synchrony

   C. Start low-volume ventilation at 6 mL/kg (approximately 450 mL)

   D. Pull endotracheal tube back approximately 2 cm

   E. Increase PEEP to 10 mm Hg

12. A 74-year-old man with hypertension, hyperlipidemia, coronary artery disease (prior 3-vessel coronary artery bypass 12 years prior), and COPD (on home oxygen) was admitted to the neuro-ICU following a large left middle cerebral artery ischemic stroke that was treated with both intravenous tissue plasminogen activator and thrombectomy. He was intubated prior to arrival to the emergency department given concerns of acute respiratory distress and inability to protect his airway. On hospital day 3, the patient had substantial improvement in his neurologic examination, but he required increased doses of norepinephrine to maintain systolic BP and mean arterial pressure goals in attempt to maintain cerebral perfusion. His current settings are as follows: pressure support with inspiratory pressure 8 mm Hg, PEEP 10 mm Hg, spontaneous RR 14 breaths/min, average tidal volume of 550 mL, FiO_2 40%, minute ventilation 7.8 L/min, and inspiratory-to-expiratory ratio 1:2. You are concerned his pressure requirement may be due to his invasive ventilation. What ventilator change can be made to potentially improve the patient's hemodynamics?

A. Decrease the PEEP from 10 mm Hg to 5 mm Hg

B. Decrease the inspiratory pressure from 8 mm Hg to 5 mm Hg

C. Change from pressure support to volume support and maintain the same minute ventilation

D. Increase the inspiratory-to-expiratory ratio to 1:4

Answers and Explanations

1. **C.** Residual neuromuscular blockade puts patients at risk for respiratory complications and is a common occurrence in the postanesthesia care unit and ICU. Clinically significant residual paralysis cannot be excluded by any combination of clinical criteria, and a quantitative assessment of the response to nerve stimulation should be assessed. The most common method to accomplish this is train-of-4 (TOF) stimulation of the ulnar nerve at the wrist; this consists of a series of 4 supramaximal stimuli given every 0.5 seconds. Each stimulus in the sequence causes the muscle to contract, and the "fade" provides the basis for evaluation; that is, dividing the amplitude of the fourth response by the amplitude of the first response provides the TOF ratio. It is difficult to exclude residual block using subjective evaluation of the tactile or visual TOF ratio (qualitative monitoring). Objective (quantitative) neuromuscular monitoring devices must be used to reliably detect clinically significant residual neuromuscular blockade. A quantitative train-of-4 ratio of 0.9 is the best indicator of return of neuromuscular function prior to extubation.

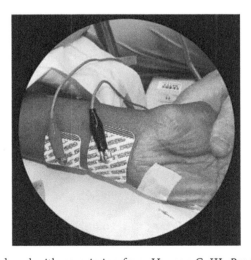

Reproduced with permission from Hanson C, III. *Procedures in Critical Care*. New York, NY: McGraw-Hill, 2009.

2. **A.** Evaluation of the lung parenchyma is based on the presence of different artifact patterns, all of which emanate from the pleural line. The arrow indicates A-lines, which are present in normal lung and represent reverberation artifacts at parallel intervals underlying the highly echogenic pleural line. B-lines are vertical, laser-like reverberation artifacts that arise from the pleural line and extend to the bottom of the image without fading. Multiple B-lines in a lung field represent increased interstitial fluid. Ultrasonographic characteristics of pneumothorax include loss of visualization of sliding between the visceral and parietal pleura (lung sliding) and visualization of the point where the normal lung pattern replaces the pneumothorax pattern (absent A-lines and lung sliding), known as "lung point." Pleural effusions appear as hypoechogenic structures accumulated in dependent areas of the chest where areas of collapsed lung can usually be seen within the effusion. Finally, lung infiltrates or consolidations are seen as hyperechoic areas with punctiform elements or "hepatization" with presence of static or dynamic air bronchograms.

3. **D.** Tracheostomy tubes can typically be changed after 5 to 7 days of the surgical procedure, when there is a mature tract from the skin to the airway. If a tracheostomy tube becomes dislodged before there is a mature tract, the standard and safe approach is to proceed with oral tracheal intubation. In an acutely hypoxic patient, this should be done without delay. Attempts at immediately replacing the tracheostomy tube are not recommended given the higher likelihood of extratracheal placement, especially in the presence of distorted anatomy and obesity. Once the airway is again secured and the patient has recovered, the surgeon can replace the tracheostomy tube in a controlled fashion.

4. **D.** Occult PEEP, or auto-PEEP, refers to the presence of continued airflow at the end of expiration

resulting in positive alveolar pressure even though the proximal airway pressure falls to atmospheric (zero) pressure. Occult PEEP can be detected on the flow tracing by noting the presence of airflow at the end of expiration as the ventilator flow waveform for this patient demonstrated. It can be quantified by measuring pressure during an end-expiratory pause. There are many causes of reduce expiration time and flow that lead to increased auto-PEEP including:

- Increased lung compliance
- High expiratory resistance due to airway or circuit problem, such as asthma or COPD, which requires mechanical ventilation and high minute ventilation. Increasing external PEEP in these situations will make it more difficult for air to leave the lungs.

5. **A.** Noninvasive positive-pressure ventilation (NPPV) has proven efficacy in the treatment of patients with hypercapnic respiratory failure resulting from an acute exacerbation of COPD. It is also beneficial in patients with cardiogenic pulmonary edema, but not in the presence of ischemia or shock as depicted in choice B; this patient is in cardiogenic shock with a metabolic acidosis and should be intubated. NPPV is unlikely to benefit the patient with mild disease, as presented in choice C. Absolute contraindications to NPPV are cardiac and respiratory arrest. Relative contraindications include the inability to control secretions, vomiting, and hemoptysis, as in choice D, because of aspiration risk.

6. **C.** Compliance is the change in volume divided by the change in pressure. Decreased lung compliance is a prominent feature of ARDS.

- Dynamic compliance is the tidal volume divided by the dynamic change in pressure (peak inspiratory pressure minus PEEP).
- Static compliance is the tidal volume divided by the static pressure differential (plateau pressure minus PEEP); in this example, $450/(30 - 15) = 30$.

  Normal respiratory system compliance is 100 mL/cm H_2O and should be greater than 50 mL/cm H_2O in mechanically ventilated patients. Compliance can be used to determine the best PEEP setting. The optimal level of PEEP is associated with the highest compliance. Low lung volume (insufficient PEEP) and overdistention (too much PEEP) are associated with a lower compliance than best PEEP.

7. **C.** Steroids have been studied for both prevention and treatment of ARDS. Systematic reviews and meta-analyses have produced ambiguous findings and, currently, routine use of steroids is not recommended. See Table 25-1 for management strategies in patients with ARDS.

Table 25-1. Strategies That Demonstrated Effectiveness in the Management of Patients With Severe Acute Respiratory Distress Syndrome (ARDS)

Management Strategies	Reported Benefits
Mechanical ventilation with tidal volumes restricted to 6 mL/kg predicted body weight	• Decrease in mortality compared with higher tidal volumes
Early, short-term use of neuromuscular blockade	• Reduces mortality • Reduces mechanical ventilation days without an associated increase in intensive care unit–acquired weakness
Prone positioning	• Shown to improve extubation rates and mortality in patients with severe ARDS

8. **D.** Placement of a tracheostomy is thought to allow a more secure and manageable airway, earlier and safer enteral feeding, easier oral care, and enhanced patient comfort while reducing sedation needs and facilitating mobilization. When no longer needed, tracheostomy tubes are downsized and removed to allow the stoma to heal by secondary intention without the need for a second procedure. Several studies, including a meta-analysis, showed that timing of tracheostomy did not alter mortality or increase the risk for hospital-acquired pneumonia. Given the lack of validated tools to predict difficulty weaning and ventilator dependency, the selection of patients for tracheostomy remains a subjective decision. Percutaneous techniques have been associated in meta-analyses with a trend toward fewer complications and cost-effectiveness by releasing surgical resources.

9. **D.** It is important to recognize that airway pressure is a poor surrogate of lung stress because it ignores the effect of chest recoil. This concept is especially relevant when managing mechanically

ventilated patients with ARDS and comorbidities such as obesity. Transpulmonary pressure (TPP) is the net distending pressure applied to the lung by contraction of the inspiratory muscles or by positive-pressure ventilation.

TPP = alveolar pressure (P_{alv}) − pleural pressure (P_{pl})

The positioning of an esophageal catheter is required to measure the esophageal pressure, which is clinically used as a surrogate for P_{pl} and allows calculation of the TPP. TPP measurement allows partitioning of lung compliance from chest wall compliance; by doing so, the clinician is able to determine optimal PEEP, avoiding lung overdistention and cyclic recruitment/derecruitment, both of which are associated with ventilator-induced lung injury.

In selected patients, the use of a mechanical ventilation strategy based on measurements of TPP has been shown to significantly improve oxygenation and respiratory system compliance.

10. **C.** Negative-pressure pulmonary edema (NPPE) is a well-described cause of acute respiratory failure that is diagnosed in the presence of evidence of intense inspiratory effort against an obstructed airway such as laryngospasm or obstructed endotracheal tubes. Patients with NPPE generate very negative airway pressures, which augment transvascular fluid filtration and precipitate interstitial and alveolar edema. Supportive care should be directed at relieving the upper airway obstruction and, in severe cases, institution of lung-protective positive-pressure ventilation and diuresis. Resolution of the pulmonary edema is usually rapid, in part because alveolar fluid clearance mechanisms are intact. Other presented causes of noncardiogenic pulmonary edema do not usually have such an acute presentation associated with airway obstruction, and they tend to have greater severity.

11. **E.** The chest x-ray shown demonstrates pulmonary edema. Given the neurologic insult with a high-grade subarachnoid hemorrhage, the likelihood of neurogenic pulmonary edema is high. This typically occurs minutes to hours after a severe central nervous system insult and will resolve in days. The pathophysiology is not fully understood, but it is thought to be in part due to increased systemic

vascular resistance from sympathetic surge due to the brain injury. The increased vascular resistance increases the pulmonary capillary pressure and then endothelial injury. The pulmonary edema that results appears the same as cardiogenic edema, but there is normal left ventricular cardiac function. The neurogenic pulmonary edema is responsive to PEEP, and although it would also respond to diuresis, attempts to obtain large negative total body balance can result in low cardiac filling and cerebral perfusion in a patient who likely has poor cerebral autoregulation. Although neuromuscular blockade and low lung volume ventilation are beneficial in ARDS, they play little role in management of neurogenic pulmonary edema.

12. **D.** The patient likely has increased pressor requirements because of auto-PEEP due to his COPD and invasive ventilation. Auto-PEEP results in increased intrathoracic pressure and reduces the preload of the right and left ventricles. The clues to suggest auto-PEEP are:

- Exhalation that continues until the next breath starts
- A delay between the start of inspiratory effort and the drop-in airway pressure
- Failure of peak airway pressure to change when external PEEP is applied
- In paralyzed patients, reduction of plateau pressure after prolonged exhalation

The treatment of auto-PEEP is multifactorial, and there are several approaches, including increasing the expiratory time, decreasing tidal volume, reducing ventilator demand (treat pain/anxiety), reducing flow resistance (frequent suctioning, bronchodilators, large-bore endotracheal tube), and continuing application of PEEP.

Although it seems somewhat counterintuitive, PEEP still maintains patency of collapsed airways that are not involved with auto-PEEP, and allowing these to remain open will create increased expiratory flow (this is similar to pursed lip breathing seen in COPD).

REFERENCES

Acute Respiratory Distress Syndrome Network. Ventilation with lower tidal volumes as compared with traditional tidal volumes for acute lung injury and the acute respiratory distress syndrome. *N Engl J Med.* 2000;342: 1301-1308.

Baumann A, Audibert G, McDonnell J, et al. Neurogenic pulmonary edema. *Acta Anaesthesiol Scand.* 2007;51:447-455.

Bhattacharya M, Richard H. Kallet RH, et al. Negative-pressure pulmonary edema. *Chest.* 2016;150(4):927-933.

Bouhemad B, Zhang M, Lu Q, Rouby JJ. Clinical review: bedside ultrasound in critical care practice. *Crit Care.* 2007;11:205.

Delaney A, Bagshaw SM, Nalos M. Percutaneous dilational tracheostomy in critically ill patients: a systematic review and meta-analysis. *Crit Care.* 2006;10:R55.

Diaz-Reganon G, Minambres E, Ruiz A, et al. Safety and complications of percutaneous tracheostomy in a cohort of 800 mixed ICU patients. *Anaesthesia.* 2008;63:1193-1203.

Engels PT, Bagshaw SM, Meier M, Brindley PG. Tracheostomy: from insertion to decannulation. *Can J Surg.* 2009;52:427-433.

Forel JM, Roch A, Papazian L. Paralytics in critical care: not always a bad guy. *Curr Opin Crit Care.* 2009;15:59-66.

Guerin C, Reignier J, Richard JC, et al. Prone positioning is severe acute respiratory distress syndrome. *N Engl J Med.* 2013;368:2159-2168.

Hess DR, Kacmarek RM. *Essentials of Mechanical Ventilation.* 3rd ed. New York, NY: McGraw-Hill; 2014

Imber DA, Pirrone M, Zhang C, et al. Respiratory management of perioperative obese patients: a literature review. *Respir Care.* 2016;61(12):1681-1692.

Kelly CR, Higgins AR, Chandra S. Noninvasive positive-pressure ventilation. *N Engl J Med.* 2015;372:e30.

Krodel DJ, Bittner EA, Abdulnour R, et al. Case scenario: acute postoperative negative pressure pulmonary edema. *Anesthesiology.* 2010;113:200-207.

Lichtenstein DA. Ultrasound in the management of thoracic disease. *Crit Care Med.* 2007;35:250-261.

Lim WJ, Mohammed Akram R, Carson KV, et al. Non-invasive positive pressure ventilation for treatment of respiratory failure due to severe acute exacerbations of asthma. *Cochrane Database Syst Rev.* 2012;12:CD004360.

Mughal MM, Dulver DA, Minai OA, et al. Auto-positive end-expiratory pressure: mechanisms and treatment. *Cleveland Clinic J Med.* 2005;72:801-809.

Murphy GS, Brull SJ. Residual neuromuscular block: lessons unlearned. Part I: definitions, incidence, and adverse physiologic effects of residual neuromuscular block. *Anesth Analg.* 2010;111:120-128.

Murphy GS, Szokol JW, Avram MJ, et al. Postoperative residual neuromuscular blockade is associated with impaired clinical recovery. *Anesth Analg.* 2013;117:133-141.

Papazian L, Forel JM, Gacouin A, et al. Neuromuscular blockers in early acute respiratory distress syndrome. *N Engl J Med.* 2010;363:1107-1116.

Peigang Y, Marini JJ. Ventilation of patients with asthma and chronic obstructive pulmonary disease. *Curr Opin Crit Care.* 2002;8:70-76.

Pepe PE, Marini JJ. Occult positive end-expiratory pressure in mechanically ventilated patients with airflow obstruction: the auto-PEEP effect. *Am Rev Respir Dis.* 1982;126:166-170.

Ranieri VM, Guiliani R, Cinnella G, et al. Physiologic effects of positive end-expiratory pressure in patients with chronic obstructive pulmonary disease during active ventilator failure and controlled mechanical ventilation. *Am Rev Respir Dis.* 1993;140:1-3.

Simon RP. Neurogenic pulmonary edema. *Neurol Clin.* 1993;11:309-323.

Slutsky AS, Ranieri M. Ventilator-induced lung injury. *N Engl J Med.* 2013;369:2126-2136.

Steinberg KP, Hudson LD, Goodman RB, et al. Efficacy and safety of corticosteroids for persistent acute respiratory distress syndrome. *N Engl J Med.* 2006;354:1671-1684.

Talmor D, Sarge T, Malhotra A, et al. Mechanical ventilation guided by esophageal pressure in acute lung injury. *N Engl J Med.* 2008;359:2095-2104.

Tobin MJ, Perez W, Guenther SM, et al. The pattern of breathing during successful and unsuccessful trials of weaning from mechanical ventilation. *Am Rev Respir Dis.* 1986;134:1111-1118.

Villar J, Kacmarek RM, Pérez-Méndez L, Aguirre-Jaime A. A high positive end-expiratory pressure, low tidal volume ventilatory strategy improves outcome in persistent acute respiratory distress syndrome: a randomized, controlled trial. *Crit Care Med.* 2006;34:1311-1318.

Wang F, Wu Y, Bo L, et al. The timing of tracheotomy in critically ill patients undergoing mechanical ventilation: a systematic review and meta-analysis of randomized controlled trials. *Chest.* 2011;140:1456-1465.

Ward NS, Dushay KM. Clinical concise review: mechanical ventilation of patients with chronic obstructive pulmonary disease. *Crit Care Med.* 2008;36:1614-1619.

26

Effects of Critical Illness in the Surgical Intensive Care Unit

Avneep Aggarwal, MD and Abraham Sonny, MD

Questions

1. A 57-year-old man is admitted from an outside hospital to your intensive care unit (ICU) in shock. Past medical history is significant for Crohn disease and a recent flare in the past month requiring prednisone. He underwent a laparoscopic cholecystectomy 1 week prior to transfer and has been having increasing abdominal pain for the past 3 days. Despite fluid resuscitation, he still requires norepinephrine and vasopressin infusions to maintain mean arterial pressure (MAP) >65 mm Hg. There is suspicion of relative adrenal insufficiency. Which of the following interventions is the best next step?

   A. Measure baseline total cortisone level
   B. Initiate hydrocortisone treatment
   C. Adrenocorticotropic hormone (ACTH) stimulation test
   D. Assay of cellular activity of cortisol

2. How do the Centers for Medicare and Medicaid Services in the United States define prolonged mechanical ventilation?

   A. 7 days of mechanical ventilation for at least 12 hours per day
   B. 14 days of mechanical ventilation for at least 6 hours per day
   C. 14 days of mechanical ventilation for at least 12 hours per day
   D. 21 days of mechanical ventilation for at least 6 hours per day

3. A 68-year-old woman is admitted to ICU for postoperative management after undergoing an emergent laparotomy for perforated duodenal ulcer. She is being weaned off mechanical ventilation. Which of the following is an essential criterion before initiating a spontaneous breath trial?

   A. Awake and alert patient
   B. Arterial blood gas (ABG) with pH of 7.20
   C. Ability to initiate an inspiratory effort
   D. Core temperature ≤38°C
   E. On PS with fraction of inspired oxygen (FiO_2) of 60% and positive end-expiratory pressure (PEEP) of 12 cm H_2O

4. A 33-year-old woman was admitted to the ICU with severe respiratory failure due to H1N1 influenza. She had a prolonged ICU stay complicated by acute kidney injury, delirium, and difficult weaning. Laboratory results showed the following: triiodothyronine (T_3) 50 ng/dL (normal 75-200 ng/dL); thyroxine (T_4) 2.4 μg/dL (normal 4.6-11.2 μg/dL); thyroid-stimulating hormone (TSH) 1.8 mU/L (normal 0.4-4.0 mU/L); and reverse T_3 (rT_3) 34 ng/dL (normal 10-24 ng/dL). Based on these lab values, which of the following is most appropriate to recommend at this time?

A. Administer combination T_4-T_3 (liothyronine) therapy.

B. Administer half the expected full replacement dose of synthetic T_4 (levothyroxine).

C. No thyroid hormone replacement treatment is required.

D. Evaluate for resistance to TSH.

5. A week ago, a 47-year-old man had a bowel perforation and underwent partial small bowel resection and anastomosis. His postoperative course was complicated by anastomotic leak requiring reexploration and massive bowel edema. His abdominal wound was closed by a vacuum-assisted wound closure device. Which of the following is a disadvantage of this kind of abdominal wound closure?

A. Decreased wound closure rate

B. Increased enterocutaneous fistula formation

C. Increased dressing changes required

D. Decreased removal of edema fluid

6. A 78-year-old woman is admitted to ICU after a fall, and proximal left hip fracture is seen on radiograph. She also complains of increasing fatigue and weight loss over the past 6 months. On further evaluation, she is found to be moderately frail by the Clinical Frailty Scale. Which of the following hormonal changes is associated with a decline in neuromuscular reserve in frailty?

A. Increased dehydroepiandrosterone sulfate (DHEA-S)

B. Increased cortisol

C. Increased growth hormone

D. Increased insulin-like growth factor-1 (IGF-1)

7. A 54-year-old man with ulcerative colitis, diabetes mellitus, coronary artery disease, hypertension, and hypercholesterolemia was admitted to the ICU after a total colectomy for toxic megacolon. On arrival in the ICU, he was in septic shock and required vasopressors and stress-dose steroids. His ICU course was complicated by prolonged mechanical ventilation and delirium. It is noted that the patient had marked muscle wasting and diffuse weakness of his extremities more proximally than distally. His muscle strength was graded as 2 to 3 on a scale of 5 proximally and 0 to 2 distally. His sensory examination was normal. His reflexes were hypoactive throughout. The muscles of the neck and respiratory system were not weak, and there were no other significant findings on neurologic assessment. Serum creatinine kinase is elevated to 1600 U/L. Nerve conduction studies showed low-amplitude motor responses, normal sensory responses, and no change on repetitive nerve stimulation. What is the most likely diagnosis?

A. Guillain-Barré syndrome

B. Critical illness myopathy

C. Rhabdomyolysis

D. Critical illness polyneuropathy

8. A 44-year-old woman presented for treatment with complaints tracing back almost 6 months ago after her discharge from an ICU. Her ICU admission was due to severe asthma leading to respiratory failure and a week of mechanical ventilation. Her main complaints included mixed hallucinations, irritability, feeling suffocated and choked, inability to perform everyday tasks, and depressed mood. No psychic symptomatology was evident before the event to her or her family. Which of the following is the most important predictor of posttraumatic stress disorder after ICU stay?

A. Length of ICU stay

B. Severity of critical illness

C. Spontaneous awakening trials

D. Use of benzodiazepines

9. A 52-year-old woman, who is postoperative day 4 from a total abdominal hysterectomy, is admitted to the ICU with fever and hypotension. Her past medical history is significant for hypertension, diabetes mellitus, moderate protein-calorie malnutrition, and anemia of chronic disease. On admission, her blood pressure is 74/40 mm Hg, pulse rate is 104 bpm, temperature is 39°C, and respiratory rate is 24 breaths/min. She is emergently intubated and is volume resuscitated but still requires norepinephrine and vasopressin to maintain MAP >65 mm Hg. On physical exam, her abdomen is soft and appropriately tender, but no bowel sounds are auscultated. Which of the following is a contraindication for initiation of enteral nutrition in this patient?

A. Absence of bowel sounds

B. Diabetes mellitus

C. Circulatory shock

D. Not passing flatus

10. Which of the following statements regarding end-of-life care discussion is true?

A. Physicians have been shown to underestimate survival rate in terminally ill patients.

B. More than 70% of elderly patients in the United States require a surrogate decision maker at the end of life.

C. Utilization of life-sustaining interventions at the end of life is not influenced by race.

D. Adult children proxies have been found to be more accurate than spouses.

Answers and Explanations

1. B. Suboptimal cortisol production during septic shock has been termed functional or relative adrenal insufficiency. The adrenal suppression in critically ill patients is often reversible, and there is no consensus about indications for its treatment or diagnostic criteria. Also, there is no consensus over what cortisol level is normal in septic shock, what constitutes an adequate response to ACTH, and what dose of synthetic ACTH should be used for stimulation testing. Adrenal suppression should be suspected when critically ill patients do not respond to volume resuscitation, especially in patients who have recently been on steroid treatment. There is a possibility that glucocorticoid resistance exists at receptor level and assay of cellular activity of cortisol can be used to assess it, but it is still experimental and not clinically relevant.

As per the available evidence at present, there is no advantage of steroids in patients with severe sepsis not in septic shock. In patients with refractory septic shock, it is reasonable to administer hydrocortisone therapy. ACTH stimulation test is not recommended prior to initiating steroid therapy in these patients because it cannot reliably differentiate between responders and nonresponders to therapy.

2. D. Prolonged mechanical ventilation (PMV) is defined by the Centers for Medicare and Medicaid Services in the United States as greater than 21 days of mechanical ventilation for at least 6 hours per day. PMV is associated with increased healthcare cost, morbidity, and mortality. Rationale is that by 21 days, most easily reversible conditions have been addressed, and continued requirement for mechanical ventilation usually signals a more persistent chronic condition. It has been observed that the majority of patients who are transferred to the long-term acute care hospital setting receiving mechanical ventilation had received ventilation for at least 21 days.

3. C. Patients receiving mechanical ventilation for respiratory failure should undergo a formal assessment of discontinuation if the following criteria are met:

- The cause of the respiratory failure has improved
- Adequate oxygenation with partial pressure of oxygen (Pao_2)/FiO_2 ≥150 or oxygen saturation (SpO_2) ≥90% on FiO_2 ≤40% and PEEP ≤5 cm H_2O
- No acidosis (ie, pH >7.25)
- Hemodynamic stability (not on vasopressors or very low dose of vasopressor required)
- Able to initiate an inspiratory effort

Additional criteria that are helpful (optional) in supporting a decision to initiate spontaneous breathing trial include:

- Awake and alert or easily arousable patient
- Adequate hemoglobin
- Not febrile
- Maximum inspiratory pressure < –30 cm H_2O

4. C. Acute, nonthyroidal illness can be associated with low plasma levels of free T_3 caused by inhibition of T_4 to T_3 conversion, leading to an increase in reverse T_3 (rT_3). It is commonly identified in critically ill patients and is also known as low T_3 and/or T_4 syndrome. Previously, these patients were thought to be euthyroid, and the term sick euthyroid syndrome was used to describe the laboratory abnormalities. Plasma TSH levels can be useful in distinguishing primary (elevated TSH) from secondary/central hypothyroidism (reduced TSH), but TSH measurements alone are not reliable in critically ill patients. In critically ill patients, TSH can be within low to normal range and is mostly without a circadian rhythm. In these cases, it has been suggested to get measurement of a full thyroid panel including a total T_4, a free T_4, and a T_3.

There is no evidence of benefit of treatment with T_3, T_4, or TSH if there are no other clinical signs of hypothyroidism. Most of the available evidence suggests it is potentially harmful to give thyroid hormone to patients with nonthyroidal illness who have low serum T_4 or T_3 concentrations.

Resistance to TSH is characterized by high serum TSH concentrations and normal or low serum T_4 and T_3 concentrations. This patient does not have lab values suggestive of resistance to TSH.

5. **B.** Negative-pressure wound therapy is a therapeutic technique using a vacuum dressing to promote healing in acute or chronic wounds, complicated abdominal injuries, evisceration, and abdominal compartment syndrome. The therapy involves the controlled application of subatmospheric pressure to the local wound. It helps in increasing blood flow to the affected area, reduce edema and excess fluid, and increase wound contraction to allow for enhancement of wound granulation. Main advantages of vacuum-assisted wound-closure devices include reduced frequency of dressing changes, improved patient comfort, improved efficiency of wound closure, and improved removal of edema. It helps in abdominal wall reconstruction later by providing a nonedematous clean tissue bed. The main disadvantages of these devices include increased risk of bleeding and increased rates of new enterocutaneous fistula formation.

6. **B.** The concept of frailty has been defined as a multidimensional syndrome characterized by the loss of physical and cognitive biologic reserves that predisposes to the accumulation of deficits and increased vulnerability to minor stressors and risk for adverse outcomes, including disability, hospitalization, postoperative complications, and death. The Clinical Frailty Scale is a rapid frailty screening tool that is scored between 1 (very fit) and 7 (severely frail) based on self-report of comorbidities and the need for help with activities of daily living (ADLs). Multiple age-related hormone changes have been associated with frailty, including decreased DHEA-S, growth hormone, IGF-1, and 25(OH)-vitamin D and increased catabolic hormone (cortisol) levels. DHEA-S likely plays a direct role in maintaining muscle mass, and therefore, decline in DHEA-S contributes to muscle decline. In addition, decreased growth hormone and IGF-1 have been associated with decreased muscle strength and decreased mobility.

7. **B.** Prolonged treatment in an ICU and, particularly, prolonged mechanical ventilation are associated with a loss of muscle mass and a marked reduction in muscle strength, which is referred to as ICU-acquired weakness. ICU-acquired weakness is a result of a number of pathophysiologic mechanisms. The most common form of ICU-acquired myopathy is critical illness myopathy (CIM). The most common presenting features are flaccid quadriparesis especially affecting proximal muscles and failure to wean from mechanical ventilation. Extraoccular muscle weakness is rare. An elevation in serum creatinine kinase is common. Diagnostic electrophysiologic findings for CIM include reduction of amplitude of muscle compound action potentials, absence of a decremental response on repetitive nerve stimulation, and near-normal sensory nerve amplitudes. Muscle biopsy will show histopathologic findings of myopathy with myosin loss. Sensation remains normal and help in differentiating it from neuropathies such as critical illness polyneuropathy and Guillain-Barré syndrome (GBS). Critical illness polyneuropathy should be suspected in a critically ill patient especially if complicated by multiorgan failure and difficult weaning. Electrophysiologic findings suggestive of critical illness polyneuropathy include decrease in both sensory and motor nerve amplitudes. GBS is characterized by a rapidly progressive polyneuropathy with weakness or paralysis. The essential clinical features of GBS are progressive, mostly symmetric muscle weakness and absent or depressed deep tendon reflexes. Critically ill patients can develop rhabdomyolysis from infectious causes or medication-related causes.

8. **D.** Posttraumatic stress disorder (PTSD) has been described as "the complex somatic, cognitive, affective, and behavioral effects of psychological trauma." PTSD is characterized by intrusive thoughts, nightmares and flashbacks of past traumatic events, hypervigilance, and sleep disturbance, all of which lead to considerable social, occupational, and interpersonal dysfunction. A 2015 meta-analysis found clinically important PTSD symptoms occurred in one-fifth of critical illness survivors at the 1-year follow-up. Risk factors for PTSD symptoms were benzodiazepine use, early memories of frightening ICU experiences, and

pre-ICU comorbid psychopathology. Neither the severity of critical illness nor length of ICU stay was predictive of PTSD.

9. **C.** Gastrointestinal dysfunction is common in the ICU depending on various preexisting medical comorbidities and use of medications. Bowel sounds and passing of flatus are not required as a prerequisite for initiation of enteral nutrition. Bowel sounds only indicate gut contractility but do not reflect absorptive capacity or mucosal integrity. Circulatory shock and use of multiple vasopressors increase risk of subclinical ischemia to intestinal mucosa, and enteral nutrition is usually withheld until the patient is hemodynamically stable. Guidelines discourage early enteral nutrition in critically ill patients who are both hemodynamically unstable and have not had their intravascular volume fully resuscitated, since such patients may be predisposed to bowel ischemia. Hemodynamic instability by itself, unless severe, is not a contraindication for enteral nutrition if there is evidence for adequate volume resuscitation and tissue perfusion. Although diabetes does increase the risk of gastroparesis, it is not a contraindication to enteral feeding. Other contraindications to enteral nutrition include bowel obstruction, severe ileus, major upper gastrointestinal bleeding, intractable vomiting or diarrhea, and gastrointestinal ischemia.

10. **B.** It has been observed that the majority of elderly patients (>70%) in the United States require a surrogate decision maker to decide end-of-life care decisions. Evidence also suggests that many surrogate decision makers have difficulty in determining what the wishes of their loved one might be, and almost 30% of surrogates incorrectly predict the treatment preferences of patients. Evidence shows that physicians are often poor at prognostication for individual patients. They have been shown to be overoptimistic regarding prognosis in terminally ill patients and tend to overestimate survival rates. In addition, nonwhite patients have been found to use more life-sustaining interventions at the end of life compared to white patients. Family relationships have been found to make an impact on the accuracy of proxies. Spouse proxies have been found to be more accurate than adult children of patients to predict the wishes of their loved one. Well-functioning families with less conflict are associated with higher accuracy about the patient's true wishes.

REFERENCES

Annane D, Bellissant E, Bollaert PE, et al. Corticosteroids for treating sepsis. *Cochrane Database Syst Rev.* 2015;1:CD002243.

Clegg A, Young J, Iliffe S, et al. Frailty in elderly people. *Lancet.* 2013;381:752.

Cooper MS, Stewart PM. Corticosteroid insufficiency in acutely ill patients. *N Engl J Med.* 2003;348:727-734.

Curtis RJ, Isaac M. What factors influence a family to support a decision withdrawing life support? *Evid-Based Pract Crit Care.* In press.

Fischer JE. A cautionary note: the use of vacuum assisted closure systems in the treatment of GI cutaneous fistula may be associated with higher mortality from subsequent fistula development. *Am J Surg.* 2008;196:1-4.

Fliers E, Bianco AC, Langouche L, Boelen A. Thyroid function in critically ill patients. *Lancet Diabetes Endocrinol.* 2015;3:816-825.

Frost DW, Cook DJ, Heyland DK, Fowler RA. Patient and healthcare professional factors influencing end-of-life decision-making during critical illness: a systematic review. *Crit Care Med.* 2011;39(5):1174-1189.

Kaptein EM, Sanchez A, Beale E, Chan LS. Clinical review: thyroid hormone therapy for postoperative nonthyroidal illnesses: a systematic review and synthesis. *J Clin Endocrinol Metab.* 2010;95:4526-4534.

Keh D, Trips E, Marx G, et al. Effect of hydrocortisone on development of shock among patients with severe sepsis: the HYPRESS randomized clinical trial. *JAMA.* 2016; 316(17):1775-1785.

Kessler RC, Rose S, Koenen KC, et al. How well can posttraumatic stress disorder be predicted from pre-trauma risk factors? An exploratory study in the WHO World Mental Health Surveys. *World Psychiatry.* 2014;13:265-274.

Khalid I, Doshi P, DiGiovine B. Early enteral nutrition and outcomes of critically ill patients treated with vasopressors and mechanical ventilation. *Am J Crit Care.* 2010;19:261-268.

Lacomis D. Electrophysiology of neuromuscular disorders in critical illness. *Muscle Nerve.* 2013;47:452-463.

Latronico N, Bolton CF. Critical illness polyneuropathy and myopathy: a major cause of muscle weakness and paralysis. *Lancet Neurol.* 2011;10:931-941.

Lone NI, Walsh TS. Prolonged mechanical ventilation in critically ill patients: epidemiology, outcomes and modelling the potential cost consequences of establishing a regional weaning unit. *Crit Care.* 2011;15:R102.

MacIntyre NR, Cook DJ, Ely EW Jr, et al. Evidence-based guidelines for weaning and discontinuing ventilatory support: a collective task force facilitated by the American College of Chest Physicians, the American Association for Respiratory Care, and the American College of Critical Care Medicine. *Chest.* 2001;120:375S.

MacIntyre NR, Epstein SK, Carson S, et al. Management of patients requiring prolonged mechanical ventilation:

report of a NAMDRC consensus conference. *Chest.* 2005;128:3937-3954.

Marquardt DL, Tatum RP, Lynge DC. *Postoperative Management of the Hospitalized Patient.* 6th ed. New York, NY: WebMD; 2007.

McClave SA, Taylor BE, Martindale RG, et al. Guidelines for the provision and assessment of nutrition support therapy in the adult critically ill patient: Society of Critical Care Medicine (SCCM) and American Society for Parenteral and Enteral Nutrition (A.S.P.E.N.). *JPEN J Parenter Enteral Nutr.* 2016;40:159.

McDermid RC, Stelfox HT, Bagshaw SM. Frailty in the critically ill: a novel concept. *Crit Care.* 2011;15(1):301.

Meade M, Guyatt G, Cook D, et al. Predicting success in weaning from mechanical ventilation. *Chest.* 2001;120:400S.

Multz AS, Aldrich TK, Prezant DJ, et al. Maximal inspiratory pressure is not a reliable test of inspiratory muscle strength in mechanically ventilated patients. *Am Rev Respir Dis.* 1990;142:529-532.

Parker AM, Sricharoenchai T, Raparla S, et al. Posttraumatic stress disorder in critical illness survivors: a metaanalysis. *Crit Care Med.* 2015;43:1121-1129.

Parks SM, Winter L, Santana AJ, et al. Family factors in end-of-life decision-making: family conflict and proxy relationship. *J Palliat Med.* 2011;14(2):179-184.

Silveira MJ, Kim SY, Langa KM. Advance directives and outcomes of surrogate decision making before death. *N Engl J Med.* 2010;362(13):1211-1218.

Walston J, Hadley EC, Ferrucci L, et al. Research agenda for frailty in older adults: toward a better understanding of physiology and etiology: summary from the American Geriatrics Society/National Institute on Aging Research Conference on Frailty in Older Adults. *J Am Geriatr Soc.* 2006;54:991-1001.

27

Cardiovascular Diseases

Christina Anne Jelly, MD and Abraham Sonny, MD

Questions

1. A 70-year-old woman presents to the emergency department with sudden-onset chest and upper back pain and was found to have a type B aortic dissection for which she is being medically managed in the intensive care unit with close hemodynamic monitoring. She initially arrived with hypertension and tachycardia but has now become hypotensive. Bedside transthoracic echocardiogram is shown below. Which of the following is true regarding cardiac tamponade?

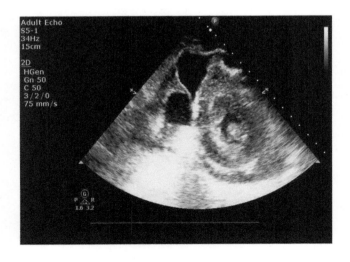

A. Pericardial fluid volume is predictive of clinical hemodynamic status.

B. Pericardiocentesis is indicated in all cases of cardiac tamponade.

C. Echocardiographic evidence of diastolic right atrial collapse is a specific finding of tamponade physiology.

D. Echocardiographic evidence that the inferior vena cava (IVC) fails to collapse during spontaneous respiration is a specific finding of tamponade physiology.

E. Intrapericardial pressure increases exponentially as pericardial fluid volume increases.

2. A 65-year-old man with past hypertension, hyperlipidemia, peripheral vascular disease, and extensive tobacco use who underwent femoral-femoral bypass grafting was found to have ST-segment elevations upon emergence of anesthesia and was taken urgently for cardiac catheterization. Compared to acute coronary syndromes in the nonsurgical population, which of the following best describes perioperative myocardial infarctions?

A. Perioperative myocardial infarctions are more likely to be associated with acute plaque rupture rather than supply-demand mismatch.

B. Perioperative myocardial infarction is more likely to manifest with ischemic symptoms.

C. Management of perioperative myocardial infarction is the same as with acute coronary syndrome (ACS) in the nonsurgical setting, except that antifibrinolytic therapy is absolutely contraindicated.

D. Troponin levels have been shown to predict increased long-term mortality in patients with perioperative myocardial infarction.

3. A 77-year-old woman with metastatic breast cancer presented for palliative vertebroplasty for persistent back pain due to vertebral metastases. The case was performed under conscious sedation. Postoperatively, the patient developed hypotension with a systolic blood pressure in the 60s. She was administered a fluid bolus and immediately transferred to the intensive care unit. Electrocardiogram (ECG) showed ST-segment depression in V_3-V_6. A troponin T was sent, which came back as 0.12 μg/L. Bedside ultrasonography demonstrated left ventricular segmental hypokinesis with mild to moderate reduction in ejection fraction. Which of the following is the most appropriate agent for treating this patient's hypotension?

A. Epinephrine

B. Norepinephrine

C. Phenylephrine

D. Milrinone

E. Levosimendan

4. A 72-year-old man with active tobacco use, severe chronic obstructive pulmonary disease, hypertension, and hyperlipidemia underwent open repair of a fractured femur. On postoperative day 2, the patient develops hypotension, tachycardia, and hypoxemia, and the intensive care triage team is called to evaluate. On arrival, the patient's blood pressure is 88/47 mm Hg, his heart rate is 104 bpm, and his oxygen saturation is 92% on 6-L face mask. Electrocardiogram reveals sinus tachycardia with no ST-T segment changes. What is the most appropriate next step?

A. Ventilation/perfusion lung scan

B. Spiral computed tomography (CT) of the pulmonary arteries

C. Cardiac catheterization

D. Point-of-care transthoracic cardiac ultrasound

E. Initiate thrombolytic therapy

5. An otherwise healthy 45-year-old man is admitted to the intensive care unit after a thoracotomy and right middle and upper lobectomy for lung cancer. He develops atrial fibrillation with rapid ventricular response postoperatively. His heart rate is 145 bpm, and his systolic blood pressure is 68 mm Hg. He appears somnolent but is able to follow commands. What is the most appropriate next step?

A. Begin immediate defibrillation

B. Initiate synchronized electrical cardioversion with 120 J

C. Initiate pharmacologic cardioversion with intravenous (IV) digoxin

D. Attempt rate control only because cardioversion would be contraindicated in the absence of anticoagulation

E. Administer IV adenosine

6. A 60-year-old man with a history of nonischemic cardiomyopathy who received a heart transplant 3 years ago is admitted to the intensive care unit after undergoing an emergent exploratory laparotomy due to gastric ulcer perforation. He is extubated at the end of the case, and an hour after arrival to the surgical intensive care unit, he develops progressive substernal and upper abdominal discomfort. What is the most appropriate next step?

A. Obtain an electrocardiogram to evaluate for myocardial ischemia

B. Perform bedside echocardiography to assess left ventricular function

C. Modify pain regimen to comfort and consider thoracic epidural placement

D. Call for a cardiology consult for emergent cardiac catheterization

7. Which of the following is true regarding methylene blue in the setting of refractory hypotension due to septic shock?

A. Methylene blue has been found to reduce overall doses of vasopressors when administered in patients with septic shock.

B. Methylene blue has been found to increase oxygen delivery in patients with septic shock by converting hemoglobin to methemoglobin.

C. Cardiac output and systemic vascular resistance exhibit a dose-dependent increase with escalating doses of methylene blue.

D. Improved survival has been associated with patients receiving methylene blue in early sepsis compared to late sepsis.

8. According to the Surviving Sepsis Guidelines, which of the following would be the most appropriate next-line agent for the treatment of septic shock when norepinephrine is insufficient to maintain a mean arterial pressure of ≥65 mm Hg?

A. Milrinone

B. Dopamine

C. Epinephrine

D. Phenylephrine

E. Dobutamine

Answers and Explanations

1. E. Point-of-care ultrasound is the modality of choice to quickly and safely evaluate patients with suspected tamponade physiology. Cardiac tamponade occurs when pericardial fluid disturbs cardiac function leading to decreased cardiac output and, in severe situations, complete hemodynamic collapse. Echocardiographic evidence of cardiac tamponade is characterized by collapse of the right atrium and ventricle during diastole. Right atrial collapse is not a specific finding for cardiac tamponade as it may also be found in patients with pleural effusions and severe dehydration. Failure of the IVC to collapse with respirations may be found in cardiac tamponade, but is also found in patients who have elevated right-sided pressures due to volume overload, pulmonary embolism, or valvular heart disease. Estimation of pericardial fluid volume is not generally predictive of clinical hemodynamic compromise as chronic pericardial effusions may expand the pericardium over time and not lead to significant tamponade. The concern in this patient is a type B dissection extending proximally into the ascending aorta leading to a retro type A dissection. Pericardiocentesis should be used with caution in cardiac tamponade secondary to aortic dissection, and the preference is for definitive surgical management. The correct answer is choice E as pericardial fluid has an exponential pressure-volume relationship.

2. D. Patients presenting for noncardiac surgery with or at risk of cardiac disease have an approximately 3.9% risk of suffering a major perioperative cardiac event. In medical patients with fatal myocardial infarctions, approximately 70% were associated with ruptured coronary plaques, as opposed to 50% in the perioperative population. Patients with perioperative myocardial infarctions are far less likely to experience ischemic symptoms, as the usual clinical picture is obscured by anesthesia, incisional pain, respiratory or gastrointestinal complications, sedation, or analgesia. The management of perioperative myocardial infarction is the same as for myocardial infarctions in medical patients. However, caution must be exercised before initiating antifibrinolytic, antiplatelet, or anticoagulation therapy, and they are only absolutely contraindicated in special situations, such as after neurosurgery. Finally, mortality has been shown to be higher among patients with marked troponin elevations compared with patients with minor troponin elevations.

3. B. This patient is likely in cardiogenic shock from left ventricular dysfunction caused by myocardial ischemia. The American College of Cardiology/American Heart Association (ACC/AHA) guidelines recommend norepinephrine for treatment of severe hypotension in the setting of myocardial infarction. Norepinephrine is a potent α_1-adrenergic agonist with β-agonist activity, making it both a potent vasopressor and a less potent direct inotrope. Inotropic agents such as epinephrine or milrinone increase contractility, potentially worsening ischemia. In comparison to norepinephrine, phenylephrine results in greater coronary vasoconstriction, which may worsen ischemia.

Dopamine and dobutamine have also been recommended for treatment of cardiogenic shock in the setting of ischemia. However, they are not preferred in the presence of severe hypotension.

4. B. This patient has a high pretest probability for the presence of pulmonary emboli, which may be calculated using the Modified Wells Score. Given the patient's recent surgery, heart rate, and high suspicion for pulmonary embolism in this setting, his Wells Score would be 6, and as such, further diagnostic imaging is indicated. In hemodynamically unstable patients, CT of the pulmonary arteries should be performed because it has 97% sensitivity for detecting emboli. Echocardiography is not recommended as a routine imaging test for diagnosis of pulmonary embolism but may be considered if the patient is critically ill and deemed too ill for transport to the CT scanner. Thrombolytic therapy may be considered in this patient, but given the risk of administration in the setting of his recent surgery, administration should be delayed until definitive diagnosis of pulmonary embolism is made on CT.

Ventilation/perfusion scanning may be considered in hemodynamically stable patients with renal failure to avoid contrast administration. Cardiac catheterization may be considered after the diagnosis of pulmonary embolism has been ruled out and if the clinical picture is more suggestive of cardiac ischemia.

Pulmonary Embolism Wells Score

Symptoms of deep venous thrombosis (DVT)	3 points
No alternative diagnosis better explains illness	3 points
Tachycardia >100 bpm	1.5 points
Immobilization (>3 days) or recent surgery (4 weeks)	1.5 points
Prior history of DVT or pulmonary embolism	1.5 points
Hemoptysis	1.5 points
Presence of malignancy	1.5 points

Interpretation of Wells Score

Score	Risk	Mean Probability
<2	Low	3.6
2-6	Moderate	20.5
>6	High	66.7

5. **B.** Prompt electrical cardioversion is indicated in patients with severe symptoms. The patient is awake and conversant and, moreover, does not have ventricular tachycardia or ventricular fibrillation; thus, immediate defibrillation would be inappropriate. Synchronized electrical cardioversion with 120 to 200 J is the most appropriate response for a patient who is unstable. Pharmacologic cardioversion may also be attempted, but an agent, such as digoxin, would not be expected to have an immediate effect. Electrical cardioversion is contraindicated in patients who have had atrial fibrillation of unknown duration or for more than 48 hours in the absence of anticoagulation. This is the first episode of atrial fibrillation in this patient; thus, he would be a candidate for either pharmacologic or electrical cardioversion without prior anticoagulation.

Adenosine is effective for managing reentrant arrhythmias using the atrioventricular node; however, this agent has no role in the management of atrial fibrillation due to its short duration of action.

6. **A.** It is likely that substernal and upper abdominal discomfort in a patient after an exploratory laparotomy with an incision extending up to the xiphoid process is primarily inflammatory in nature and related to the surgical incision. However, in a post–cardiac transplant patient, there must be a high suspicion for myocardial ischemia given the high incidence of cardiac allograft vasculopathy in transplant recipients. In the transplanted heart, sympathetic, parasympathetic, and sensory innervation are severed. One clinical manifestation of this is a higher resting heart rate in donor heart recipients due to the absence of vagal modulation. However, cardiac reinnervation, particularly of sympathetic nerves, may occur within 6 to 12 months after cardiac transplantation in up to 30% of cases. Moreover, cardiac sympathetic nerves have been proposed as the primary transmission pathway for cardiac pain. As such, chest pain in cardiac transplant patients should not be dismissed as noncardiac in origin, and the first step is to obtain an electrocardiogram. Cardiac transplant recipients often have baseline electrocardiogram abnormalities, and thus, electrocardiography alone has a poor specificity for detecting myocardial ischemia, but a baseline should be obtained prior to further diagnostic testing, including echocardiography. Cardiac catheterization would not be appropriate at this time given his recent surgery and the need for systemic anticoagulation for cardiac catheterization.

7. **A.** Methylene blue, a selective inhibitor of guanylate cyclase involved in nitrous oxide–mediated vasodilation, has enjoyed much attention due to its ability to antagonize profound, refractory hypotension in vasoplegic states, such as postoperative vasoplegia syndrome and other distributive shock states such

as anaphylaxis and septic shock. Improved survival with methylene blue has been found in rat models of late sepsis, not early sepsis, and this difference has not borne out in human studies. Several small observational studies have found beneficial effects on hemodynamic parameters, such as raising mean arterial pressure and lowering dependence on vasopressor therapy. However, no consistent beneficial effect has been found on oxygen delivery, cardiac output, or morbidity or mortality.

8. C. Per the 2011 Surviving Sepsis Guidelines, norepinephrine is the first-line vasopressor to maintain a mean arterial pressure of ≥65 mm Hg in a patient presenting with septic shock. Epinephrine may be used as an additional agent to maintain adequate arterial blood pressure or as an alternative agent. Vasopressin may also be added as an adjunct to norepinephrine to reduce to norepinephrine dose. Milrinone is an inodilator (agent with both positive inotropic and vasodilator effects) and would be an inappropriate choice in a patient with septic shock in the setting of normal cardiac function. Dopamine use in septic shock has been associated with the development of malignant tachyarrhythmias and is thus not recommended unless in highly selected patients. Phenylephrine is not recommended in the treatment of septic shock except as salvage therapy or when serious arrhythmias develop from norepinephrine.

Dobutamine may be appropriate as an inotrope to be administered in conjunction with a vasopressor in the following 2 settings: patients with myocardial dysfunction and patients who exhibit evidence of hypoperfusion despite achieving adequate mean arterial pressure.

REFERENCES

Agnelli G, Becattini C. Current concepts: acute pulmonary embolism. *N Engl J Med.* 2010;363:266-274.

Dawood MM, Gutpa DK, Southern J, et al. Pathology of fatal perioperative myocardial infarction: implications regarding pathophysiology and prevention. *Int J Cardiol.* 1996;57:37-44.

Dellinger RP, Levy MM, Rhodes A, et al. Surviving sepsis campaign: international guidelines for management of severe sepsis and septic shock: 2012. *Crit Care Med.* 2013; 41:580-637.

Goodman A, Perera P, Malilhot T, et al. The role of bedside ultrasound in the diagnosis of pericardial effusion and cardiac tamponade. *J Emerg Trauma Shock.* 2012;5:72-75.

Hosseinain L, Weiner M, Levin MA, et al. Methylene blue: magic bullet for vasoplegia? *Anesth Analg.* 2016;122:194-201.

January CT, Wann LS, Apert JS, et al. 2014 AHA/ACC/HRS guideline for the management of patients with atrial fibrillation: executive summary: a report of the American College of Cardiology/American Heart Association Task Force on Practice Guidelines and the Heart Rhythm Society. *J Am Coll Cardiol.* 2014;64:2246-2280.

Kostopanagiotou G, Smyrniotis V, Arkadopoulos N, et al. Anesthetic and perioperative management of adult transplant recipients in nontransplant surgery. *Anesthes Analg.* 1999;89(3):613-622.

Lucassen W, Geersing GJ, Erkens PM, et al. Clinical decision rules for excluding pulmonary embolism: a meta-analysis. *Ann Intern Med.* 2011;155:448-460.

Lucreziotti S, Foroni C, Fiorentini C. Perioperative myocardial infarction in noncardiac surgery: the diagnostic and prognostic role of cardiac troponins. *J Intern Med.* 2002;252:11-20.

Nagdev A, Stone MB. Point-of-care ultrasound evaluation of pericardial effusions: does this patient have cardiac tamponade? *Resuscitation.* 2011;82:671-673.

Naghavi M, Libby P, Falk E, et al. From vulnerable plaque to vulnerable patient: a call for new definitions and risk assessment strategies: part I. *Circulation.* 2003;108:1664-1672.

Overgaard C, Dzavik V. Inotropes and vasopressors: review of physiology and clinical use in cardiovascular disease. *Circulation.* 2008;118:1047-1056.

Pollack A, Nazif T, Mancini D, et al. Detection and imaging of cardiac allograft vasculopathy. *J Am Coll Cardiol Img.* 2013;6:613-623.

Reynolds H, Hochman JS. Cardiogenic shock: current concepts and improving outcomes. *Circulation.* 2008;117:686-697.

Stark RP, McGinn AL, Wilson RF. Chest pain in cardiac-transplant recipients–evidence of sensory reinnervation after cardiac transplantation. *N Engl J Med.* 1991;324: 1791-1794.

Tran TP, Khoynezhad A. Current management of type B aortic dissection. *Vasc Health Risk Manag.* 2009;5:53-63.

Wells PS, Anderson DR, Rodger M, et al. Derivation of a simple clinical model to categorize patients probability of pulmonary embolism: increasing the models utility with the SimpliRED D-dimer. *Thromb Haemost.* 2000;83: 416-420.

28

Renal Diseases

Jamie Sparling, MD and Abraham Sonny, MD

Questions

1. A 69-year-old man with stage III chronic kidney disease undergoes cerebral angiography. Which of the following interventions is most likely to prevent contrast nephropathy?

   A. Hypo-osmolar contrast media
   B. Fenoldopam infusion
   C. Intravenous (IV) hydration with sodium bicarbonate
   D. Mannitol infusion
   E. Furosemide bolus

2. A 74-year-old woman presents to the emergency department (ED) with new-onset hemoptysis and altered mental status. She is emergently intubated and admitted to the intensive care unit (ICU). Chest x-ray shows a speculated mass in the right upper lobe, and initial laboratory evaluation reveals the following values:

Sodium	134 mEq/L	Blood urea nitrogen (BUN)	10 mg/dL
Potassium	4.3 mEq/L	Creatinine	1.0 mg/dL
Chloride	100 mEq/L	Glucose	87 mg/dL
Bicarbonate	23 mEq/L	Calcium	14.8 mg/dL

What is the most important next step in management?

   A. Sodium chloride infusion
   B. Pamidronate infusion
   C. Calcitonin infusion
   D. Intravenous (IV) furosemide bolus
   E. Glucocorticoids

3. A 56-year-old woman is in postoperative day 2 from pelvic debulking for ovarian carcinoma. She has had 4 recent hospitalizations due to complications related to her chemotherapy and has ongoing diarrhea, for which stool cultures and *Clostridium difficile* antigen testing was sent today. Her postoperative course is notable for vasopressor requirement, which resolved on postoperative day 1, and postoperative anemia requiring transfusion of 3 units of packed red blood cells. Arterial blood gas analysis and basic metabolic profile show the following:

pH	7.28
$Paco_2$	35 mm Hg
Pao_2	97 mm Hg
Sodium	138 mEq/L
Potassium	4.2 mEq/L
Chloride	104 mEq/L
Bicarbonate	16 mEq/L
Albumin	4.6 g/dL

Which of these acid-base disturbances is most consistent with the values above?

A. Anion gap acidosis
B. Non–anion gap acidosis
C. Respiratory alkalosis with metabolic compensation
D. Mixed anion gap and non–anion gap metabolic acidosis
E. Combined metabolic and respiratory acidosis

4. A 33-year-old man is brought to the ED after he was found unconscious in the street. Glasgow coma scale score is 8. Arterial blood gas is sent while he is on the way to the computed tomography (CT) scanner for a noncontrast head CT. The blood gas shows the following:

pH	7.17
$Paco_2$	56 mm Hg
Pao_2	78 mm Hg
Sodium	140 mEq/L
Potassium	4.0 mEq/L
Chloride	102 mEq/L
Bicarbonate	20 mEq/L

Which of the following acid-base disturbances is most consistent with the values above?

A. Anion gap acidosis
B. Non–anion gap acidosis
C. Mixed anion gap and non–anion gap metabolic acidosis
D. Combined non–anion gap metabolic and respiratory acidosis
E. Combined anion gap metabolic and respiratory acidosis

5. A 64-year-old man is found unconscious in his apartment 36 hours after being last seen well. Noncontrast head CT shows epidural hematoma. He is intubated for airway protection in the ED and brought to the ICU. Foley catheter is placed, draining a scant amount of tea-colored urine. Initial laboratory findings are as follows:

Sodium	144 mEq/L	Creatinine	2.4 mg/dL
Potassium	5.3 mEq/L	Glucose	52 mg/dL
Chloride	104 mEq/L	Calcium	10.2 mg/dL
Bicarbonate	20 mEq/L	Creatinine kinase	15,438 IU/L
BUN	28 mg/dL		

What is the best next step in management?

A. Initiation of continuous renal replacement therapy
B. Aggressive IV hydration
C. IV mannitol
D. IV furosemide
E. IV bicarbonate

6. A 63-year-old woman is postoperative day 2 following an endovascular abdominal aortic aneurysm repair. The procedure was prolonged and technically difficult, with an estimated blood loss of 1 L. She initially required vasopressors upon arrival in the ICU but was successfully weaned on postoperative day 2 after adequate fluid resuscitation. She is now maintaining mean arterial pressure of 70 to 75 mm Hg, but urine output has dropped to 3 to 5 mL/h. She received furosemide 40 mg IV without improvement in urine output. Laboratory analysis includes the following values:

Sodium, serum	140 mEq/L
BUN, serum	43 mg/dL
Creatinine, serum	4.3 mg/dL
Sodium, urine	40 mEq/L
BUN, urine	86 mg/dL
Creatinine, urine	17 mg/dL
Osmolarity, urine	310 mOsm/kg

Which of the following is the most likely etiology of this patient's acute kidney injury?

A. Volume depletion
B. Acute tubular necrosis
C. Acute interstitial nephritis
D. Acute glomerulonephritis
E. Ureteral obstruction

7. A previously healthy 29-year-old man presents with 2 days of flank pain, gross hematuria, and fever. He is febrile to 39.2°C, is found to have a neutrophil-predominant leukocytosis, and is hypotensive to 70/40 mm Hg. CT of the abdomen and pelvis shows bilateral nephrolithiasis, an obstructing 5-mm stone at the right ureteropelvic junction, and right hydronephrosis with surrounding fat stranding. He is admitted to the ICU where he is treated with 4 L of lactated Ringer's and ceftriaxone 1 g IV, but he still requires norepinephrine 6 µg/min to maintain mean arterial pressure (MAP) >65 mm Hg. His serum creatinine has risen from 1.2 mg/dL at admission to 2.4 mg/dL 6 hours later. What is the most appropriate next step in management?

A. Urgent bedside percutaneous nephrostomy
B. Placement of a Foley catheter
C. Continue aggressive fluid resuscitation
D. Broaden antibiotic coverage to vancomycin and meropenem
E. IV furosemide

8. Which of the following scenarios constitutes acute kidney injury (AKI)?

A. A 59-year-old woman with pyelonephritis whose creatinine rises from 0.8 to 1.0 mg/dL over a 24-hour period
B. An 85-year-old man whose glomerular filtration rate (GFR) drops from 40 to 30 mL/min/1.73 m^2 during a heart failure exacerbation
C. A 14-year-old, 40-kg girl whose urine output is 15 mL/h for 4 hours intraoperatively
D. A 44-year-old, 60-kg woman whose urine output is 35 mL/h for 8 hours following cerebral angiography with IV contrast
E. A 39-year-old man with a perforated gastric ulcer whose creatinine rises from 1.0 to 1.8 mg/dL 48 hours after his admission

9. A 73-year-old woman with a history of heart failure with reduced ejection fraction (35%), depression, and chronic obstructive pulmonary disease (COPD) and who is a former smoker presents with fever and purulent cough. She denies thirst and reports voiding moderate amounts of clear yellow urine. On physical exam, her jugular venous pulsation is seen at 2 cm above the sternal notch with the bed at 45°. She is found to have a left upper lobe opacity on chest x-ray. Her initial laboratory analysis includes the following values:

Sodium, serum	128 mmol/L
Sodium, urine	40 mmol/L
Osmolarity, urine	143 mOsm/kg
Glucose	91 mg/dL

Complete blood count is notable for a white blood cell count of 18,000/µL. Complete metabolic panel is within normal limits. What is the most likely etiology of this patient's hyponatremia?

A. Primary polydipsia

B. Low sodium intake

C. Syndrome of inappropriate antidiuretic hormone

D. Hypoalbuminemia

E. Heart failure

10. A 67-year-old man arrives to the surgical ICU intubated after a 9-hour robotic-assisted retropubic prostatectomy. He received 7 L of normal saline during the procedure, and he is making approximately 0.6 mL/kg/h of urine. Estimated blood loss was approximately 500 mL. He currently requires positive end-expiratory pressure of 10 cm H_2O and fraction of inspired oxygen (FiO_2) of 0.8 in order to maintain oxygen saturation above 93%. Chest x-ray is shown below. What is the most appropriate next step in management?

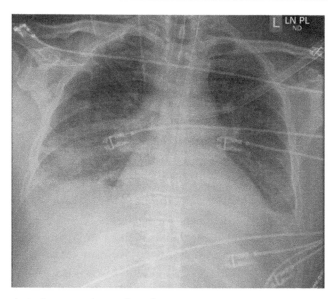

Anterior-posterior project chest x-ray.

A. Administer IV furosemide

B. Initiate broad-spectrum antibiotics

C. Extubate to non-rebreather mask

D. Withdraw the endotracheal tube 3 cm

E. Administer 500-mL bolus of 5% albumin

Answers and Explanations

1. **C.** Patients with preexisting kidney impairment are at increased risk for contrast nephropathy. IV hydration helps to maintain renal perfusion, and sodium bicarbonate further reduces free radical production in the renal medulla, mitigating the effects of the contrast. Use of iso-osmolar contrast media, compared with nonionic hypo-osmolar contrast media, reduces incidence of acute kidney injury (AKI) following administration. Although it increases renal blood flow and creatinine clearance, fenoldopam has not been shown to improve outcomes, and it further predisposes the patient to hypotension and resultant decrease in renal perfusion. Mannitol administration does not significantly reduce the incidence of AKI, whereas furosemide increases the incidence of AKI following contrast administration.

2. **A.** This woman presents with severe hypercalcemia, which often manifests with altered mental status, gastrointestinal complaints (constipation, anorexia, nausea, vomiting), renal dysfunction, and generalized weakness. Hypercalcemia may be a presenting sign of a number of malignancies including squamous cell carcinomas of the lung, as suggested by her chest x-ray. The most imperative intervention is to treat the accompanying dehydration prior to initiation of a loop diuretic to increase renal calcium clearance. Bisphosphonates and calcitonin may be initiated as a second-line therapy in patients with persistent hypercalcemia once they have undergone aggressive hydration and diuresis. Glucocorticoids may also be given as an adjunctive treatment but are reserved for cases in which an inflammatory condition is suspected, such as granulomatous disease or lymphoma. Hemodialysis is used in patients in whom the previous therapies are contraindicated or in those who fail all the above measures.

3. **D.** In order to determine the acid-base disturbance in this clinical scenario, begin by determining the primary disturbance, which in this case is an acidosis. Both the bicarbonate and partial pressure of carbon dioxide ($Paco_2$) are reduced, indicating that there is a metabolic acidosis. Next, calculate the anion gap:

$$\text{Anion gap (AG)} = [Na^+] - ([Cl^-] + [HCO_3^-])$$
$$AG = 138 - (104 + 16) = 18$$

The anion gap is elevated (normal value is approximately 8-12 mmol/L), indicating the presence of an anion gap acidosis. Now, we must evaluate whether a second process is involved by calculating the delta ratio.

$$\text{Delta ratio} = \Delta\,AG/\Delta\,[HCO_3^-]$$
$$= (AG - \text{normal AG})/(24 - [HCO_3^-])$$
$$\text{Delta ratio} = (18 - 12)/(24 - 16) = 6/8$$
$$\text{Delta ratio} < 1$$

A delta ratio <1 indicates a fall in the bicarbonate greater than that explained by the anion gap. Thus, both an anion gap and non-anion gap metabolic acidosis are present in this patient, likely explained by the combination of a lactic acidosis secondary to under-resuscitation, combined with bicarbonate loss from her diarrhea.

4. **E.** Begin by determining the primary disturbance, which in this case is an acidosis. The bicarbonate is reduced, whereas the $Paco_2$ is elevated, indicating the presence of both metabolic and respiratory processes.

Next, calculate the anion gap:

$$\text{Anion gap (AG)} = [Na^+] - ([Cl^-] + [HCO_3^-])$$
$$AG = 140 - (102 + 20) = 18$$

The anion gap is elevated (normal value is approximately 8-12 mmol/L), indicating the presence of an anion gap acidosis. The pneumonic MUDPILES can assist with recalling the differential diagnosis for anion gap metabolic acidosis (methanol, uremia, diabetic ketoacidosis, paraldehydes, isoniazid, lactate, ethanol, salicylate). Further laboratory workup is warranted, including serum and urine toxicology panels, as well as serum osmolarity in order to calculate the osmolar gap. The patient's elevated $Paco_2$ is likely due to hypoventilation, which may occur secondary to intoxication or as a result of a primary cerebral process in this patient.

Practical tip: In comparison to arterial blood gas (ABG) values, venous blood gas (VBG) values generally have a lower Pao_2, pH, and $Paco_2$. Venous pH can be reliably estimated and is typically decreased by 0.03, when compared with ABGs. Studies showed large confidence intervals in comparing ABG and VBG values for Pao_2, $Paco_2$, and bicarbonate, which limit the accurate estimation.

5. **B.** This patient has both clinical and laboratory findings consistent with rhabdomyolysis. Rhabdomyolysis-associated acute kidney injury (AKI) is induced through a combination of hypovolemia, myoglobinuria, and metabolic acidosis. In this case, the patient was likely immobile for a significant time period prior to presentation, resulting in limb ischemia and muscle degeneration. Myoglobin is released into the systemic circulation, causing direct cytotoxic effects on the nephron. Initial management of rhabdomyolysis includes aggressive IV hydration, targeting a urine output of 200 to 300 mL/h. Continuous renal replacement therapy (CRRT) has been shown to reduce serum myoglobin, potassium, BUN, and creatinine levels, but it does not have a mortality benefit. CRRT may be considered if life-threatening electrolyte abnormalities occur secondary to the AKI, but this patient's mild hyperkalemia would not warrant such an aggressive intervention in the absence of electrocardiogram (ECG) changes. Mannitol may be added if IV hydration is not sufficient to produce the targeted rate of urine output; however, it may worsen the patient's hypovolemia and should be used with caution. Furosemide similarly may worsen the patient's prerenal state. Finally, alkalinization of the urine through bicarbonate administration is thought to mitigate the toxic effects of myoglobin, but bicarbonate can paradoxically create an acidic intracellular environment and may predispose to respiratory failure by increasing $Paco_2$.

6. **B.** This clinical scenario poses a number of possible etiologies for the patient's AKI. In a patient who was known to be hypotensive following a surgical procedure with substantial blood loss, it is important to first establish whether the AKI is prerenal or intrinsic renal to guide further fluid resuscitation. Calculation of urine indices may help to make this determination.

The fractional excretion of sodium (FeNa) is calculated below. A value <1% favors prerenal etiologies, whereas a value >1% favors intrinsic renal etiologies due to loss of renal concentrating ability.

$$FeNa\ (\%) = (urine\ Na/urine\ Cr)/(serum\ Na/serum\ Cr) \times 100$$
$$FeNa\ (\%) = (40/17)/(140/4.3) \times 100 = 7.2\%,\ or >1\%$$

However, the interpretation of the FeNa is limited in scenarios where the patient has received diuretics or IV fluids (eg, normal saline), as in this patient's case. In these situations, calculation of the fractional excretion of urea (FeBUN) is helpful. A value >50% is consistent with intrinsic renal etiologies, whereas a value <35% favors prerenal etiologies.

$$FeBUN\ (\%) = (urine\ BUN/urine\ Cr)/(serum\ BUN/serum\ Cr) \times 100$$
$$FeBUN\ (\%) = (86/17)/(43/4.3) \times 100 = 51\%,\ or >50\%$$

Other indices that point toward an intrinsic renal etiology in this patient include:
- Urine osmolarity <350 mOsm/kg
- Urine sodium >30 mEq/L
- Urine creatinine/serum creatinine <20 (17/4.3 = 4 in this case)
- Urine BUN/serum BUN <3 (86/43 = 2 in this case)

This patient has several possible sources of acute tubular necrosis (ATN) including intraoperative or postoperative ischemia from hypotension and vasopressor use, and contrast administration during her endovascular procedure. Additional findings that would support a diagnosis of ATN include muddy brown casts on urine sediment.

7. **A.** This young man has AKI secondary to a postrenal obstruction, in this case the obstructing stone at the right ureteropelvic junction. He is in septic

shock from pyelonephritis likely due to an infected stone. The increase in creatinine is due to postrenal obstruction that has not yet been relieved. The appropriate next step is a bedside percutaneous nephrostomy to relieve the hydronephrosis and drain the infected kidney. Placement of a Foley catheter would relieve postrenal obstruction at the level of the bladder or ureter (eg, benign prostatic hypertrophy, neurogenic bladder), but not in the scenario described for this patient. In the absence of compelling culture data, there is no indication to broaden antibiotic coverage given the patient's clinical improvement. IV furosemide would not improve this patient's renal function until the obstruction is relieved.

8. **E.** The Acute Kidney Injury Network (AKIN) has published the following criteria for diagnosis of acute kidney injury:

- Abrupt (within 48 hours) reduction in kidney function currently defined as an absolute increase in serum creatinine of 0.3 mg/dL or more (≥26.4 μmol/L), *or*
- A percentage increase in serum creatinine of 50% or more (1.5-fold from baseline), *or*
- A reduction in urine output (documented oliguria of <0.5 mL/kg/h for >6 hours)

More recently, the Kidney Disease: Improving Global Outcomes (KDIGO) group has offered a similar definition of AKI but with staging criteria for the severity of AKI. These criteria have not yet been broadly validated. Unlike previous classification systems, such as the RIFLE criteria (risk, injury, failure, loss of kidney function, and end-stage kidney disease), GFR is not used as a criterion in either AKIN or KDIGO AKI definitions; this is due to the fact that estimates of GFR during AKI are less reliable.

Only answer choice E meets the criteria for AKI. Answer choices A to D all illustrate scenarios where patients at are risk of developing AKI, but they do not currently meet criteria.

9. **C.** This patient presents with a moderate hyponatremia. Whereas traditional approaches to classification of hyponatremia relied upon assessment of the clinical volume status, more recent approaches incorporate laboratory analysis of renal water and sodium handling to provide a straightforward, reliable, and pragmatic analysis.

The first step is to exclude pseudohyponatremia and nonhypotonic hyponatremia. Pseudohyponatremia can occur in cases with high triglycerides, cholesterol, or protein, because they reduce the aqueous fraction of blood. Although the question stem does not specifically state these values, the clinical scenario does not point toward one of these etiologies. Nonhypotonic hyponatremia can occur in cases of hyperglycemia or in the presence of mannitol or glycine. These osmotically active compounds draw free water from the intracellular to the extracellular compartment and thus cause a dilutional hyponatremia.

In the absence of either pseudohyponatremia or nonhypotonic hyponatremia, determine the urine osmolarity. If it is below 100 mOsm/kg, the urine is maximally dilute, indicating that the intake of hypotonic fluids exceeds the kidneys' capacity for free water excretion. This can occur in primary polydipsia, in low solute intake, or with use of hypotonic IV fluids.

If the urine osmolarity is ≥100 mOsm/kg, determine the urine sodium. In cases of low effective arterial volume (eg, congestive heart failure, cirrhosis, nephrotic syndrome, hypoalbuminemia), the urine sodium will be low (<30 mmol/L) indicating maximal reabsorption of sodium. If urine sodium is high (≥30 mmol/L), consider syndrome of inappropriate antidiuretic hormone (SIADH), cerebral salt wasting, salt wasting nephropathies, or specific medication effects.

SIADH is a diagnosis of exclusion. It is associated with a number of specific drugs (eg, anticonvulsants, antidepressants, opiates, antibiotics), pneumonia, COPD, central nervous system infection, subarachnoid hemorrhage, and malignancies of the lung, pancreas, and brain.

The case presented fits with a diagnosis of SIADH, likely secondary to the patient's pneumonia. A urine osmolarity >100 mOsm/kg argues against primary polydipsia (choice A) or low sodium intake (choice B). A high urine sodium (>30 mmol/L) argues against causes with low effective arterial volume, including hypoalbuminemia (choice D) or heart failure (choice E).

10. **A.** This patient arrives to the surgical ICU with respiratory compromise secondary to volume overload; acute diastolic heart failure resulting in pulmonary edema is common among elderly patients

who receive large volumes of crystalloid perioperatively, even in the absence of a known preoperative diagnosis. In addition, the length of procedure and patient positioning (eg, Trendelenburg or flex positioning) can contribute to upper airway and facial edema, compromising the airway upon extubation. For this reason, extubation at this time would be premature and places the patient at risk for hypoxemia and airway collapse. In this patient, the best next step is administration of IV furosemide, a loop diuretic. Recent evidence points toward continuous goal-directed furosemide infusion as safe and effective alternative to intermittent boluses. The other options listed would be poor choices. There is no indication of an infectious process to prompt antibiotic coverage. The endotracheal tube is correctly positioned 2 to 5 cm above the carina. Additional IV fluids at this time would worsen his pulmonary edema.

REFERENCES

Acute Kidney Injury Work Group. Kidney Disease: Improving Global Outcomes (KDIGO). Clinical practice guideline for acute kidney injury. *Kidney Int.* 2012;2:1-138.

Aspelin P, Aubry P, Fransson SG, et al. Nephrotoxic effects in high-risk patients undergoing angiography. *N Engl J Med.* 2003;348:491-499.

Ball SG, Iqbal Z. Diagnosis and treatment of hyponatraemia. *Best Pract Res Clin Endocrinol Metab.* 2016;30:161-173.

Chang CH, Lin CY, Tian YC, et al. Acute kidney injury classification: comparison of AKIN and RIFLE criteria. *Shock.* 2010;33:247-252.

Chavez L, Leon M, Einav S, et al. Beyond muscle destruction: a systematic review of rhabdomyolysis for clinical practice. *Crit Care.* 2016;20:135.

Gill N, Nally J, Fatica R. Renal failure secondary to acute tubular necrosis: epidemiology, diagnosis, and management. *Chest.* 2005;128:2847-2863.

Longnecker D, Brown DL, Newman MF, Zapol W, eds. *Anesthesiology.* 2nd ed. New York, NY: McGraw-Hill; 2012.

Mehta RL, Kellum JA, Shah SV, et al. Acute kidney injury network: report of an initiative to improve outcomes in acute kidney injury. *Crit Care.* 2007;11:R31.

Moe SM. Disorders involving calcium, phosphorus, and magnesium. *Prim Care.* 2008;35:215-237.

Navaneethan SD, Singh S, Appasamy S, et al. Sodium bicarbonate therapy for prevention of contrast-induced nephropathy: a systematic review and meta-analysis. *Am J Kidney Dis.* 2009;53:617-627.

Scharman EJ, Troutman WG. Prevention of kidney injury following rhabdomyolysis: a systematic review. *Ann Pharmacother.* 2013;47:90-105.

Shim HJ, Jang JY, Lee SH, et al. The effect of positive balance on the outcomes of critically ill noncardiac postsurgical patients: a retrospective cohort study. *J Crit Care.* 2014;29:43-48.

Stewart AF. Clinical practice. Hypercalcemia associated with cancer. *N Engl J Med.* 2005;352:373-379.

Thadhani R, Pasqual M, Bonventre JV. Acute renal failure. *N Eng J Med.* 1996;334:1448-1460.

Upadya A, Tilluckdharry L, Muralidharan V, et al. Fluid balance and weaning outcomes. *Intensive Care Med.* 2005; 31:1643-1647.

Yeh D, Van Der Wilden GM, Cropano C, et al. Goal-directed diuresis: a case-control study of continuous furosemide infusion in critically ill patients. *J Emerg Trauma Shock.* 2015;8:34-38.

Zeng X1, Zhang L, Wu T, et al. Continuous renal replacement therapy (CRRT) for rhabdomyolysis. *Cochrane Database Syst Rev.* 2014;6:CD008566.

Zoungas S, Ninomiya T, Huxley R, et al. Sodium bicarbonate therapy for prevention of contrast-induced nephropathy: a systematic review and meta-analysis. *Ann Intern Med.* 2008;148:284-294.

29

Intra-Abdominal Diseases

Ahmad Abou Leila, MD and Somnath Bose, MD

Questions

1. A 43-year-old man is admitted to emergency department (ED) following a motor vehicle accident. He is alert, awake, and oriented; primary survey demonstrates right upper quadrant bruises, periumbilical hematoma, and significant tenderness to palpation. There is no evidence of any other penetrating injuries. Vital signs upon admission to ED are as follows: blood pressure (BP) 107/85 mm Hg, heart rate (HR) 102 bpm, respiratory rate (RR) 25 breaths/min, and temperature of 37.5°C. Chest x-ray shows a right-sided pleural effusion. No intra-abdominal free fluid is appreciated on focused assessment with sonography for trauma (FAST) exam. Computed tomography (CT) of the abdomen with intravenous (IV) contrast shows subcapsular hematoma of approximately 40% of surface area with liver contrast blush but with no other injuries noted. His past medical history is significant for hypertension that is well controlled on metoprolol XL 50 mg daily. What is the best next management step?

A. Surgical exploration and control of bleeding
B. Laparoscopic exploration
C. Liver angiography and embolization
D. Admit to intensive care unit (ICU) for monitoring and serial abdominal exam
E. Endoscopic retrograde cholangiopancreatography (ERCP)

2. A 51-year-old male patient with a past medical history significant for obesity, low back pain, and recent knee replacement presented to ED with severe respiratory distress that required intubation. He was subsequently transferred to the ICU for further workup and management. A CT pulmonary embolism protocol was negative; however, it revealed bilateral multifocal pneumonia. He was started on broad-spectrum antibiotics pending speciation of a bronchoalveolar lavage, which was sent on admission. His ICU course was remarkable for difficulty weaning from the ventilator. On ICU day 4, despite being on sedation, he started complaining of abdominal pain. On examination, he appeared tachycardic and hypotensive with a BP of 80/40 mm Hg. The rest of the physical examination was unrevealing. This was soon followed by 2 episodes of melena. Home medications include prednisone 10 mg daily, ibuprofen 400 mg daily, and pantoprazole 40 mg daily. Follow-up labs reveal the following: hemoglobin 6 g/dL, partial thromboplastin time 25 seconds, and international normalized ratio 1.4. X-ray of kidneys, ureter, and bladder was negative for evidence of free air. Which of the following is the best initial management of this patient?

   A. Stop all sedation
   B. Nasogastric tube insertion
   C. IV proton pump inhibitors
   D. Administration of 1 unit of fresh frozen plasma
   E. Blood transfusion, with target hemoglobin of >9 g/dL

3. Which of the following endoscopic findings is associated with the highest risk of massive rebleeding?

   A. Greater curvature ulcer
   B. Fundus ulcer
   C. Anterior wall duodenal ulcer
   D. Lesser curvature ulcer
   E. Pyloric ulcers

4. A 35-year-old man was rushed to the ED after being evacuated from a fire accident in his garage. Upon admission to the ED, he was intubated and mechanically ventilated with assist-control ventilation with set rate of 12 breaths per minute fraction of inspired oxygen (FiO_2) 40%, tidal volume 300 mL, respiratory rate 15 breaths/min, and positive end-expiratory pressure (PEEP) 5 cm H_2O. Primary survey showed second-degree facial burn and third-degree burns on the anterior abdominal wall and bilateral thighs. Vital signs were as follows: BP 150/85 mm Hg, HR 143 bpm, temperature 35.4°C, and oxygen saturation (SpO_2) 97%. Arterial blood gas revealed the following: pH 7.21, partial pressure of carbon dioxide ($Paco_2$) 57 mm Hg, and partial pressure of oxygen (Pao_2) 205 mm Hg. Which of the following circumstances is most associated with abdominal compartment syndrome (ACS) in this case?

   A. Burn surface area >50% of total surface area
   B. Resuscitation phase
   C. Polyuric phase
   D. Burn-associated pancreatitis
   E. Resuscitation with colloids (blood product)

5. A 57-year-old woman with past medical history of type 2 diabetes and paraplegia due to thoracic epidural abscess was admitted to the ICU with necrotizing fasciitis in the sacral area. The patient was started empirically on vancomycin 1.25 g IV every 12 hours, piperacillin plus tazobactam 3.375 g IV every 6 hours, and clindamycin 600 mg IV every 8 hours. On day 3 in the ICU, the patient had 10 episodes of nonoffensive watery diarrhea with changes in her vitals as follows: mean arterial pressure (MAP) 50 mm Hg and HR 120 bpm. Stool polymerase chain reaction (PCR) for *Clostridium difficile* was positive. A CT of the abdomen was completed, which demonstrated toxic megacolon, no free air, mild liver congestion, and splenomegaly. Surgical consult was obtained, and she underwent emergent exploratory laparotomy and subtotal colectomy with diversion colostomy. Which of the following is the most appropriate management for this patient?

   A. Start patient on IV metronidazole
   B. Discontinue oral (PO) antibiotics after subtotal colectomy
   C. Repeat *C difficile* PCR to monitor for treatment
   D. Start patient on PO vancomycin and IV metronidazole
   E. Continue *C difficile* treatment for 7 days

Questions 6 and 7

A 34-year-old woman was brought to ED by her roommates after she had a mechanical fall and witnessed seizures. On admission, the patient was found to be stuporous and was hyperventilating with blood oozing from the left nares. Skin exam showed some petechial hemorrhage on the anterior abdominal wall. Vitals were as follows: HR 110 bpm, BP 90/55 mm Hg, SpO_2 93%, and RR 30 breaths/min. CT abdomen revealed mild ascites, mild nodularity of liver parenchyma, normal pancreas, and mild hydronephrosis of right kidney. The patient was admitted with acute liver failure and remained hypotensive, with MAP <50 mm Hg. A central venous catheter was inserted, and the patient was started on norepinephrine at rate of 10 μg/min. Laboratory findings were pertinent for thrombocytopenia, INR 1.7, acute renal injury with elevated anion gap metabolic acidosis, and elevated transaminases (aspartate aminotransferase [AST] 456 IU/L and alanine aminotransferase [ALT] 561 IU/L).

6. Which of the following is the correct step in management of this patient?
   A. Determine the model for end-stage liver disease (MELD) score
   B. Emergent liver transplantation
   C. Start empiric antibiotics
   D. Emergent continuous venovenous hemodialysis
   E. Start patient on benzodiazepine infusion for agitation

7. The patient was intubated for airway protection due to poor mental status and started on propofol infusion at 25 μg/kg/min. Propofol was titrated to a bispectral index (BIS) value of 40 to 60. Two hours later, sedation was discontinued for accurate assessment of neurologic status. The patient remained confused and did not follow any commands. Over the course of the next hour, she became increasingly agitated and started pulling at lines and devices. She had an episode of witnessed tonic-clonic seizure, which lasted for 10 seconds. Serum ammonia level was elevated at 254 μmol/L. Which of the following is the most correct step in management of this patient's encephalopathy?

A. Start patient on hypertonic saline
B. Start patient on methylprednisone
C. Administer lorazepam for seizure control
D. Continue lactulose until the point of diarrhea
E. Insert intracranial pressure monitors

8. A 62-year-old man with a past medical history significant for hypertension and diastolic heart failure was admitted to the ICU with severe epigastric pain that lasted for 5 hours. The patient described his pain as severe, sharp pain that radiates to his right shoulder and was associated with 3 episodes of nonbloody nonbilious vomiting. Physical exam showed an anxious, diaphoretic patient, with epigastric tenderness and mild abdominal distention. Vital signs were as follows: BP 156/61 mm Hg, HR 130 bpm, temperature 38.1°C, SpO_2 92% on a FiO_2 of 70%, and RR 26 breaths/min. A CT of the abdomen showed diffuse pancreatic edema, retroperitoneal fat stranding, normal liver, gallstones, and dilated loops of small bowel. Labs were pertinent for elevated AST 123 IU/L, ALT 115 IU/L, amylase 200 IU/L (normal 25-85 IU/L), and lipase 630 IU/L (normal 0-160 IU/L). What is the best next step in the management of this patient?

   A. Resuscitate with 500 mL/h of normal saline solution for the first 24 hours
   B. Admit for ERCP in next 24 hours
   C. Consider early total parenteral nutrition (TPN)
   D. Urgent cholecystectomy
   E. Order MRCP

Answers and Explanations

1. **C.** The patient presents with examination findings consistent with liver injury, and the CT of the abdomen with IV contrast confirms this diagnosis and shows the extent and severity of damage. The treatment approach in case of intraparenchymal hematomas without hemoperitoneum is to follow up the hematoma with serial physical exam and imaging (Table 29-1). The blush noted on CT scan is consistent with active bleeding within the liver, and active bleeding requires operative management. Methods include single pure suture, deep mattress suture, debridement, anatomic hepatectomy, hepatic arterial ligation, gauze packing, liver-coated mesh method, or embolization. The patient has a grade II liver injury (Table 29-2) that requires angiography and embolization.

Table 29-1. Management of Liver Injury Dictated by Clinical and Computed Tomography (CT) Findings

Hemodynamically stable	Nonoperative:
	• **Serial abdominal exam and CT of abdomen**
	• **Angiography and embolization are considered if patient is stable and CT scan shows contrast blush or evidence of ongoing bleeding**
	• **Grade III and above liver lacerations require embolization combined with surgical intervention**
Hemodynamically unstable	Operative
	• Exploratory laparotomy; staged approach is considered for severely acidotic patients. Simple packing can be done initially. Definitive surgery done when patient is stable
	• Endoscopic retrograde cholangiopancreatography considered in management of biloma drainage; percutaneous drainage is considered for liver abscess

Table 29-2. American Association for the Surgery of Trauma Classification of Liver Trauma

Grade	Description
I	Hematoma: subcapsular, <10% surface area
	Laceration: capsular tear, <1 cm parenchymal depth
II	Hematoma: subcapsular, 10%-50% surface area or intraparenchymal <10 cm diameter
	Laceration: capsular tear, 1-3 cm parenchymal depth, <10 cm length
III	Hematoma: subcapsular >50% surface area of ruptured subcapsular or parenchymal hematoma or intraparenchymal >10 cm or expanding
	Laceration: capsular tear >3 cm parenchymal depth
IV	Laceration: parenchymal disruption involving 25%-75% of hepatic lobe or involving 1-3 segments
V	Laceration: parenchymal disruption involving >75% of hepatic lobe or involving >3 segments
	Vascular: juxtahepatic venous injuries (retrohepatic vena cava/central major hepatic veins)
VI	Vascular: hepatic avulsion

Modified from Moore EE, Cogbill TH, Jurkovich GJ, et al. Organ Injury Scaling: Spleen and Liver (1994 Revision). *J Trauma* 1995; 38(3):323-324.

2. **C.** The most common reason for melena in critically ill patients is an upper gastrointestinal (GI) bleed. Patients on mechanical ventilation are at the highest risk of developing upper GI bleeding. The patient has multiple risk factors including being on mechanical ventilation and history of nonsteroidal anti-inflammatory drug (NSAID) and steroid use, all of which contribute to the risk of developing an upper GI bleeding. Symptomatic posthemorrhagic anemia in combination with the risk factors warrants urgent workup and management of GI bleeding. Nasogastric or orogastric lavage is not required in patients with upper GI bleeding for diagnosis, prognosis, visualization, or therapeutic effect. Patients with upper GI bleeding should generally undergo endoscopy within 24 hours of diagnosis, following resuscitative efforts to

optimize hemodynamic parameters and other medical problems.

Pre-endoscopic IV proton pump inhibitors (PPIs; eg, 80-mg bolus followed by 8 mg/h infusion) may be considered to decrease the proportion of patients who have higher risk of stigmata of hemorrhage at endoscopy and who receive endoscopic therapy. However, PPIs do not improve clinical outcomes such as further bleeding, surgery, or death. IV infusion of erythromycin (250 mg approximately 30 minutes before endoscopy) should be considered to improve diagnostic yield and decrease the need for repeat endoscopy. Restrictive transfusion strategies targeting a hemoglobin >7 g/dL have been shown to be associated with better outcomes as compared to a more liberal approach.

3. **D.** In a recent systematic review, several factors were identified as independent predictors of rebleeding:

- Hemodynamic instability
- Comorbid illnesses
- Active bleeding at endoscopy
- >2-cm ulcer size
- Ulcer location in either the posterior duodenum or lesser curvature of the stomach

It seems reasonable to consider early elective operative intervention in patients who are at high risk of recurrent bleeding. Lesser curvature ulcers are at high risk of bleeding because of proximity to arcade of vessels from the left gastric artery. Endoscopic features associated with rebleeding are listed in Table 29-3.

Table 29-3. Endoscopic Features Associated With Rebleeding

Finding	Risk of Rebleeding
Active bleeding vessel	85%-90%
Nonbleeding visible vessel	35%-55%
Presence of thrombus	30%-40%
Flat pigment spot	5%-10%
Clean-based ulcer	5%

4. **C.** Intra-abdominal hypertension (IAH) in burn patients generally occurs within 48 hours after injury, during the initial resuscitation period,

whereas abdominal compartment syndrome (ACS) usually occurs after the acute phase, during subsequent septic episodes. ACS typically occurs when resuscitation volumes are >275 mL/kg during the first 24 hours or total body surface area burned is >60%. After this, when patients reach the polyuric or diuretic phase, the IAH/ACS risk decreases. However, if patients develop sepsis, the risk for IAH/ACS increases again, and those not progressing spontaneously to the flow phase may need intervention. Moreover, the choice of resuscitation fluid among critically ill patients with burns may have a clinical importance. Randomized studies have shown that hypertonic lactated saline (HLS) or plasma-based resuscitation requires less fluid and is associated with a lower risk of IAH and ACS (Table 29-4).

Table 29-4. Risk Factors for Intra-abdominal Hypertension

High-volume fluid resuscitation	Pancreatitis
Septic shock	Decreased abdominal wall compliance
Hemorrhagic shock	Large or circumferential torso burn
Large surface area burn	Ventral hernia repair with tight abdominal wall closure
Prone positioning	Increased abdominal content
Large neoplasm	Tense ascites in patients with cirrhosis

5. **D.** Oral (PO) therapy must be used whenever possible, because IV metronidazole has no established role, and IV vancomycin has poor penetration in the gut mucosa. In mild to moderate cases, PO metronidazole is enough if there is no history of *C difficile*. In severe cases with *C difficile* and white blood cells >15,000/μL or creatinine >50% from baseline, PO vancomycin should be added to the regimen.

In severe complicated cases (toxic megacolon, hypotension, perforation), PO vancomycin plus IV metronidazole should be given. Vancomycin is also considered in any patient >65 years old. Repeat *C difficile* PCR during treatment or to monitor for the resolution of the disease is not recommended as the utility of the results has not been demonstrated. *C difficile* treatment should be continued in patients undergoing subtotal colectomy with preservation of rectum. Overall, *C difficile* treatment should continue for 10 to 14 days.

6. **C.** The management of acute liver failure has 2 main components: identifying the etiology of liver failure and reversing it and organ support to improve survival and prevent further liver damage. Determination of the etiology of the liver failure should involve a thorough physical exam and lab testing. Altered mental status and coagulopathy are common features on physical exam; however, jaundice is an infrequent finding and usually is a late sign, and hepatic failure secondary to Wilson disease may not show jaundice. Ascites is late sign in hepatic failure; early ascites in liver failure is associated with Budd-Chiari syndrome. CT of the abdomen is essential to examine the liver vessels and liver parenchyma and extrahepatic structures. Liver biopsy is necessary when autoimmune hepatitis is suspected. Supportive therapy in the setting of liver failure is complex as multiple organ systems can have dysfunction. As seen in this patient, patients may require intubation for altered mental status, management of agitation and encephalopathy with propranolol, and possible intracranial pressure monitoring. Central vascular catheter placement is needed for large volume resuscitation and potential use of hemodialysis and vasopressors. Early administration of empiric antibiotics is needed given that up to 80% of acute liver failure patients develop bacterial infections. Attempts to correct coagulopathy should be attempted. Liver transplant should be performed when stable, and minimal pressor support should be given when severe hypotension is resolved.

7. **A.** The patient in this question presented with fulminant liver failure. Patients presenting with such acute presentation are at highest risk for development of cerebral edema (serum ammonia >150 μmol/L, grade 3/4 hepatic encephalopathy), which could lead to disastrous complications including herniation and death. Prophylactic induction of hypernatremia with hypertonic saline to a sodium level of 145 to 155 mEq/L is recommended (Level 1 recommendation). Intracranial pressure (ICP) monitoring is recommended in acute liver failure patients with high-grade hepatic encephalopathy, in centers with expertise in ICP monitoring, and in patients awaiting and undergoing liver transplantation evaluation. However in this case, the patient is coagulopathic, and risk of potential intracranial hemorrhage may outweigh the benefits of ICP monitoring. Routine ICP monitoring has not been shown to confer any mortality benefit and is used only after a careful assessment of the risk-benefit ratio. In early stages of encephalopathy, lactulose may be used either orally or rectally to affect a bowel purge, but should not be administered to the point of diarrhea, and may interfere with the surgical field by increasing bowel distention during liver transplantation. Role of rifaximin, neomycin, and other nonabsorbable antibiotics is unclear in the acute setting. Corticosteroids should not be used to control elevated ICP in patients with acute liver failure. Seizure control is better achieved using short-acting benzodiazepine or propofol infusion.

8. **E.** In the absence of cholangitis and/or jaundice, magnetic resonance cholangiopancreatography (MRCP) or endoscopic ultrasound (EUS), rather than diagnostic ERCP, should be used to screen for choledocholithiasis if highly suspected. In this particular case, the patient has gallstones, which raises the concern of pancreatitis due to gallstone disease. ERCP within 24 hours of admission is recommended in patients with acute pancreatitis and concurrent acute cholangitis. Aggressive hydration, defined as 250 to 500 mL/h of isotonic crystalloid solution, should be provided to all patients, unless cardiovascular and/or renal comorbidities exist. Early aggressive IV hydration is most beneficial in the first 12 to 24 hours and may have little benefit beyond this period. In this patient, who has heart failure and signs of fluid intolerance, fluid titration for physiologic goals is recommended. Patients with acute pancreatitis and concurrent gallstones should be offered cholecystectomy before discharge to prevent recurrent episodes of acute pancreatitis. In acute pancreatitis, enteral nutrition is always recommended first. TPN should be avoided unless the enteral route is not available, not tolerated, or not meeting caloric requirements.

REFERENCES

Bardou M, Martin J, Barkun A. Intravenous proton pump inhibitors: an evidence-based review of their use in gastrointestinal disorders. *Drugs.* 2009;69:435-448.

Bernal W, Wendon J. Acute liver failure. *N Engl J Med.* 2014;370:1170-1171.

Cohen SH, Gerding DN, Johnson S, et al. Clinical practice guidelines for *Clostridium difficile* infection in adults: 2010 update by the society for healthcare epidemiology of America (SHEA) and the infectious diseases society of America (IDSA). *Infect Control Hosp Epidemiol.* 2010; 31:431-455.

Cook DJ, Fuller HD, Guyatt GH, et al. Risk factors for gastrointestinal bleeding in critically ill patients. Canadian Critical Care Trials Group. *N Engl J Med.* 1994;330:377-381.

Detry O, Arkadopoulos N, Ting P, et al. Intracranial pressure during liver transplantation for fulminant hepatic failure. *Transplantation.* 1999;67:767-770.

Elmunzer BJ, Young SD, Inadomi JM, et al. Systematic review of the predictors of recurrent hemorrhage after endoscopic hemostatic therapy for bleeding peptic ulcers. *Am J Gastroenterol.* 2008;103:2625-2632.

Goyal H, Singla U. Infectious Diseases Society of America or American College of Gastroenterology guidelines for treatment of *Clostridium difficile* infection: which one to follow? *Am J Med.* 2015;128:e17.

Holden A. Abdomen: interventions for solid organ injury. *Injury.* 2008;39:1275-1289.

Ivy ME, Atweh NA, Palmer J, et al. Intra-abdominal hypertension and abdominal compartment syndrome in burn patients. *J Trauma.* 2000;49:387-391.

Laine L, Jensen DM. Management of patients with ulcer bleeding. *Am J Gastroenterol.* 2012;107:345-360.

Lee CW, Sarosi GA. Emergency ulcer surgery. *Surg Clin North Am.* 2011;91:1001-1013.

Letoublon C, Morra I, Chen Y, et al. Arterial embolization in the management of blunt hepatic trauma: indications and complications. *J Trauma.* 2011;70:1032-1036.

Maluso P, Olson J, Sarani B. Abdominal compartment hypertension and abdominal compartment syndrome. *Crit Care Clin.* 2016;32:213-222.

McClave SA, Taylor BE, Martindale RG, et al. Guidelines for the provision and assessment of nutrition support therapy in the adult critically ill patient: Society of Critical Care Medicine (SCCM) and American Society for Parenteral and Enteral Nutrition (A.S.P.E.N.). *JPEN J Parenter Enteral Nutr.* 2016;40:159-211.

Oda J, Ueyama M, Yamashita K, et al. Hypertonic lactated saline resuscitation reduces the risk of abdominal compartment syndrome in severely burned patients. *J Trauma.* 2006;60:64-71.

Stravitz RT, Kramer AH, Davern T, et al. Intensive care of patients with acute liver failure: recommendations of the U.S. Acute Liver Failure Study Group. *Crit Care Med.* 2007;35:2498-2508.

Tenner S, Baillie J, DeWitt J, et al. American College of Gastroenterology guideline: management of acute pancreatitis. *Am J Gastroenterol.* 2013;108:1400-1415.

Villanueva C. Gastrointestinal bleeding: blood transfusion for acute upper gastrointestinal bleeding. *Nat Rev Gastroenterol Hepatol.* 2015;12:432-434.

30

Infectious Diseases

Maurice Francis Joyce, MD, EdM and Edward Bittner, MD, PhD, MSEd

Questions

1. An otherwise healthy, 75-year-old woman sustained a left ankle fracture and underwent an open reduction internal fixation 4 days ago. She received cephalexin for 4 days after surgery. She subsequently develops diarrhea and mild diffuse abdominal pain. Her white blood cell (WBC) count is 14.2×10^9 cells/L. Stool studies are pending. What is the most appropriate initial treatment regimen?

    A. Oral metronidazole

    B. Intravenous metronidazole

    C. Intravenous vancomycin

    D. Fecal transplantation

    E. Use of as-needed loperamide

2. An 85-year-old man who underwent an exploratory laparotomy and patch repair of a perforated duodenal ulcer 8 days ago remains intubated and mechanically ventilated for hypoxemic respiratory failure. He is febrile, and his WBC count is 17×10^9 cells/L. The bedside nurse notes copious, thick respiratory secretions. Respiratory cultures are pending. Based on this presentation, what is the most likely causative agent?

    A. *Streptococcus pneumoniae*

    B. *Klebsiella pneumoniae*

    C. *Staphylococcus aureus*

    D. *Mycoplasma pneumoniae*

    E. *Enterococcus faecalis*

3. A 62-year-old woman in the intensive care unit (ICU) remains intubated and mechanically ventilated after undergoing a coronary artery bypass graft (CABG) and mitral valve replacement. On postoperative day 3, she is diagnosed with pneumonia and remains hypoxemic, and respiratory cultures grow *Pseudomonas aeruginosa*. Administration of which of the following medications would have most likely prevented this pneumonia?

    A. Intravenous dexamethasone

    B. Oral chlorhexidine

    C. Intravenous pantoprazole

    D. Intravenous clindamycin

    E. Oral famotidine

4. A 58-year-old man is admitted to the ICU following an exploratory laparotomy, washout, Hartmann procedure, and diverting ileostomy for perforated diverticulitis. The patient is afebrile and hemodynamically stable, and his WBC count is now within normal limits. The surgeon reported that there was effective source control of the intra-abdominal infection. When should systemic antibiotic therapy be discontinued postoperatively?

A. Postoperative day 1

B. Postoperative day 4

C. Postoperative day 8

D. Postoperative day 10

E. Postoperative day 14

5. An 84-year-old woman is admitted to the ICU with acute mental status changes. Her vital signs are as follows: temperature 38.5°C, heart rate (HR) 112 bpm, noninvasive blood pressure (NIBP) 90/62 mm Hg, respiratory rate 26 breaths/min, and oxygen saturation 95%. Laboratory analysis is remarkable for a WBC count of 15×10^9 cells/L. Her urine is noted to be dark and turbid. Urine and blood cultures have been sent. The patient undergoes fluid resuscitation, resulting in an HR of 84 bpm and NIBP of 110/68 mm Hg. However, her urine output is 10 mL/h for 3 hours. What is the best description of this patient's clinical condition?

A. Systemic inflammatory response syndrome (SIRS)

B. Sepsis

C. Severe sepsis

D. Septic shock

6. A 42-year-old man becomes febrile and has a WBC count of 18×10^9 cells/L on postoperative day 6. Blood cultures that were drawn from a left subclavian central venous catheter are positive. What measure would have most likely prevented this complication?

A. Povidone-iodine skin preparation

B. Landmark technique for line insertion

C. Hand washing prior to line insertion

D. Choice of internal jugular vein site

E. Use of biopatch film at insertion site

7. An 86-year-old woman is admitted to the ICU following an exploratory laparotomy, small bowel resection, and lysis of adhesions for a small bowel obstruction. Her ICU course is complicated by severe hyperactive delirium requiring multiple doses of intravenous haloperidol and development of a hospital-acquired pneumonia treated with antibiotics. Which antibiotic is most likely contributing to her current clinical condition?

A. Cefepime

B. Metronidazole

C. Levofloxacin

D. Vancomycin

8. A 76-year-old man with a history of type 2 diabetes mellitus was admitted to the ICU following an exploratory laparotomy, small bowel resection, and left inguinal hernia repair for an incarcerated left inguinal hernia. Two days following admission, the nurse notes a localized area of erythema on his right thigh. On examination, the area is ill-defined and indurated with central patches of dusky blue discoloration. There is subcutaneous crepitus on palpation. He is febrile, mildly tachycardic, and has a blood pressure of 90/52 mm Hg. What is the next best step in the management of this patient?

A. Observation

B. Urgent computed tomography scan

C. Emergent surgical consult

D. Intravenous antibiotics

E. Start vasopressors to maintain mean arterial pressure >70 mm Hg

Answers and Explanations

1. **A.** Based on this patient's clinical presentation and history of antibiotic exposure, the most likely diagnosis is *Clostridium difficile* infection. First-line therapy for mild to moderate *C difficile* infection is oral metronidazole because it is effective and cost efficient, although oral vancomycin is an acceptable alternative. Intravenous metronidazole is not recommended for monotherapy. Intravenous vancomycin is not a treatment modality for *C difficile* infection as it does not achieve detectable levels throughout the colon. Fecal transplantation is generally reserved for severe infection or refractory, treatment-resistant infection. Loperamide is not appropriate treatment in the setting of infectious diarrhea.

2. **C.** Based on this patient's clinical presentation, the most likely diagnosis is a ventilator-associated pneumonia (VAP). VAP is the most common healthcare-associated infection in critical care units and is a leading cause of morbidity and mortality. Microorganisms that are responsible for VAPs may differ based on specific intensive care unit (ICU) populations, although the most common etiologic agents are antibiotic-resistant nosocomial organisms. *Staphylococcus aureus* and *Pseudomonas aeruginosa* account for a large proportion of VAPs. *Klebsiella pneumoniae* can cause VAPs, although must less frequently. *Streptococcus pneumoniae* and *Mycoplasma pneumoniae* are less frequently associated with VAPs and more frequently the etiologic organisms in community-acquired pneumonia.

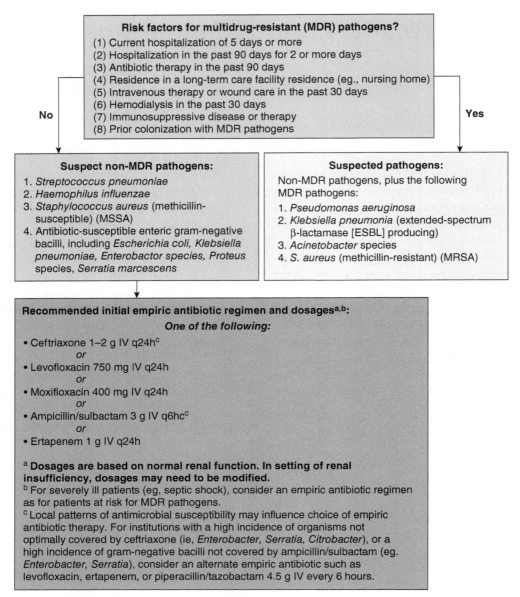

Risk factors for multidrug-resistant (MDR) pathogens?
(1) Current hospitalization of 5 days or more
(2) Hospitalization in the past 90 days for 2 or more days
(3) Antibiotic therapy in the past 90 days
(4) Residence in a long-term care facility residence (eg., nursing home)
(5) Intravenous therapy or wound care in the past 30 days
(6) Hemodialysis in the past 30 days
(7) Immunosuppressive disease or therapy
(8) Prior colonization with MDR pathogens

No   Yes

Suspect non-MDR pathogens:
1. *Streptococcus pneumoniae*
2. *Haemophilus influenzae*
3. *Staphylococcus aureus* (methicillin-susceptible) (MSSA)
4. Antibiotic-susceptible enteric gram-negative bacilli, including *Escherichia coli, Klebsiella pneumoniae, Enterobactor species, Proteus* species, *Serratia marcescens*

Suspected pathogens:
Non-MDR pathogens, plus the following MDR pathogens:
1. *Pseudomonas aeruginosa*
2. *Klebsiella pneumonia* (extended-spectrum β-lactamase [ESBL] producing)
3. *Acinetobacter* species
4. *S. aureus* (methicillin-resistant) (MRSA)

Recommended initial empiric antibiotic regimen and dosages[a,b]:
One of the following:

• Ceftriaxone 1–2 g IV q24h[c]
    or
• Levofloxacin 750 mg IV q24h
    or
• Moxifloxacin 400 mg IV q24h
    or
• Ampicillin/sulbactam 3 g IV q6h[c]
    or
• Ertapenem 1 g IV q24h

[a] **Dosages are based on normal renal function. In setting of renal insufficiency, dosages may need to be modified.**
[b] For severely ill patients (eg, septic shock), consider an empiric antibiotic regimen as for patients at risk for MDR pathogens.
[c] Local patterns of antimicrobial susceptibility may influence choice of empiric antibiotic therapy. For institutions with a high incidence of organisms not optimally covered by ceftriaxone (ie, *Enterobacter, Serratia, Citrobacter*), or a high incidence of gram-negative bacilli not covered by ampicillin/sulbactam (eg. *Enterobacter, Serratia*), consider an alternate empiric antibiotic such as levofloxacin, ertapenem, or piperacillin/tazobactam 4.5 g IV every 6 hours.

Reproduced from Lee K. *The NeuroICU Book*. New York, NY: McGraw-Hill 2012. Adapted in part from American Thoracic Society, Infectious Diseases Society of America. Guidelines for the management of adults with hospital-acquired, ventilator-associated, and healthcare-associated pneumonia. *Am J Respir Crit Care Med* 2005; 171(4): 388-416.

3. B. Prevention of VAP in the ICU is a major priority, as there is significant morbidity and mortality associated with its occurrence. Multiple prophylactic strategies have been demonstrated to be effective including oropharyngeal decontamination with chlorhexidine and head of bed elevation. Intravenous dexamethasone would not prevent or treat a VAP. Proton pump inhibitor administration has been demonstrated to be associated with increased rates of VAP. H₂-receptor blockers, such as famotidine, are used for gastrointestinal prophylaxis and would not prevent pneumonia. Most *Pseudomonas* strains, an aerobic gram-negative organism, are resistant to clindamycin.

4. B. The duration of systemic antibiotic therapy following adequate source control of an intra-abdominal infection has been a topic of controversy. Recent literature suggests that with adequate source control, systemic antibiotic therapy should be limited to 3 to 5 days. It is important to note that an individualized approach should be taken in patients without adequate source control and in patients who remain in septic shock.

5. **C.** SIRS is present when 2 or more of the following criteria are met: temperature >38°C or <36°C; respiratory rate >24 breaths/min; HR >90 bpm; and WBC count >12 × 10^9/L or <4 × 10^9/L or >10% bands. Sepsis is characterized as SIRS with a proven or suspected infectious etiology. Severe sepsis is defined as sepsis with signs of dysfunction in 1 or more organ systems. Septic shock is defined as sepsis with hypotension that is refractory to fluid resuscitation.

6. **C.** Evidence-based measures to decrease the incidence of central line–associated bloodstream infections (CLABSI) include: (1) procedure(s) to ensure compliance with infection prevention practices, such as a checklist; (2) hand hygiene prior to catheter insertion; (3) maximal sterile barrier precautions during insertion; (4) chlorhexidine skin preparation; and (5) avoidance of use of the femoral vein in controlled, planned insertions. Subclavian central venous catheters have a lower risk of infection as compared to internal jugular central venous catheters. Landmark technique, as opposed to ultrasound-guided line insertion, does not reduce the risk of a CLABSI.

7. **C.** Fluoroquinolones are underrecognized but significant contributors to delirium in the ICU. Cefepime is associated with delirium but more commonly is associated with hypoactive delirium. Metronidazole and vancomycin are not associated with hyperactive delirium.

8. **C.** Based on this patient's clinical presentation, the most likely diagnosis is necrotizing fasciitis. Necrotizing fasciitis is a surgical emergency due to its rapid expansion and associated high morbidity and mortality. The mainstay of treatment is emergent widespread debridement and broad-spectrum systemic antibiotics. Most commonly, these infections are polymicrobial in nature.

REFERENCES

Alagiakrishnan K, Wiens CA. An approach to drug induced delirium in the elderly. *Postgrad Med J.* 2004;80:388-393.

Ashraf M, Ostrosky-Zeichner L. Ventilator-associated pneumonia: a review. *Hosp Pract.* 2012;40:93-105.

Bagdasarian N, Rao K, Malani PN. Diagnosis and treatment of *Clostridium difficile* in adults: a systematic review. *JAMA.* 2015;313:398-408.

Bhattacharyya S, Darby RR, Raibagkar P, et al. Antibiotic-associated encephalopathy. *Neurology.* 2016;86:963-971.

Dellinger RP, Levy MM, Rhodes A, et al. Surviving Sepsis Campaign: international guidelines for management of severe sepsis and septic shock: 2012. *Crit Care Med.* 2013;41:580-637.

Fugate JE, Kalimullah EA, Hocker SE, et al. Cefepime neurotoxicity in the intensive care unit: a cause of severe, underappreciated encephalopathy. *Crit Care.* 2013;17:R264.

Hunter JD. Ventilator associated pneumonia. *BMJ.* 2012;344: e3325.

Marschall J, Mermel LA, Fakih M, et al. Strategies to prevent central line-associated bloodstream infections in acute care hospitals: 2014 update. *Infect Control Hosp Epidemiol.* 2014;35:S89-S107.

Rattan R, Allen CJ, Sawyer RG, et al. Patients with complicated intra-abdominal infection presenting with sepsis do not require longer duration of antimicrobial therapy. *J Am Coll Surg.* 2016;222:440-446.

Sartelli M, Catena F, Ansaloni L, et al. Duration of antimicrobial therapy in treating complicated intra-abdominal infections: a comprehensive review. *Surg Infect.* 2016;17:9-12.

Ustin JS, Malangoni MA. Necrotizing soft-tissue infections. *Crit Care Med.* 2011;39:2156-2162.

Winters BD, Berenholtz SM. Chapter 11: Ventilator-associated pneumonia: brief update review. Making Health Care Safer II: An Updated Critical Analysis of the Evidence for Patient Safety Practices. Agency for Healthcare Research and Quality (US). 2013. https://archive.ahrq.gov/research/findings/evidence-based-reports/ptsafetyII-full.pdf. Accessed June 29, 2017.

31

General Trauma, Hemorrhage, and Burn

Vicki Sein, MD and Edward Bittner, MD, PhD, MSEd

Questions

1. A 70-kg man sustains a gunshot wound to the left groin. Paramedics report a large-volume blood loss at the scene but are unable to quantify the amount. On arrival, he is anxious and combative, his blood pressure is 100/76 mm Hg, and his pulse rate is 130 bpm. Which of the following is the best estimate of his blood loss?

   A. 500-mL blood loss

   B. 1000-mL blood loss

   C. 1250-mL blood loss

   D. 2000-mL blood loss

   E. 2500-mL blood loss

2. A 34-year-old man is involved in a motor vehicle collision and sustains a large laceration to his forehead and an open femur fracture. Per report, the paramedics noted a large amount of blood at the scene. On arrival, he is anxious and combative, his blood pressure is 90/50 mm Hg, and his pulse rate is 130 bpm. Which of the following is the most appropriate initial resuscitation fluid?

   A. Blood and crystalloid

   B. Crystalloid

   C. Blood

   D. Crystalloid and albumin

   E. Albumin

3. A 75-kg man is burned in a gas station explosion. He has a first-degree burn on his face; second-degree burns to his entire chest, anterior abdomen, and left arm; and a third-degree circumferential burn on his right arm and anterior portion of his right leg. What is his total body surface area burned that would be used in the calculation of his initial resuscitation fluid?

   A. 36%

   B. 45%

   C. 50%

   D. 54.5%

   E. 60%

4. A 76-year-old man is rescued from a building fire. On initial evaluation, he has second-degree burns to the right half of his face, has soot in the oropharynx, and is coughing up carbonaceous sputum. He has audible stridor. He requires supplemental oxygen via face mask. What is the most appropriate next step?

A. Bronchoscopy to evaluate the possibility of inhalation injury

B. Immediate intubation

C. Computed tomography (CT) scan to evaluate bronchial thickening

D. Measurement of carboxyhemoglobin levels

E. Observation

5. A 100-kg man is burned in a house fire. He sustains second- and third-degree burns to 30% of his body. He presents to the hospital 3 hours after injury and has received 1 L of crystalloid from emergency medical services (EMS). What should be the rate of intravenous (IV) fluid administration when he arrives at the hospital?

A. 250 mL/h

B. 500 mL/h

C. 1000 mL/h

D. 1500 mL/h

E. 2000 mL/h

6. A 45-year-old man is a restrained driver in a high-speed motor vehicle crash. After initial assessment and resuscitation, a CT scan shows a liver laceration with active extravasation and a contained partial transection of the thoracic aorta. His vitals after transfusion of 2 units of packed red blood cells are as follows: heart rate 110 bpm, blood pressure 92/54 mm Hg, and respiratory rate 20 breaths/ min. What would be the next appropriate step in his management?

A. Immediate endovascular repair of the thoracic aorta

B. Immediate open surgical intervention for the aortic transection

C. Admission to the floor for observation

D. Admission to the intensive care unit for blood pressure management

E. Percutaneous endovascular embolization of the liver laceration

7. A 70-year-old woman suffers a fall from standing height at home. She is brought to the emergency department and found to have a comminuted femur fracture. Her past medical history is significant for systolic heart failure (last ejection fraction on echocardiogram: 45%), diabetes mellitus, hypertension, and hyperlipidemia. She is admitted to the floor for observation and preoperative assessment for surgical fixation of her fracture. On the day after admission, she acutely becomes tachycardic, tachypneic, and hypoxic and has an altered mental status. On examination, a petechial rash is noted across her chest. What is the most likely etiology of her acute decompensation?

A. Congestive heart failure exacerbation

B. Pneumonia

C. Hypoglycemia

D. Fat embolism

E. Pulmonary embolism

8. A 37-year-old man is brought in by EMS. His friends called 911 after he was found weak and confused in his tent with a kerosene tent heater on. He also complained of severe headache, nausea, vomiting, and palpitations. On presentation to the emergency department, his vital signs are as follows: heart rate 120 bpm, blood pressure 110/76 mm Hg, respiratory rate 20 breaths/min, oxygen saturation 97% on 2 L nasal cannula. What is the next most appropriate treatment?

A. Administration of methylene blue

B. Administration of naloxone (Narcan)

C. Administration of 100% fraction of inspired oxygen (FiO_2)

D. Administration of hydroxocobalamin

E. Wean supplemental oxygen

9. An 80-kg man is involved in a motor vehicle collision during which he suffers a grade 4 splenic laceration, a grade 4 liver laceration, and multiple rib
fractures. He is taken to the operating room shortly
after presentation where he undergoes a splenec-
tomy and repair of his liver laceration. During the
first 24 hours in the hospital, he receives 3 L of crystalloid, 4 units of packed red blood cells, and 3 units
of fresh frozen plasma. His chest x-ray from the
morning of hospital day 2 is shown below, and he
remains intubated. His ventilator settings are volume control: tidal volume 650 mL, positive end-
expiratory pressure (PEEP) 10 cm H_2O, frequency
20, and FiO_2 80%. Peak and plateau pressures are
37 cm H_2O and 32 cm H_2O, respectively. Arterial
blood gas results on those settings are as follows:
pH 7.31, partial pressure of carbon dioxide
44 mm Hg, and partial pressure of oxygen 77 mm Hg.
What is the next best step in management?

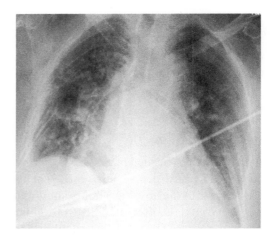

A. Reduce the respiratory rate to 18 breaths/min
B. Increase FiO_2 to 100%
C. Reduce the tidal volume to 480 mL
D. Increase the tidal volume to 700 mL
E. Reduce PEEP to 8 cm H_2O

Answers and Explanations

1. D. This patient is in class 3 hemorrhage shock, as evidenced by his tachycardia and hypotension. He is anxious and combative, but not yet lethargic, as is seen in class 4 hemorrhagic shock. Estimated blood loss in class 3 hemorrhagic shock is 1500 to 2000 mL, or 30% to 40% of the blood volume. This question focuses on the classification of hemorrhagic shock. Hemorrhagic shock can be divided into 4 classes as shown in Table 31-1.

Table 31-1. Classes of Hemorrhagic Shock

Class of Shock	Blood Volume Lost	Findings
I	<15% of blood volume <750 mL	Normal heart rate, blood pressure, capillary refill, pulse pressure Slightly anxious affect
II	15%-30% of blood volume 750-1500 mL	Normal mean arterial pressure (MAP), increased diastolic blood pressure (DBP), mild tachycardia Mildly anxious
III	30%-40% of blood volume 1500-2000 mL	Reduced MAP, systolic blood pressure (SBP), DBP, tachycardia >120 bpm Anxious and confused
IV	>40% of blood volume >2000 mL	Severely reduced MAP, SBP, DBP, tachycardia >140 bpm Confused to lethargic

2. A. This patient is in class 3 hemorrhage, as evidenced by his tachycardia and hypotension. He is anxious and combative, but not yet lethargic, as is seen in class 4 hemorrhagic shock. The appropriate resuscitation fluid in class 3 hemorrhagic shock is a combination of crystalloid and blood.

3. B. This patient has a 45% total body surface area (TBSA) burn, when taking into account his second- and third-degree burns. The "rule of 9s" can be used to provide an estimate of the TBSA burned. The front of the face counts for 4.5%, the entire chest and anterior abdomen together is 18%, the left arm is 4.5%, circumferential burn to the right arm is 9%, and the anterior portion of the leg is 9%. First-degree burns are not included in the rule of 9s estimation.

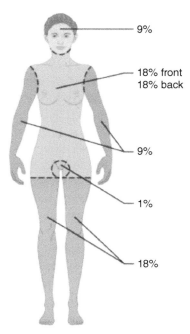

9%

18% front
18% back

9%

1%

18%

4. B. In an elderly individual who has sustained an inhalation injury, the first best option is to secure the airway. In this case, the severity of his potential injury is evidenced by the burns on his face, as well as his carbonaceous sputum. This patient may need evaluation via bronchoscopy to evaluate and follow airway damage, but this would not be the first step. Observation in this situation would be inappropriate. However, without overt signs of inhalation injury, 24 hours of close observation would be appropriate.

5. **C.** This patient has a 30% TBSA burn. The Parkland formula is commonly used to estimate fluid resuscitation for a patient sustaining a major thermal injury:

$$4 \times \% \text{ TBSA burned} \times \text{weight (kg)} =$$
$$\text{Volume of fluid resuscitation in 24 hours}$$

- Half is given in the first 8 hours.
- The remainder is given in the next 16 hours.

For this patient, the estimated fluid needs are: $4 \times 30\% \times 100$ kg = 12,000 mL. Thus, 6000 mL should be administered in the first 8 hours. Since the patient received 1 L of fluid already and the injury occurred 3 hours earlier, the initial hourly rate should be 5000/5 = 1000 mL/h.

6. **E.** The actively bleeding liver laceration is the priority for initial management in this case. This question focuses on the management of a multisystem trauma patient. This patient has 2 life-threatening injuries: a liver laceration that is actively bleeding and a blunt injury to the thoracic aorta, which is contained. The first injury to address is the injury that causes the greatest threat to life, which is bleeding from the liver laceration. Blunt thoracic aortic injuries can initially be managed with heart rate and blood pressure control. Delayed endovascular repair of the thoracic aortic injury is appropriate in the setting of a contained rupture.

7. **D.** The patient's clinical deterioration is most consistent with fat embolism syndrome. Fat embolism syndrome occurs in patients who have sustained blunt trauma and patients with long bone fractures. It can also occur after fat grafting. The classic presentation of fat embolism syndrome is acute respiratory insufficiency, altered mental status, and dermatologic findings of a petechial rash. While all 3 findings are not always present, suspicion should be high in trauma patients, especially those with long bone fractures. Management is supportive; lung-protective ventilation should be initiated, as well as immobilization of the fracture.

8. **C.** This patient has carbon monoxide toxicity. This is indicated by his use of the kerosene tent heater, weak and confused state, headache, nausea, and palpitations. Oxygen saturation on pulse oximetry will be normal in these circumstances.

Oxygen should be administered at 100% FiO_2 to displace the carbon monoxide molecules from hemoglobin. Even though the patient has a good oxygen saturation on pulse oximeter, this level will be falsely elevated in the setting of carbon monoxide toxicity. Hyperbaric oxygen has been used but is not available in all centers. Methylene blue is used as treatment for methemoglobinemia, which this patient does not have. Hydroxocobalamin is used to treat cyanide toxicity, and naloxone (Narcan) is used in opioid toxicity.

9. **C.** This patient has acute respiratory distress syndrome. On chest x-ray, diffuse bilateral pulmonary infiltrates are shown, and his arterial partial pressure of oxygen (PaO_2)-to-FiO_2 ratio is 96. The next appropriate step would be to institute lung-protective ventilation and decrease his tidal volume to 6 mL/kg. Diuresis may not be appropriate in his acute posttrauma setting, as he may still be intravascularly depleted. Increasing his FiO_2 or tidal volume would not be appropriate in this situation. This patient does not have any other clinical evidence of infection, and empiric antibiotics are not indicated.

REFERENCES

American College of Surgeons Committee on Trauma. Shock. In: *Advanced Trauma Life Support ATLS Student Course Manual.* Chicago, IL: American College of Surgeons Committee on Trauma; 2012:73.

di Eusanio M, Folesani G, Berretta P, et al. Delayed management of blunt traumatic aortic injury: open surgical versus endovascular repair. *Ann Thorac Surg.* 2013;95:1591-1597.

Guo R, Fan E. Beyond low tidal volumes: ventilating the patient with acute respiratory distress syndrome. *Clin Chest Med.* 2014;35:729-741.

Guzman JA. Carbon monoxide poisoning. *Crit Care Clin.* 2012;28:537-548.

Kasten KR, Makley AT, Kagan RJ. Update on the critical care management of severe burns. *J Intensive Care Med.* 2011;26:223-236.

Pham TN, Cancio LC, Gibran NS. American Burn Association practice guidelines burn shock resuscitation. *J Burn Care Res.* 2008;29:257-266.

Rittayamai N, Brochard L. Recent advances in mechanical ventilation in patients with acute respiratory distress syndrome. *Eur Respir Rev.* 2015;24:132-140.

Shaikh N. Emergency management of fat embolism syndrome. *J Emerg Trauma Shock.* 2009;2:29-33.

Walker PF, Beuhner MF, Wood LA, et al. Diagnosis and management of inhalation injury: an updated review. *Crit Care.* 2015;19:351.

32

Neurocritical Care in the Surgical Intensive Care Unit

Jamel Ortoleva, MD and Edward Bittner, MD, PhD, MSEd

Questions

1. A 50-year-old man with history of anxiety, depression, alcohol abuse, chronic pain, and hyperthyroidism presents with altered mental status and fever. His medications are sertraline, propylthiouracil, acetaminophen, clonazepam, and tramadol. Exam reveals a combative male mumbling incoherently. He appears diaphoretic. His vital signs are temperature of 105°F, pulse of 130 bpm, blood pressure of 190/80 mm Hg, respiratory rate of 35 breaths/min, and oxygen saturation of 89%. He is treated with intravenous (IV) haloperidol for his agitation. He subsequently has a seizure and is intubated for airway protection. Which of the following is the most appropriate treatment for this patient?

   A. Administer dantrolene
   B. Discontinue tramadol
   C. Administer IV methylprednisolone
   D. Administer fentanyl pain control
   E. Start broad-spectrum antibiotics

2. A 72-year-old man with a history of coronary artery disease, diabetes, chronic obstructive pulmonary disease, and depression presents with confusion, productive cough, fever, gastrointestinal upset, and diffuse infiltrates on chest x-ray. Several other people who live in his building presented with similar symptoms. Vital signs are oxygen saturation of 93% on 2 L/min nasal cannula, heart rate of 95 bpm, blood pressure of 115/40 mm Hg, respiratory rate of 25 breaths/min, and temperature of 103°F. His urine *Legionella* antigen is positive. Which laboratory values would be most helpful in the workup of his altered mental status?

   A. Serum electrolytes
   B. Complete blood count (CBC) with differential
   C. Arterial blood gas
   D. Liver function panel
   E. Serum lactate

3. A 45-year-old man with a history of alcohol and cocaine abuse, depression, and hypertension presents with confusion and a severe headache. Vital signs are as follows: temperature 98°F, pulse 65 bpm, blood pressure 220/110 mm Hg, respiratory rate 26 breaths/min, and oxygen saturation 96%. Pupils are equal in size, round, and sluggishly reactive. He is moving all extremities. What is the best next step in this patient's management?

   A. Thrombolysis

   B. Stat head computed tomography (CT)

   C. Head of bed elevation and ensuring a stable airway

   D. Nicardipine infusion

   E. Administration of mannitol

4. A 70-year-old man with a history of insulin-dependent type 2 diabetes, hypertension, and anxiety was admitted to the intensive care unit (ICU) 5 days ago with sepsis due to a urinary tract infection. His home medications include glyburide, lisinopril, and lorazepam. Over the past 2 days, he has had progressive lethargy and, on exam, has developed grimacing, rigidity, limbs that retain any position into which they are manipulated by examiner, and fixed gaze. Vital signs are as follows: temperature 98°F, pulse 65 bpm, blood pressure 140/90 mm Hg, respiratory rate 26 breaths/min, and oxygen saturation 96% on 2 L nasal cannula. He has not received antipsychotic medication, and lorazepam was discontinued on admission given his confusion at the time. Head CT and brain magnetic resonance imaging (MRI) are unremarkable; electroencephalogram (EEG) demonstrated diffuse slowing over the past 24 hours. What is the next best step in management?

   A. Broaden antibiotic coverage

   B. Administer empiric dose of lorazepam

   C. Administer vitamin B_{12} injection

   D. Monitor motor evoked potentials

   E. Administer dantrolene

5. A 66-year-old woman with a history of hypertension, macular degeneration, and frequent urinary tract infections presents after a fall. She is treated for pneumonia and receives surgery for a femur fracture. Postoperatively, her mental status has not returned to baseline according to a relative who last saw her 6 months ago. Over this 6-month interval, outside records indicate she has developed progressive gait instability, memory impairment, and intermittent urinary frequency. Vital signs are within normal limits. Vitamin B_{12}, CBC, and urinalysis are within normal limits. What is the best next step?

   A. Noncontrast head CT

   B. Lumbar puncture

   C. EEG

   D. Restart antibiotics

   E. Start donepezil

6. An 84-year-old man was admitted to the surgical ICU after undergoing surgical repair of a hip fracture. His medical history is notable for mild dementia, hypertension, prior stroke with residual aphasia, and a 15-pound weight loss in the past 4 months. For the past 2 nights, he has been confused, agitated, and difficult to reorient. During the day, he is oriented and does not complain of urinary symptoms. He is afebrile, and infectious workup has been negative. His neurologic exam is nonfocal. Which of the following is the best next step in management?

   A. Head CT

   B. Vitamin B_{12} level

   C. Urine analysis

   D. Frequent day-night reorientation

   E. Thyroid function panel

7. A 45-year-old man with alcoholic cirrhosis presents to the hospital with altered mental status after not taking his lactulose for the past 8 days. Which of the following is most likely to transiently improve the mental status of this patient?

   A. Haloperidol

   B. Flumazenil

   C. Kayexalate

   D. Day-night orientation

   E. Empiric IV lorazepam 2 mg

8. A 64-year-old man with Mobitz type I heart block and Parkinson disease with dementia is postoperative day 2 from a pneumonectomy. He is delirious in the ICU and combative despite attempts to reorient him. Which of the following medications would be most appropriate for the treatment of his agitation?

A. Midazolam

B. Haloperidol

C. Quetiapine

D. Donepezil

E. Dexmedetomidine

9. A 57-year-old woman with a history of morbid obesity, anxiety on clonazepam, and postoperative nausea and vomiting is confused and agitated 1 day after undergoing a laparoscopic gastric bypass. Her temperature is 103.6°F, pulse is 140 bpm, blood pressure is 93/52 mm Hg, respiratory rate is 20 breaths/min, and oxygen saturation is 92% on room air. Her right pupil is larger than the left and minimally reactive to light. Review of her medications notes that she has a scopolamine patch behind her right ear and received 0.5 mg of lorazepam 1 hour ago. What is the next best step in management for this patient?

A. 5 mg of IV haloperidol

B. Abdominal exam

C. 1 mg of IV lorazepam

D. 2 mg of IV morphine

E. Noncontrast head CT

Answers and Explanations

1. **B.** This patient likely has serotonin syndrome (SS). SS is clinical entity characterized by the triad of altered mental status, neuromuscular abnormalities, and autonomic hyperactivity. Patients with SS can present with a spectrum of clinical signs and symptoms ranging from mild tremors and gastrointestinal upset to muscle rigidity, seizures, and severe hyperthermia. The mechanism is thought to be due to excess levels of serotonin generally brought on by combinations of medications with pro-serotonergic effects. Multiple drugs have been associated with the development of SS, usually in combination, including selective serotonin reuptake inhibitors, methylene blue, fentanyl (and other phenylpiperidine narcotics), linezolid, trazodone, and tramadol. The differential diagnosis for patients presenting with SS-like signs and symptoms includes thyroid storm, neuroleptic malignant syndrome, malignant hyperthermia, catatonia, and central fever. Administration of dantrolene does not treat SS, and neuroleptic malignant syndrome is unlikely since haloperidol administration followed symptom development. Methylprednisolone could be part of a treatment for thyroid storm to reduce thyroxine (T_4) to triiodothyronine (T_3) conversion, but the symptoms are more consistent with SS. As fentanyl is a causal agent for SS, it is not an ideal analgesic for this patient. Infection is unlikely given the clinical presentation, and therefore, antibiotics are not indicated.

2. **A.** This patient likely has a Legionnaires' disease. Signs and symptoms of Legionnaires' disease include high fever (>38.8°C), cough, chills, shortness of breath, and diarrhea with nausea and vomiting. Laboratory findings include liver function test abnormalities, hyponatremia, myoglobinuria, elevated erythrocyte sedimentation rate (ESR), and chest imaging with diffuse infiltrates. Altered mental status in the setting of *Legionella* infection is common, usually attributed to inflammation and associated toxins from the infection. However, it is important to remember that electrolyte derangement can result in altered mental status and is a reversible cause. Legionella infection is known to result in hyponatremia, which is an important cause of confusion. Specifically, in 1 recent study, 44% of 27 patients with *Legionella* infection had a serum sodium <130 mmol/L. The etiology of hyponatremia in Legionnaires' disease has been attributed to syndrome of inappropriate antidiuretic hormone (SIADH), direct renal effects, or the effects of other natriuretic peptides. Patients recovering from *Legionella* infection can also suffer from slow recovery with neurologic and neuromuscular abnormalities. Recommended treatment for Legionnaires' disease is levofloxacin 750 mg for 5 to 10 days or azithromycin 500 mg for 3 to 5 days.

3. **C.** This patient is likely suffering from a spontaneous intracranial hemorrhage (ICH), the second most common type of stroke. History and clinical findings consistent with this diagnosis include the history of cocaine abuse and hypertension (the most important risk factor for ICH), the severe headache and confusion, severe hypertension, and sluggish pupils. That being said, it is still possible he is having an ischemic stroke. Ensuring a stable airway is of utmost importance in these patients (patients with a Glasgow coma scale [GCS] score ≤8 should be intubated). Thrombolysis could be fatal if this patient has an ICH. Obtaining a stat head CT is important but, as with any medical emergency, the ABCs (airway, breathing, and circulation) are paramount. A nicardipine infusion will likely be necessary if head CT confirms ICH but would not be the first intervention. Mannitol would be useful if he has signs of elevated intracranial hypertension and concern for herniation

but would not be instituted before head of bed elevation.

4. **B.** This patient is likely suffering from catatonia. Patients presenting with severe (or malignant) catatonia can manifest autonomic instability, high fevers, waxy flexibility, negativism, posturing, mannerism, stereotypy, rigidity, mutism, and fixed gaze. These patients can have the same presentation as neuroleptic malignant syndrome; however, they have not been exposed to neuroleptics. A clear cause is uncommonly identified, but catatonia related to benzodiazepine withdrawal has been described. A lorazepam trial has been described to be diagnostic in patients with catatonia. A response to therapy with benzodiazepines gives an indication that the syndrome is likely to be catatonia. The overall response rate to lorazepam in catatonia has varied between 50% and 80%.

Infection is unlikely given the stability of vital signs and finding of rigidity. Subacute combined degeneration is unlikely since he is not complaining of difficulty walking or issues with proprioception, and thus, vitamin B_{12} treatment is unlikely to be beneficial. Diffuse peripheral neuropathy is unlikely after a 6-day ICU admission, and motor evoked potentials are unlikely to assist in diagnosis or treatment. Neuroleptic malignant syndrome is unlikely since the patient is afebrile and did not receive antipsychotic medications.

5. **A.** This patient's history and presentation are consistent with a diagnosis of normal-pressure hydrocephalus (NPH), which is a rare but important cause of potentially reversible cognitive decline. Peak age of onset is typically 60 to 69 years old. Symptoms are classically gait disturbance, cognitive dysfunction, and urinary incontinence. Gait disturbance with 1 of the other 2 common symptoms should prompt consideration of the diagnosis. Diagnosis is made with a combination of typical symptoms, a noncontrast head CT scan demonstrating an Evan's index (the ratio of largest biventricular diameter to biparietal diameter) of at least 0.3, and a lumbar puncture demonstrating normal cerebrospinal fluid (CSF) pressure (normally 70-245 mm H_2O with the patient on the side). Ventriculoperitoneal shunt can alleviate symptoms of NPH, but dementia does not always resolve. Of note, failure of a ventriculoperitoneal shunt can occur, especially in patients with NPH due to a CSF-secreting tumor (about 40% of cases). Consequently, lumbar puncture should be preceded by CT of the head to exclude elevated intracranial pressure and risk of herniation. Restarting antibiotics is unlikely to improve this patient's symptoms since there is no evidence of infection. Donepezil may be of assistance if this patient has Alzheimer dementia, but progressive deterioration in ambulation is inconsistent with the diagnosis.

6. **D.** This patient is likely suffering from delirium referred to as "sundowning syndrome." Sundowning syndrome commonly occurs in elderly patients, and baseline cognitive impairment is a risk factor. It is likely brought on by circadian rhythm disturbance and is likely potentiated in this case by the inflammation associated with the patient's urgent procedure, sedative medications, and the ICU setting (an environment in which time of day is not always clear to patients). Treatment for sundowning syndrome begins with reorientation and facilitating sleep hygiene. Melatonin and ramelteon administration may also facilitate sleep. A head CT may be indicated, but this patient has no clear focal deficits. A vitamin B_{12} deficiency would be unlikely to account for his symptoms. Thyroid disease can result in dementia and altered mental status, but symptoms are usually not periodic in nature.

7. **B.** Hepatic encephalopathy is a complex toxic metabolic syndrome seen in patients with acute liver injury, liver cirrhosis, and, rarely, a portosystemic shunt. A number of factors have been implicated in the pathogenesis of hepatic encephalopathy including the accumulation of ammonia, false neurotransmitter synthesis, astrocyte swelling, inflammation, and oxidative stress. The definitive treatment is orthotopic liver transplant. Medical management starts with identifying the underlying cause of the acute deterioration and treatment with lactulose and rifaximin.

The benzodiazepine receptor antagonist flumazenil has been used for treatment of hepatic encephalopathy in a number of observational studies and randomized trials. Response to treatment, when it occurs, is seen within a few minutes after intravenous administration in most patients; however, two-thirds of patients who responded deteriorated 2 to 4 hours later.

Kayexalate is used for the treatment of hyperkalemia and is not recommended in the treatment of hepatic encephalopathy.

8. C. Over 50% of patients in the ICU may satisfy criteria for delirium during their stay. Risk factors for delirium in elderly patients can be divided into modifiable and nonmodifiable categories. Potentially modifiable risk factors include hearing or vision impairment, immobilization, medications (eg, benzodiazepines, narcotics, corticosteroids), acute neurologic disease, acute physiologic insults, metabolic derangement, surgery, ICU admission, pain, emotional distress, and sleep dysregulation. Nonmodifiable risk factors include cognitive impairment, age over 65, prior episodes of delirium, history of neurologic disease, male gender, chronic hepatic or renal disease, and a large number of comorbidities. Nonpharmacologic treatment of delirium includes reorientation, ear plugs to reduce noise at night, sleep-wake reorientation, ensuring appropriate pain control, and, as a last resort, restraints. Pharmacologic treatments for delirium include antipsychotic medications, benzodiazepines (although this class of medications frequently increases the duration and risk of delirium), and dexmedetomidine (to reduce the risk of delirium). Given this patient's history of Parkinson disease, haloperidol is not an ideal choice since dopamine blockade may worsen his symptoms. However, quetiapine is a reasonable choice in this context.

Donepezil is used for treatment of Alzheimer disease but does not currently have a role in the management of delirium. Dexmedetomidine is an α_2-agonist that acts centrally and is generally well suited to treat difficult-to-control agitation. However, given this patient's history of heart block, dexmedetomidine is not the best option as it has been associated with cases of worsening heart block.

9. B. This patient is most likely to have an acute intra-abdominal process (such as an anastomotic leak) resulting in a toxic-metabolic cause of delirium. Vital signs are most suggestive of an acute inflammatory process. Benzodiazepine withdrawal is less likely given she was treated with lorazepam an hour ago. On exam, her large right pupil is most likely the result of the scopolamine patch in place on the same side. Anticholinergic syndrome resulting from the scopolamine patch can occur but is unlikely given the duration of therapy. The patient's fever and inflammatory signs are concerning, and her abdomen should be examined. A noncontrast head CT may be warranted to assess for intracranial abnormalities given her pupillary changes and delirium, but the otherwise nonfocal exam makes this diagnosis less likely.

REFERENCES

Boyer EW, Shannon M. The serotonin syndrome. *N Engl J Med.* 2005;352:1112-1120.

Carroll R, Matfin G. Endocrine and metabolic emergencies: thyroid storm. *Ther Adv Endocrinol Metab.* 2010;1:139-145.

Cunha B, Burillo A, Bouza E. Legionnaires' disease. *Lancet.* 2016;387:376-385.

de Oliveira Manoel AL, Goffi A, Zampieri FG, et al. The critical care management of spontaneous intracranial hemorrhage: a contemporary review. *Crit Care.* 2016;20:272.

Fiumefreddo R, Zabrosky R, Haeuptle J, et al. Clinical predictors for *Legionella* in patients presenting with community-acquired pneumonia to the emergency department. *BMC Pulm Med.* 2009;9:4.

Fong TG, Tulebaev SR, Inouye SK. Delirium in elderly adults: diagnosis, prevention and treatment. *Nat Rev Neurol.* 2009;5:210-220.

Frederick RT. Current concepts in the pathophysiology and management of hepatic encephalopathy. *Gastroenterol Hepatol.* 2011;7:222-233.

Girard TD, Ely EW. Delirium in the critically ill patient. *Handb Clin Neurol.* 2008;90:39-56.

Goulenok C, Bernard B, Cadranel JF, et al. Flumazenil vs. placebo in hepatic encephalopathy in patients with cirrhosis: a meta-analysis. *Aliment Pharmacol Ther.* 2002;16:361-372.

Hatta K, Kishi Y, Wada K, et al. Preventive effects of ramelteon on delirium: a randomized placebo-controlled trial. *JAMA Psychiatry.* 2014;71(4):397-403.

Inouye SK, Westendorp RGJ, Saczynski JS. Delirium in elderly people. *Lancet.* 2014;383:911-922.

Kandiah PA, Kumar G. Hepatic encephalopathy: the old and the new. *Crit Care Clin.* 2016;32:311-329.

Khachiyants N, Trinkle D, Son SJ, et al. Sundown syndrome in persons with dementia: an update. *Psychiatry Invest.* 2011;8:275-287.

Kim P, Louis C, Muralee S, et al. Sundowning syndrome in the older patient. *Clin Geriatr.* 2005;13:32-36.

Knopman DS, Petersen RC, Cha RH, et al. Incidence and causes of nondegenerative nonvascular dementia: a population-based study. *Arch Neurol.* 2006;63:218-221.

Lonergan E, Luxenberg J, Areosa Sastre A, et al. Benzodiazepines for delirium. *Cochrane Database Syst Rev.* 2009;4:CD006379.

Northoff G. What catatonia can tell us about top-down modulation: a neuropsychiatric hypothesis. *Behav Brain Sci.* 2002;25:555-577.

Pasin L, Landoni G, Nardelli P, et al. Dexmedetomidine reduces the risk of delirium, agitation and confusion in critically ill patients: a meta-analysis of randomized controlled trials. *J Cardiothorac Vasc Anesth.* 2014;28:1459-1466.

Qureshi AI, Mendelow AD, Hanley DF. Intracerebral haemorrhage. *Lancet.* 2009;373:1632-1644.

Qureshi A, Palesch YY, Barsan WG, et al. Intensive blood pressure lowering in patients with acute cerebral hemorrhage. *N Engl J Med.* 2016;375:1033-1043.

Relkin N, Marmarou A, Klinge P, et al. Diagnosing idiopathic normal-pressure hydrocephalus. *Neurosurgery.* 2005;57:S4-S16.

Saddawi-Konefka D, Berg SM, Nejad S, et al. Catatonia in the ICU: an important and underdiagnosed cause of altered mental status. A case series and review of the literature. *Crit Care Med.* 2014;42:e234-e241.

Schuetz P, Haubitz S, Christ-Crain M, et al. Hyponatremia and anti-diuretic hormone in Legionnaires' disease. *BMC Infect Dis.* 2013;13:585.

Shprecher D, Schwalb J, Kurlan R. Normal pressure hydrocephalus: diagnosis and treatment. *Curr Neurol Neurosci Rep.* 2008;8:371-376.

Suraweera D, Sundaram V, Saab S. Evaluation and management of hepatic encephalopathy: current status and future directions. *Gut Liver.* 2016;10:509-519.

Unal A, Bulbul F, Alpak G, et al. Effective treatment of catatonia by combination of benzodiazepine and electroconvulsive therapy. *J ECT.* 2013;29(3):206-209.

Vasselon P, Weiner L, Rossi-Pujo F, et al. Unilateral mydriasis due to scopolamine patch. *Int J Clin Pharm.* 2011;33: 737-739.

Volpi-Abadie J, Kaye AM, Kaye AD. Serotonin syndrome. *Ochsner J.* 2013;13:533-540.

33

Anesthesia in the Surgical Intensive Care Unit

Connie Wang, MD and Abraham Sonny, MD

Questions

1. A previously healthy 24-year-old, 75-kg woman developed hypertension, hypercarbia, and hyperthermia after induction of anesthesia with midazolam, fentanyl, propofol, and succinylcholine. Malignant hyperthermia (MH) was suspected, and she was given an initial intravenous (IV) bolus dose of dantrolene. An intraoperative creatinine kinase was measured as 23,000 U/L, and potassium was measured as 5.7 mEq/L. After the patient was stabilized, she was transported to the intensive care unit (ICU) for monitoring. Which of the following statements about MH is correct?

   A. Patients with MH should be monitored for 12 hours in the postoperative period.

   B. MH is caused by an abnormality in ryanodine receptors in skeletal muscle.

   C. One should monitor for hypokalemia in MH.

   D. A negative screen of the *RYR1* and *CACNA1S* genes rules out MH susceptibility.

2. A 33-year-old man with a 4-day history of third-degree burns to the bilateral lower extremities and back was admitted to the ICU for stabilization. The patient has a planned extensive excision and grafting procedure in the operating room. He complains of active gastroesophageal reflux symptoms with nausea. Which neuromuscular blocking agent should be used for rapid sequence intubation?

   A. Cisatracurium

   B. Succinylcholine

   C. Rocuronium

   D. Atracurium

3. A 29-year-old gunshot wound patient underwent an exploratory laparotomy complicated with bile leak and sepsis. The patient was administered norepinephrine infusion for hypotension and propofol infusion for sedation. A triglyceride level was checked on day 6, which returned as 989 mg/dL. On day 7, the patient developed metabolic acidosis, rhabdomyolysis, and acute renal failure requiring dialysis. The next day, the patient developed cardiac arrest and died. Which of the following statements regarding this syndrome is true?

   A. A prolonged propofol infusion of ≥2 mg/kg/h increases the risk of propofol infusion syndrome.

   B. Elderly patients are more susceptible.

C. Propofol infusion syndrome is thought to be due to failure of the mitochondrial respiratory chain.

D. Cardiac failure is often one of the first signs of this syndrome.

4. A 78 year-old woman with a history of recurrent kidney stones is admitted to the ICU with sepsis due to urinary tract infection. A central line is placed in the left internal jugular vein due to abnormal anatomy on the right side. Which of the following is more likely to occur with placement of left-sided central lines when compared with right-sided central lines?

A. Lymphatic injury

B. Arterial puncture

C. Pneumothorax

D. Air embolism

5. A 58-year-old, 124-kg man with a history of chronic obstructive pulmonary disease and cervical spine fusion is admitted to the ICU for respiratory distress. After being placed on bilevel positive airway pressure for an hour, his arterial blood gas showed little improvement: pH 7.27, partial pressure of carbon dioxide 74 mm Hg, and partial pressure of oxygen 75 mm Hg on fraction of inspired oxygen (FiO_2) 100%. Based on this blood gas analysis, it was decided to intubate the patient. After administration of propofol and rocuronium, the patient was unable to be bag and masked with an oral airway in place. Subsequent attempts to intubate after direct laryngoscopy were unsuccessful. What is your next step?

A. Perform a cricothyrotomy

B. Wait until the patient has spontaneous breathing efforts

C. Use video-assisted laryngoscopy

D. Insert a supraglottic airway

6. A 64-year-old man with a past medical history of hypertension, hyperlipidemia, and diabetes type 2 is scheduled for a routine ventral hernia repair under general anesthesia. He has no known allergies. Anesthesia is induced with midazolam, fentanyl, propofol, and rocuronium. The patient is uneventfully intubated. While the surgeons are cleaning the skin with chlorhexidine, the patient suddenly develops severe wheezing, high peak airway pressures, and hypotension. Anaphylaxis is suspected. The patient is adequately treated with fluids, epinephrine, steroids, and H_2 blockers. He is transported to the ICU intubated for monitoring. Which of the following agents is most likely to have caused anaphylaxis?

A. Propofol

B. Rocuronium

C. Chlorhexidine

D. Fentanyl

7. A 19-year-old patient was brought to the emergency department after a motor vehicle crash, intubated for poor mental status, and transported to the ICU for stabilization. It was signed out to the ICU team that etomidate and rocuronium were administered for intubation due to hemodynamic instability. Which of the following may occur due to administration of etomidate?

A. Adrenal suppression

B. Tachycardia

C. Thrombocytopenia

D. Hallucinations

8. A 24-year-old woman with a history of severe scoliosis is transported to the ICU after a Harrington rod placement procedure. She experienced massive blood loss and fluid resuscitation in the operating room, resulting in inability to extubate. She is transported to the ICU, where she is sedated with propofol infusion. Ketamine infusion was added for sedation and pain control. Which of the following is true about ketamine?

A. Ketamine is a strong mu-opioid receptor agonist.

B. Ketamine causes bronchodilation.

C. Ketamine causes dry mouth.

D. Ketamine does not depress myocardial function.

9. An 88-year-old man with history of unsteady gait fell, resulting in a head strike, 3 broken ribs, and a hip fracture. Computed tomography (CT) of the head in the emergency room showed an acute subdural hematoma without midline shift. He is transported to the ICU for stabilization and monitoring. After 1.5 hours, the patient becomes increasingly tachypneic, bradycardic, and confused and unable to protect his airway. The decision is made to intubate, after which the CT scan would be repeated. Which anesthetic agent used for induction of anesthesia is most likely to increase intracranial pressure?

A. Propofol

B. Thiopental

C. Etomidate

D. Ketamine

10. A previously healthy 30-year-old postpartum woman is admitted to the ICU for treatment of severe chorioamnionitis. She is intubated, and a right subclavian central line is placed under ultrasound guidance, after which a norepinephrine infusion is initiated. After 10 minutes, the patient becomes increasingly tachycardic, hypoxic, and hypotensive. Examination reveals diminished breath sounds on the right hemithorax. The patient's blood pressure is now 74/32 mm Hg. What is the best next step in management of the patient?

A. Give a bolus of norepinephrine

B. Place a large-bore needle into the second intercostal space

C. Obtain a chest x-ray

D. Switch to broader coverage antibiotics

Answers and Explanations

1. **B.** Malignant hyperthermia (MH) is an autosomal dominant disease of hypermetabolism in the skeletal muscle that is triggered by all potent volatile anesthetics and depolarizing muscle relaxants. MH is caused by abnormalities in ryanodine receptors in skeletal muscle that cause an abnormal buildup of myoplasmic calcium, which leads to an immense metabolic reaction. This could result in increased metabolic acidosis, increased carbon dioxide production, increased heart rate, hyperthermia, hyperkalemia, increased creatine kinase, myoglobinemia, myoglobinuria, and muscle rigidity. Multisystem organ failure can also develop. The most common initial signs of MH are hypercarbia, masseter muscle rigidity, and sinus tachycardia. The most frequent clinical signs include hyperthermia, sinus tachycardia, and hypercarbia. The caffeine halothane contracture assays done on muscle biopsies remain the most reliable tests for MH. Molecular genetic testing that identifies mutations in the *RYR1* and *CACNA1S* genes confirms the diagnosis of susceptibility to MH; however, a negative screen of the *RYR1* and *CACNA1S* genes does not rule out MH susceptibility.

   When MH is suspected, all potent halogenated anesthetics and depolarizing muscle relaxants should be discontinued, and the patient should be hyperventilated. Further administration of succinylcholine should be avoided. General anesthesia should be maintained with IV nontriggering anesthetics. An IV dantrolene bolus of 2.5 mg/kg should be given through a large-bore IV. A blood gas should be obtained to determine the degree of metabolic acidosis and to determine serum potassium concentration. When the patient has stabilized, he or she should be transferred to the ICU for monitoring for at least 24 hours. The maintenance dose of dantrolene should be 1 mg/kg every 4 to 6 hours for at least 24 hours or to maintain an infusion of dantrolene at 0.25 mg/kg/h for at least 24 hours. Dantrolene may be needed for more than 24 hours, if clinically indicated.

2. **C.** Rapid sequence induction is a technique used to secure the airway in patients who are at risk of aspiration of stomach contents. Rapid sequence induction is usually carried out with an induction agent and a fast-acting muscular relaxant, and intubation is attempted without mask ventilation to decrease aspiration risk. Since bag and mask ventilation is not attempted, the muscle relaxant used for rapid sequence intubation needs to be quick in onset, typically within a minute of administration. Succinylcholine and rocuronium are the only quick-onset muscle relaxants used in clinical practice. In normal muscle, succinylcholine-induced depolarization causes serum potassium to increase by approximately 0.5 mEq/L. After a major burn, upregulation of acetylcholine receptors occurs, and life-threatening hyperkalemia can result. Succinylcholine *should not* be used from 24 hours and up to at least 18 months after a burn injury.

   Rocuronium can be used for rapid sequence induction, and it can be reversed with sugammadex. In burn patients, a dose up to 1.2 mg/kg can be used for rapid sequence induction because of the upregulation of acetylcholine receptors leading to increased resistance to nondepolarizing muscle relaxants. Studies showed that dose escalation of rocuronium shortened the onset time, prolonged the duration of action, and improved intubating conditions in burned patients.

   On the contrary, cisatracurium and atracurium have slow onset of action and are not ideal neuromuscular blocking agents for rapid sequence intubation.

3. **C.** Propofol infusion syndrome is a rare syndrome that occurs in patients who are being treated with high doses and long durations of propofol infusion. It is thought that the syndrome may be caused by impaired mitochondrial fatty acid metabolism that can be precipitated by propofol. Risk factors include being maintained on a propofol infusion of

4 mg/kg/h for ≥48 hours, younger age, low carbo-hydrate intake, catecholamine infusion, corticos-teroids, and acute neurologic injury. The clinical features of propofol infusion syndrome include 1 or more of the following symptoms: metabolic acidosis, rhabdomyolysis, hyperlipidemia, hepatomegaly with hepatic steatosis, cardiac arrhythmias, and myocardial failure. Increasing serum lipid concentration is an early sign of propofol infusion syndrome. Cardiac failure is often a late sign.

4. **A.** Central venous access comes with multiple possible complications. Pneumothorax is a possible complication of central line placement, especially with subclavian vein catheterization. There is also a risk of bloodstream infections, thrombosis, hematoma, misplacement into the carotid artery or arterial puncture, and air embolism. Patients should be placed in Trendelenburg position before placement of a central line to minimize risk for air embolism. The thoracic duct empties into the left subclavian vein. Thus, left-sided internal jugular or subclavian venous cannulation carries an increased risk of damage to the thoracic duct, leading to lymphatic injury. Teichgraber and colleagues, in their case report, describe inadvertent penetration of the thoracic duct by the guidewire during left subclavian vein catheterization.

5. **D.** The difficult airway algorithm is a stepwise way of using different techniques during a difficult to intubate and difficult to ventilate situation. If anticipating a difficult airway situation, one should consider an awake intubation. If the patient has an unanticipated difficult airway after induction of anesthesia, the initial step would be to call for help. One can consider returning to spontaneous ventilation or awakening the patient if a long-acting muscle relaxant was not used. In this case, rocuronium was used, which prohibited both of the aforementioned options. If facemask ventilation is not adequate, attempt to insert an emergency noninvasive airway such as a supraglottic airway (SGA). Laryngeal mask airway (LMA) is a type of SGA device. If SGA is inadequate, then an emergency invasive airway should be established. If mask ventilation is successful, alternative approaches to intubation should be considered such as video-assisted laryngoscopy, a different laryngoscope blade, fiberoptic

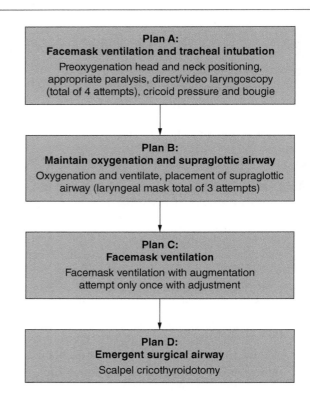

Plan A:
Facemask ventilation and tracheal intubation
Preoxygenation head and neck positioning, appropriate paralysis, direct/video laryngoscopy (total of 4 attempts), cricoid pressure and bougie

Plan B:
Maintain oxygenation and supraglottic airway
Oxygenation and ventilate, placement of supraglottic airway (laryngeal mask total of 3 attempts)

Plan C:
Facemask ventilation
Facemask ventilation with augmentation attempt only once with adjustment

Plan D:
Emergent surgical airway
Scalpel cricothyroidotomy

intubation, light wand, nasal intubation or other intubating devices.

6. **B.** The incidence of anaphylaxis in the perioperative setting is 1 in 1000 to 20,000 procedures. Although it is rare, it is an event that can lead to perioperative morbidity and mortality. The diagnosis is made initially with respiratory signs such as bronchospasm and increased peak airway pressures if the patient is intubated. Hypotension and cardiovascular collapse can occur as well. One should look for a rash on the body. The most common agents used in the perioperative setting that cause anaphylaxis include neuromuscular blockers, latex, and antibiotics. Hypnotics, opioids, chlorhexidine, local anesthetics, and protamine can be less commonly involved. Acute treatment of anaphylaxis includes removing the allergen (if possible), increasing oxygen to 100%, administering IV fluid boluses (may require many liters due to vasodilation), administering IV epinephrine in escalating doses every 2 minutes, giving H_1 and H_2 antagonists, administering corticosteroids, and treating bronchospasm. One can consider starting an epinephrine infusion. When the patient is stabilized, send a serum tryptase level and monitor for 24 hours.

7. **A.** Etomidate is one of the IV anesthetic agents that can be used in the induction of general anesthesia. Etomidate is a modulator at γ-aminobutyric acid A (GABA$_A$) receptors. It is a drug that is known for maintaining blood pressure, especially in a hemodynamically unstable patient or a patient with severe cardiovascular or cerebrovascular disease. Myocardial contractility and cardiac output are usually unchanged. One of the downsides of etomidate is the known suppression of the adrenal synthesis of cortisol. In a dose-dependent way, etomidate inhibits adrenal mitochondrial 11-β-hydroxylase, which converts 11-deoxycortisol to cortisol. Its use in patients with sepsis is controversial. Etomidate can also burn upon injection and cause myoclonic jerks. Etomidate does not cause thrombocytopenia. Tachycardia and hallucinations can be side effects of ketamine.

8. **B.** Ketamine is a medication that can be used both as an anesthetic and for pain control. Ketamine mainly binds to *N*-methyl-D-aspartate (NMDA) receptors and is a weak agonist of mu- and kappa-opioid receptors. Even though it is a direct myocardial depressant and also causes vascular smooth muscle dilatation, the drug also increases circulating catecholamines. Thus, it is often an agent used in the induction of anesthesia for patients with hemodynamic instability because ketamine could cause increased sympathetic activity such as increased blood pressure, heart rate, and cardiac output. However, in patients who have depleted catecholamine stores, ketamine will cause hypotension and decreased cardiac output due to its direct myocardial depressant properties. Ketamine is a good medication to use for both induction of anesthesia as well as pain control because it maintains respirations and laryngeal reflexes. It is a useful agent for maintaining spontaneous respiration, but the drug is also a stimulator of salivary secretions. Thus, the risk of aspiration is still present. Ketamine is also a powerful bronchodilator and can be used in patients with asthma.

9. **D.** For patients with intracranial hypertension, the most important goals are to maintain cerebral perfusion and oxygenation. Clinical signs including bradycardia, irregular respirations and hypertension with widening pulse pressure represent the **Cushing's triad** which is a physiological response to increase intracranial pressure. Measures to reduce intracranial pressure (ICP) include positioning the patient with the head up 30°, ensuring the head is inline to prevent jugular outflow obstruction, hyperventilating to decrease partial pressure of carbon dioxide to 30 to 35 mm Hg, and administering mannitol/hypertonic saline. Draining cerebrospinal fluid and decompressive craniectomy can also be performed. When choosing an anesthetic agent for induction, it is important to choose one that does not increase cerebral metabolic rate of oxygen. Propofol, etomidate, and barbiturates decrease cerebral blood flow and can be titrated according to the patient's hemodynamics and mental status. Ketamine has the potential to increase cerebral metabolic rate of oxygen and ICP; thus, it should be avoided in patients with intracranial hypertension.

10. **B.** Pneumothorax is a common complication of central line placement. The incidence of pneumothorax ranges from 1% to 6.6%. If unrecognized, a pneumothorax can progress to a tension pneumothorax. A tension pneumothorax is a buildup of air within the pleural space. It allows air to enter the lung but not to return. Positive-pressure ventilation can worsen the tension pneumothorax. A tension pneumothorax can be diagnosed by absent breath sounds, deviation of the trachea away from the side of the tension, and shift of the mediastinum.

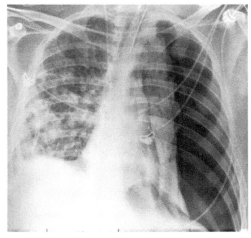

Anterior-posterior chest x-ray demonstrating a large left sided pneumothorax. There is increased lucency in the left hemithorax. Reproduced with permission from Salardini A, Biller J. *The Hospital Neurology Book*. New York, NY: McGraw-Hill, 2016.

Increasing hypoxia, tachypnea, tachycardia, hypotension, and increased peak airway pressures can occur. The treatment of tension pneumothorax is emergent needle thoracostomy prior to imaging. A large-bore needle is inserted into the second intercostal space in the mid-clavicular line for emergent decompression. A chest tube may be placed subsequently.

REFERENCES

Apfelbaum JL, Hagberg CA, Caplan RA, et al. Practice guidelines for management of the difficult airway: an updated report by the American Society of Anesthesiologists Task Force on Management of the Difficult Airway. *Anesthesiology*. 2013;118(2):251-270.

Bazin JE. Effects of anesthetic agents on intracranial pressure. *Ann Fr Anesth Reanim*. 1997;16(4):445-452.

Capacchione J, Larach M, Sambuughin N, Voelkel M, Muldoon S. Malignant hyperthermia. In: Longnecker DE, Brown DL, Newman MF, Zapol WM, eds. *Anesthesiology* (2nd ed). New York, NY: McGraw-Hill; 2012.

Dewachter P, Mouton-Faivre C, Emala CW. Anaphylaxis and anesthesia: controversies and new insights. *Anesthesiology*. 2009;111(5):1141-1150.

Harbin KR, Norris TE. Anesthetic management of patients with major burn injury. *AANA J*. 2012;80(6):430-439.

Kam PC, Cardone D. Propofol infusion syndrome. *Anaesthesia*. 2007;62(7):690-701.

Kornbau C, Lee KC, Hughes GD, Firstenberg MS. Central line complications. *Int J Crit Illn Inj Sci*. 2015;5(3):170-178.

Kurdi MS, Theerth KA, Deva RS. Ketamine: current applications in anesthesia, pain, and critical care. *Anesth Essays Res*. 2014;8(3):283-290.

Riazi S, Larach MG, Hu C, Wijeysundera D, Massey C, Kraeva N. Malignant hyperthermia in Canada: characteristics of index anesthetics in 129 malignant hyperthermia susceptible probands. *Anesth Analg*. 2014;118(2):381-387.

Teichgraber UK, Nibbe L, Gebauer B, Wagner HJ. Inadvertent puncture of the thoracic duct during attempted central venous catheter placement. *Cardiovasc Intervent Radiol*. 2003;26(6):569-571.

Thompson Bastin ML, Baker SN, Weant KA. Effects of etomidate on adrenal suppression: a review of intubated septic patients. *Hosp Pharm*. 2014;49(2):177-183.

Tsotsolis N, Tsirgogianni K, Kioumis I, et al. Pneumothorax as a complication of central venous catheter insertion. *Ann Transl Med*. 2015;3(3):40.

PART 5
Cardiac Critical Care

34

Cardiovascular Critical Care

James L. Gentry III, MD, Erich L. Kiehl, MD, Menhel Kinno, MD, MPH, Jay Patel, MD, Matthew R. Summers, MD, and Venu Menon, MD

Questions

1. A 60-year-old man with a history of rheumatic heart disease with a prior mechanical mitral valve replacement and a history of heparin-induced thrombocytopenia is admitted with transient ischemic attack. The patient's international normalized ratio (INR) on admission is 1.2 (goal, 2.5-3.5), and he undergoes a transesophageal echocardiogram, which reveals the presence of a small thrombus on his mechanical mitral valve. Given the patient's thrombus and subtherapeutic INR, anticoagulation is to be resumed. What medication should be used to systemically anticoagulate the patient?

   A. Enoxaparin
   B. Heparin
   C. Dabigatran
   D. Argatroban
   E. Warfarin

Questions 2 and 3

A 45-year-old woman with a history of multiple sclerosis (MS) with chronic right leg weakness and obesity is admitted MS flare. During her hospital admission, she develops acute-onset chest pain and shortness of breath. Her vitals are remarkable for a heart rate of 140 bpm, blood pressure of 84/50 mm Hg despite intravenous fluids, respiratory rate of 30 breaths/min, and oxygen saturation of 90% on 6 L via nasal cannula. Troponin T is 0.6 ng/mL (elevated), B-type natriuretic peptide (BNP) is 500 pg/mL (elevated), and electrocardiogram shows sinus tachycardia with a new right bundle branch block. A point-of-care echocardiography is obtained and shows right ventricle dilation, right ventricular systolic pressure of 45 mm Hg (normal <35 mm Hg), and akinesia of the mid-free wall with hypercontractility of the apex.

2. What is the most likely diagnosis?
   A. Severe pulmonary hypertension
   B. Anterior ST-segment elevation myocardial infarction
   C. Pericarditis
   D. Massive pulmonary embolism
   E. Stress-induced cardiomyopathy

3. The appropriate diagnosis is confirmed for this patient. What is the appropriate next step in management?

A. Alteplase followed by heparin infusion

B. Subcutaneous enoxaparin and alteplase

C. Rivaroxaban

D. Heparin bolus and infusion

E. Percutaneous balloon angioplasty and stent placement

4. A 40-year-old man with a history of Marfan syndrome presents with acute-onset sharp chest pain radiating to his back and transient slurred speech. The patient's heart rate is 130 bpm, and blood pressure is 84/50 mm Hg. A chest computed tomography (CT) scan reveals the presence of a dissection flap in the proximal ascending aorta extending into the aortic arch including the proximal left common carotid artery and a small pericardial effusion. A point-of-care transthoracic echocardiography was performed, confirming the above diagnosis including showing the presence of partial diastolic collapse of the right ventricle and dilated inferior vena cava. In addition to establishing central venous access and fluid resuscitation, what is the appropriate next step in management to reduce his risk of long-term mortality?

A. Intravenous sodium nitroprusside

B. Large-volume pericardiocentesis to drain the pericardial effusion

C. Cardiothoracic consult for emergent surgery

D. Intravenous heparin bolus and infusion

E. Intravenous metoprolol

5. A 65-year-old man with history of former tobacco abuse and hypertension presents with acute-onset tearing back pain. His vitals are remarkable for a heart rate of 95 bpm and a blood pressure of 200/110 mm Hg. CT with contrast of the chest reveals the presence of an aortic dissection originating distal to the origin of the left subclavian artery and extending distally to the left common iliac artery. The patient denies any abdominal pain, reports good urine output, and denies motor or sensory symptoms in his lower extremities. What is the appropriate next step in management?

A. Intravenous metoprolol

B. Intravenous sodium nitroprusside

C. Emergent coronary angiography followed by surgical repair

D. Intra-aortic balloon pump

E. Consultation to vascular surgery for emergent open or endovascular repair

6. A 19-year-old woman with no prior medical history is admitted with right-sided weakness and tingling. She underwent magnetic resonance imaging (MRI) of the brain and was diagnosed with a small acute left middle cerebral artery infarct. She has no allergies, and her only medication is an oral contraceptive. The workup for the etiology of her stroke was unremarkable including hypercoagulable workup, bilateral lower extremity Dopplers ultrasound negative for a deep vein thrombosis, and normal magnetic resonance angiogram of her neck. To further evaluate the etiology of her embolic stroke of unknown significance, she undergoes a transesophageal echocardiogram, which reveals the presence of a patent foramen ovale (PFO). What is the appropriate next step in management?

A. Undergo percutaneous closure of the PFO

B. Undergo open-heart surgery for closure of the PFO

C. Initiate aspirin and warfarin

D. Initiate aspirin only

E. Discontinue oral contraceptives and initiate aspirin

7. A 68-year-old woman with history of former tobacco abuse presents with substernal chest pain, dyspnea, and lightheadedness. The patient states the onset of her symptoms was 3 to 4 hours following her husband's funeral. Her electrocardiogram (ECG) shows inferior T-wave inversions. Cardiac biomarkers are mildly elevated with troponin T of 0.4 ng/mL (normal range <0.010-0.029 ng/mL), and creatine kinase (CK)-MB of 15.6 ng/mL (normal range 0-8.8 ng/mL). An echocardiogram is obtained, which reveals a left ventricular ejection fraction of 40% with akinesis of the apex. Which of the following is the best diagnostic test to confirm the diagnosis?

A. Stress echocardiogram

B. Cardiac stress positron emission tomography

C. Cardiac MRI

D. Coronary angiogram

E. No additional testing is indicated as this is takotsubo cardiomyopathy

8. A 29-year-old woman with a stable moderate-sized circumferential pericardial effusion is admitted with an intractable migraine associated with persistent nausea and vomiting. On admission, her blood pressure is 80/40 mm Hg, she has pulsus paradoxus of 10 mm Hg, jugular venous pressure is 4 cm H_2O, and she has muffled heart sounds. An ECG is obtained and shown below. What is the appropriate next step in management?

A. Synchronized cardioversion

B. Emergent pericardiocentesis

C. 1-L normal saline bolus

D. Amiodarone 150 mg intravenous bolus followed by an infusion

E. Obtain transthoracic echocardiogram

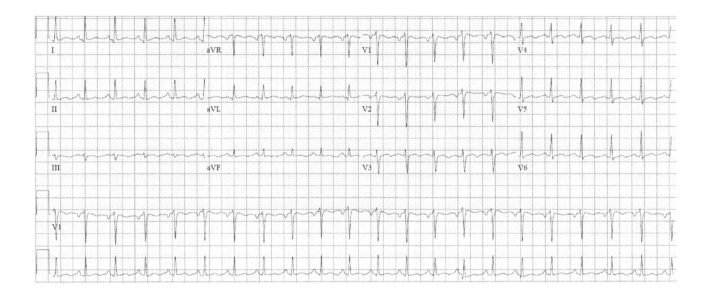

9. A patient with no past medical history is admitted with 24 hours of balance and coordination deficits and is found to have a cerebellar infarct on MRI. No identifiable cause for his stroke is identified after undergoing CT imaging of his brain and neck arteries, hypercoagulable workup, 48 hours of cardiac telemetry, and transthoracic echocardiogram. A cryptogenic stroke is presumed, but prior to establishing this diagnosis, the patient undergoes a transesophageal echocardiogram. Agitated saline is administered, as shown in the figure: panel A represents before and panel B represents 2 beats after opacification of the right atrium. What percentage of patients in the general population have this cardiac anomaly?

A. 10%

B. 25%

C. 40%

D. 55%

E. 70%

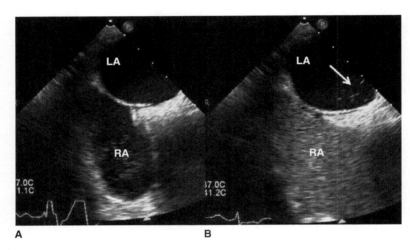

LA, left atrium; RA, right atrium.

10. A 78-year-old man is admitted with a right middle cerebral artery ischemic stroke. As part of his workup for the cause of his stroke, he has the following results: white blood cell count 9000/μL, hemoglobin 8.0 g/dL, platelets 250,000/μL, sodium 134 mmol/L, potassium 4.4 mmol/L, blood urea nitrogen 30 mg/dL, creatinine 2.0 mg/dL, glucose 96 mg/dL, calcium 12.0 mg/dL, low-density lipoprotein 116 mg/dL, triglycerides 143 mg/dL, and hemoglobin A1c 5.4%. His ECG (panel A) and transthoracic echocardiogram (panel B), a parasternal long axis view of the left ventricle in end-diastole showing increased thickness of the interventricular septum (IVSd) at 1.7 cm (normally <1.0 cm) and that of the posterior wall at 1.9 cm (normally <1.0 cm) are included below. What is the most likely diagnosis?

A. Cardiac amyloidosis

B. Primary pulmonary hypertension

C. Mitral stenosis

D. Cardiac sarcoidosis

E. Infective endocarditis

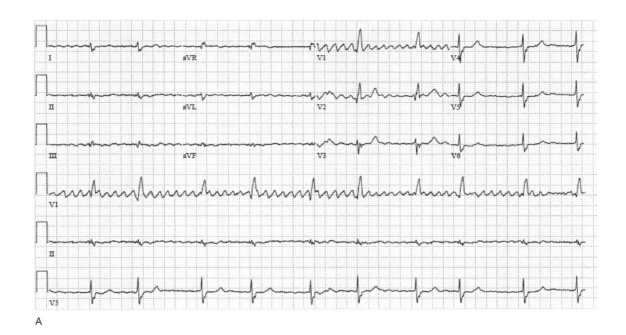

A

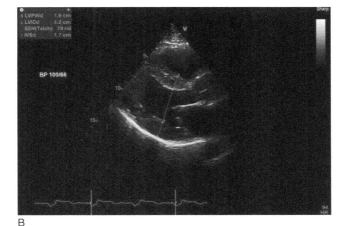

B

11. A 76-year-old man with history of a deep vein thrombosis on dabigatran (150 mg by mouth twice daily; last dose was taken 10 hour earlier) presents to the emergency department (ED) with a headache after a fall off a ladder that was associated with a brief episode of loss of consciousness. Upon presentation, his Glasgow Coma Scale score was 15, but on repeat evaluation, it has decreased to 12. A head CT scan is performed showing the presence of an acute left occipital subdural hematoma (maximum thickness of 10 mm). What is the appropriate next step in management?

   A. Supportive management
   B. Intravenous vitamin K, 10 mg injection
   C. Intravenous fresh frozen plasma, 1 unit
   D. Intravenous idarucizumab, 2 doses of 2.5 g given 15 minutes apart
   E. Andexanet alfa, 400 mg bolus over 15 minutes followed by 480-mg infusion over 2 hours

12. A 74-year-old man presents to the ED with progressive fatigue and dyspnea. His past medical history is significant for nonobstructive coronary artery disease (based on a cardiac catheterization 5 years ago), diabetes mellitus, and chronic obstructive pulmonary disease with active tobacco abuse. The below ECG is obtained in triage. Available notes state all prior ECGs were "normal." You are now seeing the patient. Which of the following is the best next step in management?

   A. CT pulmonary angiogram
   B. Observation
   C. Chest x-ray
   D. Emergent cardiac catheterization
   E. None of the above

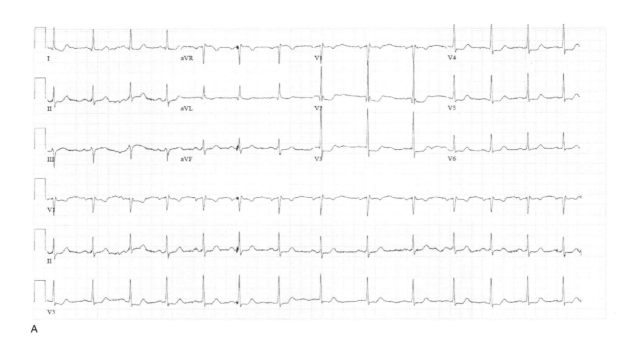

A

13. An 85-year-old woman presents to her local ED shortly after suffering a syncopal episode that occurred while walking with her walker. On history, she endorses increasing fatigue with exertion for the past several months. She denies any other prodrome preceding her syncopal episode. Her physical exam is significant for a pulse of 65 bpm, blood pressure of 100/60 mm Hg with negative orthostatics, mid-peaking 2/6 systolic murmur heard best over the right sternal border, no noticeable trauma, and a completely nonfocal neurologic exam. Her only medical history is hypertension and hyperlipidemia, for which she takes lisinopril and pravastatin. Intake ECG is shown below. For which of the following disease states do you have the highest clinical suspicion?

A. Dehydration

B. Intracranial hemorrhage

C. Coronary artery disease

D. Bradyarrhythmia

E. Aortic stenosis

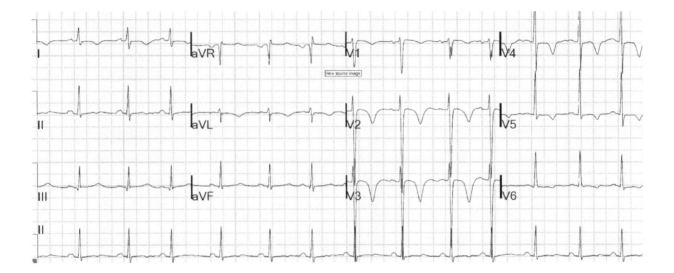

14. An 18-year-old male college freshman with no past medical history is admitted to the neuro-intensive care unit (ICU) for continuous electroencephalogram monitoring following repeated syncopal episodes associated with loss of bladder function and tongue biting. Following a 24-hour observation period, no concerning epileptiform discharges are noted. However, the patient is noted to have multiple pre-syncopal episodes that correspond to an irregularly irregular narrow-complex tachycardia.

The patient's baseline ECG is shown below. What is the most appropriate next step in management?

A. Anticoagulation

B. Cardioversion

C. Initiation of β-blocker

D. Further prolonged electroencephalogram monitoring

E. Catheter ablation

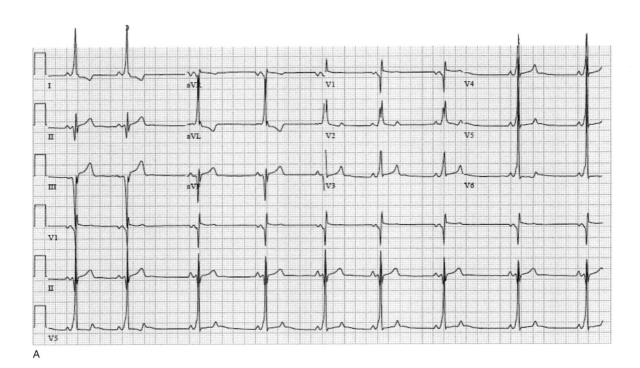

A

15. A 55-year-old man admitted to the neurology service with focal neurologic changes in the setting of hypertension to > 200 mm Hg systolic and admitted cocaine use is now back to his prior baseline several days into his hospitalization. Without warning, he develops chest pain, and an electrocardiogram is obtained (shown below). Which of the following available medications is most likely to safely resolve the patient's symptoms most rapidly?

A. Intravenous metoprolol

B. Adenosine

C. Intravenous amiodarone

D. Digoxin

E. Intravenous lorazepam

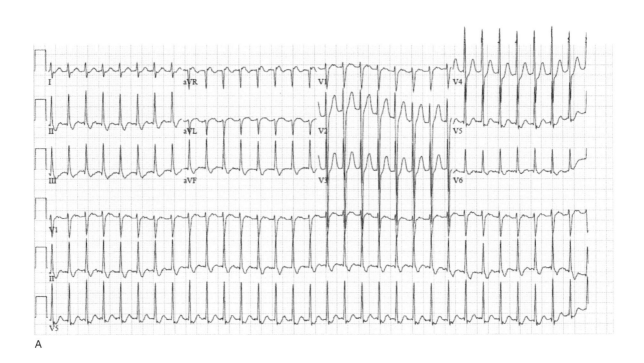

A

16. A 55-year-old woman with a past medical history of coronary artery bypass grafting arrives in your ED following resuscitated out-of-hospital cardiac arrest. The arrest was witnessed with bystander cardiopulmonary resuscitation provided and total time to return of spontaneous circulation (ROSC) estimated between 15 and 20 minutes. Per the emergency medical services report, there was never a shockable rhythm. The patient's initial arterial blood gas reveals a pH of 7.02 and a lactic acid of 12 mmol/L. Neurologic exam reveals reactive pupils and present gag reflex but no clear purposeful movement. As the on-call intensivist, per the most recent consensus guidelines, what is the most appropriate next step in management?

A. Immediate coronary angiography

B. Withdrawal of care given acidemia and prolonged anoxic time

C. External hypothermia with a target temperature of 34°C to 36°C

D. Intravascular hypothermia with a target temperature of 32°C to 34°C

E. Either C or D

17. You are alerted by a nurse that her patient, who is currently receiving therapeutic hypothermia following an in-hospital cardiac arrest, is experiencing significant ST elevation on telemetry, confirmed by an ECG (shown below). She has marked the leads that concern her. What is the next best step in management?

A. No additional intervention
B. Immediate cardiac catheterization
C. Pharmacologic treatment for hyperkalemia
D. Discontinue hypothermia
E. Pacemaker placement

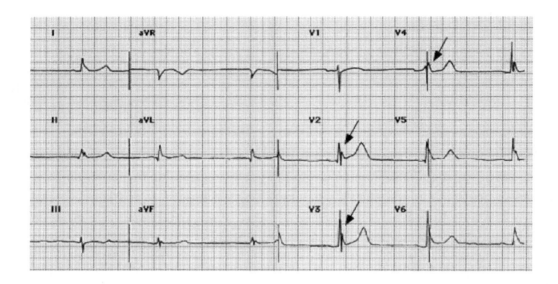

18. A 44-year-old woman is admitted to the neurology service with an exacerbation of her relapsing-remitting multiple sclerosis. In the setting of high-dose steroid administration, she has developed gastritis, which has caused profound nausea. To combat this, she has been receiving scheduled ondansetron injections every 4 hours for the past few days. The rapid response team is activated on this patient in response to concerning telemetry changes, and the following ECG is obtained (shown below). While in this rhythm, she is conscious but somnolent, and blood pressure is 80 mm Hg systolic. She is subsequently cardioverted back to normal sinus rhythm. Postcardioversion ECG reveals a heart rate of 55 bpm and a QTc interval of 515 milliseconds. Other than her multiple sclerosis medications, her only other medication is metoprolol for high blood pressure. Which of the following is an appropriate next treatment?

A. Intravenous magnesium

B. Discontinuation of β-blockade

C. Temporary pacing

D. Isoproterenol

E. All of the above

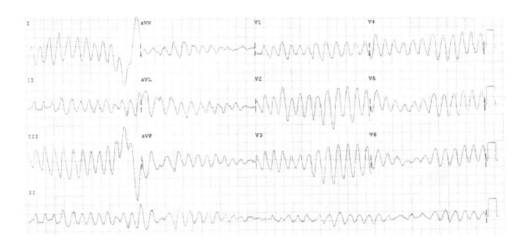

19. A 66-year-old man is admitted to the neurology ICU after a large right middle cerebral artery stroke. Poststroke workup includes both carotid ultrasound and magnetic resonance angiography without evidence of significant carotid atherosclerosis, a transesophageal echocardiogram with no evidence of thrombus or shunt, and 72 hours of telemetry monitoring revealing only scattered premature atrial and ventricular contractions. He is eventually discharged to an acute rehab facility with a diagnosis of cryptogenic stroke. Which of the following is most likely to identify the etiology of the patient's stroke?

A. 30-day patient-triggered wearable event monitor

B. Multiweek wearable continuous patch monitor

C. 48-hour Holter monitor on discharge

D. Implantable loop recorder

E. None of the above

20. A 77-year-old man with past medical history of systolic heart failure with biventricular dysfunction (left ventricular ejection fraction 20%) and atrial arrhythmias compliant with apixaban presents to the ED with worsening shortness of breath and palpitations starting 12 hours ago. The patient reports a clear timing of symptom onset. The patient's heart rate is 80 bpm with frequent spikes to 105 bpm, blood pressure is 105 mm Hg systolic (which he states is a little low for him), and he is hypoxic to 87%, corrected on 2 L via nasal cannula. On exam, the patient has elevated jugular venous pressure, bibasilar crackles, increased abdominal distention, and 2+ bilateral pitting edema to the mid-shin. The following ECG is obtained (shown below). Which of the below interventions will worsen the patient's decompensated heart failure?

A. Direct current cardioversion

B. Intravenous diltiazem

C. Intravenous diuresis

D. Oral amiodarone loading

E. Digoxin loading

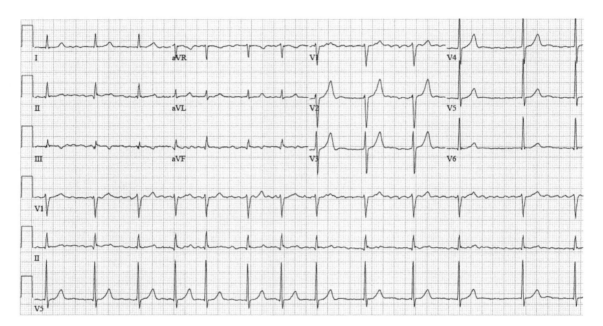

21. A 34-year-old woman with a past medical history of epilepsy is admitted to the epilepsy monitoring unit for loading with a new antiepileptic drug. At this point, she becomes unresponsive, and the rapid response team is activated. On arrival to the bedside, the patient is having convulsions. A telemetry strip (shown below) is obtained. What is the next best management strategy?

A. Synchronized cardioversion

B. Intravenous adenosine

C. Intravenous amiodarone

D. Defibrillation

E. None of the above

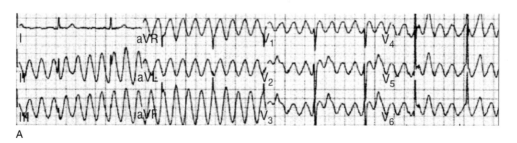

A

22. An 85-year-old man with a past medical history of coronary artery disease with multiple past bypasses and stents, as well as an implantable defibrillator, is admitted to the neurology floor following a transient ischemic accident. The patient presses his nursing call button to report acute-onset chest pain. The following ECG is obtained (see below). Vitals obtained by the bedside nurse reveal a blood pressure of 85 mm Hg systolic. The patient reports feeling slightly lightheaded but is able to follow commands and answer appropriately to questions. Which of the following is (are) the appropriate next step(s)?

A. Adenosine

B. Synchronized cardioversion

C. Antitachycardia pacing

D. Defibrillation

E. Both B and C

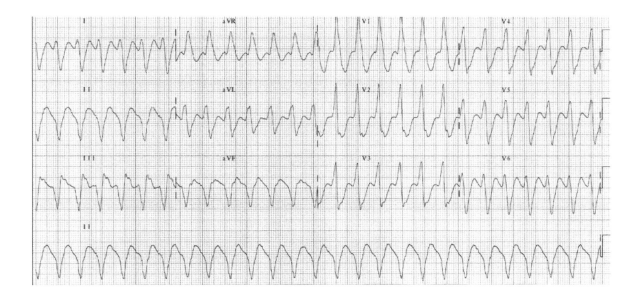

23. A 78-year-old woman is admitted to the neurology ICU following a transient ischemic attack. Since admission, she has been newly diagnosed with atrial fibrillation, felt to be the trigger for her ischemic event. For her atrial fibrillation, warfarin has been initiated as well as metoprolol with subsequent dose up-titration for rate control. You are called by the patient's nurse due to recurrent episodes of transient lightheadedness but no frank syncope. A representative telemetry strip from 1 of the symptomatic episodes is shown below. What is the most likely cause of the patient's symptoms?

A. Sinus node dysfunction

B. Atrioventricular (AV) node dysfunction

C. Infra-Hisian block

D. β-Blocker overdose

E. Intracranial pathology

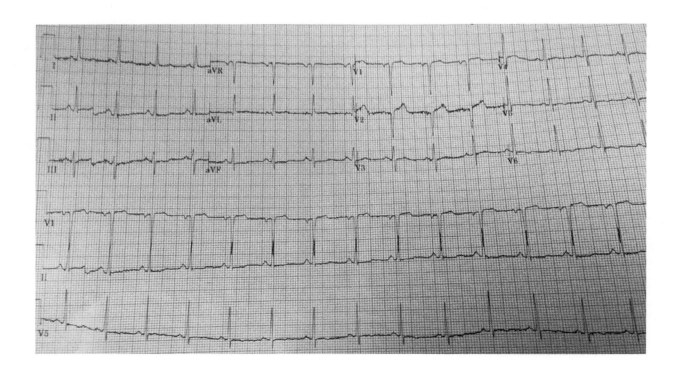

Questions 24 and 25

A 64-year-old right-handed man with ischemic cardiomyopathy (left ventricular ejection fraction of 35%), status post an implantable cardioverter-defibrillator, endovascular aortic aneurysm repair, hypertension, atrial fibrillation on dabigatran, remote stroke, and normal-pressure hydrocephalus with ventriculoperitoneal (VP) shunt presented with new-onset seizure and fall witnessed by emergency medical services. Head CT was performed on arrival and revealed bilateral acute-on-chronic subdural hematomas with mild mass effect. Intravenous loading with levetiracetam was initiated, and anticoagulation was reversed. The patient was intubated for respiratory distress, and a chest CT was obtained (see figures below). On hospital day 2, he developed a fever to 40.3°C, and blood cultures grew methicillin-sensitive *Staphylococcus aureus* in 4 bottles.

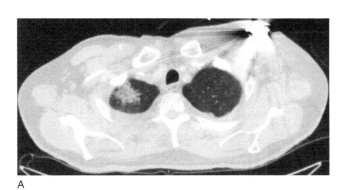

A

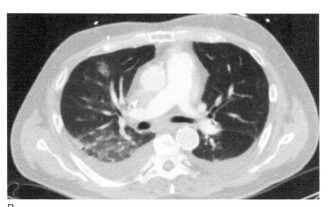

B

24. Which of the following is the next best step in management of this patient?

A. CT of the abdomen and pelvis

B. Bedside electroencephalogram monitoring

C. Transthoracic echocardiogram

D. Transesophageal echocardiogram

E. VP shunt study

25. Findings from the transesophageal echocardiogram are shown below and reveal an independently mobile mass adherent to the pacemaker lead. What is the next best step in management?

A. Intravenous vancomycin alone

B. Intravenous nafcillin alone

C. Oral nafcillin alone

D. Intrashunt nafcillin alone

E. Intravenous nafcillin followed by extraction of intracardiac leads and generator

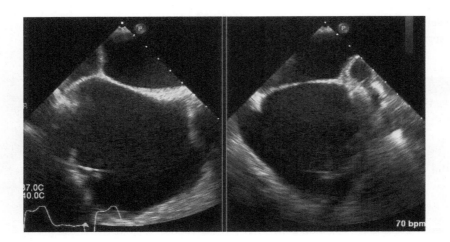

26. A 45-year-old woman with history of hypertension presents to the ED with substernal chest pain that began shortly after a heated argument with her husband. The initial ECG tracing is shown below. Coronary angiogram from 1 year ago was normal. Vital signs reveal a heart rate of 115 bpm, blood pressure of 80/55 mm Hg, respirations of 16 breaths/min, and oxygen saturation of 98%. Her exam reveals a systolic murmur heard best over the right sternal border that worsens with Valsalva maneuver. Lungs are clear to auscultation. Jugular venous pressure is 2 cm H_2O. Laboratory studies reveal a serum creatinine of 2.2 mg/d and troponin T of 1.2 ng/dL (normal 0-0.029 ng/mL). Left heart catheterization was performed showing normal coronary arteries, and the ventriculogram is shown below. Transthoracic echocardiogram shows left ventricular outflow tract obstruction with a peak gradient of 70 mm Hg. What is the next best step in management?

A. Norepinephrine infusion

B. Intra-aortic balloon pump

C. Phenylephrine infusion

D. Intravenous saline

E. Dobutamine infusion

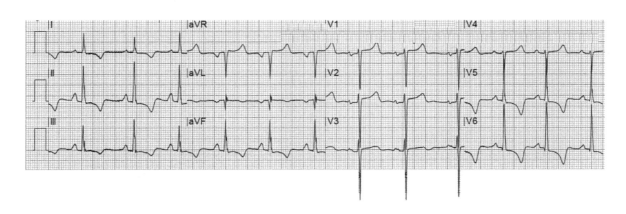

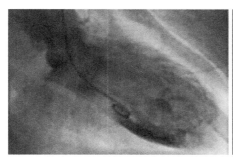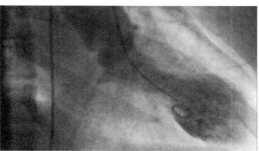

27. A 52-year-old man who is admitted to the general neurology floor receives intravenous penicillin for a urinary tract infection. Thirty minutes after his first dose, he develops marked stridor and a diffuse rash. His blood pressure is 70/43 mm Hg with a heart rate of 115 bpm and associated lightheadedness. Intravenous saline bolus is administered. What is the next best step in management?

    A. Vasopressin intravenously at 0.03 U/min

    B. Norepinephrine intravenously at 5 µg/kg/min

    C. Epinephrine 1:1000 intramuscularly at 0.5 mg

    D. Epinephrine 1:1000 intravenously at 1 mg

    E. Epinephrine 1:10,000 intravenously at 0.05 mg

28. A 45-year-old man with hypertrophic cardiomyopathy was admitted to the general neurology floor for intermittent episodes of lightheadedness and near syncope. He had been working intensely on his farm on a hot summer day. On admission, his blood pressure was 95/63 mm Hg and heart rate was 110 bpm. Metoprolol was held given borderline systemic blood pressures, and intravenous fluids were administered at a rate of 75 mL/h. Twelve hours later, the patient develops marked lethargy,

and vitals reveal a blood pressure of 70/50 mm Hg. What is the next best step?

    A. Initiate dobutamine infusion

    B. Initiate epinephrine infusion

    C. Initiate phenylephrine infusion

    D. Initiate intra-aortic balloon counterpulsation

    E. Initiate norepinephrine infusion

29. A 75-year-old man with nonischemic cardiomyopathy, permanent pacemaker for complete heart block, and chronic renal failure presents with lethargy and hypotension. Exam discloses rales in both lung fields, elevated jugular venous pressure, an S_3 on cardiac auscultation, abdominal distension, and lower extremity edema. His vitals show a blood pressure of 86/53 mm Hg and pulse of 60 bpm. His extremities are cool to the touch. What is the next best step in management?

    A. Initiate norepinephrine infusion

    B. Obtain an echocardiogram

    C. Increase the lower rate limit on the pacemaker

    D. Place a Swan-Ganz catheter

    E. Administer intravenous fluid bolus

30. A 93-year-old left-handed woman is admitted to the ICU after experiencing an acute ischemic stroke. Her vitals show a heart rate of 43 bpm and blood pressure of 184/98 mm Hg. She has no light-headedness or any other symptoms. Her laboratory exam is normal. An ECG is obtained and shown below. What is the next best step in management?

A. Administer atropine
B. Administer epinephrine
C. Administer dopamine
D. Initiate temporary transvenous pacing
E. Place transcutaneous pads and manage conservatively

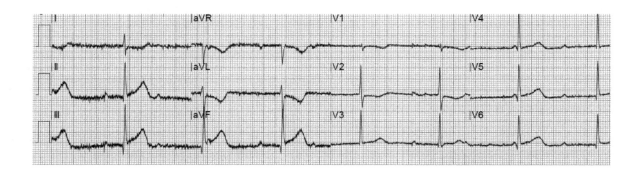

31. You are performing advanced cardiac life support on an 83-year-old man who was found to be pulseless. Chest compressions were initiated immediately upon arrival, and a rhythm check identified ventricular fibrillation. You have delivered one 200-J shock and notice that the patient is now in normal sinus rhythm on the defibrillator monitor. What is the next best step in management?

A. Immediately perform a pulse check
B. Perform a neurologic evaluation
C. Obtain a 12-lead ECG looking for any ST-segment elevations
D. Immediately resume chest compressions
E. Immediately check for a blood pressure

Questions 32 and 33

A 32-year-old man collapses at the grocery store and is unconscious. You witness the collapse and immediately arrive at his side to assist. You notice that he is pulseless and without spontaneous respirations. You initiate chest compressions after alerting bystanders to retrieve the automated external defibrillator (AED) and call 911. One minute later, the AED arrives at your side.

32. What is the next best course of action?

   A. Immediately use the AED

   B. Continue compressions for a total of 5 minutes prior to using the AED

   C. Continue compressions for a total of 2 minutes prior to using the AED

   D. Give 2 breaths first, then use the AED

   E. Finish 1 cycle of compressions and breaths before using the AED

33. After using the AED on the patient, you resume chest compressions. What is the correct compression-to-ventilation ratio for this patient without an advanced airway?

   A. 15:1

   B. 15:2

   C. 30:1

   D. 30:2

   E. 45:1

34. A 54-year-old man with known nonischemic cardiomyopathy with a prior left ventricular ejection fraction of 25% presents to the ED with altered mental status and confusion. On arrival, he is hypotensive with a blood pressure of 84/52 mm Hg and has sinus tachycardia with 125 bpm. He has a temperature of 38.4°C, a respiratory rate of 22 breaths/min, and oxygen saturation of 95% on room air. On examination, he is somnolent and oriented to person but not to place on time. Examination otherwise reveals faint bibasilar crackles, an S_3 gallop with a grade 2 out of 6 holosystolic murmur at the cardiac apex, and warm extremities. Jugular venous distension is not noted. Laboratory examination reveals a white blood cell count of 14×10^9/L with a neutrophilic predominance, a creatinine of 1.6 mg/dL, bicarbonate of 14 mg/dL, and lactate of 4.2 mg/dL. On review with the patient's wife, she noted that he was recently discharged from an outside hospital for decompensated heart failure and received intravenous diuretics. In the ED, he is given 250 mL of intravenous normal saline with only slight improvement in his blood pressure and is thus started on intravenous norepinephrine infusion at 5 µg/kg/min and admitted to the ICU. On arrival, he has a blood pressure of 95/54 mm Hg (mean arterial pressure [MAP] of 68 mm Hg) and has sinus tachycardia to 130 bpm. A pulmonary artery catheter (Swan-Ganz catheter) is placed and reveals the following hemodynamics:

- Right atrium: 4 mm Hg (mean)
- Right ventricle: 45/5 mm Hg
- Pulmonary artery: 45/14 mm Hg (mean: 25 mm Hg)
- Pulmonary capillary occlusion pressure: 8 mm Hg
- Mixed venous oxygen saturation: 69%
- Cardiac index (by Fick method): 2.8 L/min/m^2
- Systemic vascular resistance: 985 dynes·s·cm^{-5}

Based on these values, what is the next appropriate step in management?

A. Continue vasopressor support as needed to maintain MAP >65 mm Hg

B. Start volume resuscitation with intravenous normal saline

C. Start intravenous dobutamine at 5 µg/kg/min given cardiogenic shock

D. Correct tachycardia with intravenous metoprolol

E. Contact cardiology for placement of a mechanical support device

35. A 62-year-old man presented to the ED with confusion after being evaluated by a home health nurse. He had a recent complicated hospitalization 3 months prior wherein he suffered an acute ST-segment elevation myocardial infarction and received a drug-eluting stent to his proximal left anterior descending artery. During his stay, he required an intra-aortic balloon pump but was able to be titrated onto oral medications. His postinfarct echocardiogram revealed a left ventricular ejection fraction of 30%. On arrival to the ED, he was confused, with a blood pressure of 105/58 mm Hg, a heart rate of 110 bpm, and ECG demonstrating sinus tachycardia with anterior Q waves but no ischemic ST changes. He was afebrile with a respiratory rate of 28 breaths/min and oxygen saturation of 92% on room air. Further examination revealed bibasilar crackles with jugular venous distension and cool extremities. Laboratory examination was notable for a white blood cell count of 12×10^9/L with a creatinine of 1.8 mg/dL, elevated transaminases, and a lactate of 5.0 mg/dL. Chest x-ray showed bilateral pulmonary edema. He was admitted to the ICU.

A pulmonary artery catheter (Swan-Ganz catheter) was placed and revealed the following hemodynamics:

- Right atrium: 16 mm Hg (mean)
- Right ventricle: 45/16 mm Hg
- Pulmonary artery: 45/32 mm Hg (mean: 36 mm Hg)
- Pulmonary capillary occlusion pressure: 28 mm Hg
- Mixed venous oxygen saturation: 45%
- Hemoglobin: 12 g/dL

Based on these values, what is the next appropriate step in management?

A. Volume resuscitation with intravenous normal saline

B. Intravenous dobutamine at 5 µg/kg/min

C. Intravenous furosemide infusion

D. Intravenous sodium nitroprusside or nitroglycerine

E. Activation of the cardiac catheterization lab for emergent coronary angiogram and placement of an intra-aortic balloon pump

36. A 60-year-old man presents to the ED with somnolence and confusion. He has a history of atrial fibrillation (on antiarrhythmic therapy with amiodarone) and sick sinus syndrome (status post a dual-chamber permanent pacemaker) in addition to long-standing, nonischemic cardiomyopathy with an ejection fraction of 40%. On arrival to the EDD, he was confused, with a blood pressure of 85/50 mm Hg, a heart rate of 65 bpm, and an ECG demonstrating sinus rhythm without pacing. He had a temperature of 38.3°C with a respiratory rate of 27 breaths/min and oxygen saturation of 92% on room air. Further examination reveals right lower lobe rhonchi and egophony. There is mild jugular venous distension, and extremities are warm. Laboratory examination is notable for a white blood cell count of 18×10^9/L with a creatinine of 1.4 mg/dL, elevated transaminases, and a lactate of 3.0 mg/dL. Chest x-ray shows a right lower lobe opacity. He is given 2 separate 500-mL intravenous fluid boluses with improvement in his blood pressure to 94/54 mm Hg and is thereafter admitted to the ICU. Shortly after arrival, his mean arterial pressures drop again and are intermittently below 65 mm Hg. Heart rate is 61 bpm (sinus). Another 500-mL intravenous fluid bolus is given, and a Swan-Ganz catheter is placed demonstrating the following:

- Right atrium: 11 mm Hg (mean)
- Right ventricle: 35/11 mm Hg
- Pulmonary artery: 35/18 mm Hg (mean: 23 mm Hg)
- Pulmonary capillary occlusion pressure: 14 mm Hg
- Mixed venous oxygen saturation: 58%
- Hematocrit: 31%

Based on these values, what is the next appropriate step in management?

A. Start an intravenous norepinephrine infusion at 5 µg/kg/min

B. Start intravenous dobutamine infusion at 5 µg/kg/min

C. Give additional intravenous fluid resuscitation

D. Start intravenous sodium nitroprusside or nitroglycerine

E. Increase the backup atrial pacing rate to 90 bpm

37. A 42-year-old woman with a history of peripartum cardiomyopathy and a known left ventricular ejection fraction of 25% presents to the ED after an internal defibrillator shock. She is status post primary prevention internal cardiac defibrillator placement with subsequent upgrade to a biventricular device. Interrogation of the device is concerning for multiple ventricular tachycardia (VT) episodes (at 200 bpm) with failed antitachycardia pacing and subsequent delivered shocks. She reports nonadherence with her heart failure medications over the 2 preceding weeks. On presentation, she has a blood pressure of 96/52 mm Hg with a heart rate of 105 bpm. She is afebrile with a normal respiratory rate and oxygen saturation on room air. On exam, she is lethargic with cool extremities and has faint bibasilar crackles and an elevated jugular venous pressure. Laboratory exam is notable for normal electrolytes but acute kidney injury (creatinine 1.5 mg/dL from a previous normal value) and mild elevation in transaminases. She has a lactate of 3.2 mg/dL. Chest x-ray reveals mild pulmonary edema. Her ECG on arrival shows a biventricular paced rhythm. While awaiting transfer to the ICU, she again has multiple episodes of apparent monomorphic VT with multiple subsequent shocks and 1 episode of degeneration into ventricular fibrillation with a failed defibrillation. Cardiopulmonary resuscitation is initiated, and she is bolused with intravenous amiodarone and intubated. A subsequent defibrillation is successful, but the patient continues to have sustained episodes of VT that are poorly tolerated. Intravenous procainamide is initiated, and the patient is sedated and paralyzed with improvement in the frequency of VT, but not cessation. A Swan-Ganz catheter is placed and reveals a cardiac index of 1.2 L/min/m². What is the next appropriate step in management?

A. Emergent ventricular tachycardia ablation

B. Intravenous metoprolol

C. Emergent referral for cardiac transplantation

D. Intra-aortic balloon counterpulsation

E. Start intravenous dobutamine infusion at 2.5 μg/kg/min

38. A 69-year-old man presents to the ED with acute chest discomfort. His ECG shows anterolateral ST-segment elevations. He is taken emergently for primary percutaneous coronary intervention and successfully receives a drug-eluting stent to the proximal left anterior descending artery. Despite complete revascularization, the patient remains hypotensive at 92/55 mm Hg with a heart rate of 95 bpm and frequent runs of nonsustained ventricular tachycardia. A pulmonary artery catheter is placed and demonstrates the following:

- Right atrium: 15 mm Hg (mean)
- Right ventricle: 52/15 mm Hg
- Pulmonary artery: 55/30 mm Hg (mean: 38 mm Hg)
- Pulmonary capillary occlusion pressure: 28 mm Hg
- Mixed venous oxygen saturation: 51%
- Cardiac index (by Fick method): 1.7 L/min/m²

What is the next appropriate step in management?

A. Intravenous fluid resuscitation

B. Intravenous dobutamine at 5 μg/kg/min

C. Intravenous norepinephrine at 5 μg/kg/min

D. Mechanical circulatory support

E. Consideration for heart transplantation

39. A 60-year-old man presents to the ED with acute chest discomfort. An ECG is obtained and is shown below.

The patient is given aspirin 81 mg by mouth, ticagrelor 180 mg by mouth, and 1 inch of transdermal nitroglycerine and is taken emergently to the cardiac catheterization lab where coronary angiography demonstrates a total occlusion of the proximal right coronary artery. While preparing for coronary intervention, the patient becomes hypotensive (70/45 mm Hg) and bradycardic (40 bpm) with AV block. Intravenous fluids and a temporary transvenous active-fixation ventricular pacemaker is placed at the same time as successful placement of a proximal right coronary artery drug-eluting stent. The patient stabilizes and is transferred to the cardiac ICU. At the end of the procedure, the patient is only intermittently pacing at a backup rate of 50 bpm and is normotensive. Shortly after transfer to the ICU, the patient again becomes hypotensive to 78/54 mm Hg with consistent ventricular pacing at 50 bpm. A 12-lead ECG obtained with pacing temporarily suspended shows no new ST elevations and complete heart block. Bedside echocardiogram demonstrates severe reduction in right ventricular

systolic function and absence of a pericardial effusion. Intravenous fluids are given, and a pulmonary artery catheter is placed demonstrating the following:

- Right atrium: 20 mm Hg (mean)
- Right ventricle: 42/20 mm Hg
- Pulmonary artery: 42/26 mm Hg (mean: 32 mm Hg)
- Pulmonary capillary occlusion pressure: 12 mm Hg
- Mixed venous oxygen saturation: 51%

Based on these values, what is the next appropriate step in management?

A. Increase the backup temporary pacemaker rate

B. Start intravenous dobutamine at 5 μg/kg/min

C. Insert an atrial pacemaker wire and set AV pace at a rate of 90 bpm

D. Give additional intravenous fluid resuscitation

E. Reactivate the cardiac catheterization laboratory for emergent coronary angiogram and place a percutaneous mechanical support

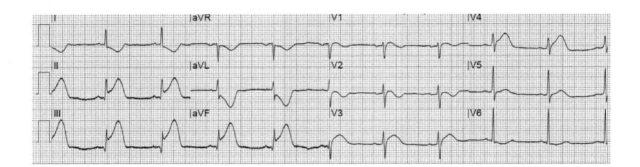

40. Which of the following scenarios warrants consideration for intra-aortic balloon counterpulsation?

A. A 45-year-old man in cardiogenic shock who is status post aortobifemoral bypass grafts

B. A 62-year-old man with refractory ventricular tachycardia and severe aortic insufficiency

C. A 55-year-old woman with fulminant myocarditis with cardiogenic shock and disseminated intravascular coagulation with severe anemia and platelets of 10,000/μL

D. A 79-year-old man with cardiogenic shock with workup revealing a large abdominal aortic intramural hematoma

E. An 82-year-old woman with delayed presentation of acute myocardial infarction found to have acute mitral regurgitation from papillary muscle rupture with leukocytosis to 22,000/μL, temperature of 38.5°C, and concern for aspiration pneumonia

41. A 39-year-old woman with progressive dyspnea presents to the ED and is found to have fulminant pulmonary edema by exam that is confirmed by chest x-ray. She is normotensive but has sinus tachycardia (110 bpm) with a respiratory rate of 32 breaths/min and an oxygen saturation of 84% on room air. Labs demonstrate an elevated NT-pro-BNP but normal creatinine and other end-organ function. She is given a bolus of intravenous furosemide for presumed acute decompensated heart failure. She is placed on 100% FiO_2 but has refractory hypoxemia with oxygen saturation of 86% and subsequent arterial partial pressure of oxygen of 62 mm Hg. She develops progressive tachypnea and then becomes anxious and altered and is intubated in the ED for refractory hypoxemia and perceived inability to cooperate with noninvasive positive-pressure ventilation. After stabilization in the ICU, she is found to have a left ventricular ejection fraction of 15% with concern for viral myocarditis given a preceding viral prodrome by collateral history. A right heart catheterization demonstrates elevated filling pressures but preserved cardiac indices. She is maintained on pressure-assisted ventilation with a positive end-expiratory pressure of 10 mm Hg. Although her hypoxemia improves over the next day with intravenous diuresis, her hemodynamics decline with low cardiac indices despite appropriate pulmonary catheter–tailored therapy. What is the next appropriate step in management?

A. Emergent cardiac transplantation

B. Decrease positive end-expiratory pressure

C. Decrease FiO_2

D. Mechanical circulatory support

E. Emergent right ventricular endomyocardial biopsy

42. A 52-year-old woman with long-standing hypertension presents to the ED with acute dyspnea. On arrival, she has a blood pressure of 224/120 mm Hg and a heart rate of 110 bpm. Chest examination reveals bilateral rales. There are no focal neurologic deficits, and she has no chest or back pain. Laboratory examination reveals a creatinine of 1.4 mg/dL but is otherwise unremarkable. While awaiting treatment, she reports severe midscapular back pain. Chest CT with contrast is obtained and is shown below. What is the next appropriate step in management?

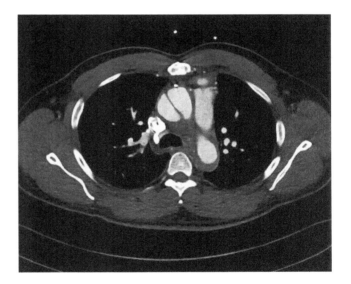

A. Intravenous sodium nitroprusside with goal of reducing blood pressure by 20% within the first hour

B. Oral captopril with goal of reducing blood pressure over next several hours

C. Intravenous furosemide

D. Mechanical circulatory support

E. Intravenous metoprolol followed by intravenous nitroprusside with the goal of rapidly lowering heart rate and systolic blood pressure to between 100 and 120 mm Hg

43. A 61-year-old woman presents to the ED for evaluation after a syncopal event. Her medical history includes hypertension, dyslipidemia, type 2 diabetes mellitus, and epilepsy for which she was previously managed with antiepileptic drugs. For the past few years, she has been observed off antiepileptic therapy. She notably had gastroenteritis the day prior to presentation and was taking ondansetron and promethazine concurrently for symptom relief.

Her family reports the current episode occurred at rest, while seated, and was not associated with tonic-clonic movement, tongue biting, or postictal state. Her initial vital signs are unrevealing, as is the initial workup including blood counts, chemistries, and CT of the brain. Initial ECG is shown below (panel A).

A historical ECG for comparison is also available (panel B).

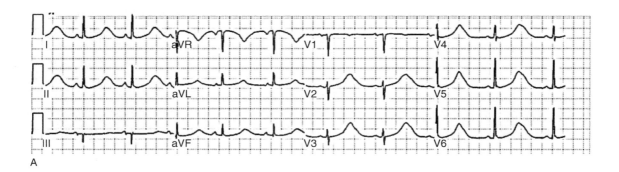

A

Levetiracetam is administered given the concern for a seizure. Her heart rhythm suddenly converts to the following rhythm (panel C).

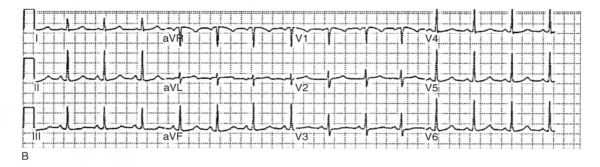

B

What is the next best step in management?

A. Defibrillation, regardless of the blood pressure
B. Intravenous amiodarone bolus and infusion
C. Intravenous magnesium sulfate injection
D. Intravenous metoprolol tartrate injection
E. Careful observation

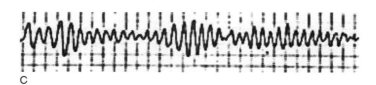

C

44. A 50-year-old man presents to the ED with a "racing heart" and mild dyspnea with exertion. His medical history includes hypertension and hyperlipidemia, for which he takes amlodipine and simvastatin, and he is a former 30-pack-year cigarette smoker. His symptoms began a "few" days ago when he noted early fatigue and shortness of breath during his usual evening walk.

He is well appearing on exam, with an irregular pulse at 115 bpm. His blood pressure is 134/72 mm Hg, respiratory rate is 16 breaths/min, and oxygen saturation is 99% on room air. An ECG demonstrates atrial fibrillation (AF) with rapid ventricular response.

He is given intravenous metoprolol, which slows his heart rate. One hour later, he is noted to be in sinus rhythm with a heart rate of 70 bpm. What is the most appropriate action regarding AF management moving forward?

A. Perform transesophageal echocardiogram and begin anticoagulation

B. Initiate oral anticoagulation with a vitamin K antagonist or novel oral anticoagulant (NOAC)

C. Perform transesophageal echocardiogram and consider anticoagulation if AF recurs

D. Given the patient's overall stroke risk, there is no need for anticoagulation

E. Placement of a percutaneous left atrial appendage occlusion device

45. A 76-year-old man is in the ICU after having a subdural hematoma evacuated. He has a history of hypertension, dyslipidemia, and type 2 diabetes mellitus, which is controlled with oral medications. He develops progressive confusion and dysarthria, and initial investigation demonstrates a large subdural hematoma with midline shift, prompting urgent surgery. He has a successful, well-tolerated procedure and now is intubated and sedated; a nicardipine infusion for tight blood pressure control is administered.

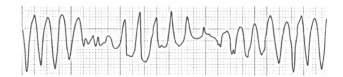

In the first few hours postoperatively, he sustains multiple episodes of a wide-complex tachycardia, which is shown below.

Between episodes, a 12-lead ECG is obtained and notable for normal sinus rhythm at 52 bpm and no ST-segment elevation, but deep, inverted T waves are present. His QTc is measured at 630 milliseconds.

Currently, after administering empiric magnesium sulfate and repeating electrolyte measurement, what is the next most appropriate step in management?

A. Discontinue the intravenous nicardipine infusion as it is the likely cause of the dysrhythmia

B. Administer intravenous β-blockade

C. Start intravenous amiodarone bolus and infusion

D. Start intravenous isoproterenol or call cardiology service for temporary pacemaker placement

E. Careful observation without further intervention

46. A 66-year-old woman presents to the ED with general fatigue and mild shortness of breath. Her medical history includes hypertension, paroxysmal atrial fibrillation, and a prior ischemic stroke attributed to atrial fibrillation with no residual neurologic deficits. Her medications include hydrochlorothiazide, metoprolol, digoxin, and warfarin. One week ago, she noted flulike symptoms with fatigue, coughing and sneezing, and general aches, which resulted in poor oral intake. She experienced progressive fatigue and shortness of breath with minimal exertion over the past 2 days. Despite poor oral intake, she maintained strict medication compliance.

On exam, she is noted to be afebrile, with blood pressure of 138/92 mm Hg, heart rate of 34 bpm, and normal oxygen saturation on 2 L via nasal cannula. She is mildly diaphoretic but is generally comfortable appearing. The rest of the exam is notable only for a slow, regular heart rhythm. Her labs are notable for sodium of 121 mmol/L, potassium of 5.2 mmol/L, carbon dioxide of 19 mmol/L, blood urea nitrogen of 65 mg/dL, creatinine of 2.2 mg/dL, glucose of 104 mg/dL, calcium of 9.8 mg/dL, and INR of 4.5. An ECG is obtained and is shown below. What is the likely cause of this patient's current condition?

A. A myocardial infarction causing complete heart block

B. Digoxin toxicity

C. β-Blocker toxicity

D. An acute cerebrovascular accident

E. Sick sinus rhythm

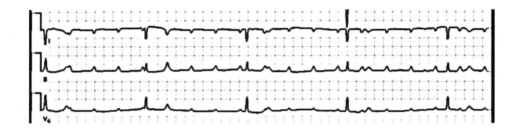

47. A 22-year-old man presents with general fatigue and an episode of syncope. He has no medical history and does not smoke, drink alcohol, or use recreational drugs. He works on a farm in rural Connecticut. He had flulike symptoms 4 weeks ago with a rash on his leg. His symptoms improved without intervention a few days afterward. He felt fatigued over the past 2 days and presented after he "blacked out" while working. An ECG is obtained and is shown below. What is the most appropriate treatment for this patient?

A. Intravenous steroids alone

B. Intravenous steroids and permanent pacemaker

C. Intravenous antibiotics and permanent pacemaker

D. Intravenous antibiotics and temporary pacemaker

E. Intravenous steroids and temporary pacemaker

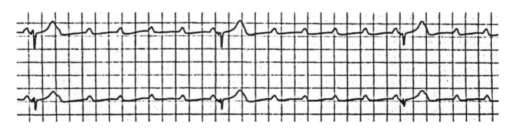

48. A 71-year-old man is being discharged after hospital observation following a transient ischemic attack. His medical history includes hypertension, diastolic heart failure, and chronic kidney disease. He presented with slurred speech and right-sided hemiplegia, which resolved by the time he arrived to the ED. His ECG demonstrated atrial fibrillation at a heart rate of 82 bpm, which was a new diagnosis.

His weight is 59 kg. His serum creatinine is 2.0 mg/dL. A transthoracic echocardiogram demonstrates normal left ventricular size and function, moderate left atrial dilation, and moderate mitral regurgitation. He does not want to have frequent blood draws. What is the most appropriate anticoagulant?

A. This patient does not require ongoing anticoagulation

B. Warfarin, dose adjusted for INR with goal of 2.0 to 3.0

C. Oral apixaban 5 mg twice daily

D. Oral rivaroxaban 20 mg daily

E. Oral apixaban 2.5 mg twice daily

49. A 72-year-old woman is evaluated for continued, progressive fatigue and generalized weakness. One year ago, she was hospitalized for an ischemic stroke attributed to new-onset atrial fibrillation. She has no residual deficits from the stroke. During her hospitalization, she was noted to be in atrial fibrillation, which was initially treated with β-blockers and cardioversion, which was unsuccessful. Ultimately the patient was discharged on metoprolol, warfarin, and amiodarone. In addition, she takes metformin, amlodipine, and low-dose aspirin for diabetes mellitus and hypertension.

On exam, she is noted to have a pulse of 62 bpm and blood pressure of 105/62 mm Hg. She is in no distress, has a flat affect, and is slow to answer questions. Her skin is cool and dry, and she has nonpitting edema of the lower extremities. Her heart sounds are regular with absence of murmurs, gallops, or rubs. What is the most likely explanation for her symptoms?

A. Amiodarone-induced hypothyroid state

B. Amiodarone-induced hyperthyroid state

C. Chronic subdural hematoma in the setting of anticoagulation

D. Persistent atrial fibrillation with poor rate control

E. Major depressive disorder

50. A 50-year-old man is being discharged after hospital observation following a transient ischemic attack. His medical history includes hypertension, for which he takes amlodipine. He presented with slurred speech and left-sided hemiplegia, which resolved by the time he arrived to the ED. His ECG demonstrated atrial fibrillation at a heart rate of 113 bpm, which is a new diagnosis.

His weight is 90 kg. Exam is notable for a diastolic opening snap followed by a diastolic rumble. His serum creatinine is 0.8 mg/dL. A transthoracic echocardiogram demonstrates normal left ventricular size and function, moderate left atrial dilation, and moderate mitral stenosis.

What is the most appropriate anticoagulant?

A. This patient does not require ongoing anticoagulation

B. Oral warfarin, dose adjusted for INR goal of 2.0 to 3.0

C. Oral apixaban 5 mg twice daily

D. Oral rivaroxaban 20 mg daily

E. Oral dabigatran 150 mg twice daily

51. An 80-year-old woman is admitted to the ICU following evacuation of a subdural hematoma. Her comorbidities include hypertension, dyslipidemia, chronic systolic heart failure (left ventricular ejection fraction is 30%), and impaired glucose intolerance for which she takes aspirin, atorvastatin, lisinopril, and carvedilol.

Currently, she is intubated and sedated with blood pressure of 110/72 mm Hg and heart rate of 64 bpm. Her lungs are clear to auscultation, heart rate and rhythm are regular without murmur or gallops, and extremities are warm without edema.

Given her current medical state, what is the most appropriate management of her comorbid heart failure?

A. Discontinue carvedilol until she is discharged

B. Add digoxin to improve cardiac inotropy in the setting of acute illness

C. Increase lisinopril and start eplerenone

D. Continue lisinopril and carvedilol

E. Add amiodarone to prevent ventricular tachyarrhythmias in the setting neurologic surgery

Answers and Explanations

1. D. The 2014 American College of Cardiology/ American Heart Association (ACC/AHA) valve guidelines recommend the use of bridging anticoagulation in patients with a mechanical mitral valve replacement (class I). Argatroban is an intravenous direct thrombin inhibitor that is indicated for use as anticoagulation for prophylaxis and treatment of thromboembolic disease in patients with heparin-induced thrombocytopenia. Heparin use is contraindicated because of the patient's history of heparin-induced thrombocytopenia. Similarly, enoxaparin is also contraindicated as there is significant cross-reactivity with this drug and heparin. The 2014 ACC/AHA valve guidelines also recommend against (class III) the use of anticoagulants therapy with oral direct thrombin inhibitors (including dabigatran) or anti-Xa agents (rivaroxaban, apixaban, and edoxaban) in patients with a mechanical valve prosthesis. This recommendation against use of novel oral anticoagulants (NOACs) comes from data from the RE-ALIGN randomized control trial, which showed excess thromboembolic and bleeding events in patient treated with dabigatran compared to warfarin. Lastly, the onset of anticoagulation with warfarin is delayed and will not be therapeutic for at least 4 to 5 days.

2. D. The right ventricle is relatively thin walled compared to the left ventricle and is unable to tolerate acute increases in afterload such as a pulmonary embolism. This results in right ventricular dilation and systolic dysfunction. The echocardiographic finding of akinesia of the mid-free wall and hypercontractility of the apex is known as McConnell's sign and has been found to be a specific (up to 94%) for the diagnosis of acute pulmonary embolism. Elevations in cardiac biomarkers such as troponin and BNP have been associated with worse outcomes, with any elevation in troponin being associated with a 5-fold increase in short-term mortality.

3. A. This patient is hemodynamically unstable related to the massive pulmonary embolism. Patients with a massive pulmonary embolism associated with hypotension (systolic blood pressure <90 mm Hg for >15 minutes) should be treated with thrombolytic therapy if they do not have a high bleeding risk. The use of heparin alone only prevents further thrombus formation while the body works to dissolve the thrombus. Warfarin takes at least 2 days to see a significant anticoagulant effect and thus should not be started as initial therapy. In contrast, fibrinolytic therapy accelerates the resolution of embolic burden, leading to improved right ventricular function, more rapid lowering of pulmonary artery pressures, and improvement in arterial oxygenation and hemodynamics. The recommended dose for alteplase is 100 mg (10 mg intravenous bolus followed by 90 mg intravenous infusion over 2 hours). If thrombolytic therapy is contraindicated in a patient with hemodynamic instability, emergent pulmonary artery thrombectomy should be considered.

4. C. The patient has a type A dissection with neurologic symptoms and associated cardiac tamponade and will require emergent surgery for aortic repair. Although patients presenting with strokes have higher association with in-hospital adverse events, the patients who undergo surgery have superior long-term survival as well as a higher rate of reversal of neurologic deficits. Cardiothoracic surgery consultation is essential because the timing of surgery is of utmost importance as the mortality rates increase 1% to 2% per hour during the first several hours, with an overall surgical mortality rate of approximately 25%. Removal of a large volume of pericardial fluid can result in a significant rise in stroke volume and exacerbate the dissection, which could result in acute decompensation. If performed, a small-volume pericardiocentesis should only be performed in the setting of impending hemodynamic collapse as a bridge to emergent surgery. Although impulse control with a reduction in heart rate and systolic blood pressure are extremely important to help prevent progression of the aortic dissection, the patient is hypotensive and would be unable to tolerate intravenous metoprolol or sodium nitroprusside. Lastly, the patient needs emergent surgery, and there is no role for systemic anticoagulation prior to cardiac surgery.

5. **A.** The patient has an uncomplicated type B dissection, and this should be managed medically while monitoring for indications for early surgery, including evidence of malperfusion such as bowel ischemia, renal failure, or spinal neurologic deficits. Surgery can also be considered for persistent pain despite adequate impulse control. When initiating impulse control, β-blockers (eg, metoprolol) should be initiated first to avoid an increase in cardiac contractility linked with use of vasodilators (eg, sodium nitroprusside) alone. There is no role for emergent coronary angiography or emergent aortic repair because type B dissections are typically medically managed, except as stated earlier.

6. **E.** The significance of finding a patent foramen ovale (PFO) on a transesophageal echocardiogram as part of an evaluation for a cryptogenic stroke or transient ischemia attack (TIA) in the absence of a concurrent thromboembolism remains unclear. To reduce the patient's risk of a recurrent stroke or TIA, she should first discontinue her oral contraceptives, which put her at an increased thromboembolic risk. Given the absence of an identified thromboembolism, there is no indication for initiation of anticoagulation. However, antiplatelet therapy should be initiated and is a class I indication in patients with an ischemic stroke or TIA not on anticoagulation. PFO closure is also not recommended (class III) in the absence of a deep vein thrombosis (DVT). However, transcatheter PFO closure can be considered (class IIb) in the presence of a cryptogenic stroke, PFO, and a DVT depending on the patient's risk of a recurrent DVT. In patients who develop a recurrent cryptogenic stroke despite optimal medical therapy, PFO closure should be considered, and the Amplatzer PFO Occluder was recently approved by the US Food and Drug Administration (FDA) on October 28, 2016.

7. **D.** Stress-induced cardiomyopathy, or takotsubo cardiomyopathy, is a well-established cardiomyopathy that can mimic a myocardial infarction. It is usually triggered by a stressful or emotional exposure, which results in exposure to high concentration of catecholamines. It typically occurs in middle-aged women and is usually fully reversible. However, the diagnosis is one of exclusion after confirming the absence of coronary artery stenosis to explain the wall motion abnormality. Mental stress has also been found to trigger increases in sympathetic tone, blood pressure, blood viscosity, endothelial dysfunction, and platelet agreeability, which can result in plaque rupture, thrombosis, and thus a myocardial infarction. Without defining the coronary anatomy, the diagnosis of stress-induced cardiomyopathy cannot be confirmed. A coronary angiogram was performed in this case and revealed severe stenosis of the mid left anterior descending artery. The patient underwent subsequent revascularization with recovery of her left ventricular ejection fraction.

8. **C.** Pericardial tamponade is a clinical diagnosis defined by Beck's triad of hypotension, muffled heart sounds, and distended neck veins (elevated jugular venous pressure; normal = 8 cm H_2O). It occurs when the intrapericardial pressure exceeds the intracardiac filling pressures, thus impairing venous return. This results in underfilling of the left ventricle and subsequent decreased cardiac output and hypotension. Tamponade typically occurs in cases with rapidly accumulating effusions, while slow accumulating moderate to large pericardial effusions are often well tolerated. However, patients can develop an entity known as low-pressure tamponade in the setting of a preexisting pericardial effusion that only becomes hemodynamically important in the setting of a decrease in intravascular blood volume (eg, dialysis, dehydration, acute blood loss, or diuresis). This diagnosis can create confusion because it is not always associated with the classic findings of elevated jugular venous pressure and/or elevated pulsus paradoxus (normal <10 mm Hg). The treatment of choice in this condition is fluid resuscitation to increase the

intravascular blood volume before proceeding with an invasive procedure such as a pericardiocentesis. Although an echocardiogram could be used to confirm a low intravascular pressure, fluid resuscitation should not be delayed while obtaining such an evaluation. The patient's ECG shows a sinus tachycardia, which is a compensatory response, and there is no role for synchronized cardioversion or amiodarone.

9. **B.** The cardiac anomaly represented in the figure is a patent foramen ovale (PFO). Panel B of the figure shows the presence of agitated saline, which traversed through the PFO (white arrow).

    A PFO is a remnant of fetal circulation. Anatomic closure typically occurs within the first couple years of life but remains patent in approximately 25% of individuals in the general population. It is important to recognize that given the prevalence of PFOs, the identification of a PFO as part of the evaluation for a cryptogenic stroke may represent an incidental finding rather than the culprit etiology. Thus, it is important to continue to evaluate for alternative causes of the cryptogenic stroke such as occult atrial fibrillation, especially in older patients. Based on the results from the CRYSTAL-AF study, atrial fibrillation was detected in 30% of patients at the 3-year follow-up, with a higher likelihood in older patients.

10. **A.** Cardiac amyloidosis is infiltrative, restrictive cardiomyopathy in which abnormal proteins deposit into the myocardium. The restrictive cardiomyopathy results in diastolic dysfunction with resultant biatrial dilation, which increases the risk of developing atrial fibrillation. Cardiac amyloidosis carries a poor prognosis, but if it is caused by monoclonal expansion of plasma cells and deposition of free light chains (ie, multiple myeloma) the disease may be reversible. Thus, prompt recognition is important.

    The keys to the diagnosis in this case are the discordance between the low voltage on the ECG and severe left ventricular hypertrophy with increased echogenicity/speckled pattern of the myocardium on echocardiogram, raising suspicion of an infiltrative cardiomyopathy measurement of fractional changes in length of myocardial segments, strain. Apical sparing of the myocardial strain has emerged as a strong method in differentiating cardiac amyloidosis from other causes of left ventricular hypertrophy. Additionally, the patient has significant anemia, renal failure, and hypercalcemia secondary to multiple myeloma. These features in association are highly concerning for cardiac AL amyloidosis.

11. **D.** Idarucizumab (Praxbind) is a humanized monoclonal antibody fragment with high affinity that irreversibly binds to free and thrombin-bound dabigatran, thus neutralizing its anticoagulant effect without interfering with the coagulation cascade. In October 2015, the FDA granted approval for use of idarucizumab during emergency situations when there is a need to reverse dabigatran's anticoagulant effects based on the results of the RE-VERSE AD study. Fresh frozen plasma, recombinant factor VII, and vitamin K have no role in the reversal of anticoagulation related to dabigatran or any of the direct thrombin inhibitors (direct or indirect). Andexanet alfa is a recombinant modified human factor Xa decoy protein that was recently shown to achieve 79% effective hemostasis by substantially reducing anti–factor Xa activity in multicenter single-group study of 67 patients; however, it has yet to receive FDA approval.

    Of note, prothrombin complex concentrates (activated and unactivated) have been shown in small human trials reverse the anticoagulant effect associated with novel oral anticoagulants. However, they should only be administered in patients with severe, life-threatening bleeding if a specific reversal agent is either not available or not approved. If the patient consumed any of the novel oral anticoagulation medications within 2 to 4 hours, oral activated charcoal may be administered to minimize absorption of the drug. Hemodialysis can also be considered in patients on dabigatran but is not an option for Xa inhibitors, which are highly protein bound.

12. **D.** Although subtle, the most striking feature is up to 2 mm of ST depression in lead V_2 with some extension of ST depression throughout the precordium to lead V_5. Given the report of a prior "normal" ECG, this tracing, along with an appropriate clinical history, is consistent with an acute posterior ST-segment elevation myocardial infarction (STEMI). See leads $V_{2/3}$ (in the figure below) from the patient's prior baseline ECG for the notable difference (previously upright ST segment and T wave).

    This patient ended up having an ulcerated 90% lesion in the proximal circumflex and received a drug-eluting stent. These types of ECGs are consistently challenging clinically. The modern 12-lead

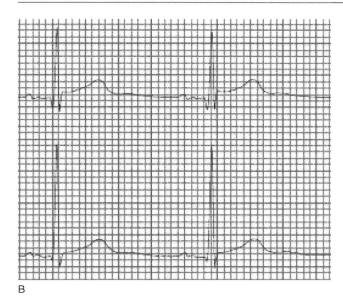

B

ECG system underrepresents the inferoposterior to posterolateral walls, the territory fed in most cases by the left circumflex system. In past literature, it has been shown that roughly 50% of circumflex occlusions present with ST elevation, 45% with ST depression, and close to 40% are electrically silent. Although non–ST-segment elevation myocardial infarctions are evenly distributed by coronary distribution in randomized controlled trials, the circumflex only represents 14% of the STEMI population in randomized controlled trials, further buffeting the point of underrecognition/non–ST-segment elevation presentation. Clinically, this has meaningful implications, with statistically significant higher cardiac enzyme release, worsened postinfarct ejection fraction, and likelihood for significant mitral regurgitation, as well as suggestion toward higher mortality compared to matched right coronary artery infarcts.

13. **C.** The ECG reveals deep, narrow T-wave inversions in V_2-V_5, but most prominently in V_2-V_4. In the correct clinical scenario (progressive fatigue with exertion) with known risk factors (hypertension, hyperlipidemia), this tracing is concerning for Wellens syndrome, which portends a high likelihood of significant stenosis in the left anterior descending artery. A prospective study of such ECG tracings with classic symptoms revealed > 50% stenosis of the left anterior descending artery in all patients, with complete or near-complete occlusion in 60% (mean stenosis 85%). Cerebral

T waves seen in the setting of subarachnoid hemorrhage or another such process that raises intracranial pressure should certainly be on the differential for such an ECG, but anecdotally, they tend to be wider, monophasic inversions (whereas Wellens variant can present as biphasic T waves with terminal inversions) and tend to extend throughout the full precordium to V_6. In addition, the given clinical information of a normal neurologic exam, no trauma (not mentioned whether patient hit her head), and no predisposing medications (anticoagulants) makes this diagnosis less likely. Although an aortic stenosis versus sclerosis murmur is described to be present, the description as mid-peaking makes *severe* symptomatic aortic stenosis much less likely. Although the given systolic blood pressure is 100 mm Hg, orthostatics are negative, thus hypotension is unlikely. Lastly, there is no evidence of either sinus node dysfunction or atrioventricular node dysfunction on the ECG to suggest a bradyarrhythmia.

14. **E.** The patient's baseline ECG shows preexcitation, otherwise known as Wolff-Parkinson-White (WPW) pattern, manifest by a short PR interval and slurred upslope of the subsequent QRS complex (delta wave). These findings are seen best in lead I and are magnified/highlighted in the figure below.

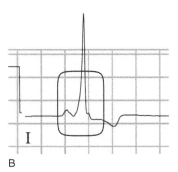

I

B

Given the patient has both the ECG pattern and clinical symptoms (tachycardia and syncope), this qualifies as WPW *syndrome*. A major hint in the question stem with regard to management approach is the "irregularly irregular" rhythm that corresponds with symptoms. This likely represents atrial fibrillation with preexcitation, which is a high-risk feature for syncope and, more importantly, mortality. Other risk factors applicable to this patient include young age and male gender. It is not uncommon to see bowel/bladder incontinence and tongue biting with cardiogenic syncope, so do not let that fool you. Catheter ablation is first-line therapy for patients at high risk for sudden cardiac death (such as this patient) or if the patient has symptomatic tachyarrhythmia. Depending on the number and location(s) of accessory pathways, sustained success with catheter ablation ranges from 85% to 100%. Although atrial fibrillation is likely present concurrently, the patient's CHADS$_2$VASc score is 0, and thus would not warrant anticoagulation. The patient is currently in sinus rhythm, and thus would not warrant cardioversion at this time. That being said, if the patients is persistently in preexcited atrial fibrillation, either urgent procainamide administration or cardioversion would be first-line therapy. β-Blockers can be used as second-line therapy in low-risk WPW patients, but are contraindicated in patients with preexcited atrial fibrillation, because they preferentially redirect conduction down the accessory pathway(s); in the wrong WPW patient, such a mistake could be fatal.

15. **B.** Although the given clinical vignette describes a patient who is high risk for acute coronary syndrome (recent cocaine use, hypertension) with clear ST changes seen on ECG (aVR elevation, diffuse upsloping ST depression), the patient's symptoms are actually attributable to his narrow-complex tachycardia. If you look closely, there

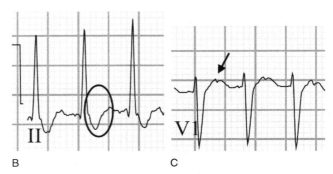

B   C

are no clear p waves before the QRS complexes, but there may be a small notch immediately *after* the S waves (buried in the ST segments), known as a retrograde p. This categorizes this supraventricular tachycardia (SVT) as a *short* RP tachycardia, of which the 2 most common subtypes are atrioventricular (AV) nodal reentrant tachycardia (AVNRT) and AV reentrant tachycardia (AVRT). Both tachyarrhythmias are often associated with ST changes that are attributable to the arrhythmia rather than ischemia, as well as a pseudo S wave in the inferior leads and a pseudo R′ in lead V$_1$, both of which are seen in this case.

Given that both AVNRT and AVRT are AV nodal–dependent pathways, adenosine, which is short acting and causes transient complete block of the AV node, is a quick diagnostic and therapeutic treatment. Intravenous metoprolol is a reasonable alternative to adenosine in most patients, but takes much longer to act (half-life of adenosine is <10 seconds) and would be relatively contraindicated

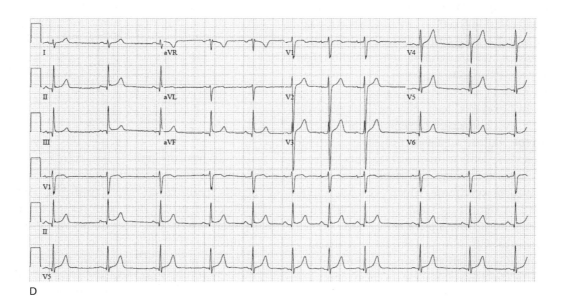

D

in a patient who recently used cocaine (unopposed α-blockade). Similarly, amiodarone and digoxin are second-line (and later) agents with much longer time to onset and inferior efficacy. With respect to intravenous lorazepam, if concerned about acute coronary syndrome or coronary vasospasm in the setting of chest pain and cocaine use, intravenous benzodiazepines are recommended, but this is not that scenario. It should be noted that if vagal maneuvers had been given as an answer choice, that would have been a reasonable alternative given their quick and noninvasive nature, but anecdotally, they are rarely effective. See the ECG (page 470) following conversion to normal sinus rhythm with adenosine administration, and note how the p wave now precedes the QRS complex (long RP interval) with no further S waves seen in the inferior leads and no R′ seen in V_1.

16. **E.** As per the most recent American Heart Association's recommendations for postcardiac arrest care, therapeutic hypothermia, preferably referred to as targeted temperature management (TTM), is a class I recommendation for all comatose patients suffering out-of-hospital cardiac arrest regardless of whether the arrest rhythm was shockable (ventricular tachycardia [VT]/ventricular fibrillation [VF]) versus nonshockable (pulseless electrical activity [PEA]/asystole). For VT/VF, the level of evidence is B, coming from multiple randomized controlled trials. For nonshockable rhythms, the level of evidence is C, based on expert opinion and evidence from meta-analyses showing more modest benefits. This recommendation is controversial, as outcomes are worse in nonshockable rhythm patients, particularly those with low pH and high lactic acid on presentation, but do not preclude patients from aggressive treatment, chiefly TTM, for at least 72 hours after arrest per the guidelines. Furthermore, a recent TTM trial showed lack of benefit of a target temperature of 33°C versus 36°C, and as such, the current guidelines specify a broad range of targeted temperature at 32°C to 36°C and do not specify administration route (internal vs external). Immediate coronary angiography is not a strong indication for non-VT/VF arrest (as opposed to VT/VF), and withdrawal of care would be considered premature at this time in the absence of a preexisting legal document expressing such wishes.

17. **A.** The noted ECG changes are J point ST elevations known as Osborn waves. They are commonly seen in patients treated with targeted temperature management and do not require intervention (hypothermia can be continued). As such, cardiac catheterization need not be performed (this is not an ST-segment elevation myocardial infarction). These are not peaked T waves from hyperkalemia (actually TTM is associated with hypokalemia). Finally, although the pictured noted heart rate is roughly 36 bpm, bradycardia is common with hypothermia, and a pacemaker is not needed.

18. **E.** The patient in question developed torsades de pointes, likely from an R-on-T phenomenon in the setting of a prolonged QTc interval that was exacerbated by ondansetron use. The offending agent should first be identified and discontinued. Magnesium can be administered to suppress early afterdepolarization. In addition, in the setting of torsades de pointes, tachycardia is preferred to bradycardia due to relative reduction in the QT interval. Discontinuation of β-blockade will begin to correct the patient's pharmacologically induced bradycardia (heart rate of 55 bpm) but will take time. In the interim, temporizing measures to induce tachycardia are reasonable, including pharmacologic methods, such as isoproterenol or dopamine, or mechanical methods, such as temporary pacing.

19. **D.** Paroxysmal atrial fibrillation is the most common cause of cryptogenic stroke that is subsequently identified in follow-up. Successful diagnosis is tied to longer duration of monitoring. The CRYSTAL-AF study randomized over 400 patients to standard of care (≥24 hours of continuous ECG monitoring) versus an implantable cardiac monitor (loop recorder). By 1 year of follow-up, atrial fibrillation was detected in 10% more patients in the loop recorder group. The other answer choices are all shorter outpatient external monitors with lower yields of diagnosis.

20. **B.** Although at first glance, there appears to be regularized atrial activity, upon close inspection with calipers, you will note there is actually irregularity present. As such, this represents coarse atrial fibrillation (not flutter) with a ventricular rate between 70 and 80 bpm (with the vignette referring to

paroxysms with rates up to 105 bpm). Clinically, the patient is in decompensated heart failure with mild hypotension, hypoxia, and evidence of volume overload with known preexisting severe biventricular systolic dysfunction. As such, the patient is in a gray area, which could be considered unstable depending on the provider. If deemed unstable (again a reasonable conclusion given heart failure decompensation), restoration of sinus rhythm via attempted electrical or pharmacologic cardioversion would be reasonable. The vignette states the patient has been compliant with his anticoagulation regimen, and as such, precardioversion transesophageal echocardiogram to rule out left atrial appendage thrombus is not needed. Electrical cardioversion is most likely to be efficacious, but attempted oral cardioversion with antiarrhythmic therapy is a reasonable alternative. It should be noted, however, that the success rate of amiodarone resulting in chemical cardioversion is rather low and that intravenous loading can actually worsen hypotension given the vasodilatory properties of the intravenous formulation diluent. If, however, the patient is deemed tenuous but "stable" (also a reasonable conclusion), diuresis targeted at clear volume overload as well as digoxin for both improved rate control and mild inotropic support

are reasonable approaches (in the inpatient setting only). Intravenous diltiazem, however, is contraindicated in this setting. The patient is already rate controlled at <110 bpm, as defined by the recent RACE II trial, and thus does not warrant more aggressive rate control. Furthermore (and more importantly), the patient is in decompensated heart failure with a known severely depressed ejection fraction. Nondihydropyridine calcium channel blockers (diltiazem and verapamil), particularly in intravenous form, are strong negative inotropes and can worsen heart failure and precipitate cardiogenic shock. Intravenous β-blockers can have a similar effect in such a scenario, although usually to a less severe degree.

21. **E.** The key to the telemetry strip is that, dependent on the lead in question, QRS complexes can be seen marching through at a regular rate. On first glance, particularly in leads II, III, aVF, aVL, and avR, you might be concerned for monomorphic ventricular tachycardia at a rate of 300 bpm. However, upon closer inspection, there is regularized ventricular activity that marches at a regular rate throughout the entire strip matched to the sinus rate clearly seen in lead I (shown in circles; see figure below).

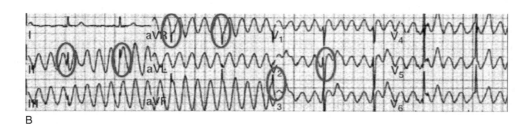

As such, this is not ventricular tachycardia nor ventricular fibrillation, but rather an artifact likely secondary to a tonic-clonic seizure. Similar artifacts can be seen with teeth brushing or Parkinson disease. The treatment would thus be abortive intravenous antiepileptic medication. No cardiac medications or procedures are indicated.

22. **E.** The rhythm in question is monomorphic ventricular tachycardia (VT) at a rate of roughly 160 bpm. Further describing the VT, it has a right bundle branch appearance (RSR′ in V_1, terminal S wave in V_6) and a rightward (positive in aVR, negative

in I/aVL), superior (negative in the inferior leads) axis. The most likely cause is reentry from scar in the apical left ventricle given the patient's clinical history. Given the patient is hypotensive and symptomatic, rhythm termination is indicated. Since the patient has a pulse and a regular rhythm, defibrillation would be inappropriate and could degenerate the rhythm into ventricular fibrillation via R-on-T phenomenon. Adenosine is similarly contraindicated in wide-complex tachycardia and acts on the AV node (thus will not terminate the rhythm). Synchronized cardioversion (after adequate analgesia and sedation if able) is a reasonable approach as per current advanced cardiac life support guidelines. Alternatively, pending patient stability, the patient's defibrillator could be used to provide "mini-shocks" at a rate slightly faster than the tachycardia cycle length as a means of terminating the rhythm without requiring a full electrical shock. This is referred to as "antitachycardia pacing," or ATP. This is an important alternative to consider because studies have shown that, in matched patient cohorts, those who receive implantable cardioverter-defibrillator shocks have increased mortality compared to patients who do not receive shocks, whereas ATP does not worsen long-term outcomes. ATP should not be administered except by an experienced provider facile with cardiac device modification, because if used inappropriately, it can similarly degenerate VT into ventricular fibrillation.

23. **A.** The telemetry strip shows atrial fibrillation with rapid ventricular response interspersed with 2 episodes of postconversion pauses with associated asystole, the second lasting longer than 5 seconds. This likely represents sinus node dysfunction, which in the presence of concurrent atrial fibrillation is referred to a tachy-brady syndrome. β-Blocker overdose is unlikely the cause of the patient's sinus pauses because there is concurrent inadequate rate control while in atrial fibrillation. AV node dysfunction is usually manifest as either a first-degree AV block (PR interval >200 milliseconds) or Wenckebach pattern. Infra-Hisian block refers to Mobitz II or complete heart block, neither of which is seen in this case. This patient has 2 indications for a permanent pacemaker: postconversion pause >5 seconds (the upper limit in atrial fibrillation vs 3 seconds of asystole in sinus rhythm) and bradycardic rhythm despite need for further intensification of AV nodal blockade. The mode of pacing the patient requires is atrial pacing (because of sinus node dysfunction), and therefore, a single chamber atrial pacemaker could be considered (as opposed to a dual-chamber pacemaker).

24. **D.** This patient has a cardiac implantable electronic device and has developed a fever and positive blood cultures. The next best step is to assess the cardiac valves and device for evidence of infection, as this would change management. Although transthoracic echocardiogram is generally the first diagnostic test of choice in most circumstances, the sensitivity is 70%, and it may be difficult to visualize a vegetation on a device lead with this imaging modality. Thus, it is reasonable to forgo transthoracic echocardiography in favor of transesophageal echocardiography, especially in cases where there is a high index of suspicion and high risk for endocarditis (eg, presence of prosthetic cardiac valves, presence of a cardiac device, or prior history of endocarditis).

25. **E.** The transesophageal echocardiogram shows a vegetation on an intracardiac lead within the right atrium. Source control, removal of all hardware (leads plus the pulse generator), and intravenous antibiotics are generally required to completely treat the infection. Narrow-spectrum antibiotics, such as nafcillin in this case, are preferred when sensitivities are known and the patient is stable.

26. **D.** This patient has takotsubo (stress-induced) cardiomyopathy with left ventricular outflow tract obstruction. She had acute-onset chest pain during an emotional setting, with T-wave inversions on her ECG and a characteristic appearance of apical ballooning with basal hyperkinesis on ventriculogram. Hypovolemia in such patients can result in marked dynamic subvalvular obstruction, resulting in hypotension, heard on physical exam here with Valsalva maneuver. Treatment of choice is to administer intravenous fluid to ensure adequate preload because this may reverse the hypotension. Norepinephrine and dobutamine infusions are incorrect because these agents will increase contractility and potentially worsen the dynamic outflow tract obstruction. Similarly, the use of intra-aortic balloon pump in the setting of left ventricular outflow obstruction is relatively contraindicated as it will increase the pressure gradient and subsequently worsen the dynamic obstruction. Phenylephrine serves to increase afterload, which can help reduce the dynamic outflow tract obstruction; however, the patient should have adequate preload before instituting this agent.

27. **E.** This patient is in anaphylactic shock and requires immediate resuscitation. Epinephrine is the vasopressor with the most evidence in anaphylaxis. While intramuscular epinephrine (1:1000 concentration at 0.5 mg) is usually the treatment of choice, intravenous epinephrine (1:10,000 concentration) at 0.05 to 0.1 mg should be administered in this case given impending cardiovascular collapse.

Epinephrine 1:1000 concentration should not be given intravenously for anaphylaxis because this may result in accidental administration of incorrect doses. As of May 2016, epinephrine concentration ratios are prohibited on drug labels due to high rates of medication errors. The ratio expression of 1:1000 equals 1 mg/mL, and 1:10,000 equals 0.1 mg/mL, and vials should be labeled as such. Vasopressin and norepinephrine are not the first-line agents of choice for anaphylactic shock but should be considered in cases refractory to epinephrine.

28. **C.** This patient has hypertrophic cardiomyopathy and likely presented in a volume-depleted state. Patients with hypertrophic cardiomyopathy are very sensitive to reduced preload. An underfilled left ventricle results in worsening left ventricular outflow tract obstruction, thus precipitating hypotension. In addition, tachycardia reduces diastolic filling time and contributes to a lower preload state. The lower preload state is also associated with increased contractility in this case as metoprolol was discontinued. Increased contractility further contributes to worsening left ventricular outflow tract obstruction. The initial treatment of choice is to administer intravenous fluids at a high rate (bolused normal saline). However, when patients are refractory to fluid boluses, vasopressors must be initiated. The vasopressor of choice in patients with hypertrophic obstructive cardiomyopathy is phenylephrine as it has virtually neutral inotropic and chronotropic effects, whereas all the other agents increase inotropy and chronotropy to some degree. The increased afterload offered by phenylephrine will serve to reduce outflow tract obstruction. In addition, this patient's metoprolol should be reinstated in order to allow for increase in diastolic filling time and reduced contractility once he is adequately hydrated and adequate systemic blood pressure is reached. Dobutamine, epinephrine, and norepinephrine will all serve to increase contractility. Intra-aortic balloon counterpulsation reduces afterload, which will actually worsen the left ventricular outflow tract obstruction. Generally, the cornerstone for management of hypertrophic obstructive cardiomyopathy is to keep contractility and heart rate low and preload high.

29. **C.** This patient is likely in cardiogenic shock as evident by altered mental status, rales, presence of S_3, and cool extremities. Review of his vitals shows that he is chronotropically incompetent; the patient's heart rate is inappropriately low for the current hemodynamic state. Cardiac output equals heart rate times stroke volume. Therefore, the simplest and least invasive intervention at this point is to increase the lower rate limit on the pacemaker, which will result in a higher heart rate. This may obviate the need for vasopressors. An echocardiogram or a right heart catheter is not immediately necessary to treat this patient because the exam findings and clinical picture are consistent with cardiogenic shock.

30. **E.** This patient has third-degree heart block with a narrow QRS complex (<120 milliseconds) escape rhythm, no symptoms, and no signs of hypoperfusion. When evaluating patients with complete heart block, the width of the escape rhythm QRS complex is important when determining the location of the complete heart block. Complete heart block in individuals with a narrow QRS escape rhythm usually originates from either within the AV node or at the level of His and is typically associated with a more stable escape rhythm between 40 and 60 bpm. In contrast, if the QRS complex escape width is wide (>120 milliseconds), the block is usually infra-Hisian and associated with heart rates of <40 bpm that are often unstable. In this case, there is no indication for atropine, vasopressors, or temporary pacing for bradycardia when the patient is asymptomatic and without evidence of end-organ dysfunction. This patient should be closely monitored in an ICU (with transcutaneous pads in place) for the development of symptoms or evidence of end-organ dysfunction while evaluating for reversible and irreversible causes of complete heart block. If the patient begins to feel symptomatic or other evidence of end-organ hypoperfusion occurs, then transcutaneous pacing should be initiated immediately (do not wait to administer atropine) while arranging for a transvenous temporary pacing wire to be placed.

31. **D.** According to the ACC/AHA guidelines, chest compressions should be resumed immediately after delivering a shock in an uninterrupted manner (without pulse or rhythm check). Even though normal sinus rhythm was noticed on the defibrillation monitor in this case, the correct answer is

to resume cardiopulmonary resuscitation (CPR) for 2 minutes. This is because cardiac output is often blunted after return of circulation and performing CPR assists the recovering heart regardless of whether there is a pulse. After the 2 minutes of chest compressions, it would be appropriate to perform a pulse check concurrently with the next rhythm check.

32. **A.** The correct answer is to use the AED as soon as it arrives since restoration of sinus rhythm is of paramount importance. There is no need to continue chest compressions as it unnecessarily delays potentially definitive therapy.

33. **D.** Per the advanced cardiac life support (ACLS) guidelines, the correct ratio of compressions to ventilation in adults without an advanced airway is 30:2. If an advanced airway is in place, then 6 to 8 breaths per minute can be delivered in an asynchronous manner (ie, do not interrupt compressions for ventilation). The compression-to-ventilation ratio for 2-rescuer child/infant CPR without an advanced airway is 15:2. If an advanced airway is in place for a child receiving CPR, then deliver 8 to 10 asynchronous breaths per minute. Other compression ratios are not appropriate.

34. **B.** Although the patient is presenting with a history of severe reduction in left ventricular systolic function, he has manifestations of septic shock, possibly from a urinary source with fever and leukocytosis after a recent admission for diuresis (when patients commonly have urinary catheters placed for accurate intake/output assessments). Although he was initially given a small intravenous fluid bolus, the pulmonary artery catheter demonstrates persistently low filling pressures and compensatory sinus tachycardia (Table 34-1). Although optimal filling pressures vary for patients, for most with longstanding histories of heart failure and dilated cardiomyopathies, higher filling pressures are often necessary for adequate preload and cardiac output. The appropriate management for this patient would be Swan-Ganz catheter–guided intravenous fluid resuscitation with titration off of vasopressors once adequate preload is obtained.

Although vasopressors are currently maintaining mean arterial pressures, the increased afterload is detrimental in the patient with chronic heart failure, and the hemodynamic profile may shift to a mixed septic and cardiogenic shock if a patient with inadequate filling pressures is managed with vasopressors (choice A). Inotropes may be required if the patient develops a mixed hemodynamic profile with a cardiogenic component, but he currently has septic shock and is underfilled, and dobutamine administration may make the patient more tachycardic and more hypotensive (choice C). Treating compensatory tachycardia in this situation with

Table 34-1. Hemodynamic Monitoring With a Pulmonary Artery Catheter: Normal Values

Location	Mean	Range
Right atrium	3 mm Hg	1-5 mm Hg
Right ventricle		
Peak systolic	25 mm Hg	15-30 mm Hg
Peak diastolic	9 mm Hg	4-12 mm Hg
Pulmonary capillary wedge pressure (PCWP)	9 mm Hg	4-12 mm Hg
Pulmonary vascular resistance	70 dyne·s·cm^{-5}	20-130 dyne·s·cm^{-5}
Systemic vascular resistance (SVR)	1100 dyne·s·cm^{-5}	700-1600 dyne·s·cm^{-5}
Mixed venous oxygen saturation (SvO$_2$)	• >75% oxygen supply > demand • 75% < SvO$_2$ > 50% Increase in demand or decrease in supply • 50% < SvO$_2$ > 30% Supply < demand, beginning of lactic acidosis • SvO$_2$ <30% suggests severe lactic acidosis and cellular death with values <25%	

intravenous β-blockers would be extremely detrimental (choice D). Recall that cardiac output is the product of heart rate and stroke volume (which is composed of preload, afterload, and contractility). In the current presentation, with inadequate preload (and thus stroke volume), the patient is maintaining a higher cardiac output with increased heart rate, and thus impairing that response would likely lead to further decompensation. Mechanical support is not indicated in the current situation where the primary issue is septic shock (choice E).

35. **D.** The patient is presenting with cardiogenic shock as a consequence of decompensated heart failure from a recent ST-segment elevation myocardial infarction and last known left ventricular ejection fraction of 30%. He has evidence of both low cardiac output (cool extremities and confusion) and volume overload (pulmonary edema and jugular venous distension) on examination and labs demonstrating end-organ dysfunction (acute renal and liver injury and elevated lactate). Hemodynamics demonstrate elevated filling pressures (pulmonary capillary wedge pressure [PCWP] of 28 mm Hg) and a mixed venous oxygen saturation of 45%. Although calculations of cardiac output and index are not given, with a normal hemoglobin, the mixed venous saturation of 45% demonstrates severely impaired cardiac output as the driver of the shock. In this case, his cardiac index is approximately 1.7 L/min/m^2. Cardiogenic shock is defined by an index of <1.8 without support or <2.2 with support and end-organ dysfunction. Also recall that the determinants of cardiac output are stroke volume and heart rate and that stroke volume is determined by preload, afterload, and contractility. In the setting of blood pressure that will likely tolerate afterload reduction via vasodilators, this is the best answer. This can be achieved by sodium nitroprusside (predominant arterial vasodilator) and to some extent by nitroglycerine (which affects predominantly preload via venodilation at lower doses and arterial vasodilation at higher doses). Ideally, the treatment strategy would involve afterload reduction as tolerated by blood pressure, then addressing preload (diuresis) and possibly contractility (ie, consideration of inotropes). It is not uncommon that all 3 parameters are being addressed at the same time.

Although intravenous diuresis (choice C) will likely be used in conjunction with afterload reduction, isolated diuresis is not the correct answer in a patient with low output. The patient has evidence of pulmonary edema and jugular venous distension on examination with a PCWP of 28 mm Hg. Diuresis will likely reduce the filling pressures and possibly increase stroke volume partially by optimizing loading conditions (preload), but will likely have a lesser effect than reducing afterload as a first strategy. In addition, with blood pressure room to tolerate afterload reduction, inotropes are also not the first step in management (choice B). Inotropes also increase myocardial consumption, thus provoking ischemia in individuals with coronary artery disease. Some might consider use of dobutamine in this situation; however, they are also associated with increased atrial and ventricular arrhythmogenicity and thus would not be our preferred management strategy unless the patient does not respond appropriately to afterload reduction. Activating the catheterization laboratory for consideration of revascularization is an important consideration in un-revascularized patients with cardiogenic shock (choice E), but the patient has a history of recent revascularization without ischemic symptoms or ECG changes. In addition, an intra-aortic balloon pump placement would not be indicated until medical therapy with afterload reduction is attempted. Finally, intravenous fluids are contraindicated in the setting of cardiogenic shock and elevated filling pressures (choice A).

36. **E.** The patient is presenting initially with septic shock from an apparent right lower lobe pneumonia. After volume resuscitation, he remains borderline hypotensive but without mounting an appropriate heart rate response (chronotropic insufficiency with relative bradycardia). This is likely occurring in the setting of chronic amiodarone use for rhythm control of atrial fibrillation. Swan-Ganz catheter–derived hemodynamics show relatively normal filling pressures with a low mixed venous oxygen saturation in the setting of sepsis. Increasing the patient's atrial rate will improve the cardiac output so as to provide cardiac compensation for the distributive shock picture. Recall that cardiac output is equal to the product of stroke volume and heart rate and that, in patients with hypotension and shock, you should pay attention not only to parameters of stroke volume (preload, afterload, and contractility), but also to whether

there is appropriate heart rate response as well as both atrial-ventricular and ventricular-ventricular synchrony (ie, the atrial rate should be increased; simply changing to VVI ventricular pacing at a higher rate may worsen hemodynamics with the consequent dyssynchrony).

Vasopressors (choice A) are an appropriate therapy for volume-refractory septic shock and may increase chronotropy as well. In the setting of significant chronotropic insufficiency and because the patient has a dual-chamber pacemaker that can be easily reprogrammed and increased afterload can be detrimental in heart failure patients, vasopressors would not be the best first-line treatment. Inotropes (choice B) and additional intravenous fluids (choice C) are not first-line treatments in this scenario but could be considered if filling pressures again become low or if the patient remains with borderline or low cardiac index despite appropriate chronotropy. Afterload reduction (choice D) would be detrimental in the setting of shock, being driven (at least initially) by pneumonia and septic shock.

37. **D.** The patient is presenting with incessant ventricular tachycardia (VT) (ie, "VT storm") in the setting of acute decompensated, presumptively nonischemic heart failure from medication nonadherence. She has evidence of both low output (cardiogenic shock with end-organ dysfunction) and volume overload decompensation and is receiving multiple, repetitive internal defibrillations. Her ventricular tachyarrhythmias are refractory to standard escalated treatment with antiarrhythmic therapy, intubation, sedation, and paralysis. She has a principle indication for an intra-aortic balloon pump (IABP) in the setting of refractory, unstable ventricular tachyarrhythmias that will also be beneficial for treating the underlying driving force behind the arrhythmias, cardiogenic shock. IABP use in medically refractory ventricular arrhythmias from underlying impaired left ventricular function has been demonstrated to be effective in stabilizing patients before definitive treatment (via heart failure treatment, catheter ablations, or transplantation). Treatment of the underlying cause of the arrhythmias (in this case, cardiogenic shock) can still occur with optimizing loading conditions via pulmonary artery catheter–tailored therapy. VT catheter ablations are generally not feasible in

emergent scenarios (choice A). Although β-blockers are part of standard medical therapy for ventricular tachyarrhythmias, in the setting of cardiogenic shock, they are contraindicated (choice B). The use of dobutamine or other inotropes may be beneficial as medical treatment for the cardiogenic shock but will increase the propensity for arrhythmias and are thus contraindicated in the setting of incessant VT (choice E). Although in some situations of incessant VT (refractory sarcoidosis), transplantation may be necessary, it is rarely considered emergent, especially in patients with prior medical nonadherence (choice C).

38. **D.** The patient is presenting with cardiogenic shock after an anterolateral ST-segment elevation myocardial infarction (STEMI) with acute left ventricular failure despite successful revascularization. The patient has hypotension precluding the optimization of loading conditions via vasodilators. Per the 2013 ACC/AHA guidelines on STEMIs, there is a class IIa (level of evidence B) indication for intra-aortic balloon counterpulsation in cardiogenic shock after STEMI and a class IIb (level of evidence C) indication for other mechanical circulatory support. Although inotropic support (choice B) is a consideration in post-STEMI cardiogenic shock and the data on the effectiveness of intra-aortic balloon counterpulsation therapy is conflicting, the use of inotropes in the setting of frequent ectopy and soon after revascularization for a STEMI with a likely large peri-infarct ischemic zone is not the best answer, especially if the patient is in a catheterization laboratory that is equipped to insert mechanical support devices. Intravenous fluids (choice A) are not indicated given the elevated filling pressures, and vasopressors (choice C) are not ideal for similar reasons to the inotropes and will further increase systemic vascular resistance/afterload. Consideration for heart transplantation (choice E) may be necessary but is not the acute treatment.

39. **C.** The patient is presenting with acute right ventricular failure in the setting of a right coronary artery STEMI (with ECG demonstrating inferior ST elevations, but also elevations in V_1 and V_2 concerning for extensive right ventricular injury). Although he underwent apparent successful primary percutaneous intervention, the patient

demonstrated features of right ventricular failure physiology around the time of the case (including a hypotensive response to nitroglycerine and intermittent heart block) before manifesting overt right ventricular failure in the cardiac ICU. Hemodynamics demonstrate an elevated right atrial and right ventricular end-diastolic pressures and low cardiac index, which are all indicative of right ventricular failure with consequent cardiogenic shock. Acute right ventricular failure and right ventricular failure physiology is a preload and synchrony-dependent state and is treated first by ensuring adequate volume. Once adequate volume is given (in this case, the right atrial pressure is 20 mm Hg), if the patient remains unstable, consideration should be made for increased atrial pacing rate (choice C). In this case, although a ventricular pacemaker was placed in the catheterization lab, simply turning up the rate (choice A) will increase chronotropy but will not maintain AV and ventriculoventricular dyssynchrony through 100% right ventricular pacing. Right ventricular failure and physiology is often worsened by ventricular pacing. Although right ventricular failure is an indication for inotropy (choice B), increasing myocardial oxygen demand so soon after an acute myocardial infarction may be detrimental by contributing to ischemia in the peri-infarct zone of ischemia despite revascularization and would not be the first-line treatment. The patient appears adequately volume resuscitated (choice D) and did not have ECG evidence of very early acute stent thrombosis on his ECG (choice E), although percutaneous right ventricular support could be considered if initial treatment of the right ventricular infarct fails.

40. **A.** Intra-aortic balloon pump (IABP) insertion can still occur in patients with severe peripheral arterial disease, including those with prior surgical revascularization, although obviously the inability to obtain access or pass guidewires precludes the insertion of intravascular devices (including IABP). Balloon pumps have been successfully placed via Dacron aortofemoral grafts as well as via alternative access sites (brachial or axillary).

Contraindications to IABP include severe aortic valvular insufficiency (choice B), given the augmented diastolic pressures will increase regurgitation; uncontrolled bleeding or severe bleeding risks (choice C); acute aortic pathology, including clinically significant aortic aneurysms (choice D); and uncontrolled sepsis (choice E).

41. **B.** The patient is on unnecessarily high positive end-expiratory pressure (PEEP) despite improving hypoxemia from intravenous diuresis. After opening hemodynamics demonstrated preserved cardiac indices and only elevated filling pressures, the patient is appropriately diuresed with initial improvement. Her cardiac indices thereafter worsen, despite improvement in filling pressures while the patient is maintained on a high PEEP. Although PEEP may be necessary to maintain or improve oxygenation in hypoxemic respiratory failure, it can markedly affect cardiac output via less predictable impacts on stroke volume (through altering loading conditions by changing lung volume and intrathoracic pressures with altered systemic venous return, right ventricular output, and left ventricular filling). This is especially true when patients are ventilated with concomitant ventricular dysfunction and in preload-dependent states (eg, right ventricular dysfunction and failure).

42. **E.** The patient initially presents with hypertensive emergency, manifesting with an elevated blood pressure and end-organ dysfunction (flash pulmonary edema and acute kidney injury). The normal treatment is intravenous blood pressure lowering with a goal of 10% to 20% reduction in the first hour and per hour thereafter (choice A). Lowering the blood pressure too quickly can result in ischemia in watershed vascular beds where autoregulation has adapted to chronically elevated pressures. This is why hypertensive urgencies (elevated blood pressure without end-organ damage) are treated with oral medications (choice B) to slowly bring down the blood pressure. One exception to this strategy is in acute aortic pathology, such as an acute type A dissection, such as shown in the figure for this question. In these situations, impulse control is achieved via intravenous injection of metoprolol followed by intravenous afterload reduction to reduce systolic blood pressures to 100 to 120 mm Hg within the first 15 to 20 minutes. Intravenous β-blockers are given first, so as to avoid compensatory tachycardia and an increased rate-pressure product that could come with isolated afterload reduction.

43. C. Brain and cardiac electrophysiology appear to be importantly connected by shared transmembrane proteins, which regulate electrical activity in both organs. Some patients with chronic epilepsy have been observed to have alterations in QTc over time, which may predispose them to polymorphic ventricular tachycardia (PMVT)/torsades de pointes. In addition, patients followed by cardiologists for long QT syndrome have a higher incidence of seizures compared to the general population. It is important to recognize the connection/overlap between cardiac and neurologic electrophysiology.

This patient has epilepsy and had a syncopal event in the setting of a prolonged QTc as demonstrated by the first ECG. She notably was taking 2 QTc-prolonging agents (ondansetron and promethazine), but does, in fact, have a prolonged QTc at baseline (approximately 510 milliseconds on the historical ECG). She experienced a tachyarrhythmia, which almost certainly represents torsades de pointes. Cardioversion or defibrillation should be reserved for patients in whom the arrhythmia persists or who are hemodynamically unstable. The first-line therapy is magnesium sulfate infusion and correction of electrolytes (ie, hypokalemia, hypocalcemia). If PMVT episodes persist, consideration of temporary atrial pacing should be considered to raise the heart rate and functionally decrease the QTc. Amiodarone, while commonly used for ventricular tachycardia, will likely lengthen the QTc and potentially worsen the dysrhythmia. β-Blockers may precipitate bradycardia, which will also functionally increase QTc.

44. B. Even though this patient has a relatively low yearly stroke risk (CHADS$_2$VASc risk score is 1 for hypertension), anticoagulation is recommended for anyone regardless of CHADS$_2$VASc score who has experienced atrial fibrillation (AF) for more than 48 hours and is cardioverted (whether spontaneously, electrically, or pharmacologically). For this reason, this patient should be placed on anticoagulation for at least 4 to 6 weeks, and the need for ongoing anticoagulation should be serially assessed. Transesophageal echocardiography is of less utility as its use is to assess for the presence of left atrial appendage thrombi, which guides appropriateness of cardioversion, and the patient already spontaneously converted back to normal sinus rhythm. Percutaneous left atrial appendage occlusion devices are only approved for patients with nonvalvular AF who are at increased risk for stroke and systemic embolism, are recommended for anticoagulation therapy, and have an appropriate rationale to seek a nonpharmacologic alternative to anticoagulation. In the above example, the patient lacks an indication to seek a nonpharmacologic alternative to anticoagulation (eg, high bleeding risk). In March 2015, the Watchman device became the only device approved for the above indication by the FDA based on the results of the PROTECT-AF and PREVAIL studies.

45. D. The patient has recurrent episodes of polymorphic ventricular tachycardia/torsades de pointes, which are the result of a prolonged QTc and exacerbated by ongoing bradycardia (heart rate was 52 bpm). This pattern of sinus bradycardia with broad, inverted T waves with prolonged QTc is a common occurrence in the setting of neurosurgery and intracranial procedures. Nicardipine may be essential in maintaining adequate blood pressure control, is not implicated in prolonging QTc, and should not be discontinued. β-Blockers may serve to worsen bradycardia, which will functionally increase the QT interval, and should be avoided in this scenario. Amiodarone, although a first-line agent for the treatment of ventricular tachycardia, should be avoided in torsades de pointes as this medication can lengthen the QTc and potentiate the problem.

In this case, isoproterenol, a pure β$_1$-agonist, is a reasonable treatment choice as it increases the heart rate, which functionally decreases the QT interval and may limit the ability of premature ventricular contractions to cause torsades de pointes. Hypotension can result from isoproterenol administration, and providers should be vigilant to watch for this. A temporary transvenous pacing system is appropriate for the same reasons as isoproterenol but will not cause hypotension and is a more durable means of therapy.

46. B. This woman likely has digoxin toxicity in the setting of acute renal injury, which likely resulted from concurrent poor oral intake and hydrochlorothiazide use. Digoxin is renally cleared; hence serum drug levels should be monitored in the setting of kidney injury. Metoprolol is not renally cleared, and although this medication should be avoided in the setting of complete heart block, this is not the likely cause of bradycardia and fatigue in this patient. Myocardial infarction and stroke are unlikely because they do not fit the presenting story and clinical picture. Sick sinus syndrome refers to bradycardia from sinoatrial node dysfunction, not AV node dysfunction.

47. **D.** The young man in the vignette has Lyme carditis resulting in complete heart block. The rhythm strip demonstrates p waves, indicating sinus rhythm at approximately 120 bpm, with dissociated narrow complex (junctional escape beats) at 21 bpm. AV conduction disturbances typically occur weeks to months after the initial untreated infection. The appropriate therapy is intravenous antibiotics, with ceftriaxone as the first-line agent. The prognosis for patients who undergo appropriate therapy is good, and AV conduction typically recovers over days to several weeks. Because the patient has symptoms and clearly has third-degree heart block, a pacemaker should be placed. This should be a temporary device as, with antibiotic treatment, the conduction disturbance is expected to resolve.

48. **E.** The patient has newly diagnosed atrial fibrillation (AF) with a $CHADS_2VASc$ score of 5, which is associated with an elevated annual stroke risk of 7.2% and thus requires anticoagulation. He wishes to be prescribed a medication that does not require blood monitoring, and there is no contraindication to a novel oral anticoagulant (NOAC). Although moderate mitral regurgitation is present, this does not fit the definition of "valvular" AF, which would require a vitamin K antagonist for anticoagulation. Valvular AF is defined by the presence of a mitral valve repair or replacement or rheumatic heart disease/mitral stenosis. Because of concomitant kidney disease, full-dose rivaroxaban should not be prescribed. Presence of 2 of the following dictate treating with dose-reduced apixaban: creatinine >1.5 mg/dL, weight <60 kg, and age >80 years. His weight and serum creatinine make dose-reduced apixaban the most appropriate option.

49. **A.** The patient was started on amiodarone, which is indicated both as a rate and a rhythm control agent in atrial fibrillation. Amiodarone, a class III antiarrhythmic drug, has multiple side effects including thyroid dysfunction (both hypo- and hyperthyroid states), as well as lung and liver toxicity. Hypothyroid states occur in approximately 5% of those treated with amiodarone; however, 25% of patients may develop subclinical hypothyroidism. The patient has a clinical syndrome consistent with a hypothyroid state. In this setting, thyroid function tests should be obtained and thyroid replacement therapy initiated in an effort to normalize hormone levels. Typically amiodarone is continued alongside thyroid hormone replacement.

50. **B.** The patient has atrial fibrillation (AF) that was diagnosed in the setting of a transient ischemic accident. With comorbid hypertension, his $CHADS_2VASc$ score is 3 with an elevated annual stroke risk of 3.2%; thus anticoagulation is indicated. Although he has no traditional contraindication to novel oral anticoagulant use, his AF is classified as "valvular" as he was found to have moderate mitral stenosis on exam and echocardiography. For this reason, the most appropriate management is to start warfarin for ongoing anticoagulation.

51. **D.** This question deals with hospitalization in the setting of comorbid chronic systolic heart failure. This patient has a normal blood pressure and heart rate and has no physical exam evidence consistent with decompensated heart failure. For this reason, it is appropriate to continue her long-term heart failure medications lisinopril and carvedilol. Close monitoring of the vital signs and kidney function is necessary during hospitalization when these are prone to fluctuation. There is no role for empiric administration of digoxin as there is no evidence of difficult-to-control atrial fibrillation or cardiogenic shock. There is no role for empiric administration of amiodarone for primary prevention of ventricular tachyarrhythmias. There is no compelling reason to perform outpatient medication adjustment (eg, increase lisinopril, add eplerenone) during acute noncardiac illness, although these may be appropriate once the patient is discharged.

REFERENCES

American Heart Association. Highlights of the 2015 American Heart Association guidelines update for CPR and ECC. https://eccguidelines.heart.org/wp-content/uploads/2015/10/2015-AHA-Guidelines-Highlights-English.pdf. Accessed on December 19, 2016.

Bater E. Cardiogenic shock. In: Jeremias A, ed. *Cardiac Intensive Care.* 2nd ed. Philadelphia, PA: Saunders; 2010:212-224.

Becattini C, Vedovati MC, Agnelli G. Prognostic value of troponins in acute pulmonary embolism a meta-analysis. *Circulation.* 2007;116(4):427-433.

Connolly SJ, Milling TJ Jr, Eikelboom JW, et al. Andexanet alfa for acute major bleeding associated with factor Xa inhibitors. *N Engl J Med.* 2016;375(12):1131-1141.

De Zwaan C, Bar FW, Janssen JH, et al. Angiographic and clinical characteristics of patients with unstable angina showing an ECG pattern indicating critical narrowing of the proximal LAD coronary artery. *Am Heart J.* 1989;117(3):657-665.

Di Eusanio M, Patel HJ, Nienaber CA, et al. Patients with type A acute aortic dissection presenting with major brain injury: should we operate on them? *J Thorac Cardiovasc Surg.* 2013;145(3):S213-S221.

Eikelboom JW, Connolly SJ, Brueckmann M, et al. Dabigatran versus warfarin in patients with mechanical heart valves. *N Engl J Med.* 2013;369(13):1206-1214.

Food and Drug Administration. Amplatzer PFO Occluder— P120021. www.fda.gov/MedicalDevices/Productsand MedicalProcedures/DeviceApprovalsandClearances/ Recently-ApprovedDevices/ucm526921.htm. Accessed December 20, 2016.

Fotopoulus GD, Mason MJ, Walker S, et al. Stabilisation of medically refractory ventricular arrhythmia by intra-aortic balloon counterpulsation. *Heart.* 1999;82(1):96-100.

Holmes DR Jr, Kar S, Price MJ, et al. Prospective randomized evaluation of the Watchman Left Atrial Appendage Closure device in patients with atrial fibrillation versus long-term warfarin therapy: the PREVAIL trial. *J Am Coll Cardiol.* 2014;64(1):1-12.

Huey BL, Beller GA, Kaiser DL, Gibson RS. A comprehensive analysis of myocardial infarction due to left circumflex artery occlusion: comparison with infarction due to right coronary artery and left anterior descending artery occlusion. *J Am Coll Cardiol.* 1988;12(5):1156-1166.

Inohara T, Kohsaka S, Fukada K, Menon V. The challenges in the management of right ventricular infarction. *Eur Heart J Acute Cardiovasc Care.* 2013;2(3):226-234.

January CT, Wann LS, Alpert JS, et al. 2014 AHA/ACC/ HRS guideline for the management of patients with atrial fibrillation: executive summary. *J Am Coll Cardiol.* 2014;130(23):2071-2104.

Kearon C, Akl EA, Blaivas A, et al. Antithrombotic therapy for VTE disease. *Chest.* 2016;149(2):315-352.

Kernan WN, Ovbiagele B, Black HR, et al. Guidelines for the prevention of stroke in patients with stroke and transient ischemic attack a guideline for healthcare professionals from the American Heart Association/American Stroke Association. *Stroke.* 2014;45(7):2160-2236.

Kim YM, Yim HW, Jeong SH, Klem ML, Callaway CW. Does therapeutic hypothermia benefit adult cardiac arrest patients presenting with non-shockable initial rhythms? A systematic review and meta-analysis of randomized and non-randomized studies. *Resuscitation.* 2012;83(2):188-196.

Krishnaswamy A, Lincoff AM, Menon V. Magnitude and consequences of missing the acute infarct-related circumflex artery. *Am Heart J.* 2009;158(5):706-712.

Larsen GK, Evans J, Lambert WE, Chen Y, Raitt MH. Shocks burden and increased mortality in implantable cardioverter-defibrillator patients. *Heart Rhythm.* 2011;8(12):1881-1886.

Lavonas EJ, Drennan IR, Gabrielli A, et al. Part 10: Special circumstances of resuscitation: 2015 American Heart Association guidelines update for cardiopulmonary resuscitation and emergency cardiovascular care. *Circulation.* 2015;132(18 Suppl 2):S501-S518.

Luecke T, Pelosi P. Clinical review: positive end-expiratory pressure and cardiac output. *Crit Care.* 2005;9(6):607-621.

McConnell MV, Solomon SD, Rayan ME, Come PC, Goldhaber SZ, Lee RT. Regional right ventricular dysfunction detected by echocardiography in acute pulmonary embolism. *Am J Cardiol.* 1996;78(4):469-473.

Neumar RW, Shuster M, Callaway CW, et al. 2015 American Heart Association guidelines update for cardiopulmonary resuscitation and emergency cardiovascular care. *Circulation.* 2015;132(18 Suppl 2):S315-S367.

Nielsen N, Wetterslev J, Cronberg T, et al. Targeted temperature management at 33° C vs. 36° C after cardiac arrest. *N Engl J Med.* 2013;369:2197-2206.

Nishimura RA, Otto CM, Bonow RO, et al. 2014 AHA/ ACC guideline for the management of patients with valvular heart disease: executive summary: a report of the American College of Cardiology/American Heart Association Task Force on Practice Guidelines. *Circulation.* 2014;129(23):2440-2492.

O'Gara PT, Kushner FG, Ascheim DD, et al. 2013 ACCF/AHA guideline for the management of ST-elevation myocardial infarction. *J Am Coll Cardiol.* 2013;61(4):78-140.

Pollack CV Jr, Reilly PA, Eikelboom J, et al. Idarucizumab for dabigatran reversal. *N Engl J Med.* 2015;373(6):511-520.

Ravindran K, Powell KL, Todaro M, O'Brien TJ. The pathophysiology of cardiac dysfunction in epilepsy. *Epilepsy Res.* 2016;127:19-29.

Reddy VY, Holmes D, Doshi SK, Neuzil P, Kar S. Safety of percutaneous left atrial appendage closure results from the Watchman Left Atrial Appendage System for Embolic Protection in Patients with AF (PROTECT AF) clinical trial and the Continued Access Registry. *Circulation.* 2011;123(4):417-424.

Rihal CS, Naidu SS, Givertz MM, et al. 2015 SCAI/ACC/ HFSA/STS clinical expert consensus statement on the use of percutaneous mechanical circulatory support devices in cardiovascular care. *J Am Coll Cardiol.* 2015;65(19):7-26.

Ruff CT, Giugliano RP, Antman EM. Management of bleeding with non–vitamin K antagonist oral anticoagulants in the era of specific reversal agents. *Circulation.* 2016;134(3):248-261.

Sanna T, Diener HC, Passman RS, et al. Cryptogenic stroke and underlying atrial fibrillation. *N Engl J Med.* 2014;370(26):2478-2486.

Saric M, Armour AC, Arnaout MS, et al. Guidelines for the use of echocardiography in the evaluation of a cardiac source of embolism. *J Am Soc Echocardiogr.* 2016;29(1):1-42.

Saver JL. Cryptogenic stroke. *N Engl J Med.* 2016;374:2065-2074.

Van Gelder IC, Groenveld HF, Crijns H, et al. Lenient versus strict rate control in patients with atrial fibrillation. *N Engl J Med.* 2010;362(15):1363-1373.

Wormser GP, Dattwyler RJ, Shapiro ED, et al. The clinical assessment, treatment, and prevention of lyme disease, human granulocytic anaplasmosis, and babesiosis: clinical practice guidelines by the Infectious Diseases Society of America. *Clin Infect Dis.* 2006;43(9):1089-1134.

Zipes DP, Camm AJ, Borggrefe M, et al. ACC/AHA/ESC 2006 guidelines for management of patients with ventricular arrhythmias and the prevention of sudden cardiac death. *Circulation.* 2006;114(10):e385-e484.

PART 6
Ethics/Professionalism

35

Ethics and Professionalism

Mohamed Osman, MD, and Michael Rubin, MD, MA

Questions

1. A 51-year-old woman with known history of hypertension and diabetes is brought to the emergency department (ED) after collapsing at a local restaurant while dinning with her family. She was found pulseless, and cardiopulmonary resuscitation (CPR) was started at the scene and continued by emergency medical services (EMS) while being transported to the ED where she has return of spontaneous circulation. Her "down time" was estimated to be around 15 minutes. She is minimally responsive to verbal stimulation, and cranial nerve exam shows no deficit. Computed tomography (CT) scan of the head on the first day shows possible decreased gray/white matter differentiation, but the findings are not definitive. Electroencephalogram (EEG) is pending. Which of the following is correct regarding neurologic prognostication in this patient?

A. The patient's exam at presentation will be no different than her exam after the first week.

B. Lack of any cranial nerve deficit indicates that the patient will have a functional recovery.

C. The family should be encouraged to wait at least 72 hours before withdrawing life-sustaining therapy as the exam may improve.

D. A unilateral do not resuscitate (DNR) order is appropriate.

E. Magnetic resonance imaging (MRI) is needed before any proper evaluation of neurologic recovery can be made.

2. A 61-year-old man is admitted to the intensive care unit (ICU) after a large left middle cerebral artery (MCA) stroke. He is intubated, comatose, and has a hemiparesis. The patient has notable brain atrophy secondary to chronic drug abuse and is not showing signs of herniation despite cerebral edema. The family informs you that he would not want to live in this condition and asks what his chances are of recovery to a "near normal life." After reviewing his case, you determine that his expected recovery to an independent state is unlikely. The family brings up the fact that he wanted to be an organ donor and is on the registry, and despite your efforts to defer the conversation to the organ procurement organization, they are asking you what conditions need to be met for him to be a donor. How would you counsel the family toward further care?

A. Since the patient is not brain dead, organ donation is not possible.

B. Since the patient has a severe neurologic injury but is not likely to progress to brain death, a declaration of death by cardiovascular criteria is necessary before organs can be recovered.

C. With the family consent, the patient can be taken for organ recovery as the dead donor rule is a principle but not an actual legal requirement.

D. The patient's history of drug abuse precludes the donation of organs, and the organ procurement organization should not be consulted.

E. No consent is needed, and the patient should be taken for living donation now.

3. A 45-year-old man is in a motor vehicle accident that results in severe head trauma. A head CT in the ED demonstrates a large subdural hematoma overlying the left frontal and parietal lobes as well as bifrontal contusions. His pupillary reflexes are intact, but he lacks corneal or gag response and has no motor response. He is admitted to the ICU after emergent decompressive hemicraniectomy. The team can adequately oxygenate him with fraction of inspired oxygen (FiO_2) of 70% and a positive end-expiratory pressure (PEEP) of 12 cm H_2O. Four days later, he has not improved, yet he is not likely to progress to brain death due to his decompression. The organ procurement organization wants to know if you think the patient is a good candidate for donation after circulatory determination of death. What is your appropriate response?

A. It would not be appropriate to comment; once a patient is a candidate for donation, the medical providers should no longer be involved in a patient's care.

B. Organ donation is not possible unless the patient is determined to be brain dead.

C. The patient has a reasonable chance of progressing to a cardiac death within 60 minutes after withdrawal of life-sustaining therapy; therefore, the patient is a good candidate.

D. Donation after circulatory determination of death can only occur if the patient is a registered organ donor.

E. Donation after cardiac death can only be performed if the patient progresses to cardiac death within 20 minutes after withdrawal of life-sustaining therapy.

4. A 78-year-old man who resides at an assisted living facility with mild dementia is brought to the hospital after discoloration is noted in his lower extremities. He is diagnosed with gangrene of the foot, and surgical amputation is recommended. He is confused to time but knows his name and that he is in a hospital. He can express an understanding of his new medical condition, understands the consequences of the disease and risks of surgery, and agrees to proceed with the amputation. His daughter, who is his legal medical power of attorney, arrives and tells you that she does not agree with the procedure and that he would not want to have the disability that would come from the surgery and believes antibiotics to be "mostly poisonous anyway." What is the best thing to do?

A. Proceed with surgery without informing the daughter

B. Cancel the surgery since the daughter has medical power of attorney

C. Transfer the patient to the service of another physician

D. Inform the daughter that her father has decisional capacity and proceed with surgery

E. Consult with psychiatry on a routine basis to evaluate the patient's dementia

5. An 82-year-old man with glioblastoma multiforme has undergone surgical resection as well as radiation and chemotherapy. He currently lives in a skilled nursing facility and has been suffering from seizures and loss of independence. He told his oncologist that he does not want to continue to suffer and that, if the time came, he would want to pass in peace. He has completed a valid out-of-hospital DNR/do not intubate (DNI) form supported by state law and hospital policy. One morning, the patient is found down at the nursing home and is brought to the ED, where he is found to have agonal breathing. While the emergency physician is preparing to intubate the patient, a nurse who is familiar with the patient from previous ED encounters brings to the physician's attention the out-of-hospital DNR/DNI form, which was sent with the patient to the hospital. The physician is unfamiliar with the form and reluctant to abide by it. What is the best course of action?

A. Intubate the patient until you can verify the status and his wishes with the family

B. Do not intubate the patient and contact his family to verify his wishes

C. Consult with the ethics committee in the hospital and defer any action until they are available

D. Intubate the patient first to secure his airway and then call the patient's primary doctor and verify the status

E. Call the in-house intensivist to evaluate the patient's respiratory status and need for intubation

6. A 28-year-old comatose male is brought to the ED after a motorcycle accident. He is found on CT imaging to have an unstable fracture of C1 with distraction injury. Neurosurgery recommends emergent surgical stabilization as there is a bone fragment that is displaced and in high proximity to the spinal cord. The patient is not accompanied by any family and only found to have an expired library card in his wallet. While social work is unable to find a next of kin, the police officer who is accompanying the patient is working on investigating the matter. What is the best way to proceed for surgical consent in this situation?

A. Proceed with surgery with the assumption of emergency consent

B. Contact the hospital ethics department to obtain assistance with the appointment of a legal guardian

C. Do not proceed with surgery; since the risk of surgery is high, written informed consent is necessary

D. Perform a "2-doctor consent"; 2 concurring physicians can always preclude the preference of a patient or their surrogate, thus circumventing the need for informed consent

E. Postpone surgery until family can be located

7. You are working in the neuro-ICU when a 57-year-old man is brought to the ED after a collapse at home. He has history of hypertension, diabetes, and atrial fibrillation for which he is on rivaroxaban. He is found to have an acute left subcortical intracerebral hemorrhage, associated with hydrocephalus, midline shift, and subfalcine herniation. At 2:00 a.m., neurosurgery consultation is called for an emergent decompression. You notice the surgeon has slurred speech, appears disinhibited, is staggering in his steps, and smells of alcohol. You ask him if he has been drinking, and he responds with a snarky glare and says that he only had "a couple or five drinks" and can handle the surgery. You are concerned about the safety of the patient and the surgeon's condition and know that a backup neurosurgeon is immediately available. What should you do?

A. Confront the surgeon, and prevent him from taking the patient to the operating room and instead call the backup surgeon

B. Call the in-house administrative supervisor and anonymously report your concerns, knowing that the surgery will have already begun operating

C. Do nothing; it is none of your business, and he is the one responsible for his actions

D. Report him via email to the state medical board in the morning and do not interfere otherwise

E. Report the physician the next day to chief of surgery at the hospital

8. A 63-year-old man is admitted to the neuro-ICU for treatment of an acute intracerebral hemorrhage found on CT after an episode of sudden headache and dizziness. On the second day of hospitalization, he is minimally arousable. Repeat CT shows increased edema around the hemorrhage and new associated hydrocephalus that requires placement of an external ventricular drain. He is accompanied in the hospital by his wife, uncle, and 2 adult children. He has assigned his eldest son, who is a medical resident, as his medical power of attorney. The patient's wife does not agree with the plan of care proposed by the rest of the family. Who is the best person to give consent for the procedure for this patient?

   A. Obtain consent from the wife, as she is next of kin.

   B. Obtain consent from the eldest son and offer the rest of the family a chance to ask questions and give their opinion.

   C. Ask the family to reach an agreement and obtain collective consent.

   D. No consent is needed; it is a bedside procedure that is commonly done in this ICU.

   E. No consent is needed, since you are very good at this procedure and no complications are expected.

9. An 87-year-old man who resides at a skilled nursing facility has acute respiratory distress, volume overload, hyperkalemia, and severe acidosis with an arterial pH of 7.1. The patient has end-stage kidney disease and has refused dialysis in the past. Nephrology consultation recommends to the patient urgent hemodialysis, which he refuses. He has decision-making capacity as evidenced by his understanding of the consequences of refusing this treatment, including death. He appears to be content with his decision and is not depressed. He reports that he has expected this from his long illness and is at peace with his fate and that he has had a long and fruitful life. Which of the following is the most appropriate management of this patient?

   A. Start dialysis and consult with the hospital's ethics department regarding this matter as the patient's decision might be an attempt at suicide

   B. Document in the chart the medical need for hemodialysis, and perform a "2-doctor" consent to override the patient's preference

   C. Call in the patient's son and discuss with him the need for the treatment to help pressure him to make the right decision

   D. Do not start hemodialysis without the patient's consent

   E. Consult psychiatry for an emergent hold for suicidality

10. The nurse calls the on-call resident to report a low serum potassium level. The resident informs the nurse that he will order a potassium replacement. Two hours later, with no replacement ordered, the nurse calls the resident again. He is surprised and says that he placed the medication order more than an hour ago. Looking back, he discovers that he placed the order in the chart of the wrong patient who has a normal potassium level and the erroneous dose was already given. Immediate recheck shows a high potassium level after replacement, and medical therapy is ordered to lower it back to normal level. No other adverse impact occurs to either patient. What is appropriate for the resident to do regarding reporting this error?

   A. The resident should report the error to his attending and not inform the quality improvement team or risk management.

   B. The resident should involve risk management or patient safety and report the error to the patient including the corrective measures that were taken.

   C. The resident should not report the error as no injury occurred.

   D. The resident should insist that the error belongs to the nurse for not checking the potassium level before administering the medication to the wrong patient.

   E. The resident should blame the pharmacy for not verifying the order.

11. You are taking care of a patient who was diagnosed with multiple sclerosis 5 years ago. He failed multiple treatment regimens in the early months of treatment, but he is now controlled with glatiramer acetate and has needed steroid therapy for exacerbation 2 times in the past 6 months. You are invited to attend a dinner for a pharmaceutical company promoting a newly approved medication for multiple sclerosis. The representative asks you if you can prescribe the medication for your patients to help

promote the medication and states that you would be compensated through "an extra hefty honorarium." What is the best way to proceed?

A. Prescribe the medication, since there is no harm and it can potentially benefit your relationship with the pharmaceutical company

B. Do not prescribe the medication under any circumstances since you ethically disagree with the marketing agenda

C. Prescribe the medication, but inform the patient that you received promotion funds from the manufacturer

D. Only prescribe the medication if you clinically think it is in the patient's best interest and avoid a quid pro quo relationship with the pharmaceutical company

E. Request a higher compensation for prescribing the medication, as doing so places you at risk of being criticized

12. A 34-year-old man is admitted to the neuro-ICU after being found down for an extended period of time (possibly 2 days). He is found on imaging to have a Hunt and Hess grade 5 subarachnoid hemorrhage (SAH) from a large basilar tip aneurysm with associated intraventricular hemorrhage and hydrocephalus and herniation of the cerebellar tonsils. On examination, he has fixed dilated pupils, no corneal response, and a weak cough and is overbreathing the ventilator. Motor exam shows extensor posturing. He is in shock on 2 vasopressors, and an external ventricular drain is placed, which shows high intracranial pressures in the 60s and bright red cerebrospinal fluid. The family asks to repair the aneurysm to reverse the damage so he can have a functional recovery. What is the best course of action?

A. Proceed with surgery and invasive medical measures as requested by the family as their autonomy requires that we follow the valid surrogate's direction

B. Explain to the family that surgery would not help achieve their goals for the patient and may lead to his demise

C. Inform the family that surgery is not indicated but you can transfer the patient to another facility that might be able to help

D. Perform the procedure as long as the patient has insurance that will pay for the procedure

E. Perform the procedure since it would serve as a training experience for your residents

13. A 61-year-old man is admitted to the ICU with status epilepticus not responsive to first-line therapy. He is intubated for airway protection. Upon further evaluation, he is found to have stage IV lung cancer with brain metastases and has failed surgical treatment as well as chemotherapy and radiotherapy over the past 2 years. He has been on dexamethasone and levetiracetam at home for 3 weeks and has been having 4 to 5 seizures daily. After several days in the ICU, he fails to have significant improvement and the family requests stopping aggressive life-supportive measures and only want comfort-directed care to be provided. The patient is terminally extubated and started on morphine infusion for comfort. His blood pressure is 87/40 mm Hg, heart rate is in the 120s, and he is breathing heavily at 32 breaths/min. What is the most appropriate management of the patient's condition?

A. Increase the rate of the morphine to achieve comfort and relieve pain without concern for hypotension

B. Avoid higher doses of opiates since they can worsen hypotension and hasten death for the patient

C. Add a paralytic to avoid the family having to watch the patient's distress

D. The patient should have been started on both morphine and midazolam drips before extubation at a high enough rate to preclude any potential sign of distress

E. Start a saline fluid infusion to counteract the hypotension and stop the morphine as comfort care cannot be provided if it expedites a patient's demise

Answers and Explanations

1. C. Neurologic prognostication after catastrophic brain injury should be postponed until at least 72 hours from the injury. It is recommended by the Neurocritical Care Society guidelines that such evaluation be based on repeated examinations over time to establish increased accuracy and that treatment should be directed to maintain physiologic stability and avoid deterioration to allow sufficient opportunity for prognostic evaluation. The society recommends using a 72-hour observation period to determine clinical response and delaying decisions regarding withdrawal of life-sustaining treatment in the interim. Exceptions can of course be made, if, for example, the patient would have preferred to have been DNR before being resuscitated by medical providers who are not aware of a previously established patient preference of advance directives.

2. B. The Uniform Determination of Death Act defines death by (1) irreversible loss of circulatory and respiratory function and (2) irreversible loss of all functions of the entire brain. The dead donor rule requires that death be declared before recovery of organs. Stated another way, the recovery of organs cannot be the proximate cause of death. This separation is meant to avoid the appearance of a conflict of interest that medical care is not being provided to favor organ recovery rather than improvement of the patient's health.

Since the patient has not progressed to brain death, the only situation that allows organ donation to occur is if it is done after declaration of circulatory death after withdrawal of life-supporting measures. The only instance in which a patient might be taken for organ procurement before cardiac death is after the declaration of brain death. Living organ donation (ie, single kidney or partial liver) is consistent with the dead donor rule as the organs recovered in these circumstances will not lead to the donor's demise.

3. C. This patient has not shown signs of progression to brain death. For donation after circulatory determination of death to occur, the patient must be expected to progress to cardiac arrest within 60 minutes of withdrawal of life-sustaining therapy. If the patient is expected to sustain cardiac function and respiration without supportive measures for a longer time, that would exclude the patient from being a candidate. A lack of corneal or gag response is a predictor of death before 60 minutes, as is a high oxygenation index (OI = [$FiO_2 \times$ Mpaw]/PaO_2), where Mpaw is mean airway pressure and PaO_2 is partial pressure of oxygen.

Regarding choice A, a patient is still under the medical provider's care until a declaration of death has been made; although the provider should not approach a family about donation, medical providers are permitted to discuss the case with the organ procurement organization.

4. D. While cognitive impairment may preclude medical decision-making capacity, such is not always the case. A very specific set of criteria must be met to have decisional capacity. Rather than just assessing a person's orientation and alertness, criteria for capacity should be analyzed. Patients must be able to (1) understand the situation, the extent of their illness, and the risks and benefits of treatments; (2) have a value system by which they are basing their decision; (3) apply a rational thought process to their decision making that is aligned with their value system; (4) have a means of communicating their preferences. A useful mnemonic for remembering these criteria is CURVES: **C**hoose and Communicate, **U**nderstand, **R**eason, **V**alue, **E**mergency, **S**urrogate.

Regarding surrogate decision makers (including those appointed as medical power of attorney), they only assume the role of decision maker if the patient has been shown to lack decisional capacity.

At that point, they must also be shown to meet criteria for decisional capacity before they will be allowed to make decisions on another's behalf.

5. **B.** The existence of a valid out-of-hospital DNR order, in jurisdictions that allow for such documents, requires physicians to respect the directive of the document and abide by the indicated patient preferences even if they themselves have not addressed the subject directly with patients. It is incumbent on each medical practitioner to be familiar with the hospital policies regarding emergency care, and lack of familiarity does not justify ignoring a valid patient preference. In this case, verification with a nurse who has previous experience with the patient corroborates a decision to not intubate. Knowingly performing a procedure against an expressed wish of a patient could lead to legal charges or a complaint to a regulatory board.

6. **A.** In the setting of an emergency where there is imminent risk of significant morbidity or mortality and the patient lacks decision-making capacity and a surrogate is not immediately available, the presumption is made that the average rational person would accept the risk needed to prevent the harm. While obtaining an ethics or risk management consult to initiate the appointment of a legal guardian might be appropriate in some circumstances, it will not occur quickly enough to meet the emergent needs of the situation.

   If time permits, informed consent should be obtained, which requires the following elements:

   - Patient or surrogate must have decisional capacity.
   - The nature of the decision/procedure must be clearly expressed.
   - Reasonable alternatives to the proposed intervention should be explained.
   - The relevant risks, benefits, and uncertainties related to each alternative must be communicated.
   - An assessment of the patient's understanding should be performed.

   While more invasive procedures often require the completion of a template written consent document, the conversation detailing the above criteria is more important.

7. **A.** Each physician has an obligation to put patient safety first, even if interceding might be unpleasant or lead to conflict. While choices B, D, and E may be valid if the surgeon was not placing a patient in immediate harm, a delay in this scenario poses a significant risk. Most institutional ethics and compliance departments provide access to an anonymous compliance line to avoid concern for retribution.

8. **B.** In this situation, the eldest son is the designated medical power of attorney named by the patient. His designation would make him the legal decision maker over the wife, who would be considered the next of kin in the absence of that designation. State law varies on the order of surrogate decision maker if there is no medical power of attorney. Often, the next of kid would be determined as follows in this order: spouse, adult children, parents, siblings, and then closest living relative. If no living relatives are available, a chaplain or close friends may be considered to provide alternative consent, depending on jurisdiction and hospital policy.

   The underlying principle is *substituted judgement*: the surrogate is required to make a decision that is in line with what the patient would most likely choose for himself or herself. If medical providers suspect that a decision is being made for ulterior motives or is not in line with the patient's previously expressed wishes, an ethics consult would be helpful in providing clarification.

9. **D.** Since the patient is refusing life-prolonging treatment, the physician must assess if the patient is making an informed decision based on an acceptance of an irreversible life-limiting illness, or if there is concern that treatment refusal is a suicidal attempt based on a severe depression. In light of the patient's lack of clinical depression, long-standing illness that is inherently life limiting, and relative higher risk of treatment with dialysis, the patient's decision should be respected. A comparable example where depression might be leading to a suicide attempt might be a young person who intentionally consumed massive amounts of potassium and who needs emergent dialysis.

10. **B.** Voluntary error reporting is integral to the safety improvement strategy of any institution.

The vast majority of errors result in no harm or have only very minimal temporary effects. Reporting errors, as well as disclosing them to the patients involved, allows for the opportunity to improve on existing processes to reduce the risk that errors will be repeated. A "just culture" of patient safety emphasizes both the importance of improvement as well as transparency. The majority of medical errors involve multiple system failures; not only did the physician make an error in this scenario, but both the nurse administering potassium to a patient without a deficit and the pharmacy not correctly verifying the order did not prevent the incorrect treatment.

11. **D.** The fiduciary relationship requires that physicians make decisions based on the best interests of the patient. Providing a new medical therapy for personal financial benefit that may be of less value to the patient is a direct violation of this principle. While receiving compensation for speaking on behalf of a pharmaceutical company is commonly practiced and justifiable, the pharmaceutical representative in this case is clearly establishing that the practitioner will be compensated not for his or her time or effort in a speaking role but for switching patients to the new medication. This violation should also be reported to the appropriate authorities.

12. **B.** Treatment of the aneurysm in this situation fulfills the definition of physiologic futility. The goal of aneurysm treatment would be to prevent further rupture and worsening in the patient's medical status. Considering the severity of the hemorrhage, poor neurologic exam, and the extended time to evaluation at hospital, the patient may not even survive such a procedure, and it would have no reasonable potential to reverse the existing damage. While repair of the same aneurysm in a patient with a better exam who has presented to the hospital earlier may also have a low chance of promoting improvement in the patient, such therapy would likely be categorized as a "potentially inappropriate treatment." Patients do have a right to choose from all reasonable available therapies, but physicians must practice some judgement to not offer interventions that lack a prospect of benefit. Available patient funding and the training opportunity should have no influence on an evaluation of the appropriateness of an intervention.

13. **A.** The doctrine of double effect morally permits an adverse secondary effect if the primary intent is a moral good and the secondary effect is proportionate. In the case of a patient with a life-limiting illness whose demise is inevitable, providing opioids for symptom relief is permitted, even if it may expedite the patient's death. The medication must be given in response to distress and not because of the *potential* for distress. Choices C and D do not allow for an assessment of the patient's need of treatment, and choices B and E incorrectly claim that the adverse effect of opioids must be avoided.

REFERENCES

Bosslet GT, Pope TM, Rubenfeld GD, et al. An official ATS/AACN/ACCP/ESICM/SCCM policy statement: responding to requests for potentially inappropriate treatments in intensive care units. American Thoracic Society ad hoc Committee on Futile and Potentially Inappropriate Treatment. *Am J Respir Crit Care Med.* 2015;191:1318-1330.

Chow GV, Czarny MJ, Huges MT, et al. CURVES: a mnemonic for determining medical decision-making capacity and providing emergency treatment in the acute setting. *Chest.* 2010;137:421-427.

Joint Position Statement of the American College of Emergency Physicians, the National Association of EMS Physicians®, the Air Medical Physician Association, the Association of Air Medical Services, and the National Association of State EMS Officials. Code of Ethics for Emergency Physicians. *Ann Emerg Med.* 2008;52:581-590.

Rabinstein AA, Yee AH, Mandrekar J, et al. Prediction of potential for organ donation after cardiac death in patients in neurocritical state: a prospective observational study. *Lancet Neurol.* 2012;11:414-419.

Richardson WC, Berwick DM, Bisgard JC. The Institute of Medicine report on medical errors. *N Engl J Med.* 2000;343:663-665.

Robertson JA. Delimiting the donor: the dead donor rule. *Hastings Center Report.* 1999;29:6-14.

Snyder L, American College of Physicians Ethics, Professionalism, and Human Rights Committee. American College of Physicians Ethics Manual: sixth edition. *Ann Intern Med.* 2012;156:73-104.

Souter MJ, Blissitt PA, Blosser S, et al. Recommendations for the critical care management of devastating brain injury: prognostication, psychosocial, and ethical management. *Neurocrit Care.* 2015;23:4-13.

PART 7
Case Vignettes

36

Case Vignettes

CLINICAL CASE VIGNETTE 1: POSTPARTUM ISCHEMIC STROKE

Rajan Gadhia, MD and Annesh B. Singhal, MD

History of Present Illness

A 42-year-old woman presented to our hospital's emergency department (ED) 3.5 hours after the onset of acute neck pain and left-sided face, arm, and leg weakness. She was 10 days postpartum after cesarean delivery of twins. She had had an uncomplicated full-term pregnancy; however, since day 3 after delivery, she had developed intermittent hypertension and headache that did not respond to labetalol treatment.

Exam

On arrival to the ED, the temperature was 37.2°C (98.9°F), blood pressure was 162/63 mm Hg, heart rate was 80 bpm, and respiratory rate was 22 breaths/min. She was alert and able to follow commands. She had a right gaze preference and left-sided neglect. There was dysarthria but no aphasia. Her pupils were normal in size, symmetric, and reactive to light and accommodation. Bilateral ptosis was present. The extraocular movements were intact. Motor exam showed left lower facial weakness and 2/5 strength in the left upper and bilateral lower limbs. She had decreased pinprick and light touch sensations on the left hemibody. The left-sided muscle reflexes were brisk, and left Babinski sign was present. The total National Institutes of Health Stroke Scale (NIHSS) score was 14. She underwent urgent brain imaging and was transferred to the neurocritical care unit for further management.

WHAT IS THE DIFFERENTIAL DIAGNOSIS?

The neurologic deficits (left hemiparesis and neglect and right gaze deviation) localize to the right cerebral hemisphere with cortical involvement. Given the abrupt onset, vascular lesions (ischemic or hemorrhagic stroke) are highest on the differential. Given her postpartum state, cerebral venous sinus thrombosis should be considered. The 1-week history of hypertension and headache prior to onset raises concern for postpartum preeclampsia with the posterior reversible encephalopathy syndrome (PRES). Demyelinating conditions and an underlying mass lesion causing a focal seizure with post-ictal Todd paralysis are less likely possibilities.

WHAT IS THE MOST APPROPRIATE INITIAL DIAGNOSTIC TEST?

Since the time from symptom onset to hospital arrival was within 4.5 hours (ie, within the time window for acute stroke treatment with intravenous thrombolysis), the most appropriate diagnostic test would be an urgent head computed tomography (CT) with CT angiography (CTA) of the head and neck arteries. Brain magnetic resonance imaging (MRI) with magnetic resonance angiography is usually more time consuming but can be considered after the CT (or instead of the CT) to more accurately delineate the ischemic lesion and enable decision making about intra-arterial clot retrieval, which

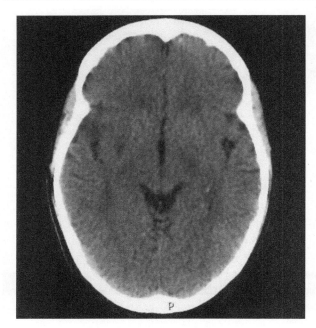

Figure 36.1-1 Initial noncontrast head computed tomography.

is another effective and approved treatment for acute ischemic stroke.

RESULTS

The head CT showed subtle hypodensity and loss of gray-white differentiation in the right insula and basal ganglia (Fig. 36.1-1). Arterial imaging findings were

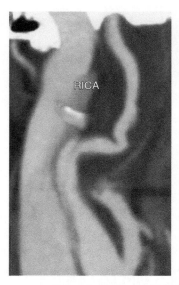

Figure 36.1-3 Computed tomography angiography of neck: right common carotid artery and right internal carotid artery (RICA) dissection with mild to moderate stenosis.

suggestive of multiple neck artery dissections: a right internal carotid artery (ICA) dissection with moderate luminal stenosis and no associated thrombus, a left ICA dissection with occlusion, and bilateral vertebral artery dissections without focal stenosis (Figs. 36.1-2 and 36.1-3). The intracranial arteries were patent without evidence for embolic occlusion in the proximal circle of Willis arteries. A brain MRI showed acute infarction involving the right middle cerebral artery (MCA) territory (Fig. 36.1-4).

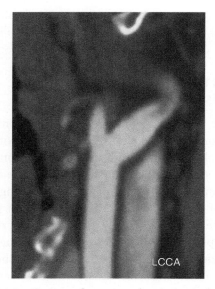

Figure 36.1-2 Computed tomography angiography of neck: left common carotid artery (LCCA) and left internal carotid artery dissection with occlusion.

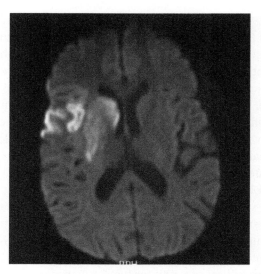

Figure 36.1-4 Magnetic resonance imaging of the brain showing an acute infarction in the right middle cerebral artery territory.

WHAT IS THE MOST APPROPRIATE ACUTE AND CHRONIC TREATMENT?

Given her recent cesarean section, the patient was deemed ineligible for intravenous thrombolysis with tissue plasminogen activator (tPA). Intra-arterial thrombectomy was not offered given the absence of embolic occlusion in the culprit arteries and the presence of arterial dissections (which confer high procedural risk). After a discussion with the patient, her family, and the acute stroke team, the patient was treated with intravenous unfractionated heparin.

Treatment of dissection for the purpose of primary or secondary stroke prevention has remained a controversial topic among vascular neurologists worldwide. The recently published CADISS trial compared the safety and efficacy of antiplatelet therapy compared to anticoagulation for secondary prevention of stroke. A total of 250 subjects (118 carotid and 132 vertebral artery dissections) were included, and 126 were randomized to antiplatelets and 124 to anticoagulation at an average of 3.65 days after symptom onset. A total of 4 strokes occurred in the 3-month follow-up period, 3 in the antiplatelet arm and 1 in the anticoagulation arm. One patient in the anticoagulation arm developed subarachnoid hemorrhage. On the basis of these data, most clinicians today prefer antiplatelet agents as chronic treatment for spontaneous extracranial cervical artery dissection.

It should be noted that randomization in the CADISS trial occurred a few days after onset, so anticoagulation (eg, intravenous heparin) may still be useful to prevent ischemic stroke in the first 4 days when stroke risk is highest in such patients. Furthermore, our patient had multiple dissections including acute contralateral arterial occlusion, which poses a higher risk for thromboembolism. Hence, our patient was treated with intravenous heparin in the acute stage.

OUTCOME

The patient remained stable with no further infarcts. Her clinical deficits resolved, except for residual facial paresis. The NIHSS score improved from 14 to 2 within 3 days. Intravenous heparin was discontinued, and she was discharged on therapeutic anticoagulation with subcutaneous enoxaparin. We planned to continue enoxaparin for 3 months, repeat vascular imaging, and switch to long-term aspirin unless there was a significant residual luminal narrowing or other high-risk features for thromboembolism.

WHAT IS YOUR FINAL DIAGNOSIS?

- Acute ischemic stroke with 4-vessel dissection

REFERENCE

CADISS Trial Investigators, Markus HS, Hayter E, et al. Antiplatelet treatment compared with anticoagulation treatment for cervical artery dissection (CADISS): a randomised trial. *Lancet Neurol.* 2015;14:361-367.

CLINICAL CASE VIGNETTE 2: WORSENING FOLLOWING CAROTID ENDARTERECTOMY

Daniel B. Rubin, MD, PhD, Saef Izzy, MD, and Guy Rordorf, MD

History of Present Illness

A 61-year-old woman with a history of hypertension, alcohol abuse, and a 50-pack-year smoking history presented to the emergency department with language deficits and subtle right-sided weakness for the past 2 weeks. The patient had been having difficulty participating in conversation, getting easily frustrated and frequently seeming confused. In addition, she noted that for the past 10 days she has been having difficulty moving her right side. On exam in the emergency department, she had deficits in naming and reading, had frequent word-finding difficulties, and could not follow 2-step commands. A mild right hemiparesis was appreciated as well. She underwent a magnetic resonance imaging (MRI) scan of the brain that demonstrated scattered foci of restricted diffusion throughout the left hemisphere of varying age (Fig. 36.2-1).

A subsequently computed tomography (CT) angiogram (CTA) of the head and neck demonstrated critical stenosis (99%) of the proximal left internal carotid artery (Fig. 36.2-2).

The patient was started on a continuous infusion of unfractionated heparin and was admitted to the inpatient neurology service. The vascular surgery service was consulted, and the following day, the patient was taken for an urgent left carotid endarterectomy.

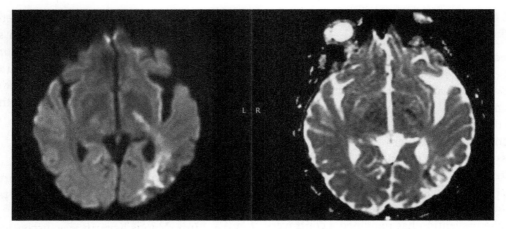

Figure 36.2-1 Magnetic resonance imaging of the brain, axial view, diffusion-weighted imaging and apparent diffusion coefficient sequences, showing scattered foci of restricted diffusion throughout the left hemisphere of varying age.

Preoperative National Institutes of Health Stroke Scale (NIHSS) score was 3 (1 point for right-sided weakness, 2 points for aphasia). Postoperatively, she was admitted to the surgical intensive care unit (ICU) for hemodynamic monitoring. Her postoperative NIHSS assessment was unchanged. She was started on aspirin 325 mg orally once a day for secondary stroke prevention. In the afternoon of postoperative day 4, the patient was found by her nurse to have suffered a sudden decline in clinical status, and the acute stroke team was activated.

Exam

At the time of postoperative day 4 acute stroke team evaluation, her temperature was 36.8°C (98.2°F),

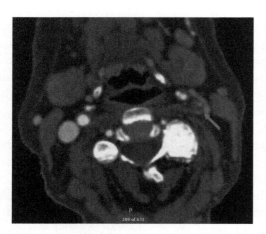

Figure 36.2-2 Computed tomography angiography of the neck showing critical stenosis (99%) of the proximal left internal carotid artery (*arrow*).

blood pressure was 212/109 mm Hg, heart rate was 78 bpm, and oxygen saturation was 97% on room air. Neurologic exam at that time was significant for global aphasia; the patient was awake and mute and followed no commands. The patient had a left-gaze preference and a right facial droop and could not move her right arm or leg. The NIHSS score was 18.

WHAT IS THE DIFFERENTIAL DIAGNOSIS?

Given the abrupt onset of neurologic symptoms referable to the left hemisphere, a vascular complication of the carotid endarterectomy must be considered. Acute stroke in the perioperative period occurs in approximately 3% to 6% of patients in trials of endarterectomy for symptomatic carotid disease; ischemic stroke after endarterectomy can occur due to atheroembolism from the operated vessel, in situ thrombus formation with subsequent embolization or acute vessel occlusion, or arterial dissection. When endarterectomy is performed in the urgent setting after acute stroke, hemorrhagic transformation must be considered as well. The patient's markedly elevated blood pressure raises the possibility of postrevascularization cerebral hyperperfusion syndrome. Similarly, cerebral hypoperfusion is an important cause of perioperative neurologic injury in carotid revascularization procedures, although this would be less likely to occur 4 days postoperatively and would be unlikely in the setting of elevated blood pressure. Because symptom onset was unwitnessed, focal or generalized seizure with subsequent postictal Todd paresis or ongoing nonconvulsive seizure activity should be on the differential as well.

WHAT WOULD YOU ORDER NEXT?

The patient was taken for a stat CT/CTA of the head and neck, which demonstrated no evidence of intracerebral hemorrhage or high-grade occlusion of either the intracranial or extracranial vasculature. As the patient was being transferred out of the CT scanner, she experienced a generalized convulsion lasting approximately 1 minute, which devolved into persistent right hemibody rhythmic shaking.

HOW WOULD YOU MANAGE THIS PATIENT GOING FORWARD?

The patient was treated immediately with 2 doses of intravenous (IV) lorazepam and was transferred to the neuro-ICU for further care. On arrival to the neuro-ICU, she was found to have ongoing right hemibody shaking and persistently altered mentation. She was treated with additional doses of IV lorazepam and 2000 mg of IV levetiracetam, with subsequent cessation of shaking movements. She was placed on continuous electro-encephalogram (EEG) monitoring that demonstrated ongoing left-sided lateralized periodic discharges but no evidence of seizure activity. A repeat MRI was obtained that showed a confluent region of T2/fluid-attenuated inversion recovery (FLAIR) hyperintensity throughout the left anterior cerebral artery (ACA) and middle cerebral artery (MCA) territories but no new foci of restricted diffusion, consistent with diffuse cerebral edema (Fig. 36.2-3). The patient's blood pressure was controlled with a continuous infusion of IV nicardipine for a goal systolic blood pressure <140 mm Hg. She was started on 750 mg of IV levetiracetam twice daily and standing methylprednisolone. Starting steroids is a controversial decision to treat this pathology and lacks strong literature support. Over the next 2 days, the patient's neurologic exam slowly improved toward baseline.

DISCUSSION

Cerebral hyperperfusion complicates approximately 1% of carotid endarterectomy cases. The classic triad of findings in this syndrome include focal neurologic deficits with or without ipsilateral headache, seizure, and intraparenchymal hemorrhage; severe cases can involve depressed level of consciousness or even coma. The mechanism underlying hyperperfusion syndrome is incompletely understood but is thought to be due to a preoperative loss of autoregulatory vasoreactivity in the cerebral arterial bed as a result of

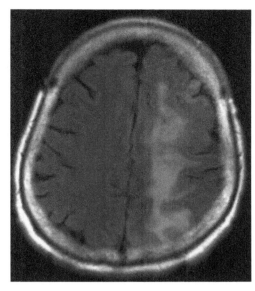

Figure 36.2-3 Magnetic resonance imaging of the brain, axial view, fluid-attenuated inversion recover (FLAIR) sequence, showing T2/FLAIR hyperintensity throughout the left anterior cerebral artery and middle cerebral artery territories.

chronic hypoperfusion. To maintain adequate perfusion in the setting of poor cerebral blood flow, arteries downstream from a highly stenotic carotid artery become tonically dilated. When the vascular territory is then reperfused by either carotid endarterectomy or stenting, the distal vasculature, which has lost its normal vasoreactivity, is unable to compensate for the increased blood flow, and the elevated cerebral perfusion causes breakdown of the blood-brain barrier with resultant neurologic dysfunction. CT scan may or may not demonstrate petechial hemorrhage or frank intraparenchymal hematoma. MRI typically demonstrates increased T2/FLAIR signal in the affected hemisphere without restricted diffusion, a pattern consistent with vasogenic edema similar to that observed in posterior reversible encephalopathy syndrome (PRES). If obtained, perfusion-weighted imaging demonstrates relative hyperperfusion of the affected hemisphere, as expected.

The highest risk time period for hyperperfusion syndrome is 2 to 7 days postoperatively. Patients at greatest risk for cerebral hyperperfusion syndrome include those with a long-standing, high-grade carotid stenosis (typically >80%), an arterially isolated cerebral hemisphere, and reperfusion surgery immediately after acute stroke. Elevated blood pressure is thought to be a proximate trigger, and so blood pressure should be monitored closely and aggressively controlled in the postoperative period to prevent the development of hyperperfusion. Once symptoms emerge, blood pressure control remains the mainstay of treatment. The specific agent best suited for blood pressure control in the setting of hyperperfusion is unclear; experts in the field advocate against the use of antihypertensives with direct cerebral vasodilatory effects, such as sodium nitroprusside or dihydropyridine calcium channel blockers, although there is no direct evidence guiding this decision making. Beyond the recommendation for aggressive blood pressure control, there exist no specific guidelines covering the use of direct monitoring of cerebral blood flow via transcranial Doppler ultrasound (TCD) or single-photon emission CT.

Seizures should be controlled using antiepileptic drugs (AEDs). There is no consensus on the need for long-term AED therapy, but as seizures are provoked by the cerebral hyperemia, AEDs can likely be discontinued following resolution of the clinical syndrome. Adjunctive treatments for cerebral edema, such as mannitol, hypertonic saline, and corticosteroids, are occasionally employed; however, there is a lack of robust evidence supporting their use. Depending on the presence of acute hemorrhage, antithrombotic regimen may need to be adjusted, and the precise timing of reinstituting

antiplatelet therapy in the setting of recent carotid intervention becomes an often challenging risk-benefit decision.

This patient was monitored in the neuro-ICU for 2 days before slowly returning to her preoperative baseline. Her antihypertensives were converted to an oral regimen prior to transfer out of the ICU, and her AEDs were subsequently discontinued on discharge.

WHAT IS YOUR FINAL DIAGNOSIS?

- Postrevascularization hyperperfusion syndrome

REFERENCES

Bouri S, Thapar A, Shalhoub J, et al. Hypertension and the post-carotid endarterectomy cerebral hyperperfusion syndrome. *Eur J Vasc Endovasc Surg.* 2011;41(2):229-237.

Karapanayiotides T, Meuli R, Devuyst G, et al. Postcarotid endarterectomy hyperperfusion or reperfusion syndrome. *Stroke.* 2005;36(1):21-26.

Wu TY, Anderson NE, Barber PA. Neurological complications of carotid revascularisation. *J Neurol Neurosurg Psychiatry.* 2012;83:543-550.

CLINICAL CASE VIGNETTE 3: RAPIDLY PROGRESSIVE QUADRAPLEGIA

Feras Akbik, MD, PhD, Starane Anthony Shepherd, MD, and Saef Izzy, MD

History of Present Illness

A 56-year-old woman with a history of left multifocal ductal carcinoma in situ breast cancer, status post bilateral mastectomies 11 years prior, diverticulitis, and ileostomy for bowel perforation presented with sudden-onset neck pain, paresthesia, and weakness. The patient was at home when she experienced acute onset of intense occipital and neck pain. The pain was quickly followed by bilateral upper extremity paresthesia with an unclear distribution. She presented to a local emergency department (ED) and, by arrival, had begun to develop bilateral upper extremity weakness. On presentation to the ED, she syncopized and required emergent intubation due to acute respiratory failure. During this intubation, she became severely bradycardic, and 0.5 mg of atropine was administered. There was a total of 3 hours between the initial prodrome of pain and flaccid quadriplegia. She was then transferred to a tertiary center with a neurocritical care unit for further management.

Exam

Vital signs on arrival to the unit were notable for a temperature of 37.6°C, blood pressure of 90/50 mm Hg, heart rate of 37 bpm, and respiratory rate of 16 breaths/min. She was on volume control ventilation at a rate of 22 with a tidal volume of 350 mL, positive end-expiratory pressure of 8 cm H_2O, and fraction of inspired oxygen of 40%. Her systemic exam was unremarkable. She could nod and communicate via yes/no questions. Cranial nerves were intact. Motor exam was notable for flaccid quadriplegia in all 4 extremities. She had diminished neck flexion and neck extension (2/5). Pinprick and temperature sensation were diminished at a level of C5 on the left upper and lower extremities and preserved on the right hemibody. Vibratory sensation was preserved throughout. Reflexes were 2+ throughout. Toes were mute. Rectal tone was absent.

WHAT IS THE DIFFERENTIAL DIAGNOSIS?

The patient presents with acute-onset quadriplegia with intact cranial nerves and mental status. The spared cranial nerves and involvement of all 4 limbs localizes to a high cervical lesion of extrinsic or intrinsic etiology. The exam localizes to an anterior cord syndrome, involving predominantly motor fibers, asymmetric involvement of the spinothalamic fibers, and relative sparing of the posterior columns. Spinal cord infarction, given the acuity of the patient's presentation, and transverse myelitis should be considered as the most likely diagnoses. However, in the absence of supporting history, an acute cord compression syndrome must be considered and emergently assessed to determine if neurosurgical intervention is warranted.

HOW WOULD YOU APPROACH THE INITIAL DIAGNOSTIC EVALUATION?

Electrocardiogram (ECG) was notable for a junctional rhythm, with heart rates consistently in the 30s. Troponins were negative. The patient underwent a noncontrast head computed tomography (CT) scan, which was unrevealing. Magnetic resonance imaging (MRI) of the brain with contrast demonstrated rare nonspecific, nonenhancing subcortical T2 hyperintensities. CT angiogram of the head and neck revealed no evidence of dissection in the posterior circulation and no evidence of intracerebral arterial disease. An MRI of the cervical spine demonstrated a T2 hyperintense lesion in the ventral cord from C2-C4 with relative sparing of the posterior columns (Fig. 36.3-1). There was no

Differential Diagnoses of a Spinal Cord Lesion

VINDICATE:

- **V**ascular
  - Spinal cord infarction
  - Spinal vascular malformations
  - Vasculitis
- **I**nfectious
  - Viral, bacterial, fungal, parasitic
- **N**eoplastic
- **D**egenerative
- **I**atrogenic/Intoxication
  - Intrathecal chemotherapy
  - Organophosphate toxicity
  - Nitrous oxide
  - Neurolathyrism
  - Cassava (konzo)
- **C**ongenital/Inherited
  - Adrenomyeloneuropathy
  - Metachromatic leukodystrophy
- **A**utoimmune/Inflammatory
  - Transverse myelitis
  - Neuromyelitis optica
  - Multiple sclerosis
  - Sarcoidosis
- **T**raumatic
- **E**ndocrine/Metabolic/Nutritional
  - Vitamin B_{12} deficiency
  - Folate deficiency
  - Copper deficiency
  - Vitamin E deficiency

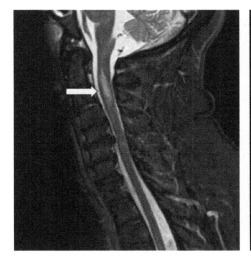 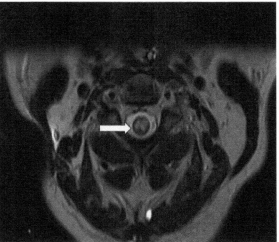

Figure 36.3-1 Magnetic resonance imaging of the cervical spine with and without contrast. T2 sequence in sagittal and axial planes showing hyperintense lesion in mostly ventral aspect of the cervical cord from C2-C4.

abnormal enhancement. The lesion exhibited restricted diffusion on diffusion-weighted imaging sequencing and was correspondingly hypointense on apparent diffusion coefficient sequencing. The thoracic spine MRI was unremarkable. Magnetic resonance angiography of the spine did not reveal a vascular abnormality. A lumbar puncture was performed, with 2 nucleated cells/microL in tube 4 and no red blood cells. Protein was 20.6 mg/dL; glucose was 145 mg/dL (serum glucose was 226).

HOW WOULD YOU APPROACH THE RADIOGRAPHIC FINDINGS?

The MRI results demonstrate a myelopathy of the upper cervical cord, corroborating the physical examination. The 2 likely diagnoses—spinal cord infarction and transverse myelitis—unfortunately have similar radiologic findings. Transverse myelitis can present with variable contrast enhancement characteristics, and lesions may be enhancing or nonenhancing. The differential diagnosis for transverse myelitis is quite broad and touches on innumerable nutritional, infectious, inflammatory, and neoplastic causes. The approach to transverse myelitis is simplified when the history, clinical time course, and presence of contrast enhancement on imaging are considered.

WHICH TREATMENT OPTIONS SHOULD BE CONSIDERED?

Corticosteroids do not play a role in the treatment of spinal cord infarction unless secondary to an inflammatory process such as vasculitis. However, because there were no contraindications to steroid therapy and due to the severity of the patient's presentation, the decision was made to administer intravenous methylprednisolone 1 g/d for a total of 3 days pending final cerebrospinal fluid (CSF) results.

Blood pressure augmentation to improve spinal cord perfusion was performed for 24 hours without any improvement seen in motor or sensory symptoms. CSF drainage via lumbar drain placement may also be considered in spinal cord infarction. CSF drainage is thought to remove resistance to microcirculatory flow and improve collateral vascular supply to the ischemic penumbra.

WHAT ARE THE NEXT MANAGEMENT STEPS?

Final CSF results did not indicate any underlying infectious or inflammatory process indicating a transverse myelitis; therefore, spinal cord infarction was thought to be the most likely diagnosis. Her ventilator support was

Diagnostic Studies to Consider in Transverse Myelitis

Serum Studies:
- Nutritional:
  - Zinc, copper, vitamin E, vitamin B_{12}
- Infectious:
  - Human immunodeficiency virus, rapid plasma reagin, Epstein-Barr virus (EBV), *Enterovirus* immunoglobulin (Ig) G/M, *Mycoplasma* IgG/M, hepatitis panel, HTLV-1 antibodies, Lyme enzyme-linked immunosorbent assay (ELISA)
  - Blood cultures
- Inflammatory:
  - Erythrocyte sedimentation rate, C-reactive protein, antinuclear antibodies, rheumatoid factor, angiotensin-converting enzyme (ACE), antineutrophil cytoplasmic antibodies, anti-Ro, anti-La, Neuromyelitis optica (NMO)
  - Chest x-ray
  - Consider computed tomography staging scans, positron emission tomography, and paraneoplastic panel
- Vascular:
  - Consider hypercoagulability profile

Cerebrospinal Fluid Studies:
- Routine studies including Gram stain, acid-fast bacilli smear and stain, India ink stain, and viral cultures
- Infectious:
  - Mycoplasma polymerase chain reaction (PCR), herpes simplex virus PCR, varicella-zoster virus PCR, *Enterovirus* PCR, EBV PCR, cytomegalovirus PCR, herpes 6/7 PCR, West Nile IgG/M, IgG/M, Lyme ELISA
- Inflammatory
  - ACE, oligoclonal bands
  - Consider paraneoplastic panel
- Neoplastic
  - Flow cytometry, cytology

Imaging:
- Magnetic resonance imaging (MRI) of brain
- MRI of cervical, thoracic spine
- Magnetic resonance angiography of spine
- Consider conventional spinal angiogram

weaned to pressure support ventilation, and she was discharged to a ventilator-dependent rehabilitation facility.

On further discussion with the patient's family, it was discovered that there was a family history of early miscarriages and a cerebral ischemic event in a family member at the age of 40. The patient's hypercoagulable panel demonstrated resistance to activated protein C, and direct genetic testing revealed that the patient was heterozygous for the factor V Leiden mutation. This mutation confers an increased risk of thrombosis. Because the patient had been discharged prior to these results, she was referred to hematology for follow-up and possible commencement of therapeutic anticoagulation.

OUTCOME

At the 2-month rehabilitation follow-up evaluation, patient was reported to be alert and oriented × 3. She was able to talk using tracheostomy valve. She was able to move her hands and her forearms in the range of 3/5. She was able to walk 12 feet with assistance. She passed the swallow test and was eating lunch with supervision.

WHAT IS YOUR FINAL DIAGNOSIS?

- Spinal cord infarction secondary to underlying hypercoagulable disorder

REFERENCES

Cheung AT, Pochettino A, McGarvey ML, et al. Strategies to manage paraplegia risk after endovascular stent repair of descending thoracic aortic aneurysms. *Ann Thorac Surg.* 2005;80(4):1280-1288.

Rabinstein AA. Vascular myelopathies. *Continuum (Minneap Minn).* 2015;21(1 Spinal Cord Disorders):67-83.

CLINICAL CASE VIGNETTE 4: KNOWN EPILEPSY PATIENT PRESENTING WITH STATUS EPILEPTICUS

Mohammad I. Hirzallah, MD, Manan Shah, MD, and Kiwon Lee, MD, FACP, FAHA, FCCM

History of Present Illness

A 42-year-old man with untreated epilepsy, alcohol abuse, alcoholic cirrhosis, and marijuana abuse presented with hematemesis. Emergency medical services estimated a total of 900 mL of frank blood in his emesis at the scene. On arrival to the emergency department, vitals were as follows: blood pressure 90/41 mm Hg, pulse 79 bpm, temperature 98.0°F, respiratory rate 26 breaths/min, and oxygen saturation of 98% on room air. Patient was jaundiced and continued to vomit bright red blood. He was started on a proton pump inhibitor infusion, octreotide, and ceftriaxone and transfused 2 units of packed red blood cells and 1 unit of fresh frozen plasma. He was emergently intubated and underwent emergent esophagogastroduodenoscopy (EGD) with hemostasis of a bleeding varix and a plan to repeat the EGD the following day.

His emergency department workup revealed an elevated gap metabolic acidosis, mild hyponatremia, acute kidney injury (creatinine 2.5 mg/dL; prior baseline 0.8 mg/dL), mild transaminitis (alanine aminotransferase 65 IU/L and aspartate aminotransferase 170 IU/L), and elevated total bilirubin of 20.2 mg/dL. A urine drug screen was positive for cannabinoid and benzodiazepine (patient had been discharged on a chlordiazepoxide taper). He had a coagulopathy with an elevated international normalized ratio (INR) of 2.1 and partial thromboplastin time (PTT) of 49 seconds. Chest x-ray demonstrated bibasilar atelectasis and a retrocardiac opacity.

On admission to the intensive care unit (ICU), the patient started having generalized tonic-clonic seizures despite being on a propofol infusion at 10 mg/kg/h for sedation.

WHAT ARE THE POTENTIAL UNDERLYING CAUSES OF SEIZURES IN THIS PATIENT?

Most adult-onset status epilepticus is secondary to an underlying symptomatic brain lesion, a toxic or metabolic disturbance, or medication non-compliance. Depending on the clinical scenario, workup for underlying etiology should be initiated as soon as possible in order to interrupt the seizure. This would include a neurologic examination, evaluation of oxygenation and respiratory status, finger stick glucose, blood work including electrolytes, a liver panel, complete blood count (CBC), and a toxicology screen. Depending on the scenario, emergent imaging and administration of glucose and thiamine should be considered.

In this patient, poor medication compliance for his underlying seizure disorder, alcohol and illicit drug abuse, and acute renal failure are all potential causes. In addition, another immediate concern would be a coagulopathic intracranial hemorrhage given elevated PTT, INR, and platelet dysfunction. The fact that this patient developed a seizure despite being on a propofol drip is particularly concerning.

WHAT IS THE NEXT STEP IN ANTIEPILEPTIC MANAGEMENT?

First-line therapy includes benzodiazepines: lorazepam (0.1 mg/kg with a maximum of 2 mg/min), midazolam 10 mg intramuscular (IM), or diazepam 10 to 20 mg IM, which is particularly useful in an out-of-hospital setting where intravenous (IV) access is not yet established. Second-line medications aim to obtain longer term seizure control once benzodiazepines interrupt the seizure. These include fosphenytoin 20 mg/kg IV and valproic acid 40 mg/kg IV. Although there are limited data for use of levetiracetam in management of status epilepticus, many providers will still use this with an initial IV load of 20 to 40 mg/kg.

The patient continued to seize for 20 minutes. During that period, he received a total of 6 mg of IV lorazepam and 1 g of IV levetiracetam, and his propofol drip was increased to 21 mg/kg/h. The patient stopped seizing but became hypotensive, and his propofol was subsequently switched to midazolam 2 mg/h. An hour later, the patient had a 1-minute generalized tonic-clonic seizure for which he was loaded with 20 mg/kg of fosphenytoin. One hour following the IV fosphenytoin load, he had a similar seizure, for which he was loaded with lacosamide 400 mg IV and a second 1 g of levetiracetam. He remained seizure free for a few hours during which a computed tomography (CT) scan of his head ruled out a spontaneous intracerebral hemorrhage (ICH). While on the CT table, the patient seized again. The midazolam drip was increased to 10 mg/h. Patient had stopped seizing clinically, but his exam was limited by heavy sedation. The facility the patient was in did not have continuous electroencephalography (EEG) capability; so a spot EEG was obtained, which demonstrated bihemispheric posterior quadrant seizures.

WHAT IS THE NEXT BEST STEP IN THIS PATIENT'S MANAGEMENT?

This patient is not clinically seizing, but his EEG demonstrates ongoing seizures. He is in refractory subclinical status epilepticus. He needs ongoing titration of anesthetic agents to achieve seizure control and continuous EEG monitoring.

If the patient continues to seize despite therapies (first- and second-line agents), then he is in refractory status epilepticus. Third-line therapy includes maximizing second-line therapy agents used initially or using a different second-line agent not initially administered. The patient is then intubated and mechanically ventilated prior to starting midazolam, propofol, or pentobarbital infusions. It is important to recognize that due to paralytics used during intubation, neurologic exam is no longer reliable to monitor seizure resolution. At that point, emergent continuous EEG monitoring should be requested. Midazolam loading dose is 0.2 mg/kg IV bolus followed by an infusion at 0.1 to 3 mg/kg/h titrated for seizure control. Propofol loading dose is 1 to 2 mg/kg followed by an infusion that can be titrated to up 12 mg/kg/h for seizure control. Pentobarbital loading dose is 5 mg/kg over 10 minutes, which can be repeated as needed until seizures stop and titrated to 1 to 5 mg/kg/h for basal infusion. With all anesthetic agents, it is important to recognize that pressor support may be needed for hypotension. Reassess whether or not the anesthetic agent is working based on clinical, electrophysiologic, and hemodynamic data and consider switching to a different agent if it is not working.

It is common to have underlying uncontrolled seizures on continuous EEG monitoring despite clinical cessation, and if there are breakthrough seizures with treatment, the vast majority are subclinical. There is some controversy with how to best manage subclinical seizures within the ICU, but for patients who present with convulsive status epilepticus who devolve into nonconvulsive status epilepticus, the aggressiveness of treatment does not differ substantially from management of status epilepticus. A major component of management is continuous EEG monitoring as this will guide titration of anesthetic medications.

An initial EEG was obtained and is shown in Figure 36.4-1.

Doses and Pharmacokinetic Features of Initial Therapy for GCSE

1. Lorazepam
- Loading Dose: 4-8 mg IV (or 0.1 mg/kg)
- Onset of Action: 3-10 min
- Duration of Effect: 12-24 h
- Elimination Half-Life: 14 h
- Main Side Effects: Sedation, respiratory depression, hypotension

2. Phenytoin
- Loading Dose: 20 mg/kg IV, maximum infusion rate 50 mg/min (25 mg/min in elderly, patients with preexisting cardiovascular conditions).
- Maintenance: 5-7 mg/kg/day in 2-3 divided doses.
- Onset of Action: 20-25 min.
- Contraindications: Heart block; caution if hepatic and renal impairment.
- Main Drug Interactions: May displace other drug that are protein bound and increase free level of other drugs. Induces hepatic metabolism of many medications, including other antiepileptic drugs (precipitates if given together with potassium, insulin, heparin, norepinephrine, cephalosporin, dobutamine).
- Main Side Effects: Cardiac arrhythmias, hypotension, hepototoxicity, pancytopenia, phlebitis, soft tissue injury from extravasation, purple glove syndrome, allergy including Stevens-Johnson syndrome.
- Target Serum Level: Total 15-25 μg/mL, free level 2-3 μg/mL (monitor free level when on valproate, benzodiazepines, other highly protein-bound medication; low albumin; or critically ill), adjustments if free level not available; total level/(Alb × 0.1) + 0.1 (in patients with renal failure: total level/[Alb × 0.2]+0.1).

3. Fosphenytoin
- Loading Dose: 20 mg/kg IV, maximum infusion rate 150 mg/min. If patient continues having seizures after 20 mg/kg, an additional 5-10 mg/kg may be given.
- Maintenance: 5-7 mg/kg/day in 2-3 divided doses.
- Onset of Action: 20-25 min (can be given faster than phenytoin but needs to be converted to phenytoin prior to onset of action, which takes ~15 min).
- Main Side Effect: See phenytoin, additionally transient pruritus from solvent. No purple glove syndrome.
- Target Serum Levels: Same as phenytoin. Serum phenytoin levels should be measured more than 2 h after IV or 4 h after IM administration to allow complete conversion to phenytoin.

4. Valproate
- Loading Dose: 40 mg/kg IV over 10 min, if still seizing, additional 20 mg/kg over ~ 5 min (max rate 6 mg/kg/min).
- Maintenance: 1 g IV q6h (infusion dose range 2-8 mg/kg/h).
- Contraindications: Severe liver dysfunction, thrombocytopenia, active bleeding.
- Major Drug Interactions: Due to interactions between phenytoin and valproic acid, it is important to follow unbound levels, especially phenytoin to avoid toxicity. In combination with phenobarbital, valproate can cause severe impaired mental status. Meropenem decreases valproate concentrations dramatically.
- Main Side Effect: Hepatotoxicity, thrombocytopenia, pancreatitis, hyperammonemic encephalopathy (consider I-camitine 33 mg/kg q8h), fibrinogen levels. Hypotension is rare but has been reported.
- Target Serum Levels: Total: 80-140 μg/mL, free: 4-11 μg/mL (only consider if toxicity suspected)

Abbreviation: GCSE, generalized convulsive status epilepticus.

Source: Reproduced from Lee K. *The NeuroICU Book*. New York, NY: McGraw-Hill Education; 2012.

WHAT IS YOUR INTERPRETATION OF THE EEG?

EEG records electrical activity from the cerebral cortex. EEG electrode placement follows standardized measurements that go beyond the scope of this book. Electrode placement is shown in the table on page 505. Basic terminology includes: Fp (fronto-polar or prefrontal), F (frontal), P (parietal), O (occipital), and C (central). The number following the letter indicates the sidedness: odd numbers for the left side, even numbers for the right side, and "z" for the central leads. EEG measures potential difference. To do so, an electrode has to be compared to a different electrode. There are multiple "montages" that compare electrodes in different configurations. We will only discuss the bipolar montage, also known as the "double banana" montage. In this montage, an electrode is compared to adjacent electrodes as indicated by the direction of the arrows in the first figure in the table on page 505.

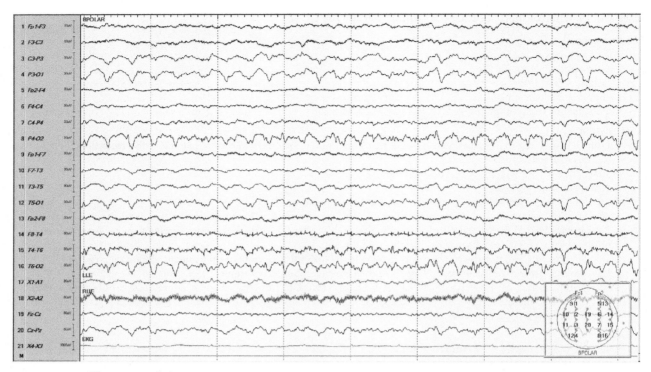

Figure 36.4-1   Electroencephalogram.

The normal EEG has several characteristics that are missing in the images in the table below from our patient. A normal EEG demonstrates normal background activity depending on the state of wakefulness. The suppression of these waveforms is what is referred to as "burst suppression" in heavily sedated patients. The images in the table below were obtained from our patient's EEG recordings.

Continuous EEG monitoring in the ICU can lead to multiple abnormal results that fall on the ictal (clearly seizure) and intra-ictal spectrum. The EEG in Figure 36.4-1 demonstrates diffuse slowing (an abnormal posterior dominate rhythm), which is most commonly due to a toxic, metabolic, or medication etiology. Also demonstrated are left-sided lateralized periodic discharges. Periodic discharges fall on the intra-ictal spectrum. Periodic discharges occur at a regular rate (measured in rate per second or Hertz) and have a specific morphology. The EEG shown has simple periodic discharges but more complex, polyphasic, spike, spike-wave, or sharp-wave complexes. The periodic discharges are commonly due to underlying brain injury and may or may not be epileptogenic.

The patient was given a total of 6 mg of lorazepam, and his midazolam drip rate was increased to 20 mg/h. A repeat EEG demonstrated a burst suppression pattern. At that point, the patient was on the following medications: levetiracetam 2000 mg every 12 hours, lacosamide 200 mg IV, phenytoin 100 mg every 8 hours, and midazolam 10 mg/h. The patient's exam showed intact brainstem reflexes (pupils round, equal, and reactive; positive corneal reflex; positive gag reflex; and intact oculocephalic reflex) with no response to noxious stimulation. On day 3, the patient had a fever with a temperature of 101°F, for which he was started on cefepime 1 g every 24 hours for pneumonia. Sputum cultures later revealed *Acinetobacter baumannii-calcoaceticus* complex. Urine cultures were negative. The patient was transferred to our hospital for continuous EEG monitoring on day 4 of his presentation.

Continuous EEG was obtained and demonstrated a diffusely slow and suppressed background in addition to slowing and epileptiform sharp waves over the right posterior temporal region consistent with an active seizure focus in that area. An MRI of the brain was obtained as part of his refractory status epilepticus workup and is shown in Figure 36.4-2.

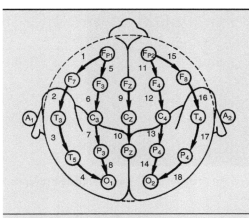

A "bipolar montage," also known as the "double banana" montage. Each electrode is compared to an adjacent electrode as indicated by the direction of the arrows. Electrode placement follows standardized measurements. Basic terminology includes: Fp (fronto-polar or prefrontal), F (frontal), P (parietal), O (occipital), and C (central). The number following the letter indicates the siddedness: odd numbers for the left side, even numbers for the right side, and "z" for the central leads.

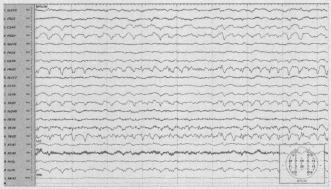

There is diffuse suppression of the EEG baseline. Superimposed epileptiform discharges are seen around the parietal (P3, P4), occipital (O2, O3), and central (C3) electrodes bilaterally.

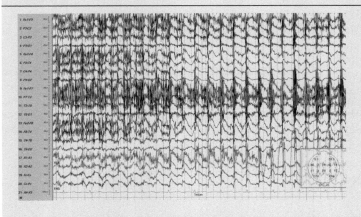

As the epileptic discharges generalize into a full-blown status epilepticus, rhythmic generalized bursts of muscle artifacts, synchronous, that are more prominent over the left hemisphere than over the right hemisphere are noted. Muscle (electromyography) artifacts have higher frequency and amplitude than EEG waves.

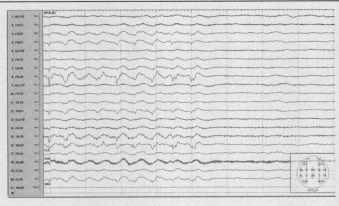

As the patient is treated with antiepileptics, the seizures abate. This image shows the transition from epileptiform discharges in the left posterior quadrant back to burst suppression. Generalized seizures typically demonstrate this pattern of evolution captured in the above 3 images: epileptiform discharges evolving into generalized seizures and then devolving as the seizure subsides.

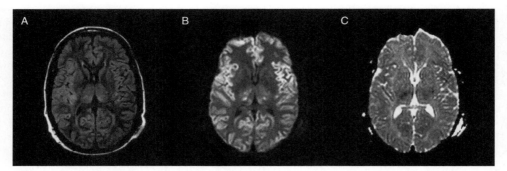

Figure 36.4-2 Magnetic resonance imaging of the brain: axial cut at the level of the thalamus. **A.** Fluid-attenuated inversion recovery sequence. **B.** Diffuse sequence. **C.** Apparent diffusion coefficient sequence.

WHAT ARE THE PERTINENT FINDINGS ON THE MRI OF THE BRAIN?

MRI was obtained and showed diffuse cortical/gray matter diffusion restriction and edema most consistent with hypoxic-ischemic injury secondary to status epilepticus. Although the patient did not have events of profound hypotension or hypoxia, his brain imaging is consistent with this finding. This is likely due to the increased metabolic demand of ongoing seizures. However, on intermittent EEG that was completed at the hospital, there was likely intermittent electrographic seizures resulting in the above findings. Further medication use was limited by hemodynamic instability, hepatic failure, and renal failure. After 3 days of continuous refractory clinical and subclinical seizures, hepatic failure, and renal failure, the family decided to terminate care given the poor prognosis. Overall prognosis of status epilepticus is poor. Predictors of poor outcomes include acute underlying medical or neurologic etiology, refractory status epilepticus, and subclinical status epilepticus. However, it should be noted that many patients do well with excellent recovery if managed timely and appropriately.

WHAT IS YOUR FINAL DIAGNOSIS?

- Super-refractory status epilepticus thought to be multifactorial: systemic infection, multisystem organ failure, and medication noncompliance
- Anoxic brain injury

REFERENCES

Brophy GM, Bell R, Claassen J, et al. Guidelines for the evaluation and management of status epilepticus. *Neurocrit Care.* 2012;17:3-23.

Chen JWY, Wasterlain CG. Status epilepticus: pathophysiology and management in adults. *Lancet Neurol.* 2006;5: 246-256.

DeLorenzo RJ, Waterhouse EJ, Towne AR, et al. Persistent nonconvulsive status epilepticus after the control of convulsive status epilepticus. *Epilepsia.* 1998;39:833-840.

Kilbride RD, Reynolds AS, Szaflarski JP, et al. Clinical outcomes following prolonged refractory status epilepticus (PRSE). *Neurocrit Care.* 2013;18:374-385.

Lai A, Outin HD, Jabot J, et al. Functional outcome of prolonged refractory status epilepticus. *Crit Care.* 2015; 19:199.

Rowan AJ, Tolunsky E. *A Primer of EEG: With a Mini-Atlas.* Oxford, United Kingdom: Butterworth-Heinemann; 2003.

Trinka E, Cock H, Hesdorffer D, et al. A definition and classification of status epilepticus: report of the ILAE Task Force on Classification of Status Epilepticus. *Epilepsia.* 2015;56: 1515-1523.

Manan Shah, MD and Stephen Katzen, MD

History of Present Illness

A 65-year-old man with a past medical history of numerous resections for a brain tumor over the past 20 years presented to the clinic with progressive deterioration of his vision. Over past 2 years, he developed progressive difficulty seeing objects in his lower fields of vision but was reluctant to get medical attention until his wife convinced him to be evaluated. He also noted subjective intermittent flashing of lights in his lower fields of vision. He admitted having similar vision problems in the past and underwent tumor resection 3 times. His last tumor resection was 4 years ago, after which he was lost to follow-up. He did not recall any further details about his tumor diagnosis. He was otherwise healthy and did not have any active medical problems.

Exam

His vital signs were unremarkable during the clinic visit. His visual acuity was 20/30 in the left eye and 20/40 in the right eye. Fundoscopic examination showed normal retinal vessels and optic discs. Patient had an old surgical incision over the occipital region of his scalp. His neurologic exam revealed inferior altitudinal defect. The rest of the neurologic exam was within normal limits.

TO WHERE CAN THE LESION BE LOCALIZED?

The patient's inferior altitudinal visual field defect serves as a marker for localization. Recalling optic pathway anatomy, this is a very unusual deficit and is usually associated with lesions involving the chiasm. Inferior quandrantopsia ("pie on the floor") is associated with a lesion distal to division of optic radiations and includes upper division traversing through parietal and occipital lobes (superior to calcarine sulcus). If the patient does not have chiasmal involvement, then a lesion affecting multiple radiations more posterior in the optic pathway should be assessed. It is possible that he had a residual visual field deficit and now has involvement of other side. Given his past history of neoplasm, a recurrence of tumor is highly likely. History of recurrence can also help in determining the type or aggressiveness of the tumor. Among other differential diagnoses, cerebral infarction is a possibility, although less likely. Given his complaints of intermittent flashes, a seizure should be considered in the differential as well, which can be from cortical irritability due to any structural abnormality.

WHAT WOULD YOU ORDER NEXT FOR WORKUP?

The patient underwent magnetic resonance imaging (MRI) of the brain with gadolinium contrast, which is shown in Figure 36.5-1. The mass also seemed to invade the posterior half of the superior sagittal sinus. Diffusion-weighted imaging and apparent diffusion coefficient sequences did not demonstrate any ischemic area. Conventional cerebral angiogram was completed, which is shown in Figure 36.5-2. Video electroencephalography (EEG) monitoring showed normal posterior dominant activity with breach rhythm on the right side. The patient did notice flashes of light during monitoring but did not have an electrographic correlate to support a seizure diagnosis.

The patient underwent an occipital craniotomy for the goal of a gross total resection of his tumor. Upon initial incision, minimal blood loss was appreciated due to the prior scar tissue present. Once the craniotomy was completed, significant dural bleeding occurred. This was stopped with bipolar cautery and dural tack up sutures. Next, the tumor was localized using a 3-dimensional intraoperative navigation system. The dura was then incised just lateral to the mass, and meticulous dissection was then undertaken. Significant bleeding occurred throughout the case and was not unexpected given the high vascularity of the mass. There were also significant adhesions to the surrounding dura and brain. A gross total resection was achieved with good hemostasis. His neurologic exam, including visual field deficits, was unchanged in the immediate postoperative period, and he was discharged to home on the third postoperative day.

WHAT IS THE DIFFERENTIAL DIAGNOSIS?

The differential diagnosis of dural-based masses includes the following:

- Meningioma (the most common primary brain tumor compared to the others listed below)
- Solitary fibrous tumor of dura (of which hemangiopericytoma is a subtype)

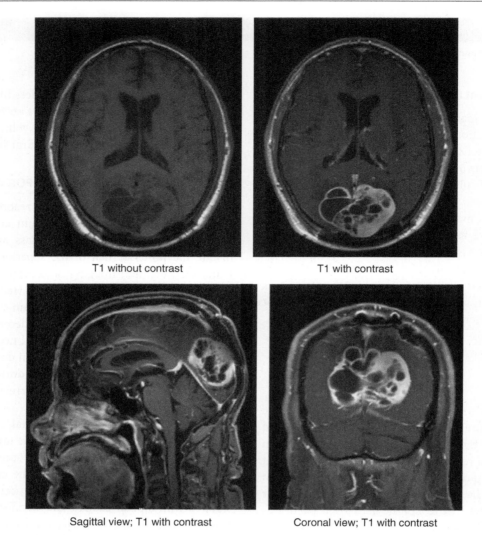

T1 without contrast   T1 with contrast

Sagittal view; T1 with contrast   Coronal view; T1 with contrast

Figure 36.5-1   Contrast magnetic resonance imaging of the brain, which showed a 4.6 × 6.9 × 5 cm, dural-based cystic mass straddling the posterior falx bilaterally, with homogenous contrast enhancement of the solid areas, causing compression of bilateral parieto-occipital lobes.

- Primary dural lymphoma
- Primary meningeal malignant melanoma
- Sarcoids
- Dural metastasis

Biopsy specimen of the patient showed hypercellular tissue with spindle-shaped cells and increased mitotic figures. It was extremely vascular with dilated "stag horn"–shaped vessels (Fig. 36.5-3). Immunohistochemical staining showed positivity toward CD34, BCL2, and vimentin, confirming the diagnosis of a rare World Health Organization (WHO) grade III anaplastic hemangiopericytoma (HPC).

First described by Stout and Murray in 1942, HPC is a rare intracranial tumor (0.4%). It is a soft tissue tumor of pericytic origin. HPC has been classified as WHO grade II and is now considered along a spectrum of a solitary fibrous tumor of the dura. It is commonly located in the supratentorial region. HPC can be difficult to distinguish from meningioma. It is clinically more aggressive, tends to occur in the younger population (30s and 40s), and has a higher recurrence rate. Its anaplastic variant is even rarer and is classified as a WHO grade III lesion. It has a strong tendency to metastasize extracranially. Histology assists in differentiating between HPC and meningioma. HPC has a classic stag horn appearance of stromal vessels, and they are reactive to vimentin, CD34, and BCL2, unlike meningioma, which is positive for epithelial membrane antigen (EMA). Gross total resection

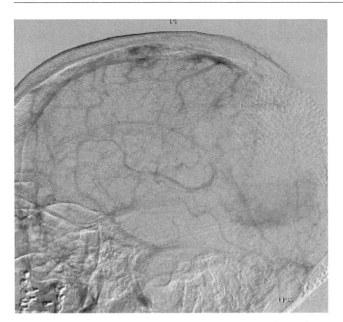

Figure 36.5-2 Digital subtraction angiogram showed an occlusion of the posterior third of the superior sagittal sinus and increased regional supply by the distal branches of the middle cerebral and middle meningeal arteries.

is first-line treatment. The use of preoperative arterial embolization can help to limit blood loss. Adjuvant radiotherapy is recommended to reduce recurrence.

WHAT IS THE NEXT STEP IN MANAGEMENT AFTER SURGERY? WOULD ONE EXPECT ANY POSTOPERATIVE COMPLICATIONS?

The patient had partial improvement in his inferior field of vision and was able to recognize shapes and movement in the inferior visual fields. He was able to return to

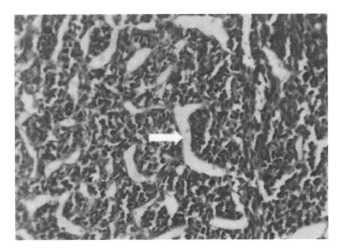

Figure 36.5-3 "Stag horn" shapes seen on biopsy specimen.

work. He was also found to have soft, nontender swelling underlying the incision. Patient had noticed this swelling 5 days postoperatively after he lifted heavy boxes at home. He denied any associated headache, fever, nausea/vomiting, or nuchal rigidity. Subsequent MRI showed a fluid collection in the deep scalp region overlying the craniotomy site, consistent with pseudomeningocele.

A pseudomeningocele refers to a cerebrospinal fluid (CSF) collection through an abnormal leak from CSF spaces of the brain and spinal cord. It is not lined by dura and is a known complication of posterior fossa surgery. It often manifests as leakage of fluid from a surgical incision and can hamper the healing of surgical wounds. This open connection can also lead to meningitis. Our patient was readmitted to the hospital and was initially managed with a lumbar drain placement and head wrap for 5 days. This treatment proved ineffective. He later underwent ventriculoperitoneal shunt placement. Two months later, his pseudomeningocele was found unchanged, after which he had catheter placement in the pseudomeningocele itself and later lumboperitoneal shunt placement. All of the above-mentioned CSF diversion strategies accelerate resolution of pseudomeningoceles by reducing the egress of CSF through the dural defect. This allows faster healing and sealing of the dural defect. Failure of conservative management ultimately requires surgical intervention with reestablishment of a watertight closure using a duraplasty. This case also stresses the importance of postoperative wound precautions, such as avoiding heavy weight lifting, keeping incisions dry, and avoiding sneezing or coughing with open mouth.

WHAT IS YOUR FINAL DIAGNOSIS?

- Recurrent anaplastic hemangiopericytoma
- Pseudomeningocele secondary to surgery

REFERENCES

Ali HS, Endo T, Endo H, Murakami K, Tominaga T. Intraspinal dissemination of intracranial hemangiopericytoma: case report and literature review. *Surg Neurol Int.* 2016; 7(Suppl 40):S1016-S1020.

Menger R, Connor DE Jr, Hefner M, et al. Pseudomeningocele formation following Chiari decompression: 19-year retrospective review of predisposing and prognostic factors. *Surg Neurol Int.* 2015;6:70.

Stout AP, Murray MR. Hemangiopericytoma: a vascular tumor featuring Zimmermann's pericytes. *Ann Surg.* 1942; 116(1):26-33.

Tommasi CD, Bond AE. Complicated pseudomeningocele repair after Chiari decompression: case report and review of the literature. *World Neurosurg.* 2016;88:688.e1-e7.

CLINICAL CASE VIGNETTE 6: WEAKNESS IN THE ICU

David P. Lerner, MD, and Matthew B. Bevers, MD, PhD

History of Present Illness

A 76-year-old right-handed woman with chronic obstructive pulmonary disease, diabetes mellitus not on insulin, stage IV chronic kidney disease, ischemic systolic cardiomyopathy, and peripheral artery disease was admitted to the intensive care unit (ICU) for progressive, symmetric diffuse weakness.

She had a complicated recent medical history. She was admitted approximately 1 month prior for a nonhealing left lower extremity ulcer. She underwent surgical intervention with left femoral artery endarterectomy and stent placement to the left superficial femoral artery. Following placement of the stent, clopidogrel and high-dose atorvastatin were started. Shortly after initiation of these medications, she developed hematemesis and was found to have a duodenal ulcer that was treated endoscopically.

After discharge to a rehabilitation facility, she had progressive weakness. Initially she had difficulty with lifting her legs, and then noted the same issues with her arms, and finally noted difficulty lifting her head. Around this time, she developed difficulty swallowing solids and thin liquids, so she was readmitted to the hospital.

Exam

On admission to the ICU, the examination was pertinent for symmetric, reactive pupils, full extraocular movements, moderate facial diplegia with ability to forcibly open eyes on manual testing, transverse pucker, weakness of jaw opening/closing, moderate neck flexion and extension weakness, weak cough, and no movement in the bilateral deltoids, bicep, hip flexors, and quadriceps. There was decreased sensation to pinprick in a graded stocking distribution. There were no reflexes present. She had moderate mixed dysarthria and was able to count to 4 with a single large breath.

Her vitals on admission were as follows: heart rate 114 bpm, noninvasive blood pressure 86/52 mm Hg, respiratory rate 32 breaths/min, oxygen saturation on 6 L nasal cannula 96%. Her labs from the outside facility earlier in the day were pertinent for the following: white blood cell count 22.7×10^9 cells/dL, creatinine 2.4 mg/dL, blood urea nitrogen 38 mmol/L, and creatinine kinase 24,512 U/L (normal 60-250 U/L).

SHOULD THIS PATIENT BE INTUBATED?

In patients with neuromuscular weakness, there are multiple reasons for intubation and mechanical ventilation, with the most common being hypercarbic respiratory failure. Frequent neurologic examination and bedside pulmonary function testing can assist with determining early neuromuscular failure and need for potential noninvasive or invasive ventilation. Commonly monitored pulmonary function tests are forced vital capacity (FVC), negative inspiratory force (NIF), and maximum expiratory pressure (MEP). The "20/30/40 rule" can be used as a guideline for potential intubation (vital capacity <20 mL/kg ideal body weight, NIF <-30 cm H_2O, MEP <40 cm H_2O). These numbers are a guideline, and others use more stringent criteria of vital capacity <15 mL/kg and NIF <-20 cm H_2O.

In this patient's case, we do not have formal pulmonary function tests, but there are bedside surrogate markers that can assist with determining pulmonary function. The single breath count test is a reproducible bedside measure. Patients are instructed to take as large a single breath as possible and then count out loud to the highest number possible. In those with neuromuscular weakness the ability to count is limited due to the lower vital capacity. A count to 20 approximates an FVC of 1 L. With the patient only counting to 4, there is marked reduction in FVC. Another potential indicator for intubation is the patient's bulbar weakness. She has limited ability to swallow and clear her secretions, which is leading to ongoing aspiration.

After discussion with the patient, a joint decision was made for intubation. Anesthesia was contacted for assistance given the concern of a potential difficult airway.

WHAT ARE THE MOST APPROPRIATE INDUCTION AND PARALYTIC AGENTS FOR THIS PATIENT?

There are multiple combinations of induction and paralytic medications that can be used for intubation. Although we do not know the etiology of the patient's neuromuscular weakness, myasthenia gravis is a possibility. This disease process results from autoantibodies to the acetylcholine receptor at the neuromuscular junction with ultimate destruction of the junction and upregulation of acetylcholine receptors outside the normal neuromuscular junction. As a result, myasthenia patients typically are resistant to depolarizing agents (eg, succinylcholine). Conversely, myasthenic patients are very sensitive to nondepolarizing agents (eg, rocuronium, vecuronium) such that their use can result in loss of airway protection and respiratory drive even at low doses. In addition, the commonly used nondepolarizing agents undergo renal clearance and, in the setting of her chronic renal disease, will last substantially longer; elimination half-life is increased by 25% to 56%. Cisatracurium is another potential consideration because this nondepolarizing neuromuscular blocking agent is cleared via esterases within the bloodstream and is not affected by renal or liver failure.

Options for anesthetic induction include etomidate, fentanyl, propofol, midazolam, and ketamine; each of which has its own benefits and drawbacks. Etomidate exerts direct action on the γ-aminobutyric acid (GABA) receptor causing blockage of neuroexcitation. Etomidate has limited vasoactive properties, which can be useful in hemodynamically unstable patients, but in those with sepsis, there is increased risk of death. Given that our patient is tachycardic and hypotensive and has an elevated white blood cell count with active aspiration, there is a high likelihood of sepsis, and etomidate should be avoided. Although propofol is commonly used in the neuro-ICU because it has the property of decreasing intracranial pressure, this also comes with the complication of hypotension. Benzodiazepines, most commonly midazolam, can be used for induction, but there is the common side effect of hypotension with mean arterial pressure decreases of 10% to 25%. Our patient's already tenuous hemodynamics would preclude the use of benzodiazepines. Ketamine stimulates the N-methyl-D-aspartate (NMDA) receptors and blocks the GABA complex, resulting in a dissociative anesthetic effect. It has the side effect of increasing heart rate, mean arterial pressure, intracranial pressure, and cerebral blood flow (which typically limits its use in the neuro-ICU), but in our patient's case, it can be used in augmentation of her hemodynamics during induction. It also does not depress respiratory drive and allows for "awake" intubations.

For induction, the patient received ketamine at a dose of 2 mg/kg with 50 µg of fentanyl. No neuromuscular blockade was given due to the concern for potential myasthenia gravis. The intubation was uneventful, and the patient was placed on assist-control ventilation. After stabilization, the patient underwent nerve conduction and electromyography studies while intubated. The results are summarized in the tables below.

Nerve Conduction Study (NCS) or Right Upper Extremity (Median and Ulnar) and Right Lower Extremity (Common Peroneal and Tibial) Motor Responses

Motor NCS							
Nerve/Sites	Distance cm	Segments	Latency ms	Amplitude mV	Velocity m/s	Temp. °C	d Lat. ms
R MEDIAN-APB							
Wrist	7	Wrist-APB	4.74	**1.6**		29	
Elbow	19.5	Elbow - Wrist	8.80	1.6	48.0	29	4.06
R ULNAR - ADM							
Wrist	7	Wrist - ADM	3.18	**1.5**		29.4	
B. Elbow	18.5	B. Elbow - Wrist	6.56	0.8	54.6	29.3	3.39
A. Elbow	9	A. Elbow - B. Elbow	8.49	0.9	46.7	29.3	1.93
R COMM PERONEAL - EDB							
Ankle	8	Ankle - EDB	7.60	**0.1**		29.7	
Fib Head	17	Fib head - Ankle	10.52	0.0	58.3	29.8	2.92
Knee	8	Knee - Fib head	12.14	0.1	49.5	29.6	1.61
R TIBIAL - AH							
Ankle	8	Ankle - AH	5.63	**0.8**		29.3	
Knee	34	Knee - Ankle	14.58	0.8	38.0	29.4	8.96

Note: Bold results (amplitude) are abnormal. Not shown are normal sensory nerve conduction studies.

Electromyography (EMG) Study: Right (R) Upper Extremity (Deltoid, Bicep, Extensor Digitorum Communis [Ext. Dig.]) and Right Lower Extremity (Vastus Lateralis [Vast. Lat.] and Tibialis Anterior [Tib. Ant.]) Results

	Insertional Activity	Fibrillation	Fasciculation	Motor Unit Amplitude		Motor Unit Duration		Motor Unit Phases	Recruitment Pattern
R deltoid	Increased	2+	None	No activity		No activity		No activity	No activity
R bicep	Increased	2+	None	Few	Small	Few	Brief	Many	Early
R Ext. Dig.	Increased	2+	None	Normal		Normal		Normal	Normal
R Vast. Lat.	Increased	3+	None	No activity		No activity		No activity	No activity
R Tib. Ant.	Increased	3+	None	Normal		Normal		Normal	Normal

WHAT IS THE INTERPRETATION OF THE DATA?

Most do not have extensive training in neuromuscular disease, and interpretation of nerve conduction studies (NCS) and electromyography (EMG) studies done in the ICU can be particularly difficult. While likely appearing overly simplistic to an electrophysiologist, the following discussion is intended to give a solid foundation of knowledge that will allow for interpretation of electrodiagnostic studies.

The NCS should be interpreted first as it will assist with EMG interpretation. Again, not shown above but noted in the legend, the sensory NCSs for the patient were normal. In an NCS, there are 2 main data points: the latency/conduction velocity and the amplitude. Latency is the delay from stimulation to nerve response at the recording device, which can be used to determine the velocity at the distal portion. When stimulating 2 points on the same nerve (for the median nerve at the wrist and the elbow), the delay in electrical response at the recording device at the more proximal stimulation can be used to determine the velocity at more proximal portions of the nerve. This is best shown as a mathematical equation:

$$\text{Velocity (m/s)} = \frac{10 \times (\text{Latency}_{proximal} - \text{Latency}_{distal}\,(ms))}{\text{Distance between stimulation (cm)}}$$

The velocity of electrical conduction through the nerve is determined predominantly by myelination. The second data point of importance in nerve conduction is the amplitude. This is the voltage of the electrical impulse that is generated from the recording device. This is mainly determined by the number of axons that are able to carry signal to the recording device. The other potential amplitude generation in NCSs is the muscle itself, as motor NCSs require healthy muscle to generate a muscle contraction.

- Velocity is determined by myelin.
- Amplitude is determined by axons (for sensory and motor responses) and muscle (for motor responses).

The NCS for this patient shows a marked decrease in the amplitudes of all motor nerves with normal velocity and latencies. This is also the case with normal sensory nerve conduction velocities and amplitudes. Given the amplitude is low with motor testing, there is either a motor axon or muscle disease present.

EMG has two main components (resting potentials and activation potentials). At rest, a normal muscle should have no activity. With activation, there should be similar-appearing, simple (single or double phase) motor unit potentials that will increase in frequency when additional force is applied to approximately 10 Hz when an additional motor unit will join. Insertional activity, fasciculations, and fibrillations are markers of "resting activity." Our patient's muscles demonstrate increased resting activity given that there are fibrillations present. The motor units found in the bicep are small amplitude, brief, and polyphasic with early recruitment when applying additional force. This is consistent with a myopathic process. If this was due to a neuropathic process, there would initially just be few motor units, and a more chronic process would have motor units that are large amplitude, long, and polyphasic with delayed recruitment. This is because a single motor unit (motor nerve and the muscle fibers innervated by it) enlarges so more motor fibers are included.

Summary of Electromyography Findings in Myopathic/Neuropathic Processes

	Motor Unit			
	Amplitude	**Duration**	**Phases**	**Recruitment Pattern**
Myopathic	Low	Short	Polyphasic	Early recruitment
Early neuropathic	Normal	Normal	Normal	Delayed recruitment
Late neuropathic	High	Long	Polyphasic	Delayed recruitment

To briefly summarize, the NCS and EMG findings show that this is a diffuse but more proximal than distal, disfiguring (giving the increased insertional activity and fibrillations) myopathic process.

WHAT IS THE DIFFERENTIAL DIAGNOSIS FOR ACUTE, PROGRESSIVE, DISFIGURING MYOPATHY?

Myopathy can occur as a result of endocrine, autoimmune, infectious, or toxic etiologies. Endocrine myopathies are see in hyper-/hypothyroidism, hyper-/hypoparathyroidism, adrenal insufficiency, and diabetes mellitus. Only hypothyroidism typically has elevation in creatine kinase and true muscle breakdown. Inflammatory myopathies (dermatomyositis, polymyositis, inclusion body myositis) can commonly cause destruction and will have increased insertional activity, as seen in our patient, but typically have a more indolent course. Additional autoimmune diseases such as lupus and rheumatoid arthritis can result in myopathies. Infectious diseases can present with a profound, rapid inflammatory myopathy with common etiologies of influenza, coxsackie group B, and human immunodeficiency virus, and although uncommon, bacterial infectious diseases (*Staphylococcus aureus, Yersinia pestis, Streptococcus, Borrelia burgdorferi,* and *Legionella pneumophila*) can cause inflammatory myopathies. Toxic myopathies from lipid-lowering agents and glucocorticoids can present similar to the patient. Other less commonly encountered drugs that can result in a myopathy include alcohol, cocaine, heroin, toluene, cimetidine, colchicine, and cyclosporine. Finally, critical illness myopathy can present with flaccid quadriparesis and profound muscle breakdown.

Given the recent start of high-dose atorvastatin following her vascular intervention, there was risk of toxic myopathy, but there was also concern given the profound weakness that she may have at least a component of critical illness myopathy.

IF THE PATIENT HAS PRIMARILY CRITICAL ILLNESS MYOPATHY (CIM), WHAT PLACED HER AT RISK FOR THIS DISEASE PROCESS, AND WHAT IS HER ANTICIPATED PROGNOSIS?

There are a number of clinical factors and medications that increase the risk of CIM. Those with uncontrolled blood glucose, female sex, and higher underlying

Differential Diagnosis for Myopathy

Disease Category	Specific Disease Processes
Endocrine	Hypo-/hyperthyroid
	Hypo-/hyperparathyroid
	Adrenal insufficiency
	Diabetes mellitus
Autoimmune	Dermatomyositis
	Polymyositis
	Inclusion body myositis
	Lupus
	Rheumatoid arthritis
	Scleroderma
Infectious	Influenza
	Coxsackie group B
	Human immunodeficiency virus
	Staphylococcus aureus
	Yersinia pestis
	Streptococcus
	Borrelia burgdorferi
	Legionella pneumophila
	Protozoa
Drug induced	Alcohol
	Heroin
	Cocaine
	Statin
	Steroid
	Colchicine
	Cimetidine
	Cyclosporine
Critical illness	

disease severity, as shown by higher Acute Physiology and Chronic Health Evaluation (APACHE) III and Sequential Organ Failure Assessment (SOFA) scores, have higher odds ratios of having CIM. Other severity of illness findings, including use of renal replacement therapy and duration of mechanical ventilation, have produced mixed results on risk of CIM. The classic presentation of CIM was first described in patients with asthma exacerbation receiving high-dose intravenous steroids and neuromuscular blockade. However, since that time, multiple studies have not found increased risk of CIM in this group. Additional medications that have shown link between administration and CIM are vasopressors, but this is limited to patients in the cardiothoracic ICU. Although CIM can present with striking weakness, as is seen in our patient, recovery is anticipated. There are limited long-term follow-up reports for CIM, but in small studies, the majority of patients with CIM had complete recovery between 6 and 12 months.

Early in her hospital course, the statin was discontinued with fairly rapid decrease in her creatine kinase. She was successfully extubated and ultimated discharged from the hospital to an acute rehabilitation facility.

FINAL DIAGNOSIS

- CIM with superimposed toxic myopathy from high dose statin.

REFERENCES

Abel M, Eisenkraft JB. Anesthetic implications of myasthenia gravis. *Mount Sinai J Med.* 2002;69:31-37.

Amato AA, Russell JA, eds. *Neuromuscular Disorders* (2nd ed). New York, NY: McGraw-Hill Education; 2016.

Bartfield JM, Ushkow BS, Rosen JM, et al. Single breath counting in the assessment of pulmonary function. *Ann Emerg Med.* 1994;24:256-259.

Benson M, Junger A, Fuchs C, et al. Use of an anesthesia information management system (AIMS) to evaluate the physiological effects of hypnotic agents used to induce anesthesia. *J Clin Monit Comput.* 2000;16:183.

Blumer JL. Clinical pharmacology of midazolam in infants and children. *Clin Pharmacokinet.* 1998;35:37-47.

Chawla J. Stepwise approach to myopathy in systemic disease. *Front Neurol.* 2011;2:49.

Ebert TJ. Sympathetic and hemodynamic effects of moderate and deep sedation with propofol in humans. *Anesthesiology.* 2005;103:20-24.

Elseikh B, Arnold WD, Gharibshahi S, et al. Correlation of single-breath count test and neck flexor muscle strength with spirometry in myasthenia gravis. *Muscle Nerve.* 2016;53:134-136.

Guarneri B, Bertolini G, Latronico N. Long-term outcome in patients with critical illness myopathy or neuropathy: the Italian multicenter CRIMYNE study. *J Neurol Neurosurg Psychiatry.* 2008;79:838-841.

Hull CJ. Pharmacokinetics and pharmacodynamics of the benzylisoquinolinium muscle relaxants. *Acta Anaesthesiol Scand.* 1995;106(Suppl):13-17.

Khuenl-Brady KS, Pomaroli A, Puhringer F, et al. The use of rocuronium in patients with chronic renal failure. *Anesthesia.* 1993;48:873-875.

Langsjo JW, Kaisti KK, Aalto S, et al. Effects of subanesthetic doses of ketamine on regional cerebral blood flow, oxygen consumption and blood volume in humans. *Anesthesiology.* 2003;99:614-623.

Rabinstein AA. Acute neuromuscular respiratory failure. *Continuum (Minneap Minn).* 2015;21:1324-1345.

Shepherd S, Batra A, Lerner DP. Review of critical illness myopathy and neuropathy. *Neurohospitalist.* 2017;7:41-48.

CLINICAL CASE VIGNETTE 7: HYDROCEPHALUS

Jose R. McFaline Figueroa, MD, PhD, and Saef Izzy, MD

History of Present Illness

A 43-year-old man with a history of polysubstance abuse and chronic hepatitis B and C infection presented after being found unresponsive. He was last seen well 4 days prior, when he purchased large amounts of alcohol and locked himself in his room. On the day of presentation, neighbors called the police because they had not seen him for several days. He was found on a mattress, covered in feces and surrounded by bottles of alcohol, bupropion, and gabapentin. He was brought in by ambulance to our institution.

Exam

On arrival, he was afebrile with a heart rate of 76 bpm, blood pressure of 220/80 mm Hg, respiratory rate of 32 breaths/min, and an oxygen saturation of 100% on room air. He opened his eyes spontaneously and mumbled incomprehensibly, although occasionally, he could answer yes or no questions and follow limited commands. His pupils were equal and reactive, and he moved all his extremities against gravity and symmetrically. His exam was otherwise intact.

Initial computed tomography (CT) of the head showed ventricular debris, a poorly defined obstructive lesion in the third ventricle, and acute hydrocephalus (Fig. 36.7-1, A-C). Magnetic resonance imaging (MRI) showed transependymal flow, ventricular wall thickening, dependent areas of intraventricular restricted diffusion, and ependymal enhancement involving the anterior aspect of the left lateral ventricle, bilateral foramen of Monro, and third ventricle (Fig. 36.7-1, D-F). An external ventricular drain (EVD) was emergently placed, and he was admitted to the neurointensive care unit.

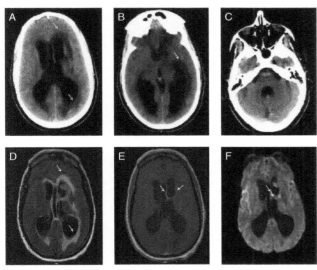

Figure 36.7-1 Neuroimaging findings on presentation. **A-C.** Noncontrast computed tomography of the head showing diffuse ventricular enlargement consistent with acute hydrocephalus. There are areas of periventricular hypodensity consistent with transependymal flow (*arrows*). **D-F.** Magnetic resonance images of the head. Diffuse ventricular enlargement is again demonstrated. **D.** Fluid-attenuated inversion recovery (FLAIR) image showing periventricular T2/FLAIR hyperintensities consistent with edema and transependymal flow (*arrows*). **E.** T1-weighted image after gadolinium contrast administration showing ependymal enhancement of the anterior horn of the left lateral ventricle and septum pellucidum (*arrows*). Splitting of the septum pellucidum corresponds to a cavum septum pellucidum vergae, a normal anatomic variant. **F.** Diffusion-weighted imaging (DWI) showing diffusion-restricting layering debris within the anterior horn of the left lateral ventricle (*arrow*). The area of DWI hyperintensity is hypointense in a corresponding apparent diffusion coefficient image (not shown).

WHAT IS THE DIFFERENTIAL DIAGNOSIS?

Enhancement of the ependyma, the epithelial cell layer that lines the ventricles and central canal of the spinal cord, is a neuroimaging finding with a differential diagnosis that includes neoplastic, inflammatory, vascular, and infectious etiologies (Table 36.7-1). Ependymal enhancement from most tumors represents extension of tumor growth from an adjacent site, as may be seen in glial tumors or primary central nervous system lymphoma, whereas metastatic disease is rare. Systemic inflammatory diseases result in ependymal enhancement through granuloma formation and may cause hydrocephalus. Subependymal hemorrhage is common in neonates, whereas traumatic intracranial hemorrhages may rarely be predominantly subependymal. Finally, infectious ventriculitis, most commonly viral and pyogenic, is a well-known cause of ependymal enhancement.

WHAT WOULD YOU ORDER NEXT FOR WORKUP?

Cerebrospinal fluid (CSF) analysis revealed a protein of 32 mg/dL (normal <45 mg/dL), glucose of 63 mg/dL (normal 45-80 mg/dL), 1100 red blood cells, and 24 total nucleated cells (76% lymphocytes, 13% neutrophils, 9% atypical lymphocytes, 2% monocytes). CSF cultures were negative. Serum galactomannan, β-glucan, cytomegalovirus, cysticercosis, and *Toxoplasma* testing, as well as CSF *Cryptococcus*, were negative. Human immunodeficiency virus (HIV) antibody and viral load were negative. CD4 count was 734 cells/L. Serum angiotensin-converting enzyme was 42 U/L (normal 8-53 U/L). CSF cytology and flow cytometry were negative. On hospital day 5, he underwent an endoscopic third ventriculostomy with biopsy, which showed acute necrotizing granulomatous inflammation with fungal organisms consistent with mucormycosis (Fig. 36.7-2).

HOW WOULD YOU MANAGE THE PATIENT NEXT?

The patient was initially started on vancomycin and cefepime for empiric bacterial meningitis coverage. After brain biopsy was positive for mucormycosis, antibiotics were transitioned to liposomal amphotericin B, and on hospital day 10, posaconazole was added. CT of the head initially showed some improvement, with decompression of the ventricles. However, the patient required multiple EVDs due to purulent CSF drainage and EVD obstruction. Sequential MRI imaging showed increasing area of ependymal enhancement, consistent

Table 36.7-1. Differential Diagnosis of Ependymal Enhancement

Neoplastic	Inflammatory	Vascular	Infectious
Primary CNS	Sarcoidosis	Subependymal hemorrhage (neonates)	CMV
Lymphoma	Histiocytosis	Arteriovenous malformation	VZV
Gliomas	Neuromyelities optica		Pyogenic
Ependymomas			Fungal
Germinomas			Toxoplasmosis
Hamartomas			Tuberculosis
(tuberous sclerosis)			
Metastases			

Abbreviations: CMV, cytomegalovirus; CNS, central nervous system; VZV, varicella-zoster virus.

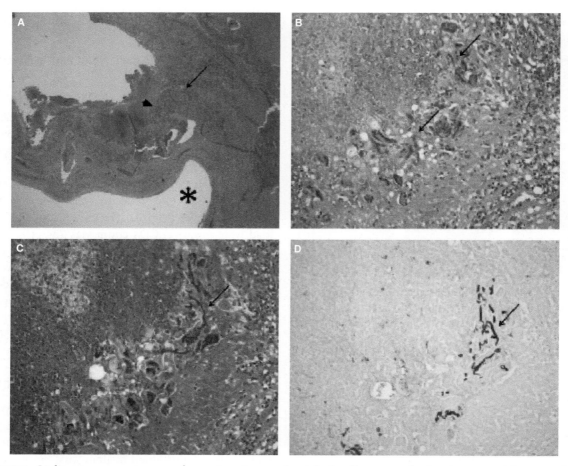

Figure 36.7-2 Light microscopy images of a postmortem periventricular tissue sample showing necrotizing granulomatous inflammation and organisms consistent with mucormycosis. **A.** Low-magnification (2×) image of a hematoxylin and eosin (HE)–stained section through the ventricular wall. There is an inflammatory infiltrate with granuloma formation (*arrow*). Asterisk denotes intraventricular space. **B.** High-power (20×) image of the HE section shown in panel A (*arrowhead*, A). Hyphael organisms are seen (*arrows*), in addition to chronic inflammation and necrosis. **C.** Periodic acid-Schiff-diastase (PAS) stain of the area shown in panel B. The hyphael organisms are strongly PAS positive. **D.** Grocott's methenamine silver (GMS) stain of the area shown in panel B. The hyphael organisms are GMS positive.

Table 36.7-2. Microbiology of Ventriculitis

Bacterial	Coagulase-negative staphylococci[*], *Staphylococcus aureus*[*], gram-negative rods, anaerobes, Nocardia species, *Listeria monocytogenes*
Viral	Cytomegalovirus, varicella-zoster virus
Fungal	*Candida* species, *Cryptococcus neoformans*, *Coccidioides immitis*, *Mucor* species
Mycobacterial	*Mycobacterium tuberculosis*
Parasites	*Toxoplasma gondii*, neurocysticercosis

Note: Asterisks denote the most common causes of nosocomial ventriculitis.

with worsening infection, despite antifungal treatment. Given the poor prognosis, the family transitioned to comfort-oriented care, and the patient died on hospital day 45.

DISCUSSION

Nosocomial ventriculitis is most commonly associated with the use of EVDs and infection by skin flora, primarily staphylococcal species. However, spontaneous infectious ventriculitis has a broad differential diagnosis, both in the immunocompromised and immunocompetent host (Table 36.7-2). Often, layering intraventricular debris leads to ventricular outflow obstruction and hydrocephalus, as in our patient. Therapy consists of supportive care, ventricular decompression with EVDs, intravenous antimicrobials, and in some cases, intraventricular antimicrobials. However, prognosis is poor, and the mortality rate is high, particularly when appropriate antibiotic coverage is delayed. Our case highlights the importance of considering these rare pathogens to provide appropriate antibiotic coverage in patients presenting with ventriculitis.

WHAT IS YOUR FINAL DIAGNOSIS?

- Ventriculitis due to mucormycosis

REFERENCES

Banker P, Sonni S, Kister I, Loh JP. Pencil-thin ependymal enhancement in neuromyelitis optica spectrum disorders. *Mult Scler*. 2012;18(7):1050-1053.

Beer R, Lackner P, Pfausler B, Schmutzhard E. Nosocomial ventriculitis and meningitis in neurocritical care patients. *J Neurol*. 2008;255(11):1617-1624.

Chen M, Zhang B, Gao C, Zheng Y, Xie L, Gao Q. Brain gadolinium enhancement along the ventricular and leptomeningeal regions in patients with aquaporin-4 antibodies in cerebral spinal fluid. *J Neuroimmunol*. 2014;269(1-2):62-67.

Cota GF, Assad ECP, Christo PP, Giannetti AV, Santos Filho JAMD, Xavier MAP. Ventriculitis: a rare case of primary cerebral toxoplasmosis in AIDS patient and literature review. *Braz J Infect Dis*. 2008;12(1):101-104.

Cuetter AC, Andrews RJ. Intraventricular neurocysticercosis: 18 consecutive patients and review of the literature. *Neurosurg Focus*. 2002;12(6):1-7.

Dettenkofer M, Ebner W, Els T, et al. Surveillance of nosocomial infections in a neurology intensive care unit. *J Neurol*. 2001;248(11):959-964.

Kleinschmidt-DeMasters BK, Mazowiecki M. Coccidioidomycosis meningitis with massive dural and cerebral venous thrombosis and tissue arthroconidia. *Arch Pathol Lab Med*. 2000;124(2):310-314.

Lozier AP, Sciacca RR, Romagnoli MF, et al. Ventriculostomy-related infections: a critical review of the literature. *Neurosurgery*. 2002;51(1):170-181.

Mongkolrattanothai K, Ramakrishnan S. Ventriculitis and choroid plexitis caused by multidrug-resistant *Nocardia pseudobrasiliensis*. *Pediatr Infect Dis J*. 2008;27(7):666-668.

Nathoo N, Narotam PK, Nadvi S, van Dellen JR. Taming an old enemy: a profile of intracranial suppuration. *World Neurosurg*. 2012;77(3-4):484-490.

Osborn AG, Daines JH, Wing SD. The evaluation of ependymal and subependymal lesions by cranial computed tomography. *Radiology*. 1978;127(2):397-401.

Schleip R, Findley TW, Chaitow L, Huijing P. *Fascia: The Tensional Network of the Human Body*. New York, NY: Elsevier Health Sciences; 2013.

Shimol SB, Einhorn M, Greenberg D. Listeria meningitis and ventriculitis in an immunocompetent child: case report and literature review. *Infection*. 2012;40(2):207-211.

Vandesteen L, Drier A, Galanaud D, et al. Imaging findings of intraventricular and ependymal lesions. *J Neuroradiol*. 2013;40(4):229-244.

Rajan Gadhia, MD, Stacy V. Smith, MD, Andrew G. Lee, MD, and Eugene C. Lai, MD, PhD

History of Present Illness

A 75-year-old man with hypertension, hyperlipidemia, and essential tremor presented to the emergency department with 3 weeks of acutely progressive diplopia, periorbital numbness, and gait instability with falls. He had been seeing a neurologist as a result of 6 months of progressive diplopia, gait instability, and fatigue without diagnosis despite extensive evaluation. Workup included a repeat magnetic resonance imaging (MRI) the day before.

Review of systems was significant for 7-pound unintentional weight loss and dizziness during ambulation. He had no history of recent travel, sick contacts, or exposure to harmful substances. He confessed to a significant remote 40-pack-year history of tobacco use, but denied any current excessive alcohol use or tobacco use.

Exam

The patient was alert and oriented to self, place, and date. His speech was fluent but with mild guttural dysarthria. His pupils were equally round and sluggishly reactive to light, from 2 mm to 1 mm. His visual acuity in each eye was 20/20, and visual fields were full to confrontation. His extraocular muscles showed an incomitant esotropia with moderate abduction deficit of the left eye consistent with a left sixth nerve palsy. There was gaze-evoked dissociated horizontal nystagmus in his right eye only during left lateral gaze. He had no ptosis or facial weakness. Sensation was symmetrical in the face. Hearing was decreased to finger rub in both ears. Other cranial nerves were intact. Muscle strength suggested symmetrical proximal weakness in the upper limbs of 3/5. His lower limb strength was 4/5 proximally and distally. He had significant dysmetria with the left upper and lower limbs. His reflexes were 2+/4 in the upper extremities and 3+/4 at the patellar. Upon standing, he leaned toward the left, with an unsteady wide-based gait. He could not perform heel, toe, or tandem walking, or the Romberg test.

WHAT IS THE ANATOMIC LOCALIZATION OF HIS MYRIAD SYMPTOMS? WHAT ARE SOME OF THE COMMON ANATOMIC CONSIDERATIONS FOR DIPLOPIA?

This patient's symptoms and neurologic findings of diplopia and ataxia localize to the brainstem and cerebellum. A subjective complaint of double vision needs further definition as monocular versus binocular and horizontal versus vertical. Monocular diplopia remains present if the fellow eye is covered and can occur in 1 or both eyes. Binocular diplopia will resolve with either eye covered. Monocular diplopia localizes to the eye itself, whereas binocular diplopia suggests misalignment of the 2 eyes. Differentiation between horizontal and vertical diplopia can help localize the lesion to a particular cranial nerve and/or extraocular muscle, especially when combined with the extraocular movement exam. In this case, the left eye esotropia on primary gaze corresponds with a horizontal diplopia that resolves with either eye covered. Left eye esotropia with inability to fully abduct the eye indicates lateral rectus weakness, due to damage to either the muscle or the nerve. A lesion to the left sixth nerve could be at the nucleus in the pons, the fascicle, or the nerve. The additional exam finding of horizontal nystagmus in the right eye during left lateral gaze indicates involvement of the left paramedian pontine reticular formation (PPRF), since this coordinates lateral gaze to abduct the ipsilateral eye and adduct the contralateral eye. The PPRF is located adjacent to the sixth nerve nucleus and fascicle and makes this the most likely location for the lesion. The lesion to these structures is likely incomplete due to the absence of a complete left lateral gaze palsy. In addition, the seventh nerve nucleus is located anterior to the sixth nucleus, and the fascicle loops around the sixth nucleus to exit the brainstem lateral to the sixth nerve. The lack of facial weakness indicates that the seventh nerve was not also involved and also suggests a punctate focal lesion.

The gait and limb ataxia suggest a more diffuse cerebellar process, in addition to the pontine lesion. The dysarthria is a nonlocalizing feature, but correlates with

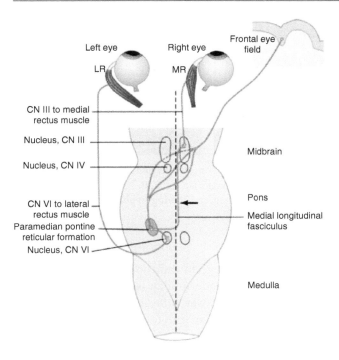

a brainstem process. The mild, symmetric motor weakness in his extremities with hyperreflexia suggests an upper motor neuron process. This could be consistent with multiple lesions and/or bilateral involvement of the motor tracts at the level of the brainstem.

Since the examination suggests specific focal involvement of the brainstem at the level of the pontine tegmentum and also indicates more diffuse cerebellar and motor pathway involvement, the patient merits further evaluation and workup at this point.

WHAT IS THE DIFFERENTIAL DIAGNOSIS TO CONSIDER GIVEN THE TIME COURSE OF HIS SYMPTOMS? WHAT FURTHER TESTING IS NECESSARY TO MAKE THE DIAGNOSIS?

Given the progressive time course of his symptoms, etiologies include vasculitis, inflammation with or without demyelination, a neurodegenerative process, toxic or metabolic processes including infection, and autoimmune pathologies. Testing should include a thorough neuro-ophthalmologic assessment to better characterize the double vision. Lab tests should be considered including serum vitamin levels, thyroid function tests, inflammatory markers, autoantibody assays, and complete blood count with differential and a metabolic panel. This patient should have imaging with gadolinium-enhanced magnetic resonance imaging (MRI), as this can help

identify inflammation or infectious etiologies that may go undetected on noncontrast imaging. Cerebrospinal fluid (CSF) analysis may reveal central nervous system (CNS) inflammation or infection.

Extensive neuromuscular workup, MRI, and CSF analysis were all normal. The patient then experienced acute exacerbation of his symptoms with new-onset dysphagia, dysarthria, and severe ataxia while undergoing a repeat MRI of the brain. Emergent evaluation with the neurovascular service revealed an ischemic lesion in the left cerebellum (not shown).

Due to progression of symptoms at his 4-week follow-up, he underwent a repeat MRI. The contrast study revealed enlargement of the ischemic lesion as well as brainstem periventricular enhancement and numerous lesions involving the pons, cerebellum, and deep ganglionic structures. More specifically, imaging showed postcontrast T1 enhancement of the pons in a "salt and pepper" distribution, with diffusion restriction and apparent diffusion coefficient (ADC) correlative hypointensity (Fig. 36.8-1). Neoplastic, paraneoplastic, inflammatory, and infectious workup was unremarkable, including computed tomography (CT) scan of the chest, abdomen, and pelvis; viral polymerase chain reaction (PCR) in serum and CSF; and CSF IgG synthesis studies.

WHAT IS THE DIAGNOSIS, AND HOW SHOULD THIS PATIENT BE TREATED?

The patient was ultimately diagnosed with chronic lymphocytic inflammation with pontine perivascular enhancement responsive to steroids ("CLIPPERS") given the characteristic imaging findings. Symptoms began to improve after a 5-day course of high-dose intravenous methylprednisolone, and he remained on steroid maintenance therapy after discharge, with a slow taper to oral prednisone alone.

The dysarthria and dysphagia resolved completely within several months. Diplopia due to a residual small esophoria occurred only intermittently, and extraocular motility exam was normal in his 9-month follow-up neuro-ophthalmologic exam. The nystagmus resolved. His gait remains slightly widened, but he no longer uses an assistive device and has returned to golfing. His repeat MRI of the brain with and without contrast showed resolution of the previously enhancing pontine lesions (Fig. 36.8-2). Due to his dramatic response to therapy, he has deferred a brain biopsy. He will remain under surveillance for both relapse and/or neoplastic disease.

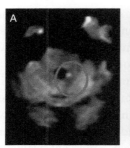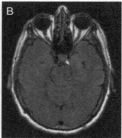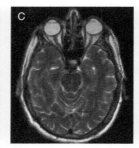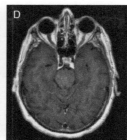

Figure 36.8-1 Initial presentation: brain magnetic resonance imaging with and without contrast. **A.** Diffusion-weighted imaging showing an area of restricted diffusion during acute exacerbation of symptoms, suggesting acute ischemia. **B.** Axial T2 fluid-attenuated inversion recovery showing hyperintense lesions in the pons. **C.** Axial T2 propeller imaging showing hyperintense lesions in the pons. **D.** Axial T1 postcontrast image showing enhancement in the pons.

CLIPPERS was first described by Pittock and colleagues in 2010. In their paper, they identified 8 patients who presented with a subacute onset of gait ataxia and diplopia, for which MRI revealed punctate and curvilinear peppering in the pons. Patients underwent CSF testing, which was negative for malignancy. Biopsy in half of the patients revealed white matter lymphocytic infiltrate with perivascular predominance. Ultimately, all patients experienced rapid improvement with intravenous methylprednisolone therapy, but also required long-term maintenance immunosuppression. One must first rule out other diagnoses in the differential, including lymphoma or other CNS neoplasm, autoimmune and inflammatory disorders, infections, and paraneoplastic syndromes. Patients with CLIPPERS are at increased risk for developing malignancy.

Interestingly, one of the core radiologic features of CLIPPERS includes absence of restricted diffusion on diffusion-weighted imaging. Our patient met the diagnostic criteria for CLIPPERS except for the acute diffusion restriction at the time of his symptom exacerbation.

However, this change in diffusion restriction also did not fit the typical pattern of an ischemic stroke since it actually progressed over time instead of resolving. In addition, his rapid response to steroid therapy is characteristic of CLIPPERS and would not occur in ischemic stroke.

The literature typically describes CLIPPERS as a steroid-dependent syndrome, but a variety of other immunosuppressive treatments have been used with varying success for long-term maintenance. In a series of 12 patients with long-term follow-up with CLIPPERS, Taieb and colleagues reported that a quarter of these patients received either rituximab or cyclophosphamide. Only 1 of these patients experienced relapse nearly 1 month after treatment. Although our patient has, to date, been treated with long-term steroids, he is also unique in his ability to tolerate tapering of his steroid without the addition of another immunosuppressant therapy. He will remain under long-term observation by multiple care teams due to the future risk of both relapse and developing a malignancy.

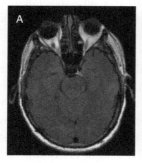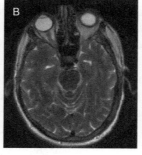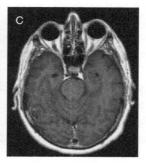

Figure 36.8-2 After steroid treatment: brain magnetic resonance imaging with and without contrast. **A.** Axial T2 fluid-attenuated inversion recovery showing resolution of hyperintense lesions in the pons. **B.** Axial T2 propeller imaging showing resolution of hyperintense lesions in the pons. **C.** Axial T1 postcontrast imaging showing resolution of enhancement in the pons.

FINAL DIAGNOSIS

- Chronic lymphocytic inflammation with pontine perivascular enhancement responsive to steroids

REFERENCES

Dalmau J, Glechman AJ, Hughes EG, et al. Anti-NMDA receptor encephalitis case series and analysis of the effects of antibodies. *Lancet Neurol.* 2008;7:198108.

Dudesek A, Rimmele F, Tesar S, et al. CLIPPERS: chronic lymphocytic inflammation with pontine perivascular enhancement responsive to steroids. Review of an increasingly recognized entity with the spectrum of inflammatory central nervous system disorders. *Clin Exp Immunol.* 2014;175:385-396.

Pittock SJ, Debruvne J, Krecke KN, et al. Chronic lymphocytic inflammation with pontine perivascular enhancement responsive to steroids (CLIPPERS). *Brain.* 2010;133: 2626-2634.

Simon NG, Parratt JD, Barnett MH, et al. Expanding the clinical, radiological and neuropathological phenotype of chronic lymphocytic inflammation with pontine perivascular enhancement responsive to steroids (CLIPPERS). *J Neurol Neurosurg Psychiatry.* 2012;83:15-22.

Taieb G, Duflos C, Renard D, et al. Long-term outcomes of CLIPPERS (chronic lymphotic inflammation with pontine perivascular enhancement responsive steroids) in a consecutive series of 12 patients. *Arch Neurol.* 2012;69: 847-855.

CLINICAL CASE VIGNETTE 9: PENETRATING TRAUMATIC BRAIN INJURY

Zachary Threlkeld, MD, and Brian L. Edlow, MD

History of Present Illness

An otherwise healthy 21-year-old man is brought to the emergency department by ambulance after suffering 2 gunshot wounds to the head. In the field, he was confused, with a Glasgow coma scale (GCS) score of 14 (E4M6V4). On arrival to the emergency department, he is found to have a GCS score of 8 (E2M5V1) and is intubated emergently for inability to protect his airway.

Exam

His vitals were as follows: noninvasive blood pressure 185/110 mm Hg, heart rate 43 bpm, temperature 36.3°C, respiratory rate 19 breaths/min, oxygen saturation 98% on 2 L nasal cannula. His primary survey was pertinent for the following:

- Penetrating injury to the left temple without evidence of an exit wound
- Orbital edema without periorbital ecchymoses
- Dried blood in left ear canal; no hemotympanum or clear otorrhea
- Blood in bilateral nares
- Lungs clear to auscultation bilaterally
- Bradycardic; no murmurs, rubs, or gallops
- Abdomen soft, nondistended, without guarding

His neurologic examination was as follows: eyes open briefly to noxious stimulation; he does not follow commands, right pupil is briskly reactive, 3 to >2 mm; left pupil is sluggishly reactive and larger, 5 to >4 mm. Eye movement testing was limited by neck stabilization in a cervical collar. Corneal reflex was present on the right but not on the left. There was a right facial droop in an upper motor neuron pattern.

He localized with the left arm and moved the left leg spontaneously. The right arm and leg did not move spontaneously or in response to noxious stimuli.

Focused assessment with sonography in trauma (FAST) did not reveal abdominal free fluid, pneumothorax, or pericardial effusion. He was hemodynamically stable. His initial noncontrast head computed tomography (CT) scan is shown in Figure 36.9-1.

WHAT IS THE MOST IMMEDIATE NEXT STEP IN MANAGEMENT?

As with any patient suffering acute trauma, the ABCs (airway, breathing, circulation) are the first step in management. This patient's airway has been secured, he is oxygenating well, and he is not hypotensive. Clinically and radiographically, there is evidence of elevated intracranial pressure (ICP) with incipient herniation. The most important next step in management is treatment of his ICP to halt and reverse herniation.

A tiered approach to treatment of elevated ICP is the standard of care. Even prior to undergoing CT scan, he should have his head of bed elevated to promote venous drainage from the intracranial compartment.

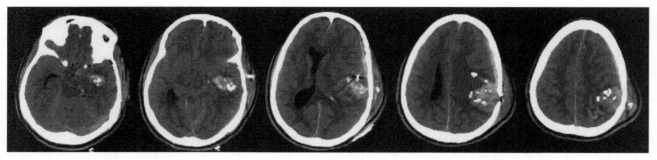

Figure 36.9-1   Noncontrast head computed tomography demonstrates an acute left-sided subdural hematoma (5-mm thickness), focal convexal subarachnoid hemorrhage, multifocal intraparenchymal hemorrhage, and intraventricular hemorrhage. There is 10-mm left-to-right midline shift at the level of the septum pellucidum, with obliteration of the left lateral ventricle and left uncal herniation. There is scattered pneumocephalus, and a 1- to 2-cm defect in the left parietal bone with fracture extending into the left temporal bone and mastoid air cells, as well as fractures of the left orbit. Numerous metallic and bony fragments are seen in the left hemisphere, including 2 large metallic-appearing hyperdensities in the left parietal extracranial soft tissue (best seen on bone window images; not shown).

Hyperventilation may reduce ICP by inducing vaso-constriction of cerebral vessels. However, hyperventilation should only be used as a temporizing measure and may cause cerebral ischemia in settings where cerebral blood flow may already be compromised. Furthermore, hyperventilation may induce reflex vasodilation and ICP elevation when normal ventilation is resumed. Current consensus guidelines recommend only avoidance of hypoventilation, with a target partial pressure of carbon dioxide of 35 to 40 mm Hg. Most importantly, hyperventilation, if used, should serve as a bridge to more definitive treatment.

Adequate sedation and analgesia are essential but frequently overlooked. Pain, discomfort, and ventilator desynchrony may elevate both blood pressure and ICP. Propofol is a common first-line sedative agent, as it may reduce ICP by decreasing the cerebral metabolic rate. Propofol also can be rapidly cleared when cessation of sedation is necessary for repeat neurologic examinations. Fentanyl is a common first-line analgesic agent, as it reduces pain, may prevent bronchospasm associated with an endotracheal tube, and is also rapidly cleared when held for a repeat neurologic examination.

Hyperosmolar therapy with mannitol or hypertonic saline is the most appropriate next treatment. In the absence of known renal dysfunction and refractory hypotension, mannitol dosed at 1 g/kg is the most appropriate initial empiric therapy for elevated ICP. It is widely available and does not require central venous access. In this case, it would be reasonable to start mannitol prior to CT scan, given the patient's rapid decline, high clinical suspicion of elevated ICP, and need to lie flat for the scan.

Given the osmotic diuresis that frequently occurs after a dose of mannitol, clinicians should consider intravenous volume repletion with isotonic or hypertonic solutions to prevent hypovolemia.

Hyperosmolar therapy may also be initiated with 23.4% hypertonic saline, typically given as a bolus of 30 mL. Due to the risk of soft tissue necrosis with extravasation of this solution, peripheral intravenous infusion should be avoided if possible. As such, it is more useful for medical management of ongoing elevations in ICP once central venous access has been obtained. Available evidence suggests that mannitol and hypertonic saline are likely equally efficacious at reducing ICP. Thus, the choice of hyperosmolar agent is guided by institutional preference, availability, venous access, renal function, and volume status.

Intravenous corticosteroids are contraindicated for the treatment of acutely elevated ICP. The MRC CRASH trial showed that steroids neither improve outcome nor reduce ICP in traumatic brain injury (TBI) and, in addition, are associated with a higher mortality rate.

Neurosurgical consultation should be sought concomitantly as the above measures are being undertaken, as this patient's rapid decline suggests that medical therapies alone may be insufficient. Cerebrospinal fluid (CSF) drainage by external ventricular drain (EVD) should be considered. Any TBI patient with an abnormal CT scan associated with coma or rapid decline in GCS is a candidate for EVD placement, which serves both to measure and treat elevated ICP via CSF diversion.

Fronto-temporo-parietal decompressive craniectomy is potentially a life-saving measure to treat elevated

ICP and should be considered in cases of elevated ICP refractory to the preceding interventions. However, although a large randomized trial has shown that fronto-temporo-parietal craniectomy may reduce ICP, shorten intensive care unit stay, and improve mortality, the intervention also increases the likelihood of severe disability or vegetative state. Bifrontal craniectomy is not recommended because it increases the likelihood of unfavorable outcome and confers no mortality benefit.

Hypothermia and barbiturate coma may be considered in cases of elevated ICP refractory to the above maximal medical and surgical therapies. Although these interventions may be effective at reducing refractory ICP elevation in selected patients, their efficacy has not been demonstrated in randomized controlled trials. Furthermore, these interventions may lead to worse outcomes when used early or prophylactically.

The patient was emergently taken to the operating room for decompressive left fronto-temporo-parietal hemicraniectomy with concomitant placement of an EVD in the right lateral ventricle. The largest bullet fragments were not removed given associated hemorrhage and proximity to cerebral vessels. The bone flap was left off. On arrival to the neurointensive care unit, sedation was withheld for neurologic examination, which revealed no eye opening or command following, equal and reactive pupils, absent left corneal reflex, absent gag, intact cough, right hemiplegia, localization with the left arm, and triple flexion in the left leg.

WHAT HEMODYNAMIC AND BRAIN PERFUSION PARAMETERS DO YOU TARGET?

All efforts share the goal of maximizing cerebral perfusion, where cerebral perfusion pressure (CPP) is defined as the difference between mean arterial blood pressure (MAP) and ICP (CPP = MAP − ICP). Although the mathematical relationship between these parameters is simple, the interplay between them is complex. It is intuitive that a higher MAP is necessary to maintain CPP in the setting of elevated ICP and that cerebral perfusion ceases as the ICP approaches the MAP. However, the relationship between CPP, MAP, and ICP can differ depending on an individual patient's cerebrovascular autoregulatory function. If cerebrovascular autoregulation is intact, hypotension induces compensatory vasodilation, which can increase cerebral blood volume and may ultimately increase ICP. If cerebrovascular autoregulation is disrupted by injury to the brain parenchyma or vasculature, hypotension may lead to a decrease in ICP, although at the expense of CPP. In either case, hypotension may lead to cerebral ischemia.

The most recent TBI guidelines recommend systolic blood pressure (SBP) of >110 mm Hg for most TBI patients, with a liberalized goal of SBP >100 mm Hg in patients age 50 to 69 years, based on a retrospective study in which optimal hypotension thresholds were derived post hoc in an age-stratified sample.

Severe TBI may be a diffuse process, often with superimposed focal lesions. As a result, elevated ICP may persist, either globally or in a specific intracranial compartment (eg, posterior fossa), even after CSF diversion and hemicraniectomy. Presumably, elevated ICP is a surrogate for ongoing secondary neurologic injury and is therefore to be aggressively monitored and avoided. Classically, the recommended goal ICP is <20 mm Hg, and this is a reasonable initial target. No randomized trial of target ICP values exists, although there is evidence to suggest that treating ICP >22 mm Hg reduces mortality and improves functional outcomes. CPP may also be targeted with a goal of 60 to 70 mm Hg. Although CPP may seem like a more physiologically relevant measure, there is little evidence to support targeting CPP or ICP preferentially. Careful monitoring and optimization of both ICP and CPP are associated with improved survival.

WHAT MEDICAL PROPHYLAXIS IS INDICATED TO AVOID COMMON SEQUELAE OF SEVERE TBI?

In addition to the tiered therapies already discussed, treatment of persistently elevated ICP demands high-quality intensive care. Avoidance of metabolic disarray, poor nutrition, fever, seizure, and other preventable complications is essential. The common thread is prevention of excess metabolic demand in an injured brain with potentially comprised metabolic supply.

Seizures are symptomatic of brain dysfunction and are an expected—but potentially preventable—sequela of severe TBI. Although prevention of seizures seems intuitively beneficial, acute seizures have never been linked to worse long-term outcomes. Still, seizures in the acute phase presumably increase metabolic demand and may increase ICP. A 7-day course of phenytoin reduces the incidence of seizures acutely, and levetiracetam has been shown to be noninferior. Longer use of prophylactic anticonvulsants may impede functional recovery and furthermore does not reduce the incidence of seizures occurring more than 7 days after the initial injury.

As with all trauma patients, the incidence of venous thromboembolism (VTE) is significantly elevated in acute TBI. Indeed, the prolonged immobility associated with TBI makes it an independent risk factor for the development of VTE among trauma patients in general. TBI patients should receive mechanical VTE prophylaxis (sequential compression devices), and chemoprophylaxis should be considered once hemorrhage stability has been demonstrated.

As with all critically ill patients, nutrition via enteral access should be initiated in a timely fashion. No benefit to intensive glycemic control has been shown, and a typical goal serum glucose is <180 mg/dL, consistent with broader critical care literature.

The patient's exam improved over the next 48 hours, and he began following commands with his left arm and leg and localizing with the right arm and leg. ICP remained well controlled with around-the-clock mannitol and CSF drainage. On day 3 of hospitalization, the patient lost the ability to follow commands and became tachycardic and febrile. He localized with both arms. ICP was borderline elevated. His oxygen requirement had not changed. Serum sodium was 140 mEq/L.

WHAT ARE THE POSSIBLE ETIOLOGIES OF HIS NEUROLOGIC DECLINE? WHAT ARE YOUR NEXT DIAGNOSTIC AND THERAPEUTIC STEPS?

Myriad complications may induce a sudden decline in mental status in a patient with severe TBI. The most worrisome is hemorrhage expansion or new infarction, which should be assessed immediately with CT of the head, particularly if the decline is focal. The finding of a borderline elevated ICP transduced from the EVD may be reassuring but should be interpreted cautiously in the setting of hemicraniectomy. Furthermore, ICPs measured by an EVD in the lateral ventricle do not always reflect regional compartmental pressures in the posterior or middle fossae. Worsening cerebral edema should be high on the differential diagnosis, particularly given the timing.

Serum sodium should be closely followed in all patients with severe TBI and cerebral edema, with aggressive treatment of hyponatremia. When sustained cerebral edema is anticipated, induced hypernatremia may be helpful. This may be achieved with continuous 3% saline infusion or with scheduled boluses of 23.4% saline (sometimes staggered with mannitol to achieve maximal medical hyperosmolar therapy). Both strategies may be used successfully, and there is little evidence to favor one over the other.

Seizure is also a consideration, and continuous electroencephalography (EEG) monitoring is helpful if available. In addition to detecting seizures and nonconvulsive status epilepticus, focal slowing and specialized quantitative EEG measures may detect ischemia from a variety of causes—even prior to its clinical manifestations.

Venous sinus thrombosis should also be considered, particularly in penetrating injury with depressed fractures. This patient's known temporal bone fracture predisposes to transverse sinus thrombosis, and extension of this thrombosis to the torcula with associated impaired venous drainage of the thalami could manifest as an acute decline in mental status.

Fever itself may cause a decline in the neurologic exam. TBI patients are subject to the same causes of fever as other critically ill patients, and consideration should be given to infection (particularly pneumonia and meningitis) and VTE. It would be reasonable to start deep vein thrombosis (DVT) prophylaxis if his intracranial hemorrhages are stable, and ultrasonography of the extremities should be considered to assess for DVT if other causes of infection have been excluded. Given the presence of a contaminated foreign body, penetrating head injury is typically treated with empiric broad-spectrum antibiotics. Even in the absence of obvious penetrating injury, TBI patients are at greater risk for meningitis due to violation of the dura, whether iatrogenic or from the trauma itself. Nevertheless, prophylactic antibiotics in nonpenetrating TBI are not recommended unless risk factors for infection are present, such as CSF otorrhea or rhinorrhea, violation of the sinuses, or retention of bone fragments.

Fevers in patients with severe central nervous system injury, particularly TBI, are frequently attributed to the central nervous system injury itself. Such "central fevers" likely reflect a combination of autonomic dysregulation and systemic inflammatory response. Symptomatic treatment with antipyretics and cooling blankets is warranted to reduce cerebral metabolic demand; furthermore, if fevers are sustained and high grade or correlated with ICP elevations, normothermia may be achieved by targeted temperature management (TTM) systems more commonly used for therapeutic hypothermia after cardiac arrest. Although effective, use of these devices may require significant sedation or even paralysis—with loss of the neurologic exam—to control shivering.

Finally, TBI patients with episodic fever, tachycardia, profuse diaphoresis, and refractory hypertension without a clear etiology may have paroxysmal sympathetic hyperactivity (PSH), or "autonomic storming." Such episodes often respond to propranolol and clonidine.

Workup of the patient's fever, including cultures of the blood, urine, and CSF, did not reveal an infectious etiology. His exam improved with induced hypernatremia and treatment of his fevers. He was started on around-the-clock acetaminophen and cooling blankets. Shivering was treated with buspirone. On day 7 of hospitalization, he again stopped following commands and was noted to have left gaze preference with right hemiplegia, while continuing to localize with the left arm. EEG revealed focal left hemispheric slowing with an increased proportion of frequencies in the delta range.

DO YOU THINK STROKE OR SEIZURE IS MOST LIKELY IN THIS PATIENT? WHAT TESTS WOULD BE MOST HELPFUL?

All of the previously discussed etiologies for sudden decline in the patient's exam still apply, although this exam change is more focal, and thus, a systemic insult such as fever or metabolic disarray is less likely. Gaze preference directed contralateral to the side of paresis suggests ischemia or may be the result of postictal dysfunction of the frontal eye fields. Deep seizures not detected by scalp EEG are a possibility, although symptomatic aphasia and hemiplegia suggest widespread cortical propagation that should be detectable.

Cerebral vasospasm should be high in the differential, particularly given the time elapsed since the injury. At day 7, the degree of cerebral edema is anticipated to decline, while the incidence of vasospasm is expected to increase. Although more classically associated with aneurysmal subarachnoid hemorrhage, vasospasm is also a well-recognized sequela of traumatic subarachnoid hemorrhage and blast-related TBI. Results of randomized controlled trials do not support the use of nimodipine for TBI, because the underlying mechanism is likely different from aneurysmal subarachnoid hemorrhage and because the potential adverse effects (eg, hypotension) can be detrimental in the setting of the impaired autoregulation frequently observed in TBI. The standard of care for symptomatic vasospasm in TBI is induced hypertension (to the extent tolerated by ICP and CPP) and, in some cases, endovascular intervention.

CT angiogram revealed severe focal stenosis of the left greater than right distal internal carotid and middle cerebral arteries (Fig. 36.9-2). Vasopressors were started to maintain SBP >160 mm Hg with improvement of his aphasia and right hemiplegia. Conventional angiogram confirmed the CT angiogram findings (Fig. 36.9-3), and intra-arterial verapamil was injected into the left internal

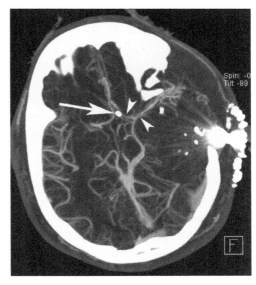

Figure 36.9-2 Computed tomography angiogram showing vasospasm (*arrowheads*). Note also the proximity of the bullet fragment (*arrow*) to the anterior and middle cerebral arteries.

carotid artery. His exam improved, his fevers resolved, and hyperosmolar therapies and sedation were weaned over the ensuing 7 days.

The patient's EVD was removed 20 days after his initial injury, and he was discharged to an inpatient rehabilitation facility. His bone flap was replaced 1 month later.

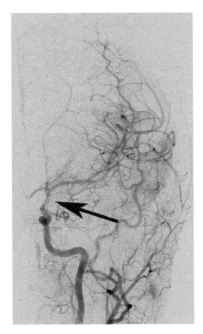

Figure 36.9-3 Conventional cerebral angiogram, anteroposterior view, after left internal carotid artery contrast injection showing vasospasm (*arrow*).

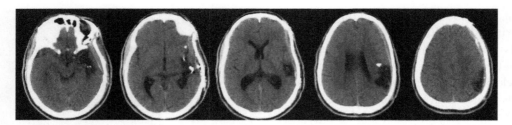

Figure 36.9-4   Noncontrast head computed tomography obtained 4 months after initial trauma.

Follow-up CT 4 months after injury is shown in Figure 36.9-4. Six months after the injury, he completed intensive inpatient and outpatient rehabilitation, was living at home, and was receiving outpatient physical and occupational therapy. The patient continues to experience decreased vision in his left eye, fatigue, and irritability, but no weakness. He now spends time with family and friends and is actively seeking employment.

FINAL DIAGNOSIS

- Severe penetrating TBI with subdural hematoma and subarachnoid hemorrhage

REFERENCES

Allen BB, Chiu YL, Gerber LM, Ghajar J, Greenfield JP. Age-specific cerebral perfusion pressure thresholds and survival in children and adolescents with severe traumatic brain injury. *Pediatr Crit Care Ced.* 2014;15(1):62-70.

Andrews PJ, Sinclair HL, Rodriguez A, et al. Hypothermia for intracranial hypertension after traumatic brain injury. *N Engl J Med.* 2015;373(25):2403-2412.

Antibiotic prophylaxis for penetrating brain injury. *J Trauma.* 2001;51(2 Suppl):S34-S40.

Baguley IJ, Perkes IE, Fernandez-Ortega JF, et al. Paroxysmal sympathetic hyperactivity after acquired brain injury: consensus on conceptual definition, nomenclature, and diagnostic criteria. *J Neurotrauma.* 2014;31(17):1515-1520.

Berry C, Ley EJ, Bukur M, et al. Redefining hypotension in traumatic brain injury. *Injury.* 2012;43(11):1833-1837.

Bower RS, Sunnarborg R, Rabinstein AA, Wijdicks EF. Paroxysmal sympathetic hyperactivity after traumatic brain injury. *Neurocrit Care.* 2010;13(2):233-234.

Carney N, Totten AM, O'Reilly C, et al. Guidelines for the management of severe traumatic brain injury, fourth edition. *Neurosurgery.* 2017;80(1):6-15.

Coester A, Neumann CR, Schmidt MI. Intensive insulin therapy in severe traumatic brain injury: a randomized trial. *J Trauma.* 2010;68(4):904-911.

Cooper DJ, Rosenfeld JV, Murray L, et al. Decompressive craniectomy in diffuse traumatic brain injury. *N Engl J Med.* 2011;364(16):1493-1502.

Gerber LM, Chiu YL, Carney N, Hartl R, Ghajar J. Marked reduction in mortality in patients with severe traumatic brain injury. *J Neurosurg.* 2013;119(6):1583-1590.

Greer DM, Funk SE, Reaven NL, Ouzounelli M, Uman GC. Impact of fever on outcome in patients with stroke and neurologic injury: a comprehensive meta-analysis. *Stroke.* 2008;39(11):3029-3035.

Hutchinson PJ, Kolias AG, Timofeev IS, et al. Trial of decompressive craniectomy for traumatic intracranial hypertension. *N Engl J Med.* 2016;375(12):1119-1130.

Inaba K, Menaker J, Branco BC, et al. A prospective multicenter comparison of levetiracetam versus phenytoin for early posttraumatic seizure prophylaxis. *J Trauma Acute Care Surg.* 2013;74(3):766-771; discussion 771-763.

Izzy S, Muehlschlegel S. Cerebral vasospasm after aneurysmal subarachnoid hemorrhage and traumatic brain injury. *Curr Treat Options Neurol.* 2014;16(1):278.

Knudson MM, Ikossi DG, Khaw L, Morabito D, Speetzen LS. Thromboembolism after trauma: an analysis of 1602 episodes from the American College of Surgeons National Trauma Data Bank. *Ann Surg.* 2004;240(3):490-496; discussion 496-498.

Langham J, Goldfrad C, Teasdale G, Shaw D, Rowan K. Calcium channel blockers for acute traumatic brain injury. *Cochrane Database Syst Rev.* 2003;4:CD000565.

Mangat HS, Chiu YL, Gerber LM, Alimi M, Ghajar J, Hartl R. Hypertonic saline reduces cumulative and daily intracranial pressure burdens after severe traumatic brain injury. *J Neurosurg.* 2015;122(1):202-210.

NICE-SUGAR Study Investigators, Finfer S, Chittock DR, et al. Intensive versus conventional glucose control in critically ill patients. *N Engl J Med.* 2009;360(13):1283-1297.

Roberts I, Yates D, Sandercock P, et al. Effect of intravenous corticosteroids on death within 14 days in 10008 adults with clinically significant head injury (MRC CRASH trial): randomised placebo-controlled trial. *Lancet.* 2004; 364(9442):1321-1328.

Sorrentino E, Diedler J, Kasprowicz M, et al. Critical thresholds for cerebrovascular reactivity after traumatic brain injury. *Neurocrit Care.* 2012;16(2):258-266.

Temkin NR, Dikmen SS, Wilensky AJ, Keihm J, Chabal S, Winn HR. A randomized, double-blind study of phenytoin for the prevention of post-traumatic seizures. *N Engl J Med.* 1990;323(8):497-502.

Ward JD, Becker DP, Miller JD, et al. Failure of prophylactic barbiturate coma in the treatment of severe head injury. *J Neurosurg.* 1985;62(3):383-388.

CLINICAL CASE VIGNETTE 10: COMPLICATIONS OF MENINGITIS

Faheem Sheriff, MD, David P. Lerner, MD, and Saef Izzy, MD

History of Present Illness

A 66-year-old woman with T11-L1 chordoma treated with multiple resections, spinal fusion, and brachytherapy 2 weeks prior to admission presented with unresponsiveness after a computed tomography (CT) myelogram (performed for staging of her malignancy). She was in her usual state of health the night prior and was found down by her friends the next morning. Of note, she had some right lower extremity weakness and difficulty with proprioception prior to admission; however, she was otherwise neurologically intact.

Exam

On arrival to the emergency department, she had a Glasgow coma scale (GCS) score of (E1M5V1). She was intubated for airway protection given her altered mentation and was admitted to the medical intensive care unit (ICU). Her vital signs on arrival to the unit were as follows: temperature 37.2°C, blood pressure 128/63 mm Hg, heart rate 81 bpm, and respiratory rate 32 breaths/min. She was on pressure support ventilation on the following settings: inspiratory pressure 10 cm H_2O, positive end-expiratory pressure 5 cm H_2O, with a fraction of inspired oxygen of 40%. Her systemic exam was only remarkable for mild nuchal rigidity. She did not have any murmurs or rubs on cardiac exam, and breath sounds were coarse anteriorly. On neurologic exam off sedation, she did not arouse to voice or noxious stimuli but did grimace and did not follow commands. Her cranial nerves were intact. She localized to pain and moved both arms spontaneously against gravity. Lower extremity tone was decreased, and there was no movement to noxious stimulation in the legs. Reflexes were present and symmetric in the upper extremities but decreased in the lower extremities. Her plantar reflexes were mute bilaterally.

WHAT IS THE DIFFERENTIAL DIAGNOSIS?

Given the abrupt onset, a vascular process is high on the differential. Seizure is also possible, but there is no clear ictal activity. Given nuchal rigidity on exam, meningeal irritation is present and could be due to an infectious process or subarachnoid hemorrhage. The temporal association with recent CT myelogram is concerning for possibility of iatrogenic meningitis. Metastases to brain or carcinomatous meningitis is another possibility, although abruptness of onset would argue against these processes; in addition, chordomas rarely metastasize to the central nervous system. Given her lower extremity weakness and loss of tone, a spinal cord or cauda equina process must be considered. Cord compression from mass effect or pathologic fractures related to her treated chordoma are important considerations but would not explain her overall neurologic presentation. Cord infarct is also part of the differential given abrupt onset.

WHAT WOULD YOU ORDER NEXT FOR WORKUP?

Her noncontrast head CT was negative. Lumbar puncture was performed and had the following profile: glucose 24 mg/dL (normal 45-80 mg/dL), total protein 2100 mg/dL (normal <45 mg/dL), and 2550 nucleated cells (83% neutrophils). The Gram stain demonstrated gram-variable rods with no growth on cultures. 16S polymerase chain reaction (PCR) testing later identified the organism as *Bacillus cereus*. Blood cultures were persistently negative. The patient was started on vancomycin and ceftazidime (later changed to meropenem); acyclovir was added while awaiting herpes simplex virus PCR results and stopped later in the course when it came back negative. Magnetic resonance imaging (MRI) of the brain performed and was notable for left middle cerebral artery and right posterior inferior cerebellar artery strokes (Fig. 36.10-1). Magnetic resonance angiogram was unremarkable. A transthoracic echocardiogram was performed with mobile densities on mitral valve thought most likely to be redundant chordae. MRI of the thoracic and lumbar spine was performed; no large epidural or cord process was seen, but imaging was limited by artifact from hardware.

The patient's ICU course was complicated by jerking movements and intermittent left gaze deviation. She received 2 mg of intravenous (IV) lorazepam and was loaded with IV levetiracetam and maintained on the same. Continuous electroencephalography showed frequent sharp-and-slow-wave discharges over the right frontal area, which became briefly periodic, consistent with lateralized periodic discharges (LPDs; Fig. 36.10-2).

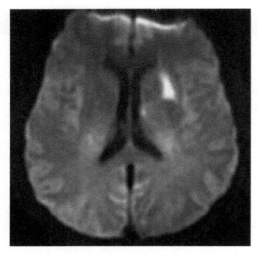

Figure 36.10-1 Magnetic resonance imaging. Diffuse weighted sequence with hyperintensity in the left basal ganglia with corresponding apparent diffuse coefficent hypointensity (not shown) consistent with acute ischemic infarction.

Repeat MRI was performed and demonstrated developing right cerebellar abscess as well as concern for venous sinus thrombosis of the right transverse, sigmoid, occipital sinuses and torcula, which was confirmed on a CT venogram (Fig. 36.10-3).

WOULD YOU ANTICOAGULATE THIS PATIENT? WOULD YOU GIVE STEROIDS TO THIS PATIENT?

Use of anticoagulation in septic venous sinus thrombosis is controversial and has been better described in cavernous sinus thrombosis patients in whom there was a trend toward decreased morbidity when anticoagulation was used early along with antibiotics. Arguments against using anticoagulation include possibility of intracranial hemorrhage, especially in cases where there are concomitant cerebral infarcts, as well as the theoretical risk of dissemination of infection by lysis of the infected thrombus. Although corticosteroids and prophylactic antiplatelet therapy have been used in infectious cerebral vasculitis, there are no randomized clinical trials that have evaluated their efficacy and safety.

After thorough risk-benefit discussion with her family and given lack of clinical improvement, heparin infusion was started (without bolus) for her venous sinus thrombosis. Steroids were withheld. Subsequently, over the next several days, the patient was noted to have improved neurologically and was able to verbalize in brief sentences and follow commands in her arms (but not her legs). She was then transferred to the floor and was stable until the following morning when she was

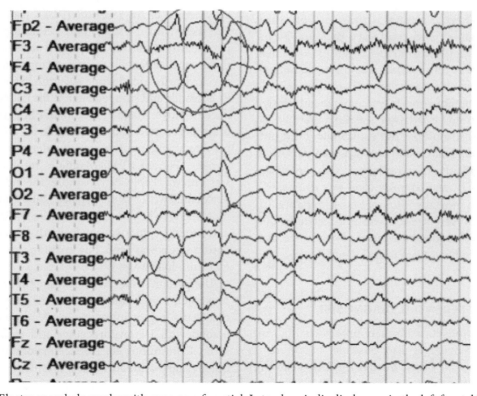

Figure 36.10-2 Electroencephalography with average referential. Lateral periodic discharges in the left frontal lobe shown.

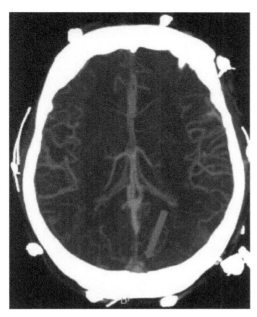

Figure 36.10-3 Computed tomography venogram showing incomplete filling of the superior saggital sinus consistent with sinus thrombosis.

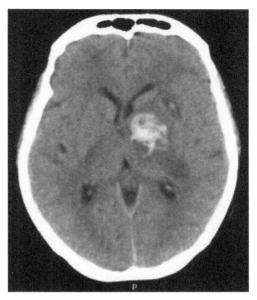

Figure 36.10-4 Noncontrast computed tomography with hyperdensity within the left basal ganglia with mild mass-effect and compression of the left lateral ventricle.

noted to be febrile to 102.1°F and only minimally arousable to noxious stimuli, have right facial droop with left gaze preference, and have inability to move her right upper extremity.

WHAT WOULD BE YOUR NEXT STEP IN MANAGEMENT OF THIS PATIENT?

Heparin was stopped, blood cultures and labs were drawn, and the patient was taken for a stat noncontrast head CT that showed a bleed in the left basal ganglia. She was reversed with IV protamine sulfate 15 mg and transferred to the neuro-ICU. Repeat CT scans showed stable bleed, thought to be secondary to hemorrhagic conversion of the ischemic stroke she had had earlier in her hospitalization (Fig. 36.10-4).

Several hours later, the patient started requiring more oxygen support. Repeat chest x-ray showed complete opacification of the left hemithorax requiring emergent intubation and bronchoscopy and mucus evacuation. She was on vasopressors for a brief period of time. After an extended discussion with her husband, the healthcare

proxy, she was transitioned to comfort measures and subsequently extubated. The family did not request an autopsy.

WHAT ARE YOUR FINAL DIAGNOSES?

- Iatrogenic meningitis due to *Bacillus cereus*
- Multifocal cerebral infarcts and venous sinus thrombosis likely due to infectious vasculitis
- Suspected cord infarct

REFERENCES

Bhatia K, Jones NS. Septic cavernous sinus thrombosis secondary to sinusitis: are anticoagulants indicated? A review of the literature. *J Laryngol Otol.* 2002;116:667-676.

Carod AJF. Clinical management of infectious cerebral vasculitides. *Expert Rev Neurother.* 2016;16:205-221.

Hall WA, Clark HB. Sacrococcygeal chordoma metastatic to the brain with review of the literature. *J Neuro-Oncol.* 1995;25:155-159.

Levins SR, Twyman RE, Gilman S. The role of anticoagulation in cavernous sinus thrombosis. *Neurology.* 1988;38: 517-522.

CLINICAL CASE VIGNETTE 11: SUBACUTE PROGRESSIVE ENCEPHALOPATHY

David P. Lerner, MD, and Steven K. Feske, MD

History of Present Illness

A 62-year-old woman was transferred to the neurologic intensive care unit from an outside hospital for further evaluation and management of change in mental status and concerning magnetic resonance imaging (MRI) of the brain. The patient had a history of subacute dementia and repeated falls. Four months before presentation, she developed progressive fluctuating confusion with paranoid ideation but was able to complete activities of daily living. One month before presentation, she suffered a mechanical fall down a flight of stairs. A noncontrast head computed tomography (CT) showed no intracranial abnormality. She was discharged to a rehabilitation facility where her memory continued to decline and she continued to fall repeatedly. She was readmitted to an outside facility for progression of her symptoms, and workup there included cardiac and metabolic testing, which was unremarkable. A brain MRI was completed and is shown in Figure 36.11-1.

Exam

On transfer, she was alert and interactive but oriented only to person. She was able to follow 1-step appendicular and axial commands. She was abulic, but her speech was otherwise normal. Cranial nerves were normal. She had a symmetric, bilateral, upper extremity high-frequency tremor present at rest and with action. Strength was full throughout, and sensation was normal. There was no ataxia. She was able to stand from a seated position without assistance, but her gait was very unsteady.

WHAT IS THE DIFFERENTIAL DIAGNOSIS?

The differential diagnosis for the initial imaging and neurologic findings, bilateral thalamic fluid-attenuated inversion recovery (FLAIR) signal hyperintensities in the setting of cognitive decline, is large and includes the following:

- Neurodegenerative diseases, such as Creutzfeldt-Jakob disease
- Inflammatory disorders, such as vasculitis
- Malignancies, such as low-grade glioma
- Toxic exposures, such as toluene inhalation
- Metabolic disorders, including Wernicke encephalopathy, Fabry disease, Wilson disease, and Leigh disease
- Infectious diseases, including encephalitis from West Nile virus, influenza, eastern equine encephalitis virus, rabies, and *Borrelia*
- Vascular disorders, including posterior reversible encephalopathy syndrome, top of the basilar syndrome, occlusion of the artery of Percheron, and thrombosis of the deep cerebral venous system

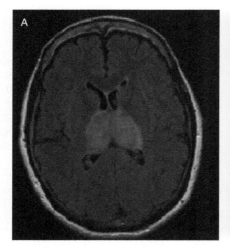 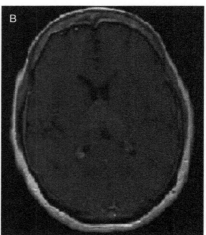

Figure 36.11-1   Magnetic resonance imaging of the brain 1.5-T magnet. **A.** Fluid-attenuated inversion recovery sequence at the level of the mid-thalamus with bilateral, symmetric hyperintensity. **B.** T1-weighted image with contrast at the same level with patchy enhancement within the bilateral anterior thalami.

WHAT WOULD YOU ORDER NEXT FOR WORKUP?

The original MRI raised concern for possible cerebral venous sinus thrombosis, but further imaging was deferred until after transfer. Cerebrospinal fluid (CSF) showed the following: protein 104 mg/dL, glucose 72 mg/dL, red blood cells 49,200 cells/μL in tube 1 and 1180 cells/μL in tube 4, and nucleated cell count 15 cells/μL in tube 1 and 5 cells/μL in tube 4. CSF 14-3-3, herpes simplex virus polymerase chain reaction (PCR), West Nile virus PCR, fungal culture, and acid-fast bacilli culture were negative.

A repeat MRI with venous imaging demonstrated right transverse sinus thrombosis and dural arteriovenous malformation with multiple feeding arteries: the posterior branch of the right middle meningeal artery, the medial tentorial artery from the cavernous carotid artery, extradural feeders from the right vertebral artery, and the bilateral occipital arteries via transosseous meningeal branches. Venous drainage was via a dilated vein of Galen, which drained retrograde into the superior cortical veins emptying into the sagittal sinus and into the basal veins emptying into the cavernous sinus and pterygoid plexus.

WOULD YOU ANTICOAGULATE THIS PATIENT?

Use of anticoagulation in venous sinus thrombosis is considered standard therapy, but this patient is a higher risk than standard for complications from anticoagulation given the dural arteriovenous fistula.

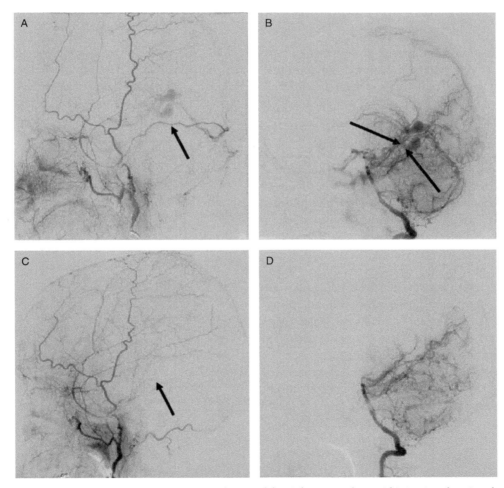

Figure 36.11-2 Digital subtraction arteriogram. **A.** Lateral view of the right external carotid injection showing the occipital artery (*arrow*) with early feeding into dural arteriovenous fistula. **B.** Lateral view of the right vertebral artery injection with early filling of a dilated vein of Galen (*arrows*). **C.** Postintervention lateral view of the right external carotid artery injection. The occipital artery (*arrow*) no longer feeds into the dural arteriovenous fistula. **D.** Postintervention lateral view of the right vertebral artery injection without filling of the dural arteriovenous fistula.

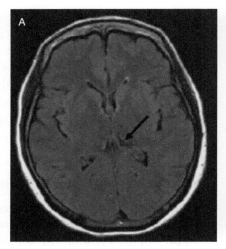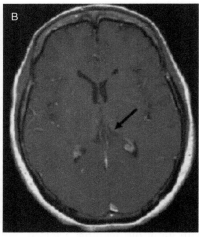

Figure 36.11-3 **A.** Fluid-attenuated inversion recovery sequence at the level of the mid-thalamus, with normal parenchymal intensity. **B.** T1-weighted image with contrast at the same level showing resolution of enhancement. Both images show a hypointensity within the posterior left thalamus consistent with evolution of hemorrhage following endovascular intervention (*arrows*).

Initial anticoagulation was deferred given her high risk for hemorrhage with potential hemorrhage into the thalami, which would result in persistent, significant neurologic injury.

HOW WOULD YOU MANAGE HER NEXT?

Embolization occurred at the point of fistulization between the artery and draining venous structures using Onyx (Covidien, Plymouth, MN) via the middle meningeal artery. After completion of the embolization, there was no longer early venous drainage from the bilateral occipital arteries and right vertebral artery (Fig. 36.11-2, C and D).

Three months after endovascular treatment, she was living in a long-term care facility. Her primary complaint was impaired long-term memory, which was thought to be due to ongoing benzodiazepine use. Her examination demonstrated normal prosody of speech; orientation to person, place, and time; and the ability to recount her medical history. She had no abnormal movements and was ambulating without assistance. Repeat imaging demonstrated resolution of the FLAIR hyperintensity within the bilateral thalami and resolution of

the enhancement. There was hypointensity within the left thalamus due to a small intraparenchymal hemorrhage following the interventional treatment of the dural arteriovenous fistula (Fig. 36.11-3, A and B).

WHAT ARE YOUR FINAL DIAGNOSES?

- Thalamic dementia due to secondary type III dural arteriovenous fistula
- Transverse sinus thrombosis

REFERENCES

Aydin K, Sencer S, Demir T, et al. Cranial MR findings in chronic toluene abuse by inhalation. *AJNR Am J Neuroradiol.* 2002;23:1173-1179.

Bartynski WS, Boardman JF. Distinct imaging patterns and lesion distribution in posterior reversible encephalopathy syndrome. *AJNR Am J Neuroradiol.* 2007;28:1320-1327.

Linn J, Danek A, Hoffmann LA, Seelos KC, Bruckmann H. Differential diagnosis of bilateral thalamic lesions. *Clin Neuroradiol.* 2007;1:1-22.

Lorenzi S, Pfister HW, Padovan C, Yousry T. MRI abnormalities in tick-borne encephalitis. *Lancet.* 1996;347:698-699.

Catherine S.W. Albin, MD, and David P. Lerner, MD

History of Present Illness

A 61-year-old woman with hypertension, diabetes, hypothyroidism, and recently diagnosed breast cancer (T2/N0/M0 grade 3, estrogen receptor/progesterone receptor negative, human epidermal growth factor receptor positive, recently treated with mastectomy and recent administration of carboplatin, paclitaxel, and trastuzumab) presented with altered mental status.

She was in her usual state of health when she acutely developed nausea, vomiting, diffuse abdominal pain, and bloody diarrhea. On arrival to the hospital, she was neurologically intact but febrile with mild hypotension. She had tenderness to abdominal palpation. Her initial laboratory data demonstrated a leukocytosis and mild acute kidney injury. She was found to have pancolitis on computed tomography (CT) of the abdomen. She was admitted to the hospital and, over the course of a week, developed pancytopenia: white blood cells decreased from 20 cells/μL to 1 cell/μL, and platelets decreased from 230 platelets/μL to 85 platelets/μL. She developed acute kidney injury that rapidly progressed to anuria. Over the same time, her neurologic status progressed from normal to mild confusion, then rapidly to somnolence, and finally coma. She was intubated both for failure to protect her airway and for increasing pulmonary edema. A day after intubation, she was noted to have 2 minutes of generalized tonic-clonic activity. She was transferred to the neurointensive care unit for further workup.

Exam

On exam, she was afebrile. She was hypotensive to 84/47 mm Hg. General exam was notable for diffuse anasarca and pulmonary crackles. Off propofol for several minutes, she was unarousable to voice or to sternal rub. Her pupils were 3 mm with minimal reactivity. Corneals were intact. The vestibulo-ocular reflex was difficult to elicit. She had a cough but no gag. To nailbed pressure, she had extensor posture in the upper extremities and had triple flexion in the lower extremities. She had a positive Babinski sign in the left toe. While off propofol, she began having rhythmic myoclonus of the orbicularis oculi, which then spread to the mouth with rhythmic mouth closure and biting on the tube.

WHAT IS THE DIFFERENTIAL DIAGNOSIS?

The differential diagnosis for seizures and a rapidly progressive encephalopathy in a neutropenic oncologic patient is broad. Causes for her depressed mental status include any etiology affecting the reticular activating system along the dorsal brainstem, a process affecting the thalamus, or a process that diffusely affects both cerebral hemispheres or results in hydrocephalus.

Given the stereotyped movement of the eyelids and mouth and the previously witnessed generalized tonic-clonic seizure, nonconvulsive status epilepticus should be a top consideration for her obtundation. The underlying cause of seizures is also a chief concern: infectious, autoimmune/parainfectious, vascular, metabolic, neoplastic, and paraneoplastic etiologies should all be considered.

In this case, the unilateral positive Babinski should raise concern for an acute structural abnormality. Although her original breast cancer seemed localized, an epileptogenic brain metastasis is a possibility. Other neoplastic-related etiologies in this case include leptomeningeal carcinomatosis (leading to seizures, and possibly acute hydrocephalus and coma) or a paraneoplastic encephalitis. Breast cancer is infrequently associated with paraneoplastic encephalitis, although this has been shown in case reports only.

Given her ongoing shock, pancolitis, and cytopenia, sepsis and infectious etiologies are also top considerations. Not only can sepsis cause a toxic-metabolic encephalopathy, but also it could lead to endocarditis-related strokes, mycotic aneurysmal bleeds, or brain abscesses, all of which might serve as a seizure focus. Given her immunosuppression, she is also at risk of infectious meningitis and encephalitis, either as result of direct bacterial/viral brain involvement or via a parainfectious, immune-mediated process. Of potential infectious etiologies, a tick-borne illness such as Rocky Mountain spotted fever or ehrlichiosis might explain her hematologic abnormalities. *Yersinia* or Whipple disease could account for both an encephalitis and the colitis; however, neither would be expected to present with this acuity. Autoantibodies to dipeptidyl-peptidase-like protein-6 (DPPX) may produce an autoimmune encephalitis that is frequently associated with diarrhea at symptom onset. The course is usually protracted.

Differential Diagnosis for Encephalopathy With (or Without) Seizures

Infectious	Herpes simplex virus (HSV)	**Paraneoplastic**	Ma1/Ma2/Ma3 (testicular, breast)
	Varicella-zoster virus (VZV)		Cv2 (thymoma, small-cell lung cancer [SCLC])
	Cytomegalovirus (CMV)		Hu (SCLC)
	Epstein-Barr virus (EBV)		GAD-65
	Enterovirus		GABA (lung)
	Human herpes virus-6 (HHV-6)		AMPAR (lung, breast)
	Adenovirus		LG1 (thymoma)
	Powassan		NMDA (ovarian)
	Eastern equine virus (EEE)		mGluR5 (Hodgkin lymphoma)
	Rabies		
	Syphilis	**Autoimmune**	Acute disseminated encephalomyelitis (ADEM)
	Lyme		Hashimoto encephalitis
	Mycoplasma		Systemic lupus erythematosus
	Toxoplasmosis		Sjögren syndrome
	Human immunodeficiency virus		Sarcoidosis
	West Nile virus		Postinfectious
	Measles		DPPX autoantibody
	Mumps		
	Treponema whipplei	**Metabolic**	Acute liver failure
	Bartonella		Acute renal failure
	Cerebral abscess		Lactic acidosis
	Bacterial meningitis		Hyper-/hypoglycemia
	Rocky Mountain spotted fever		Hyper-/hyponatremia
			Hyperammonemia
Vascular	Hypertension		Hypothyroidism
	Posterior reversible encephalopathy syndrome (PRES)		Hyper-/hypocalcemia
	Primary/secondary vasculitis		Hypercarbia
	Artery(s) of Percheron ischemic stroke		Hypoxia
	Eclampsia		Intoxication (illicit and nonillicit medications)
	Fat emboli syndrome		Withdrawal
	Intraparenchymal hemorrhage		Thrombotic thrombocytopenic purpura
	Endocarditis (merantic or infectious)		Hemolytic-uremic syndrome
Neoplastic	Primary/metastatic intraparenchymal tumor		
	Leptomeningeal carcinomatosis	**Other**	Hydrocephalus

The Shiga toxin associated with enterohemorrhagic *Escherichia coli* could cause hemolytic-uremic syndrome (HUS) and thrombotic microangiopathy, which could account for the hematologic findings and the gastroenteritis; it is also associated with both focal and generalized seizures. Herpes simplex encephalitis should be considered not only because it is a common cause of viral encephalitis, but also because it often manifests with seizures given its predilection for the temporal lobe.

The patient should also be screened for metabolic causes of seizures and encephalopathy. This workup is very broad but should include screening for hypo-/hypernatremia, hypo-/hyperglycemia, hyperammonemia, and uremia. Disseminated intravascular coagulation or heparin immune-mediated thrombocytopenia should also be investigated as causes of both strokes and intraparenchymal bleeds.

WHAT WOULD YOU ORDER NEXT?

There are several tests that should be rapidly completed to evaluate for the underlying etiology of coma and seizures. Basic imaging with a noncontrast head CT should be obtained to rule out a focal lesion (mass, hemorrhage, ischemic stroke) and may provide evidence of many other life-threatening intracranial diseases. In addition, given the patient's focal neurologic findings and coma, it is crucial to obtain imaging before proceeding with lumbar puncture (LP). Neuroimaging should be obtained prior to LP in any patient presenting with altered mentation, focal neurologic signs, concern for elevated intracranial pressure, papilledema, recent seizures, and/or impaired cellular immunity. Following imaging, LP would be appropriate given her immunosuppressed status and sepsis.

Her noncontrast head CT demonstrated symmetric hypoattenuation in the bilateral insula, mesial temporal lobes, and periventricular white matter, but no intracranial hemorrhage (Fig. 36.12-1).

The patient was urgently evaluated with continuous electroencephalography. Off propofol, she had 2 electrographic seizures (Fig. 36.12-2) and then developed near continuous multifocal periodic discharges, which, given their association with the witnessed ocular and oral stereotypies, were consistent with status epilepticus.

Magnetic resonance imaging (MRI) was completed. As shown in Figure 36.12-3, she was found to have relatively symmetric abnormal parenchymal T2 hyperintensities involving the insula, thalamus, and limbic structures.

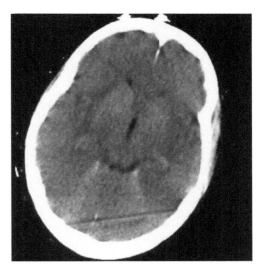

Figure 36.12-1 Axial noncontrast head computed tomography at the level of the third ventricle shows symmetric hypoattenuation in the bilateral insula, mesial temporal lobes, and periventricular white matter, but no intracranial hemorrhage.

An LP was completed, which demonstrated the following:

	Tube 1	Tube 4
White blood cells	4	3
Red blood cells	12	94
Protein	413 mg/dL (normal <45 mg/dL)	
Glucose	85 mg/dL	

HOW DO YOU INTERPRET THE LP AND MRI?

Her LP demonstrated albuminocytologic dissociation. Although classically associated with Guillain-Barré syndrome, elevated total protein may also be seen in any condition that results in cerebral edema and/or breakdown of the blood-brain barrier, and may be seen without elevated cell count in conditions such as posterior reversible encephalopathy syndrome, seizures, intracranial neoplasms, and encephalitis. The slightly elevated red blood cell count was initially concerning for thrombocytopenia-associated petechial hemorrhage into the areas of cerebral edema; however, no evidence of bleeding was seen on MRI. This was ultimately deemed secondary to a traumatic LP. The fact that the white blood cell count was not elevated should not be reassuring against infectious encephalitis. For example, in one retrospective review, nearly a quarter of patients ultimately found to have herpes simplex virus encephalitis had an initially normal cerebrospinal fluid.

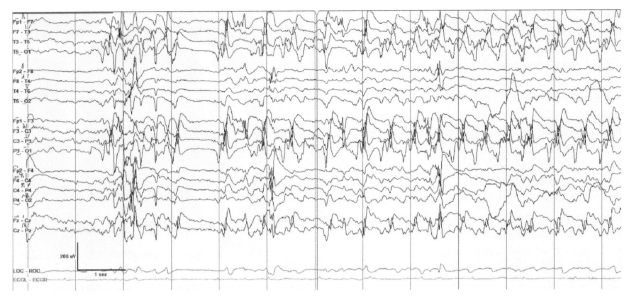

Figure 36.12-2 Electroencephalogram: Standard 10-20 lead placement with left over right double banana montage. Left-sided regular discharges at 2-Hz frequency that evolve over the course of 30 seconds (not fully shown) and then abate are consistent with an electrographic seizure.

In autoimmune limbic encephalitis, a normal cell count was reported in up to two-thirds of patients.

The MRI findings raise concern for limbic encephalitis. However, this pattern of symmetric hyperintensity and diffusion restriction in the medial temporal lobe, insula, thalamus, and deep subcortical white matter has also been seen in cases of diarrhea-associated HUS.

HOW WOULD YOU MANAGE THIS PATIENT?

The patient was initially managed with broad-spectrum antibiotics until blood cultures and the cerebrospinal fluid were negative for bacterial pathogens. While undergoing workup, her rapid test for *E coli* 0157 and Shiga toxin returned positive. This was felt to be a unifying diagnosis, and she continued to be managed with supportive care and continuous venovenous hemofiltration. Plasma exchange was not pursued in this case.

For her seizures and status epilepticus, she was initially managed with escalating doses of levetiracetam and then phenytoin. Because she was still found to have findings on the ictal-interictal continuum, intravenous propofol was used to achieve burst suppression for 3 days (Fig. 36.12-4). She was then slowly weaned off high-dose propofol and remained seizure free.

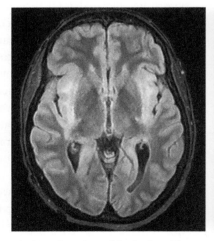 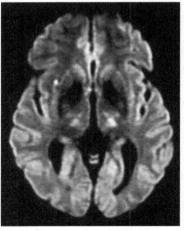

Figure 36.12-3 Magnetic resonance imaging of the brain without contrast. Left panel: Axial section at the level of thalami and insula fluid-attenuated inversion recovery sequence. Right panel: Axial section at the level of thalami and insula diffusion sequence.

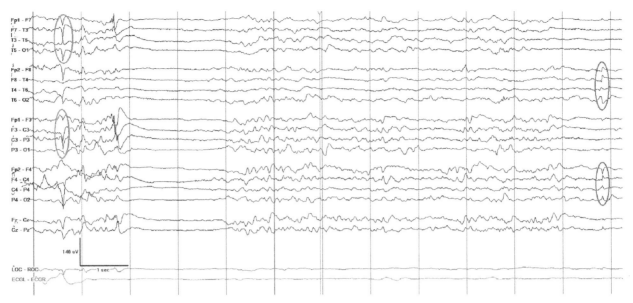

Figure 36.12-4 Electroencephalogram: Standard 10-20 lead placement with left over right double banana montage following initiation of multiple intravenous antiepileptic medications. Intermittent bilateral independent hemispheric discharges are circled.

Over a month-long hospitalization, her mental status improved, and at discharge, she was awake and responsive; she was oriented to place and able to communicate in simple phrases with her family and answer yes/no questions.

WHAT ARE YOUR FINAL DIAGNOSES?

- Encephalitis due to HUS due to *E coli* 0157
- Status epilepticus

REFERENCES

Boronat A, Gelfand JM, Gresa-Arribas N, et al. Encephalitis and antibodies to dipeptidyl-peptidase-like protein-6, a subunit of Kv4.2 potassium channels. *Ann Neurol.* 2012;73: 120-128.

Datar S, Singh TD, Fugate JE, et al. Albuminocytologic dissociation in posterior reversible encephalopathy syndrome. *Mayo Clin Proc.* 2015;90:1366-1371.

Hasbun R, Abrahams J, Jekel J, et al. Computed tomography of the head before lumbar puncture in adults with suspected meningitis. *N Engl J Med.* 2001;345:1727-1733.

Malter MP, Elger CE, Surges R. Diagnostic value of CSF findings in antibody-associated limbic and anti-NMDAR-encephalitis. *Seizure.* 2013;22:136-140.

Nathanson S, Kwon T, Elmaleh M, et al. Acute neurological involvement in diarrhea-associated hemolytic uremic syndrome. *Clin J Am Soc Nephrol.* 2010;5:1218-1228.

Sahashi K. Anti-Ma2 antibody related paraneoplastic limbic/brain stem encephalitis associated with breast cancer expressing Ma1, Ma2, and Ma3 mRNAs. *J Neurol Neurosurg Psychiatry.* 2003;74(9):1332-1335.

Saraya AW, Wacharapluesadee S, Petcharat S, et al. Normocellular CSF in herpes simplex encephalitis. *BMC Res Notes.* 2016;9:95.

Tumani H, Jobs C, Brettschneider J, et al. Effect of epileptic seizures on the cerebrospinal fluid: a systematic retrospective analysis. *Epilepsy Res.* 2015;114:23-31.

Index

Note: Page number followed by *f* indicates figure only.